T0201296

Clinical Laboratory Animal Medicine

Clinical Laboratory Animal Medicine

An Introduction

Fifth Edition

Lesley A. Colby, DVM, MS, DACLAM
Megan H. Nowland, DVM, DACLAM
Lucy H. Kennedy, DVM, DACLAM

WILEY Blackwell

This edition first published 2020

Edition History
4e 2013 John Wiley & Sons, Inc.; 3e 2007 Karen Hrapkiewicz and Leticia Medina; 2e 1998 © Iowa State University Press; 1e 1984 Iowa State University Press

Registered Office(s)
John Wiley & Sons, Inc., 111 River Street, Hoboken, NJ 07030, USA
John Wiley & Sons Ltd, The Atrium, Southern Gate, Chichester, West Sussex, PO19 8SQ, UK

Editorial Office
111 River Street, Hoboken, NJ 07030, USA

For details of our global editorial offices, customer services, and more information about Wiley products visit us at www.wiley.com.

Wiley also publishes its books in a variety of electronic formats and by print-on-demand. Some content that appears in standard print versions of this book may not be available in other formats.

Library of Congress Cataloging-in-Publication Data

Names: Colby, Lesley, A., author.
Title: Clinical laboratory animal medicine : an introduction / Lesley A. Colby, DVM, MS, DACLAM, Megan H. Nowland, DVM, DACLAM, Lucy H. Kennedy, DVM, DACLAM.
Description: Fifth edition. | Hoboken, NJ : Wiley-Blackwell, 2020. | Revision of: Clinical laboratory animal medicine : an introduction / Karen Hrapkiewicz, Lesley Colby, Patricia Denison. Fourth edition. 2013. | Includes bibliographical references and index.
Identifiers: LCCN 2019030439 (print) | LCCN 2019030440 (ebook) | ISBN 9781119489566 (paperback) | ISBN 9781119489634 (adobe pdf) | ISBN 9781119489597 (epub)
Subjects: LCSH: Laboratory animals–Diseases. | Veterinary medicine.
Classification: LCC SF996.5 .H65 2020 (print) | LCC SF996.5 (ebook) | DDC 636.088/5–dc23
LC record available at https://lccn.loc.gov/2019030439
LC ebook record available at https://lccn.loc.gov/2019030440

Cover Design: Wiley
Cover Images: Austin Thomason, Michigan Photography – University of Michigan; Amy Puffenberger, Animal Care & Use Program – University of Michigan

Set in 10/13pt Stempel Garamond by SPi Global, Pondicherry, India

SKY10079323_071024

I dedicate this book:

- To the memory of all the animals that have contributed both to my education and to the advancement of human and animal health. It has been a pleasure learning from you.
- To the animal technicians, veterinary technicians, and veterinarians who have devoted their lives to the care of laboratory animals and in support of animal welfare. It has been an honor working beside you.
- To my husband, Ben; our children, Nate and Tess; and our "special" family members (aka dogs), Troika, Ronal Danne, Tasha, and Bacca—for your incredible patience and support through all the nights, weekends, and holidays I spent studying or working over the years. Without you, I would not be who I am today.

LAC

To my husband, who supports me in all things whether large or unimportant, while reminding me not to take myself too seriously.

MHN

To Carolyn "Kit" Kestrel Leigh Kennedy, whose timely arrival made completing this book a difficult task! And to Scott and Mer, who made it possible anyways.

LHK

NOTE

The dosages given in this text are derived from published literature, but as few drugs are specifically licensed for use in the species described, the application is often extra-label and may be empirical or based on clinical experience. The authors have made every attempt to verify all dosages and references; however, despite these efforts, errors in the original sources or in the preparation of this book may have occurred. Users of this text should exercise caution and evaluate all dosages prior to use to determine that they are reasonable.

Contents

About the Authors

Lesley A. Colby, DVM, MS, DACLAM, is Associate Professor and Senior Director of Animal Resources and Operations in the Department of Comparative Medicine at the University of Washington (UW). She is Director of the UW's BSL3/ABSL3 Facility and has particular interests in biocontainment, occupational health, and facility design and management. Dr. Colby is a Diplomate of the American College of Laboratory Animal Medicine.

Megan H. Nowland, DVM, DACLAM, is an Associate Professor in the Unit for Laboratory Animal Medicine at the University of Michigan in Ann Arbor, Michigan. There, she directs the Postdoctoral Training Program in Laboratory Animal Medicine, is the Associate Attending Veterinarian and the Assistant Director for Clinical Services.

Lucy H. Kennedy, DVM, DACLAM, is an Assistant Professor in the Unit for Laboratory Animal Medicine at the University of Michigan in Ann Arbor, Michigan. She is also the Managing Director for the Unit for Laboratory Animal Medicine's Germ-Free Mouse Facility and enjoys the challenges of gnotobiotic mouse research.

Preface

The purpose of this book is to provide basic information regarding the safe and responsible conduct of animal research as well as the unique anatomic and physiologic characteristics, husbandry practices, and veterinary care of many of the animals frequently used in research: rodents, rabbits, ferrets, zebrafish, nonhuman primates, and agricultural animals. As the book name implies, we have designed the materials to be especially useful for individuals who are new to animal research as well as for those experienced in this field and expanding their knowledge of additional species. As a result, the book should be a useful resource for practicing veterinarians, veterinary students, veterinary technicians, research scientists, and others interested in learning about the field.

This, the fifth edition of the book, has been revised to include not only updated information but also new chapters on zebrafish and agricultural animals used in biomedical research. Significant changes have been made to expand and/or reorganize the non-species chapters, to refine drug dosage tables to reflect the drugs most frequently utilized for each species, and to provide recommended reading sources for additional inquiry. As in previous editions of this book, study review questions are provided for each chapter and supplemental materials are provided in an accompanying website.

This book would not have been possible without the contributions of all previous edition authors: Donald Holmes, Karen Hrapkiewicz, Leticia Medina, and Patricia Denison. We thank you for providing such a strong foundation upon which to build. We also acknowledge and thank the many individuals and vendors who provided images for inclusion in the book and website. A very special thanks to our family, friends, and colleagues for their patience and support during the writing of this text. Lastly, our heartfelt thanks to all the animals that have contributed to the remarkable advancements in biomedical research throughout the ages, without whom many of the scientific breakthroughs we now take for granted would not have been possible.

Lesley A. Colby
Megan H. Nowland
Lucy H. Kennedy

About the Companion Website

This book is accompanied by a companion Website:

www.wiley.com/go/colby/clinical

The Website includes:

- Editable chapter review exercises and answers
- Teaching PowerPoint presentations
- Images in PowerPoint

Watch for  throughout the book. These pinpoint materials that are also available on the Website.

1 Introduction to Laboratory Animal Medicine

The health and welfare of animals used in biomedical research must be supported to be consistent with contemporary ethical standards and to help ensure the scientific validity of research results. Providing this support requires individuals with expertise in many fields including basic and applied sciences, bioethics, regulatory oversight, experimental design, and laboratory animal science. Laboratory animal science is defined by the US National Library of Medicine as "[t]he science and technology dealing with the procurement, breeding, care, health, and selection of animals used in biomedical research and testing" (Box 1.1). It includes husbandry, nutrition, behavior, health care, production, and management of laboratory animals.

Laboratory animal medicine is a specialized field within laboratory animal science and a recognized specialty within veterinary medicine. At its core, laboratory animal medicine encompasses the diagnosis, treatment, and prevention of diseases in animals used in research, teaching, and testing. It emphasizes methods to prevent and minimize pain, discomfort, and distress in research animals; facilitates acquisition of biologically meaningful results; and minimizes experimental variability. The field has progressively grown and evolved in response to scientific and medical advances, shifts in the regulatory environment, and the ever-changing focus of scientific inquiry.

Diverse groups of individuals play important roles within laboratory animal medicine. Veterinarians have a variety of responsibilities within an animal care and use program that may include provision of veterinary care, management of animal care

Clinical Laboratory Animal Medicine: An Introduction, Fifth Edition.
Lesley A. Colby, Megan H. Nowland, and Lucy H. Kennedy.

Companion website: www.wiley.com/go/colby/clinical

Box 1.1

The US National Library of Medicine defines laboratory animal science as "[t]he science and technology dealing with the procurement, breeding, care, health, and selection of animals used in biomedical research and testing."

and use facilities, education of individuals who care for and use laboratory animals, assisting biomedical scientists in the selection of and humane use of animals, obtaining and interpreting biologically relevant data, and assuring compliance with regulations and policies that affect research animals. Veterinary technicians work under the supervision of a veterinarian, assisting them in carrying out these responsibilities. They often provide technical support in disease detection, including oversight of colony health monitoring programs, treatment of ill animals, blood sampling, and necropsy and tissue collection. When engaged in research or drug study positions at a pharmaceutical firm or university, they administer test products and collect data. This type of employment often requires the veterinary technician to be credentialed and have a bachelor's degree. Credentialed veterinary technicians, with sufficient education, training, and experience, and who have completed testing requirements can apply to join the Academy of Laboratory Animal Veterinary Technicians and Nurses, a specialty organization within the National Association of Veterinary Technicians in America (NAVTA). Veterinary technicians may also work in research compliance or supervise other animal facility staff such as assistant laboratory animal technicians, animal caretakers, and cagewash personnel. It should also be noted that individuals without formal veterinary training make significant contributions in support of laboratory animal medicine. For example, animal caretakers who closely observe and handle animals on a daily basis can be instrumental in detecting behavioral changes and identifying early signs of illness so that animals can be promptly assessed by veterinary personnel.

ANIMALS USED IN RESEARCH, TEACHING, AND TESTING

Biomedical Research

Remarkable advances have been made in medicine and science over the past century, such as the characterization of complex host–pathogen interactions and immune system functions, development of vaccines for polio and hepatitis B, creation of antibiotics and antivirals for infectious diseases, procedures for organ transplantation and open heart surgery, and development of drugs for chronic disorders such as diabetes and high blood pressure. Animals played a major role in each of these advances (Table 1.1). New treatment modalities for cancer, less invasive surgical approaches, and the development of equipment such as the laser and endoscopic instruments would not have been possible without the use of animals. Often, advances made in human health are also applied to the benefit of companion animals (Figure 1.1). For instance, most cancer treatments and many advanced surgical techniques and imaging modalities developed for use in humans are now routinely available to veterinary practices.

Table 1.1. Animal roles in medical discoveries and advancements

Year*	Scientist(s)	Animal(s) Used	Contribution
1901	von Behring	Guinea pig	Development of diphtheria antiserum
1904	Pavlov	Dog	Animal responses to various stimuli
1923	Banting, Macleod	Dog, rabbit, fish	Discovery of insulin and mechanism of diabetes
1924	Einthoven	Dog	Mechanism of the electrocardiogram
1945	Fleming, Chain, Florey	Mouse	Discovery of penicillin and its curative effect in various infectious diseases
1954	Enders, Weller, Robbins	Monkey, mouse	Culture of poliovirus that led to development of vaccine
1964	Block, Lynen	Rat	Regulation of cholesterol and fatty acid metabolism
1966	Rous	Rat, rabbit, hen	Discoveries concerning hormonal treatment of prostatic cancer
1970	Katz, von Euler, Axelrod	Cat, rat	Mechanism of storage and release of nerve transmitters
1979	Cormack, Hounsfield	Pig	Development of computer-assisted tomography (CAT scan)
1984	Milstein, Koehler, Jerne	Mouse	Techniques of monoclonal antibody formation
1990	Murray, Thomas	Dog	Organ transplant techniques
1997	Prusiner	Mouse, hamster	Discovery of prions, a new biological principle of infection
2003	Lauterbur, Mansfield	Clam, mouse, dog, rat, chimpanzee, pig, rabbit, frog	Discoveries concerning magnetic resonance imaging
2008	Barre-Sinoussi, Montagnier	Monkey, chimpanzee, mouse	Discovery of human immunodeficiency virus
2008	zur Hausen	Hamster, mouse, cow	Discovery of papilloma viruses causing cervical cancer
2011	Hoffman, Beutler	Fruit fly, mouse	Discoveries concerning the activation of innate immunity
2011	Steinman	Mouse	Discovery of the dendritic cell and its role in adaptive immunity
2012	Gurdon, Yamanaka	Frog, mice	Discovery that mature cells can be reprogrammed to become pluripotent
2013	Rothman, Schekman, Sudhop	Mouse, hamster	Discovery of how cells organize movement of materials into and out of cells
2014	O'Keefe, Britt, Moser	Rat	Discovery of cells that constitute the brain's "inner GPS" positioning system

(Continued)

Table 1.1. (Continued)

Year*	Scientist(s)	Animal(s) Used	Contribution
2015	Campbell, Omura, Tu	Mouse, dog, sheep, cattle, chicken, monkey	Discoveries contributing to development of novel therapies for roundworm and for malarial infections
2016	Ohsumi	Mouse	Discovery of mechanisms for cellular autophagy
2017	Rosbash, Hall, Young	Fruit flies	Discovery of molecular mechanisms controlling the circadian rhythm

Sources: National Association of Biomedical Research (https://www.nabr.org/biomedical-research/medical-progress), Foundation for Biomedical Research (https://fbresearch.org/medical-advances/nobel-prizes), and Nobel Prize (www.nobelprize.org).

* Year of occurrence or award recognition.

Box 1.2

Ex vivo experimental methods should be used in place of in vivo experimental methods whenever possible.

Significant advances have been made in the development and use of *ex vivo* ("out of the living") experimental methods which do not require the use of animals or animal-derived products. These experimental methods should be used in place of *in vivo* ("in life") experimental methods whenever possible, but only when resultant experimental findings are truly representative and predictive of the system(s) they are intended to model (Box 1.2). Unfortunately, most *ex vivo* testing systems cannot generate sufficiently comprehensive and accurate data representative of an intricate, living being. As a result, use of *in vivo* experimental methods is still required until more refined alternatives are developed and validated. In the interim, use of *ex vivo* experimental methods can be effective and valuable in refining and reducing animal use for some areas of study such as early identification of toxic or ineffective experimental compounds and modeling compound–receptor interactions.

Teaching

Animals play a valuable role in education, starting from preschool and continuing to the college and graduate levels. Although computer modeling and videos can replace select learning experiences, some personal learning styles and educational objectives are best suited to hands-on learning. Through interactions with animals, children can learn how to care for another living being. They also learn lessons in responsibility and respect. At the middle and high school levels, animal tissues may be used for hands-on experience with dissection and now-common laboratory methods such as immunoassays and molecular diagnostics. These experiences often reveal the amazing world of biology and science to young people as they learn about the complex and specialized processes that form the basis of biological functions. In college, animals are used in a variety of professional and graduate-level courses in medical and health-related fields. Surgery courses provide young veterinary surgeons a chance to hone their skills before performing them on client-owned animals. Physicians use animals to practice robotic, endoscopic, and laser surgery prior to performing them in people. Animals are used in training courses for medical personnel so they may acquire and advance their skills in emergency and critical care environments. Clinical technique courses provide veterinary students and veterinary technician students opportunities to develop the diverse range of skills necessary for the safe and humane care of their future animal patients, such as animal handling and performance of physical exams, injections, and catheterizations. It is now common for animals used for educational purposes to either be temporarily housed in a research/teaching environment and then adopted into loving homes or be pets brought in by their owners to assist with training.

Product Safety Testing

Several decades ago, consumers were subjected to publicly marketed drugs and cosmetics that were not adequately tested to assess human safety. Examples included early treatments for syphilis containing mercury and arsenic, an eyelash dye that caused blindness in numerous individuals, and an elixir marketed for use by children and that caused the death of over 100 people. These and other similar events led to the passage of the Food, Drug, and Cosmetic Act (FD&C) in 1938. Broadly speaking, the FD&C was created to safeguard and protect consumer health and safety from the sale of dangerous products. The Act is enforced primarily by the Food and Drug Administration (FDA) which requires animal testing of products when a scientifically valid, alternative testing method is not available. When animal testing is required to obtain FDA approval, the FDA requires product manufacturers and sponsors to conduct the studies in accordance with the Good Laboratory Practice for Nonclinical Laboratory Studies (21 CFR Part 58). Recently, many manufacturers have marketed cosmetic products as "cruelty-free." This unregulated labeling or advertising practice can be deceiving to consumers who may incorrectly assume that neither the product nor any product components were tested in animals. However, it is more likely that animal safety testing had been performed on individual product components (but not necessarily the final product) or that testing had been contracted by the manufacturer to be performed by an external testing group. As a consequence, consumers must be savvy in their interpretation of unregulated product labeling.

Animal Usage Statistics

According to the US Department of Agriculture (USDA) *Animal Report Animal Usage by Fiscal Year*, 792,168 animals whose use is regulated by the Animal Welfare Act were used for research, teaching, and product safety testing in the United States in 2017. It should be noted that this figure does not include the annual usage of mice, rats, birds, or fish as the USDA is not charged with regulatory oversight of these species as required by Animal Welfare Act. Rather, use of these species is regulated by other entities and the precise numbers of their use is unknown. However, it is estimated that up to 26 million animals of these species are used annually. Mice and rats

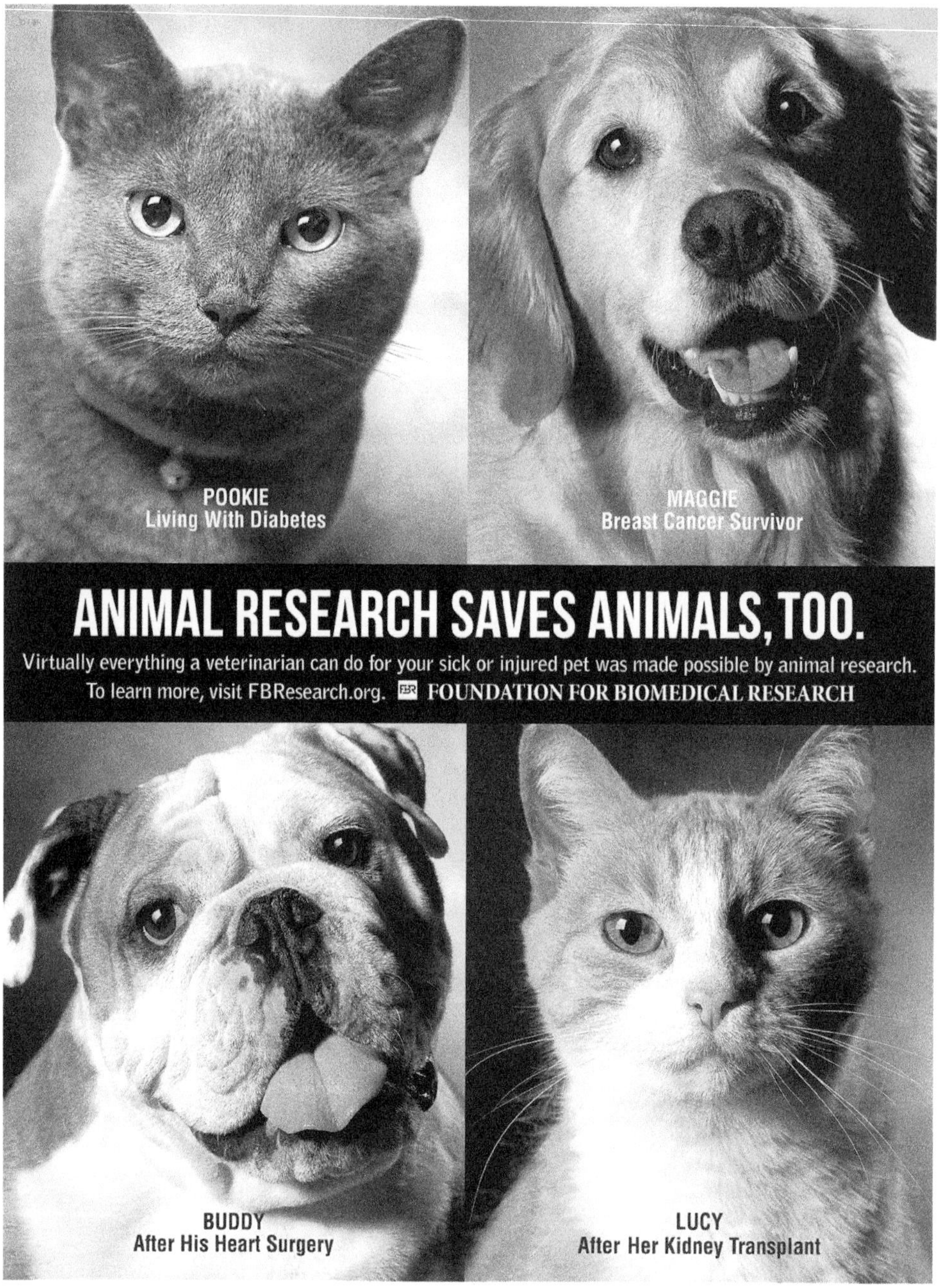

Fig 1.1. Animal research saves animals too. (*Source:* Foundation for Biomedical Research.)

account for greater than 95% of all animals used while the number of dogs, cats, and nonhuman primates combined account for less than 1% of the animals used.

With the exception of the increased use of zebrafish, the use of nonrodent animals has been declining over the past three decades primarily due to use of more refined experimental systems and an intense effort by the biomedical research community to

Box 1.3

With the exception of the increased use of zebrafish, the use of nonrodent animals has been declining over the past three decades.

decrease animal use (Box 1.3). The number of dogs used in research currently is less than one-third of its numbers in the late 1970s. The number of nonhuman primates used over the past decade has risen slightly, in part due to increasing emphasis of research into human brain function and neurodegenerative diseases such as Alzheimer's. Across all species, the majority of animals used in biomedical research are bred specifically for that purpose.

To put the numbers in perspective, approximately 12–27 million animals are used in research in the United States. All but approximately 1 million of these are mice, rats, birds, or fish. According to Speaking of Research (www.speakingofresearch.com), "we consume over 1800 times the number of pigs than the number [*of pigs*] used in research" and we consume over 340 times more chickens than the total number of animals used in biomedical research.

Funding Sources

In the United States, the National Institutes of Health (NIH) and the National Science Foundation (NSF) are the primary public granting agencies for biomedical research. The NIH, a branch of the Public Health Service (PHS), provides competitive federal grants for investigators interested in the health-related advancement of humans and animals. The NSF encourages basic research in behavior, mathematics, physics, medicine, biology, and other sciences. In addition to the NIH and NSF, funding is available from universities and colleges, state governments, industry, and private foundations. Acquiring funds to conduct research is difficult as competition for grant money is high, with only 10%–20% of submitted proposals receiving funding. Typically, a grant provides money for the primary scientist's and research team's salaries, supplies, equipment, and purchase and care of animals for a 3-year period. The primary scientist, or principal investigator (PI), is responsible for planning and coordinating all phases of the research study, including tabulating data, reporting findings to the funding agency, and publication of results. When a study yields valuable results, the funding agency may renew the grant for an additional period of time.

Regulatory Oversight and Accreditation

Multiple levels of regulation (e.g., federal, state, and local) function to provide oversight of animal research including mandating standards for animal care and use. In addition, many institutions choose to participate in voluntary assessment and accreditation programs which recognize institutions that have exceeded the minimum standards required by law and have achieved excellence in animal care and use. Chapter 2 provides additional information regarding the oversight provided by governmental and voluntary organizations.

Institutional Animal Care and Use Committee

Prior to the use of animals in research, teaching, or testing, a protocol must be submitted to and approved by the institution's Institutional Animal Care and Use Committee (IACUC) (Box 1.4). The protocol is a detailed, written description of the proposed animal care and use. It justifies the use of vertebrate animals to accomplish the study's aims, details the procedures that will be performed on the animals, and describes how the animals will be housed and cared for throughout the project. Additionally, the PI must give several assurances, including that the study does not unnecessarily duplicate previous studies, that the staff working with the animals have adequate training to accomplish the study tasks in a humane manner, that alternatives to animal use have been carefully considered, and that any activities that may induce animal pain or distress are scientifically necessary. Animal use protocols are usually approved for 3 years, may undergo an annual review by the IACUC, and must be resubmitted for full, *de novo* (anew) review every 3 years. IACUCs must formally review and approve all changes to approved protocols prior to their implementation. Moreover, IACUCs are required, at a minimum frequency (usually twice yearly), to review their institution's established program of animal care and use and physically inspect facilities where animals are housed or manipulated. Additional information about IACUCs can be found at www.iacuc.org.

Box 1.4

Prior to the use of animals in research, teaching, or testing, a protocol must be submitted to and approved by the institution's Institutional Animal Care and Use Committee (IACUC).

ETHICAL CONSIDERATIONS

The 3Rs: Replacement, Refinement, and Reduction

Two English scientists, Russell and Burch, coined the term "the 3Rs." In 1959, they examined the ethical aspects and "the development and progress of humane techniques in the laboratory" (Russel and Burch, 1959). The 3Rs represent three ethical tenets of responsible animal use: replacement, refinement, and reduction (Box 1.5). Research institutions and regulatory authorities continually strive to apply the principles of the 3Rs to ensure animals are used in an ethical manner. There is an ethical imperative that scientists use animals only when they have provided assurance to the

Box 1.5

Russel and Burch's 3Rs represent three ethical tenets of responsible animal use: replacement, refinement, and reduction.

IACUC that no nonanimal methods will allow them to achieve their scientific aim. This search for alternatives is mandated for species covered by the Animal Welfare Act (AWA; see APHIS, 2017). For species not covered by the AWA, both the Public Health Service Policy and the *Guide for the Care and Use of Research Animals* (ILAR, 2011; the *Guide*) refer to the "US Government Principles for the Utilization and Care of Vertebrate Animals Used in Testing, Research, and Training" (OLAW, 1985), which includes language about alternatives to animal use (see Chapter 2, Table 2.1). The US Government Principles also mandate using the minimum number of animals necessary to obtain valid results. This is synonymous with reduction, one of the 3Rs.

Replacement refers to replacing animals with a nonanimal alternative, such as *in vitro* ("in glass," outside of the body) screens with cell culture or computer (*in silica*) modeling, or by using the least sentient animal (e.g., rat in place of dog; fish in place of mouse) that will enable collection of meaningful and valid data. Continued advances in the sciences and testing methods have helped to spur development of animal testing alternatives. Any alternative test, however, must be validated before it can be used to replace a test currently using animals. The development and use of genetically specialized animals, such as nude and transgenic mice, has made it possible to reduce the number of other species such as dogs and cats. Environmental toxicity studies often use zebrafish rather than mice or other mammals. Alternate tests for ophthalmic safety testing have been developed using tissues obtained from slaughterhouses as well as specially designed cell and tissue culture systems. In addition, the limulus amebocyte lysate (LAL) assay has largely replaced the rabbit pyrogen test for detecting pyrogens, such as endotoxin, in injectable substances.

Refinement refers to methods that incorporate modification of a procedure to lessen animal pain and distress or enhance animal well-being. Use of less invasive procedures, provision of pain relief, provision of environmental enrichment, and decreased restraint time are examples of refinements. For example, through advanced imaging techniques, such as magnetic resonance imaging (MRI), researchers can now view structures and observe anatomic functions that once could only be accomplished during surgery or at necropsy. Investigators must constantly review the way animal studies are conducted to ensure that the methods used are the most humane and refined to minimize pain and distress. In addition, investigators work closely with laboratory animal veterinarians and the IACUC to assure that humane experimental endpoints are in place to minimize pain and distress to the greatest degree possible. The IACUC often collaborates with investigators and veterinary personnel to develop humane endpoint guidelines that help determine when an animal should be euthanized or removed from a study. Examples of humane experimental endpoints include a defined percentage of weight loss, tumor size, presence of labored breathing, or an inability to ambulate. There is a delicate balance between collecting the necessary scientific data from a study and ensuring that animal welfare is preserved. For example, it can be difficult to identify the point at which an animal should be removed from study or euthanized before it becomes significantly ill. When appropriate, the least invasive experimental methods should be used, and anesthesia or analgesia be administered to eliminate unnecessary pain and distress.

Reduction refers to using the minimal number of animals in a study while remaining consistent with sound scientific and statistical standards. Investigators must constantly strive to find ways to reduce animal numbers. Using a combination of computer-based simulators in conjunction with animal subjects, employing better statistical methods, or using one control group with multiple study groups are examples of methods used to reduce animal numbers. The number of animals used in product safety testing has been significantly reduced through validation of alternative testing methods. Experiments can be designed using multiple sections with the results derived from earlier sections used to refine the number of animals or experimental groups used in later sections. For example, a "staircase design" is often used in acute toxicology testing. This method involves administration of a limited number of drug dosages (high and low) to then determine a more precise dose range for further testing. Used with sophisticated computer-assisted computational methods, the staircase design can determine a point estimate of the lethal dose, approximate confidence intervals, and determine toxic signs for the substance tested, yet use fewer animals.

Overall, the research community must continually challenge itself to consider whether the animal research being performed is ethical and justifiable. The principles underlying the "3Rs" should be observed so that animal use in biomedical research is minimized while at the same time, data obtained from animal research is optimized. Only in that way will we be assured of continued public support for the animal research that benefits so much of society, including the health and welfare of nonhuman animals!

Animal Rights and Animal Welfare

The terms "animal rights" and "animal welfare" are not synonymous. Animal rights represents a philosophical belief that gives animals the same equality and protection as humans (Box 1.6). According to this philosophy, a field mouse has the same right to life as a human. Animal rights purports that animals should not be regarded as property. No matter how humane, animal use is viewed as exploitation and should be banned. This includes keeping dogs and cats as pets; displaying animals in zoos and aquariums; using chickens, cattle, or swine for food; and using animals in research, teaching, and testing. Furthermore, adherence to this philosophy prohibits one's use of medications including vaccines and medical treatments that were developed through animal research.

Animal welfare represents a philosophical belief that it is morally acceptable for humans to use animals provided they are treated humanely and their physical and psychological well-being is met (Box 1.7). This philosophy is based on a belief that animals can contribute to human welfare. Animals provide companionship, entertainment, labor, food, fiber, and advancement of knowledge when used in research and teaching. When animals are used, it is paramount that responsible practices of animal

Box 1.6

Animal rights represents a philosophical belief that gives animals the same equality and protection as humans.

Box 1.7

Animal welfare represents a philosophical belief that it is morally acceptable for humans to use animals provided they are treated humanely and their physical and psychological well-being is met.

welfare are adhered to, including provision of appropriate housing, handling, management, disease prevention and treatment, and, when necessary, euthanasia.

Sources of Animals Used in Biomedical Research

Animals used in research may be obtained from a variety of sources. The sale of AWA-covered species (e.g., dogs and cats) to research facilities is regulated by the USDA who licenses Class A and Class B animal dealers. USDA-licensed Class A dealers supply "purpose bred" animals, animals bred and raised specifically for use in research. Purpose-bred animals are of genetically similar backgrounds, often with defined pedigrees, and have well-documented health histories. To help ensure that these animals are accustomed to the research environment and are easy to handle, many vendors have instituted robust animal handling and socialization programs as components of their animal care programs.

A small number of animals used in research are obtained from USDA Class B dealers, who acquire animals from "random sources" such as individual owners, hobby breeders, and pounds and shelters. Although Class B dealers are subject to federal legislation under the Animal Welfare Act and are licensed by the USDA, public concern regarding acquisition of dogs and cats from Class B dealers led to the decision by NIH to discontinue funding of experiments using random source dogs and cats. Institutions do occasionally elect to obtain animals directly from random sources when purpose-bred animals do not possess the characteristics necessary for study, such as advanced age or preexisting health conditions. Acquisition of these animals is tightly regulated.

Nonhuman Primate Use

Nonhuman primates are human's closest genetic relatives. Due to this and their associated high level of sentience, their use in research should be reserved only for when another animal model cannot be used. Nonhuman primates account for less than 1% of the USDA-regulated animals used in the United States. The vast majority of nonhuman primates used are rhesus and cynomolgus macaques. Although the use of chimpanzees was invaluable in advancing human health, including for the development of vaccines for polio and hepatitis B, the NIH no longer supports the use of chimps in research and all use of chimps in research has been significantly restricted and effectively eliminated. Chimps previously used in research have been retired to designated sanctuaries or have been retired "in place" when it was reasonably expected that they would experience harm if relocated.

ORGANIZATIONS

The need for more systematic and specialized information on laboratory animal husbandry, medical care, and management of animal facilities and the desire to foster collaborative environments led to the development of several organizations that support the laboratory animal science community. The following is an introduction to some of the most important organizations and a brief description of their purpose.

American Association for Laboratory Animal Science

In 1950, the Animal Care Panel (ACP), a national professional organization dedicated to the care, production, and study of laboratory animals, was established. In 1967, the ACP became the American Association for Laboratory Animal Science (AALAS) whose mission is to advance "responsible laboratory animal care and use to benefit people and animals." AALAS is a nonprofit, professional association that serves as the principal means of communication between individuals and organizations within the field of laboratory animal science. AALAS currently has over 14,500 individual and institutional members and more than 43 local branches. AALAS produces two scientific journals, *Comparative Medicine* and *Journal of the American Association for Laboratory Animal Science*, and several technician-targeted publications including the quarterly magazine, *Laboratory Animal Science Professional.* AALAS also certifies trained technicians; promotes education through publications; supports the AALAS Learning Library, an extensive Web-based continuing education site; and hosts an annual national meeting. Scientists, veterinarians, technicians, managers, and suppliers share information through presentations, discussions, and exhibits at the annual meeting. Recently, AALAS has increased its role in public outreach and promoting the benefits of biomedical research. For further information, visit www.aalas.org.

AALAS administers the AALAS Technician Certification Program through which technicians receive certification at one of three levels: Assistant Laboratory Animal Technician (ALAT), Laboratory Animal Technician (LAT), and Laboratory Animal Technologist (LATG) (Figure 1.2). The minimum qualifications required to take each certification exam are listed in Figure 1.3. The duties of assistant laboratory animal technicians are primarily related to animal care and facility sanitation. Laboratory animal technicians are expected to have increased diagnostic and technical skills and research responsibilities. Laboratory animal technologists are frequently involved in

ALAT™ LAT™ LATG™

Fig 1.2. AALAS technician certification level logos. (*Source:* AALAS.)

Eligibility requirements

Below are the minimum eligibility requirements for each exam. To be eligible for the exam you wish to take, you must meet one of the combinations of education and work experience.

Exam		Current cert. level	Education level: HS/GED or higher	Education level: AA/AS or higher	Education level: BA/BS or higher	Lab animal work experience (years)
ALAT Exam	❑					2
	❑		•			1
	❑			•	•	0.5
LAT Exam	❑		•			3
	❑			•		2
	❑				•	1
	❑	ALAT	•			0.5*
	❑	ALAT				2**
LATG Exam	❑		•			5
	❑			•		4
	❑				•	3
	❑	LAT	•			0.5*

* Work experience must be acquired after attaining the specified certification.
** Option for those without documentation of education level.

Fig 1.3. Minimum eligibility requirements for AALAS technician certification. (*Source:* AALAS.)

supervisory capacities and conducting portions of the research study. The achievement of certification at any level denotes an individual dedicated to the pursuit of a higher standard of technical skill and knowledge. Many institutions now require or prefer AALAS certification as a prerequisite for obtaining jobs in their animal facility. Alternatively, many institutions encourage employees to pursue certification as a means of advancing their careers and offer classes as part of their training programs. AALAS offers training manuals for each of the three levels and suggests other materials appropriate for examination preparation. Employers often provide employees with financial support for the examinations and frequently reward the achievement of certification with a specific increase in salary.

AALAS also sponsors the Certified Manager of Animal Resources (CMAR) program. The CMAR designation is a sign of professionalism in the field of animal resources management. Certification requires successful completion of a series of general business management exams offered through the Institute for Certified Professional Managers (ICPM) or through AALAS as well as completion of the more specialized Animal Resources Exam offered by AALAS. Educational materials for the exams are available from ICPM and from AALAS, including AALAS' *Management Training Manual.* The minimum eligibility requirements for CMAR designation are

Table 1.2. Eligibility requirements for CMAR designation

Education Level	Total Work Experience	Total Management Experience
BA/BS	5 years	3 years
AA/AS	8 years	3 years
HS/GED	10 years	3 years

Source: AALAS.

Note: Candidates meeting these requirements who pass the Animal Resources Exam and the Certified Manager (CM) exams will achieve the status of a Certified Manager of Animal Resources and will be able to use the CMAR acronym after their names.

listed in Table 1.2. CMAR recipients must fulfill continuing education requirements to maintain their designation.

Laboratory Animal Management Association

The Laboratory Animal Management Association (LAMA) was established in 1984 with the mission of "enhancing the quality of management and care of laboratory animals throughout the world" by "promot[ing] education, knowledge exchange and professional development" of facility managers and supervisors (www.lama-online.org). The organization publishes a quarterly journal, *LAMA Review,* sponsors training sessions, and hosts an annual educational meeting. For further information, visit www.lama-online.org.

American Society of Laboratory Animal Practitioners

In August 1966, the Laboratory Animal Welfare Act became law and mandated that "adequate veterinary care" be provided to select laboratory animals. The American Society of Laboratory Animal Practitioners (ASLAP) was founded later that same year, partially in response to the Act's passage. ASLAP is a professional organization through which veterinarians engaged or interested in the practice of laboratory animal medicine can freely exchange ideas, experiences, and knowledge. In 1967, ASLAP was officially recognized as an ancillary organization of the American Veterinary Medical Association (AVMA) and in 1986, ASLAP became an affiliate of AALAS. Both veterinarians and veterinary students make up the membership of ASLAP. According to its website, the objectives of ASLAP are to (1) "provide a mechanism for the exchange of scientific and technical information among veterinarians engaged in laboratory animal practice," (2) "actively encourage its members to provide training for veterinarians in the field of laboratory animal practice at both the pre and postdoctoral levels and lend their expertise to institutions conducting laboratory animal medicine programs," (3) "encourage the development and dissemination of knowledge in areas related to laboratory animal practice," and (4) "act as a spokesperson for laboratory animal practitioners within the AVMA House of Delegates and to work with other organizations involved in the care and use of laboratory animals in representing our common interests and concerns to the scientific community and the public at large." For further information, visit www.aslap.org.

American College of Laboratory Animal Medicine

As stated in their website, the College was originally established as the American Board of Laboratory Animal Medicine in 1957 to "encourage education, training, and research in laboratory animal medicine"; to "establish standards of training and experience for veterinarians professionally involved with the care and health of laboratory animals"; and to "recognize qualified persons in laboratory animal medicine, through certification examination and other means." The name of the organization was changed to the American College of Laboratory Animal Medicine (ACLAM) in 1961. ACLAM is a specialty board recognized by the AVMA. Veterinarians who have successfully completed the comprehensive certification examination and fulfilled other stated requirements earn the right to be board certified and to be called Diplomates of the American College of Laboratory Animal Medicine. ACLAM sponsors an annual educational meeting, the ACLAM Forum, to highlight different topics of importance to the laboratory animal medicine community. In addition, ACLAM has developed a series of textbooks and programs to promote education about laboratory animal medicine. For further information, visit www.aclam.org.

National Association for Biomedical Research

The National Association for Biomedical Research (NABR) was founded in 1979. It is a national, nonprofit organization that advocates for sound public policy in support of ethical and essential animal use in biomedical research. NABR serves as a unified voice in Washington, DC, for the scientific community on legislative and regulatory matters affecting laboratory animal research.

NABR supports the responsible and humane care and use of laboratory animals and believes that only as many animals as necessary should be used; that the pain or distress animals may experience should be minimized; and that alternatives to the use of live animals should be developed and employed whenever feasible. NABR, however, recognizes "that now, and for the foreseeable future, it is not possible to completely replace the use of animals in biomedical research, and that the study of whole, living organisms is an indispensable element of biomedicine that is beneficial to both veterinary and human health." For more information, visit www.nabr.org.

Foundation for Biomedical Research

The Foundation for Biomedical Research (FBR), partner organization to NABR, was established in 1981. It is a nonprofit organization dedicated to improving the quality of human and animal health by promoting public understanding and support for the humane and responsible use of animals in biomedical research. FBR provides information to teachers, students, the media, and the general public on the essential need for animals in medical research and for scientific advancement. A wide variety of educational materials, including brochures, posters, reference papers, discussion papers, and videos to support their effort are available from the FBR (Figure 1.4). For further information, visit www.FBResearch.org.

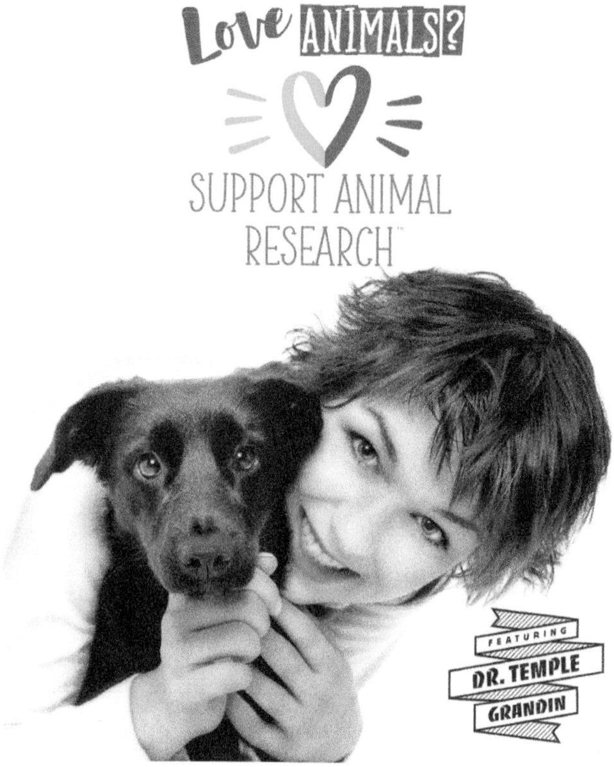

Fig 1.4. Educational brochure cover. Full brochure available on the book's accompanying website. (*Source:* Foundation for Biomedical Research.)

Institute for Laboratory Animal Research

The Institute for Laboratory Animal Research (ILAR) was founded in 1952 under the guidance of the National Research Council (NRC) of the National Academy of Sciences. ILAR functions as an advisor to the federal government, the biomedical research community, science educators and students, and the public. Its mission is "to evaluate and to report on scientific, technological, and ethical use of animals and related biological resources, and of non-animal alternatives in non-food settings, such as research, testing, education, and production of pharmaceuticals." ILAR's core values are (1) "support [of] the responsible use of animals in research, testing, and education as a key component to advancing the health and quality of life of humans and animals"; (2) promotion of "high-quality science and humane care and use of research animals based upon the principles of refinement, replacement, and reduction (the 3Rs) and high ethical standards"; and (3) fostering of "best practices that enhance human and animal welfare by organizing and disseminating information and by facilitating dialogue among interested parties." Advice on all activities of the organization is provided by the ILAR Council which is composed of experts in laboratory animal medicine, medicine, bioethics, and other biomedical sciences. ILAR prepares authoritative reports on subjects of importance to the animal care and use community, including the *Guide for the Care and Use of Laboratory Animals*. ILAR also publishes the *ILAR Journal*, a quarterly peer-reviewed publication on a variety of topics pertinent to the biomedical research community. For further information, visit www.dels.nas.edu/ilar.

As evident by the diversity of organizations listed above, those who work in laboratory animal medicine continually strive to improve the quality of animal-based biomedical research while at the same time supporting animal welfare. Numerous organizations assist individuals in this pursuit through the educational opportunities, scientific resources, and advocacy activities that they provide.

BIBLIOGRAPHY

American Association for Laboratory Animal Science (AALAS). https://www.aalas.org [accessed September 24, 2018].

American College of Laboratory Animal Medicine (ACLAM). https://www.aclam.org [accessed September 24, 2018].

American Society of Laboratory Animal Practitioners (ASLAP). https://www.aslap.org [accessed September 24, 2018].

Animal and Plant Health Inspection Service (APHIS). 2017. *The Animal Welfare Act and Animal Welfare Regulations as of January 1, 2017*. Washington, DC: US Department of Agriculture. Available at https://www.aphis.usda.gov/animal_welfare/downloads/AC_BlueBook_AWA_FINAL_2017_508comp.pdf [accessed September 19, 2018].

Animal and Plant Health Inspection Service (APHIS). 2018a. *AWA Inspection and Annual Reports*. Available at https://www.aphis.usda.gov/aphis/ourfocus/animalwelfare/sa_awa/AWA-Inspection-and-Annual-Reports [accessed September 19, 2018].

Animal and Plant Health Inspection Service (APHIS). 2018b. *Annual Report Animal Usage by Fiscal Year*. Available at https://www.aphis.usda.gov/aphis/ourfocus/animalwelfare/sa_awa/AWA-Inspection-and-Annual-Reports [accessed December 28, 2018].

Foundation for Biomedical Research (FBR). https://www.FBResearch.org [accessed September 24, 2018].

Institute of Laboratory Animal Resources (ILAR). 2009. *Scientific and Human Issues in the Use of Random Source Dogs and Cats in Research*, National Research Council. Washington, DC: National Academies Press. Available at https://grants.nih.gov/grants/olaw/random_source_dog_and_cat_report.pdf [accessed September 19, 2018].

Institute of Laboratory Animal Resources (ILAR). 2011. *Guide for the Care and Use of Laboratory Animals*, 8th ed. ILAR, National Research Council. Washington, DC: National Academies Press. Available at https://grants.nih.gov/grants/olaw/guide-for-the-care-and-use-of-laboratory-animals.pdf [accessed September 19, 2018].

Institute of Laboratory Animal Resources (ILAR). https://www.del.nas.edu/ilar [accessed September 24, 2018].

Laboratory Animal Management Association (LAMA). http://www.lama-online.org [accessed September 24, 2018].

Levin, J., and F. B. Bang. 1964. The role of endotoxin in the extracellular coagulation of limulus blood. *Bull Johns Hopkins Hosp* 115: 265–274.

Levin, J., and F. B. Bang. 1968. Clottable protein in limulus: its localization and kinetics of its coagulation by endotoxin. *Thromb Diath Haemorrh* 19(1): 186–197.

National Association for Biomedical Research (NABR). https://www.nabr.org/biomedical-research [accessed September 24, 2018].

Office of Laboratory Animal Welfare (OLAW). 1985. *US Government Principles for the Utilization and Care of Vertebrate Animals Used in Testing, Research, and Training*. Available at https://olaw.nih.gov/policies-laws/gov-principles.htm [accessed September 19, 2018].

Russell, W. M. S., and R. L. Burch. 1959. *The Principles of Humane Experimental Technique*. London: Methuen.

Speaking of Research. www.speakingofresearch.com [accessed September 13, 2018].

FURTHER READING

American Veterinary Medical Association (AVMA). 2018. *Use of Animals in Research, Testing, and Education*. Available at https://www.avma.org/KB/Policies/Pages/Use-of-Animals-in-Research-Testing-and-Education.aspx [accessed December 10, 2018].

Canadian Council on Animal Care. 2018. *Ethics in Animal Experimentation*. Available at https://www.ccac.ca/en/training/modules/core-stream/ethics-in-animal-experimentation.html [accessed December 10, 2018].

Congressional Research Service (CRS). 2018. *Enforcement of the Food, Drug, and Cosmetic Act: Select Legal Issues,* R43609. Available at https://fas.org/sgp/crs/misc/R43609.pdf [accessed September 24, 2018].

Festing, M. F. W., P. Overend, M. C. Borja, and M. Berdoy. 2002. *The Design of Animal Experiments: Reducing the Use of Animals in Research through Better Experimental Design*. Oxford: Royal Society of Medicine Press.

Interagency Coordinating Committee on the Validation of Alternative Methods (ICCVAM). 2018. *About ICCVAM*. Available at https://ntp.niehs.nih.gov/pubhealth/evalatm/iccvam/index.html [accessed December 10, 2018].

Kilkenny, C., W. J. Browne, I. C. Cuthill, M. Emerson, and D. G. Altman. 2010. Improving bioscience research reporting: The ARRIVE guidelines for reporting animal research. *PLoS Biol* 8(6): e1000412. doi:https://doi.org/10.1371/journal.pbio.1000412.

Office of Laboratory Animal Welfare (OLAW). https://olaw.nih.gov [accessed September 24, 2018].

Online Ethics Center (OEC). 2018. *The Ethics of Using Animals in Research*. Available at https://www.onlineethics.org/Resources/TeachingTools/Modules/19237/animalres.aspx [accessed December 10, 2018].

CHAPTER 1 REVIEW

Matching

Match the following with their respective descriptions:

A. AALAS
B. ACLAM
C. ASLAP
D. CMAR
E. FDA
F. FBR
G. FD&C
H. IACUC
I. ILAR
J. LAMA
K. LAT
L. NABR
M. NIH

Fill in the blank

1. ____ Organization that provides educational workshops in support of a certificate program for managers of animal facilities
2. ____ Develops guidelines and disseminates information to the federal government on scientific, technological, and ethical use of animals
3. ____ Prior to use of animals, a protocol must be approved by this committee
4. ____ Certification program for managers of animal facilities that requires applicable experience and successful completion of a series of exams
5. ____ AALAS certification level for technicians who have achieved diagnostic and technical skills
6. ____ Law created to safeguard and protect consumer health and safety from the sale of dangerous products
7. ____ Nonprofit organization that serves as the principal means of communication between individuals and organizations within the field of laboratory animal science
8. ____ Federal agency that requires animal testing of products when a scientifically valid, alternative testing method is not available
9. ____ Nonprofit organization dedicated to promoting public understanding and support for use of animals in research through the creation and distribution of educational materials
10. ____ Specialty board recognized by the AVMA
11. ____ Professional organization for veterinarians engaged or interested in the practice of laboratory animal medicine
12. ____ Nonprofit organization dedicated to advocating sound public policy that recognizes the vital role of animal use in biomedical research
13. ____ Main public granting agency for biomedical research

Below are examples of the application of the 3Rs in animal research. Indicate which of the ethical principles (Replacement, Reduction, or Refinement) is represented by each example:

(Continued)

14. ____ Delivering medications to nonhuman primates in food treats instead of by injection
15. ____ Use of corneas for an ocular irritation assay that are obtained from food animals during the meat processing process and that would otherwise be discarded
16. ____ Use of cell culture in an oncology study
17. ____ Use of the limulus amebocyte lysate assay for pyrogen testing in which blood is taken from horseshoe crabs which are then returned to the ocean
18. ____ Use of a computer model instead of a rat model
19. ____ Corrositex®, an *in vitro* assay used to assess chemicals that are potentially corrosive to skin
20. ____ Use of statistical methods to decrease the number of animals used in a study
21. ____ Use of hollow fiber bioreactors, instead of rabbit models, for monoclonal antibody production
22. ____ Housing female rabbits in groups instead of singly
23. ____ Use of fish animal model instead of a hamster animal model
24. ____ Selection of an appropriate experimental endpoint that occurs earlier in a disease course
25. ____ Use of a dose escalation study design for a drug treatment study
26. ____ Fasting a rat for 8 hours rather than 16 hours before a procedure
27. ____ Utilizing multiple areas on the back of a few pigs instead of using one spot on the back of many pigs for a skin study

Suggested Activities

Watch the video "Love, Care, Progress" produced by Association for Medical Progress at https://www.amprogress.org/love-care-progress-video. Discuss your thoughts on the use of dogs in research and the adoption of dogs previously used in research.

Utilize the Foundation for Biomedical Research website: https://fbresearch.org/biomedical-research/animal-testing-facts and the Michigan Society for Medical Research website: http://mismr.org/facts-myths-about-animal-research to initiate a discussion on common misconceptions about animal testing and research.

Review the AALAS Foundation website: https://www.aalasfoundation.org/outreach/About-Animal-Research/Animal-Rights-vs-Animal-Welfare and the AVMA website: https://www.avma.org/KB/Resources/Reference/AnimalWelfare/Pages/what-is-animal-welfare.aspx then discuss the difference between the terms Animal Rights and Animal Welfare. How do you define each term and how do these philosophical views differ? What do you believe are our responsibilities to animals? Do you believe that humans are entitled to utilize animals? If so, within what limits?

Utilize the interactive Animal Ethics Dilemma website: http://www.aedilemma.net to consider ethical dilemmas about our treatment of animals. The website provides a role-playing game through which multiple case studies can be explored and philosophical views examined.

Seek out information on organizations that you believe make significant contributions to the protection of animals. Explore the organizations' stated philosophies on the use of animals as pets, in food production, in exhibits (e.g., zoos), in research and teaching, and in entertainment. Are the organizations' philosophies and activities consistent with their public image? With your philosophy on the use of animals?

chapter 2

2

Regulations, Policies, and Principles Governing the Care and Use of Laboratory Animals

Numerous regulations, policies, and guidelines impact the care and use of animals in research, teaching, and testing. Institutions involved in animal use must follow federal regulations such as the Animal Welfare Act, the Public Health Service Policy, and the Good Laboratory Practice Act, where applicable. In addition, institutions that meet and exceed regulatory requirements may elect to pursue accreditation by an independent entity. This chapter outlines the primary federal regulatory requirements as well as other important guidelines.

ANIMAL WELFARE ACT AND REGULATIONS

Animal Welfare Act

The Animal Welfare Act (AWA), initially named the Laboratory Animal Welfare Act, was the first US federal law to regulate the handling, sale, and transport of select animal species intended for use in research (Figure 2.1) (Box 2.1). It has been amended multiple times, most recently in 2013. The US Department of Agriculture (USDA) is responsible for the administration and enforcement of the AWA. Within the USDA,

Clinical Laboratory Animal Medicine: An Introduction, Fifth Edition.
Lesley A. Colby, Megan H. Nowland, and Lucy H. Kennedy.

Companion website: www.wiley.com/go/colby/clinical

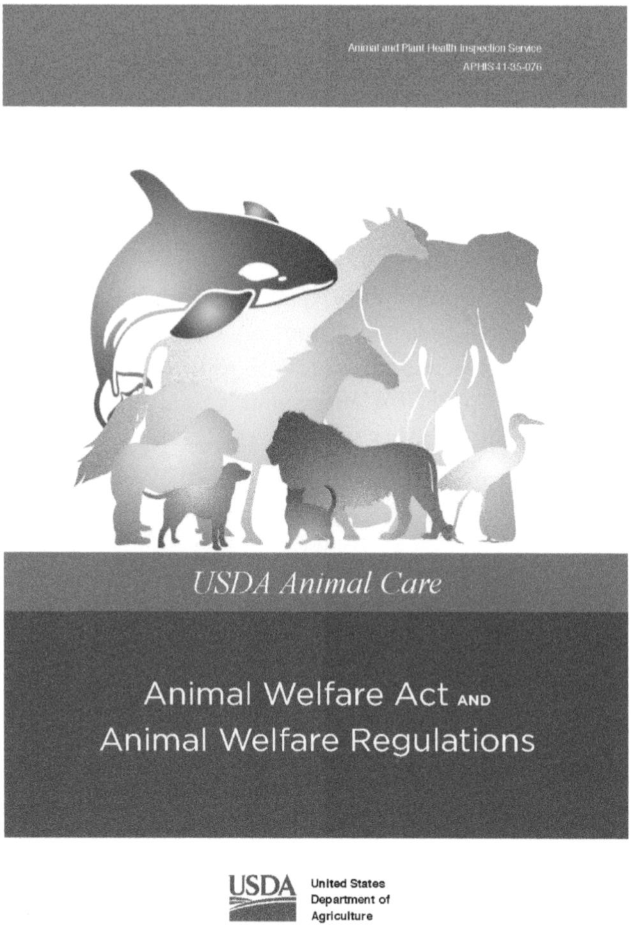

Fig 2.1. Animal Welfare Act and Regulations booklet cover (APHIS Publication No. 41-35-076). (*Source:* USDA Animal Care.)

> **Box 2.1**
>
> *The Animal Welfare Act was the first US federal law to regulate the handling, sale, and transport of select animal species intended for use in research.*

this responsibility has been delegated to the Animal Care program of the Animal and Plant Health Inspection Service (APHIS).

Passage of the Laboratory Animal Welfare Act in 1966 was largely in response to public outcry over the theft and then sale of a pet Dalmatian, "Pepper," to a research lab. The intent of the Act was to protect owners of dogs and cats from theft of their pets, prevent the sale or use of dogs and cats that had been stolen, and ensure that certain animals intended for use in research facilities were provided humane care and treatment. While the primary focus of the law was on the protection of dogs and cats, hamsters, guinea pigs, rabbits, and nonhuman primates were also mentioned. The law required licensure of individuals or corporations that bought or sold these animals for laboratory activities if the animals were transported across state lines. Organizations that used dogs or cats in biomedical activities were required to register with the USDA if they received federal funding or purchased dogs or cats transported across state lines. The legislation applied only to animals being held before or after actual research and testing, and not during their use.

In 1970, through Public Law (PL) 91-579, the Laboratory Animal Welfare Act was renamed the Animal Welfare Act (AWA) and amended to, among other things, broaden the list of regulated species to include all warm-blooded laboratory animals, extend oversight to intra- as well as interstate transportation of animals, and require animal care standards be upheld the entire time an animal is present in a research facility. The Act did not allow the Secretary of Agriculture to issue rules, regulations, or orders specific to the conduct of research. It did require, however, that every research facility demonstrate at least annually that professionally acceptable standards governing care, treatment, and use of animals were being followed. Research facilities were also required to file an annual report listing the number of animals used or held for research and stating if the animals required or received anesthetics, analgesics, or tranquilizers. Submission of this report is still required today. Completed reports must be submitted to USDA-APHIS Animal Care by December 1 and include information for the period of October 1 of the preceding year through September 30 of the current year.

AWA Amendment of 1976: In 1976, the AWA was further amended, PL 94-279, to redefine the regulation of animals during transportation and to prohibit most animal fighting activities. All carriers and intermediate handlers who were not required to be licensed under the AWA were required to register with the USDA. The Secretary of Agriculture also promulgated regulations that specifically excluded rats and mice bred for use in research, birds, horses, and farm animals intended for use as food or fiber or used in studies to improve production of food or fiber.

AWA Amendment of 1985: Major changes were made to the AWA in 1985 with the passage of the Food Security Act, PL 99-198, which contained an amendment titled, "The Improved Standards for Laboratory Animals Act." Changes included creation of Institutional Animal Care and Use Committees (IACUC) and the Animal Welfare Information Center as well as establishment of guidelines and requirements regarding surgical procedures, personnel training, animal exercise programs, and the psychological well-being of nonhuman primates. Methods used to implement each of these changes continue to evolve.

The 1985 amendment required the chief executive officer of each research facility to appoint an IACUC and specified that an IACUC must consist of at least three members, including a doctor of veterinary medicine with experience or training in laboratory animal medicine and one member who is not affiliated with the institution in any way and who can represent the general interests of the community. The IACUC is charged to act as an agent of the research facility to assure compliance with the

AWA. Once every 6 months, the IACUC is required to inspect all animal facilities and study areas and to review the research facility's program to assure that the care and use of the animals comply with regulations and standards. This includes review of the institution's formal program of veterinary care. The IACUC must submit a report of its findings to the Institutional Official of the research facility. The report must distinguish significant deficiencies, those that threaten animal health or safety, from minor deficiencies. A reasonable and specific plan with dates for correction of the deficiencies must be included in the final report. If significant deficiencies or deviations are found during the inspection and review and are not corrected in accordance with the IACUC's specifications, the USDA and other applicable federal funding agencies must be notified in writing. Recommendations to the Institutional Official regarding any aspects of the animal program, facilities, or personnel training are included in the report. The report must be signed by a quorum or majority of the committee members and must include any minority views expressed. This report must be available to the USDA, upon request. The IACUC is also required to review and, if warranted, investigate concerns involving the care and use of research animals raised by members of the public or by animal care or research personnel. Personnel must be provided a means to report concerns with anonymity and without fear of reprisal by the institution.

The IACUC must review and approve all proposed activities (protocols) involving the care and use of animals in research, teaching, or testing not less than annually. The protocol is a detailed description of the procedures or proposed activities involving the use of animals. The protocol must provide the following information: (1) the species and approximate number of animals to be used; (2) a rationale for involving animals and for the appropriateness of the species and number of animals requested; (3) a complete and detailed description of the proposed use of the animals; (4) a description of procedures and pharmacologic agents designed to assure that discomfort and pain to animals will be limited to that which is unavoidable for the conduct of scientifically valuable research; and (5) a description of the euthanasia method to be used. The protocol must provide assurance that animal discomfort, distress, or pain will be avoided or minimized. The 1985 amendment specifies that consultation with a doctor of veterinary medicine is necessary in planning any procedure that could cause pain to animals. For procedures that might cause more than momentary or slight pain or distress, a written narrative description of the methods and sources used to determine that alternatives are not available is required. The principal investigator of the protocol must also assure the committee that the proposed work does not unnecessarily duplicate previous experiments. The website http://www.aalas.org/iacuc is a useful resource for additional information regarding the function and operations of IACUCs.

The 1985 amendment required that survival surgical procedures be performed using aseptic techniques, including use of sterile instruments, masks, and surgical gloves. It also states that major survival surgery on nonrodents may be conducted only in facilities intended for that purpose. In this context, major surgery involves penetration and exposure of a body cavity or produces substantial impairment of physical or physiologic functions such as laparotomy, thoracotomy, and joint replacement. In contrast, minor surgery does not expose a body cavity and causes little or no physical impairment. Examples include peripheral vessel cannulation and suturing a wound. Further, the amendment specified that no animal may be used in more than one major operative procedure from which it recovers unless it is justified and approved by the IACUC, required as a routine veterinary procedure, or necessary to protect the health or well-being of the animal.

The 1985 amendment was the first federal legislation to mandate training of all personnel using animals in research facilities. More specifically, institutions were required to provide instruction on the care and handling of animals, humane methods of experimentation, aseptic surgery techniques, methods to minimize or eliminate the use of animals, and procedures to report deficiencies in animal care and treatment.

In addition, the amendment set standards for the exercise of dogs and an environment adequate to promote the psychological well-being of nonhuman primates. The dog exercise standards require a plan be developed, documented, and followed to provide dogs over 12 weeks of age with the opportunity for exercise. The Attending Veterinarian must approve the exercise plan. The opportunity for exercise may be provided in a number of ways, such as allowing access to a run or open area for a prescribed time and frequency or walking animals on a leash. Additional opportunity for exercise is not required for individually housed dogs provided at least twice the minimum floor space specified in the AWA. It is also not required for group-housed dogs maintained in an area that provides at least the cumulative total of floor space minimally required for each dog, if housed individually. The Attending Veterinarian may approve exemptions to this exercise plan based on the dog's health, condition, or well-being. Such exemptions must be documented and reviewed at least every 30 days by the Attending Veterinarian unless the condition for exemption is a permanent one (e.g., chronic heart failure).

The standards for environmental enhancement to promote psychological well-being of nonhuman primates require a plan be developed in accordance with currently accepted professional standards. This plan must be directed by the Attending Veterinarian, documented, and followed. At a minimum, the plan must address animal social needs, environmental enrichment of primary enclosures, special needs of individual species, use of restraint devices, and the exemption of certain primates from the standards due to health concerns or research needs.The 1985 amendment also established the Animal Welfare Information Center (AWIC) within the USDA National Agricultural Library. AWIC's mission is to provide information pertinent to employee training and to the reduction and refinement of animal use through avoidance of unnecessary duplication of animal experimentation, reduction or replacement of animal use, and minimization of animal pain and distress.

AWA Amendment of 1990: The 1990 amendment of the AWA entitled "Protection of Pets" was a component of the farm bill Food, Agriculture, Conservation, and Trade Act, PL101-624. This amendment mandated pounds and shelters, both private and public, to hold any live dog or cat for a minimum period of 5 days, not including the day of acquisition, before euthanizing or releasing the animal to a Class B USDA-licensed dealer. See Chapter 1 for further information regarding Class B dealers and random source animals.

AWA Amendment of 2002: In 2002, the Farm Security and Rural Investment Act (PL 107-171) redefined the term "animal" in the AWA to specifically exclude birds, rats of the genus *Rattus*, and mice of the genus *Mus* bred for use in research. The amendment also included verbiage to address animal fighting. It made it a misdemeanor to ship a bird in interstate commerce for fighting purposes or to sponsor or exhibit a bird in a fight when the bird had been shipped for that purpose.

AWA Amendment of 2007: The "Animal Fighting Prohibition Enforcement Act of 2007" (PL 110-22) made violation of the animal fighting provisions of the AWA a felony, punishable by up to 3 years in prison. The law also made it a felony to trade, sell, or ship select equipment designed for use in animal fighting, or to promote an animal fighting venture.

AWA Amendment of 2008: The "Food, Conservation, and Energy Act of 2008" (PL 110-246) contained a number of AWA amendments to strengthen definitions of and penalties for activities related to animal fighting. It also required regulations to limit the transport and resale of dogs unless they are at least 6 months of age, are in good health, and have all necessary vaccinations. Exemptions exist for research, veterinary treatment, or imports into Hawaii from certain countries. The monetary maximum penalty for a general violation of the act for each occurrence was also increased.

Currently, animal research facilities, animal dealers and exhibitors, operators of animal auction sales, and carriers and transporters of animals must be licensed and/or registered by the USDA (Box 2.2). Retail pet stores are exempt from this requirement unless they sell animals to a research facility or a wholesale dealer.

As part of USDA's oversight of registered entities, a USDA veterinary medical officer performs unannounced compliance inspections at least annually to ensure that entities are operating in compliance with the AWA. Inspections include assessment of facilities, husbandry practices, programs of veterinary care, records, and animal handling procedures. Reports to the USDA of a suspected violation can also trigger a visit "for cause."

Animal Welfare Regulations

The Animal Welfare Regulations (AWR) [Code of Federal Regulations, Title 9 (Animals and Animal Products), Chapter 1 (Animal and Plant Health Inspection Service, Department of Agriculture), Subchapter A (Animal Welfare), Parts 1–4] interpret the Animal Welfare Act into enforceable standards (Figure 2.1). The regulations describe

Box 2.2

Animal research facilities, animal dealers and exhibitors, operators of animal auction sales, and carriers and transporters of animals must be licensed and/ or registered by the USDA.

humane handling, care, identification, recordkeeping, treatment, and transportation of animals. Mandatory minimum animal care standards are provided for dogs, cats, guinea pigs, hamsters, rabbits, nonhuman primates, and marine mammals. These standards address feeding, watering, sanitation, lighting, ventilation, shelter from extremes of weather and temperatures, separation by species, and adequate veterinary care. Maintenance of health records is considered an important component of adequate veterinary care. As such, health records must be current, legible, and sufficiently comprehensive to demonstrate the delivery of adequate health care. An animal's health records must be held for at least 1 year after its disposition or death.

To further clarify the intent of the AWA, and to help maintain consistency in application of the regulations, the USDA periodically issues Animal Care Policies (accessible at https://www.aphis.usda.gov/aphis/ourfocus/animalwelfare/sa_publications).

PUBLIC HEALTH SERVICE POLICY ON HUMANE CARE AND USE OF LABORATORY ANIMALS

The Health Research Extension Act of 1985 (PL 99-158) provides the legislative mandate for the US Public Health Service Policy on Humane Care and Use of Laboratory Animals (PHS Policy) (Figure 2.2). The PHS Policy applies to the use of all live vertebrate animals in research and other biomedical activities wholly or partially funded by the US Public Health Service (PHS) agencies or US Department of Health and Human Services components as well as activities performed at an institution with an Animal Welfare Assurance, regardless of the source of funding. The Office of Laboratory Animal Welfare (OLAW), organizationally positioned within the National Institutes of Health (NIH), is the governmental body responsible for interpreting and implementing the PHS Policy and evaluating institutional compliance with it (Box 2.3). To facilitate compliance with the PHS Policy, OLAW provides instruction to institutions and researchers who receive PHS support.

The PHS Policy requires institutions to submit an Animal Welfare Assurance document to OLAW, fully describing each institution's program for the care and use of animals and assuring their commitment to following the "US Government Principles for the Utilization and Care of Vertebrate Animals Used in Testing, Research, and Training" (US Government Principles) (Table 2.1) and complying with the PHS Policy, the *Guide for the Care and Use of Laboratory Animals* (the *Guide*; ILAR, 2011), and the Animal Welfare Act Regulations. An institution's participation in the voluntary accreditation process of AAALAC International strongly demonstrates this commitment. The Animal Welfare Assurance document must identify the IACUC chairperson and include the names, positions, titles, and credentials of all IACUC members. Under the PHS Policy, the IACUC must maintain oversight of all animal facilities and procedures and must consist of at least five members, including at least (1) one doctor of veterinary medicine, with training or experience in laboratory animal science and medicine, who has direct or delegated program authority and responsibility for activities involving animals at the institution; (2) one practicing scientist

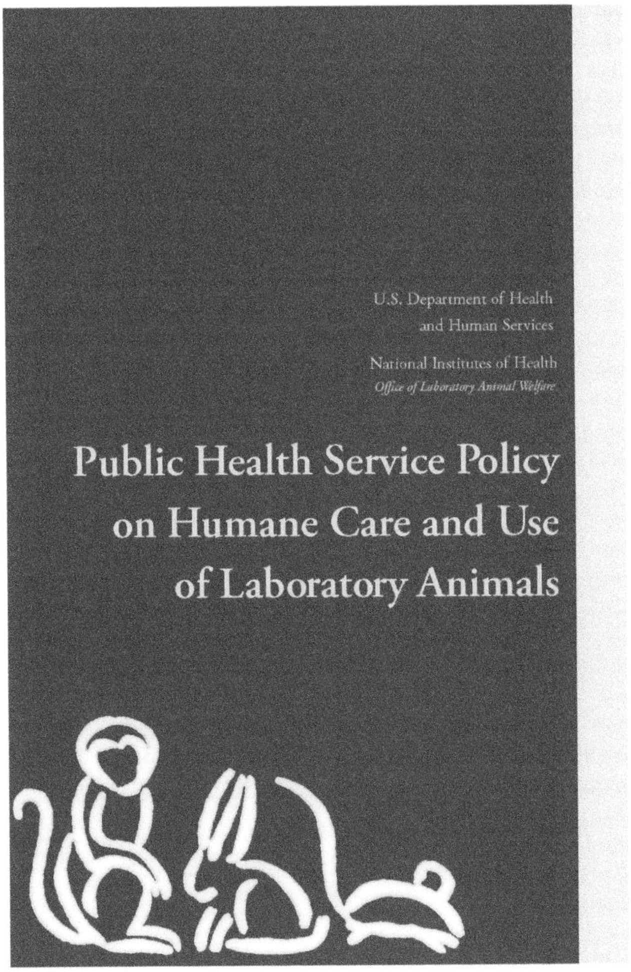

Fig 2.2. PHS Policy booklet cover (NIH Publication No. 15-8013). (*Source:* Office of Laboratory Animal Welfare, NIH.)

experienced in research involving animals; (3) one non-scientist, an individual whose primary concerns are in a nonscientific area (e.g., ethicist, lawyer, member of the clergy); and (4) one member who is not affiliated with the institution in any way other than as a member of the IACUC and who is not in the immediate family of a person affiliated with the institution. While an individual who meets the requirements of more than one category may fulfill more than one requirement, a committee may not consist of fewer than five members.

Box 2.3

The Office of Laboratory Animal Welfare (OLAW) is the governmental body responsible for interpreting and implementing the PHS Policy and evaluating institutional compliance with it.

Table 2.1. US government principles for the utilization and care of vertebrate animals used in testing, research, and training

I.	The transportation, care, and use of animals should be in accordance with the Animal Welfare Act (7 U.S.C. 2131 et seq.) and other applicable Federal laws, guidelines, and policies.
II.	Procedures involving animals should be designed and performed with due consideration of their relevance to human or animal health, the advancement of knowledge, or the good of society.
III.	The animals selected for a procedure should be of an appropriate species and quality and the minimum number required to obtain valid results. Methods such as mathematical models, computer simulation, and in vitro biological systems should be considered.
IV.	Proper use of animals, including the avoidance or minimization of discomfort, distress, and pain when consistent with sound scientific practices, is imperative. Unless the contrary is established, investigators should consider that procedures that cause pain or distress in human beings may cause pain or distress in other animals.
V.	Procedures with animals that may cause more than momentary or slight pain or distress should be performed with appropriate sedation, analgesia, or anesthesia. Surgical or other painful procedures should not be performed on unanesthetized animals paralyzed by chemical agents.
VI.	Animals that would otherwise suffer severe or chronic pain or distress that cannot be relieved should be painlessly killed at the end of the procedure or, if appropriate, during the procedure.
VII.	The living conditions of animals should be appropriate for their species and contribute to their health and comfort. Normally, the housing, feeding, and care of all animals used for biomedical purposes must be directed by a veterinarian or other scientist trained and experienced in the proper care, handling, and use of the species being maintained or studied. In any case, veterinary care shall be provided as indicated.
VIII.	Investigators and other personnel shall be appropriately qualified and experienced for conducting procedures on living animals. Adequate arrangements shall be made for their in-service training, including the proper and humane care and use of laboratory animals.
IX.	Where exceptions are required in relation to the provisions of these Principles, the decisions should not rest with the investigators directly concerned but should be made, with due regard to Principle II, by an appropriate review group such as an institutional animal care and use committee. Such exceptions should not be made solely for the purposes of teaching or demonstration.

Source: https://olaw.nih.gov/policies-laws/phs-policy.htm#USGovPrinciples.

Under the PHS Policy, the IACUC must conduct a *de novo* (anew) review of each animal use protocol at least once every 3 years. The Policy also requires that institutions maintain an occupational health program to safeguard the health of individuals associated with the conduct of animal research. In addition, institutions must provide instruction in the responsible conduct of research to all staff engaged in research or research training funded by the PHS. Areas of instruction must include data acquisition, management, sharing, and ownership; mentor–trainee responsibilities; publication practices and responsible authorship; peer review; collaborative science; research involving human subjects; research involving animals; research misconduct; conflict of interest and commitment; and compliance with existing PHS and institutional policies.

Institutions are required to establish a mechanism for the semiannual review of their animal facilities and procedures for conformance with the *Guide*. Findings of the review must be provided to the institution's designated Institutional Official who holds ultimate responsibility for the institution's animal care and use program. Review findings must also be provided to OLAW upon its request. Additionally, institutions must provide to OLAW an annual update to their Animal Welfare Assurance document, describing any changes to their animal care and use program, including changes in select personnel (e.g., IO, IACUC members). For further information regarding annual reporting, visit https://olaw.nih.gov/guidance/topic-index/animal-welfare.htm.

OTHER REGULATIONS, POLICIES, GUIDANCE DOCUMENTS, AND ORGANIZATIONS

Guide for the Care and Use of Laboratory Animals

The *Guide for the Care and Use of Laboratory Animals*, published by the Institute of Laboratory Animal Research (ILAR) of the National Academy of Sciences, was first published in 1963 and most recently revised in 2011 (ILAR, 2011). As stated by ILAR, "The purpose of the *Guide* is to assist institutions caring for and using animals in ways judged to be scientifically, technically, and humanely appropriate. The *Guide* is also intended to assist investigators in fulfilling their obligation to plan and conduct animal experiments in accord with the highest scientific, humane, and ethical principles." The *Guide* defines laboratory animals as "any vertebrate (e.g., traditional laboratory animals, farm animals, wildlife, and aquatic animals) used in research, testing, or education." It makes recommendations for humane animal care and use based on published data, scientific principles, expert opinion, and experience with methods and practices proven consistent with high-quality, humane animal care and use. *The Guide*'s recommendations carry the force of law based on the Health Research Extension Act passed by Congress in 1985.

The *Guide* is used throughout the world as a resource for laboratory animal research facilities (Box 2.4). Currently, the *Guide* is available in numerous translations, including Chinese, English, French, Japanese, Korean, Portuguese, Russian, Spanish, and Taiwanese. The *Guide* addresses the major components of an animal care and use program, including institutional policies and responsibilities; animal environment, housing, and management; veterinary medical care; and physical plant. Personnel qualifications and training, occupational health and safety of personnel,

> **Box 2.4**
>
> *The* Guide for the Care and Use of Laboratory Animals *is used throughout the world as a resource for laboratory animal research facilities.*

preventive medicine, surgery and postsurgical care, and euthanasia are addressed in detail. The *Guide* states that, unless justified for scientific or medical reasons, the method of euthanasia should be consistent with the most recent *AVMA Guidelines for Euthanasia* (AVMA, 2013).

The *Guide* encourages programs to adhere to the US Government Principles (see Table 2.1). It also clarifies that programs should function in accord with the USDA regulations, the PHS Policy, and other applicable federal, state, and local laws, regulations, and policies. Importantly, the *Guide* largely employs performance-oriented standards in addition to engineering standards. Recommendations that are performance-oriented direct the user to achieve a specific goal but do not specify the methods used to achieve that outcome. This approach allows flexibility and professional judgment and tends to result in greater enhancement of animal well-being. Engineering standards are specific and generally science-based, giving an exact requirement that must be met. When performance and engineering standards are balanced, programs achieve higher levels of care and use because professional judgment can be used to apply standards to meet a variety of situations. To download a free copy of the *Guide*, visit http://www.nap.edu/catalog.php?record_id=12910.

Guide for the Care and Use of Agricultural Animals in Research and Teaching

The *Guide for the Care and Use of Agricultural Animals in Research and Teaching*, commonly referred to as the *Ag Guide,* was first published in 1988 under the title of *Guide for the Care and Use of Agricultural Animals in Agricultural Research and Teaching*. In the third (2010) and most recent edition of the document (Figure 2.3), the title was changed to remove the second use of the word "agricultural" to reflect the understanding that agricultural animals' needs as well as the basic requirements to maintain their welfare are not dictated by the objective of their use (e.g., biomedical versus agricultural research) (FASS, 2010).

The *Ag Guide* is maintained by a joint committee of the American Dairy Science Association (ADSA), the American Society of Animal Science (ASAS), and the Poultry Science Association (PSA). It is intended to supplement applicable federal and state laws, regulations, and policies and the *Guide for the Care and Use of Laboratory Animals* (ILAR, 2011) as they pertain to the use of agricultural animals. It is science-based and provides guidelines for husbandry, veterinary care, facility construction and maintenance, and institutional policies for agricultural animals. Similar to the *Guide*, the *Ag Guide* endorses the US Government Principles and emphasizes the use of performance-oriented standards in place of more rigid and less-adaptable engineering standards. The *Ag Guide* is based on the premise that "Farm animals have certain needs and requirements and these needs and requirements do not necessarily change because of the objectives of the research or teaching activity" (FASS, 2010). The *Ag Guide* is not intended to pertain to animals produced on farms and ranches for commercial purposes. AAALAC International uses the *Ag Guide* for relevant program assessment and accreditation purposes. To download a copy of this publication, visit https://www.asas.org/ag_guide_3rded/HTML5/index.html.

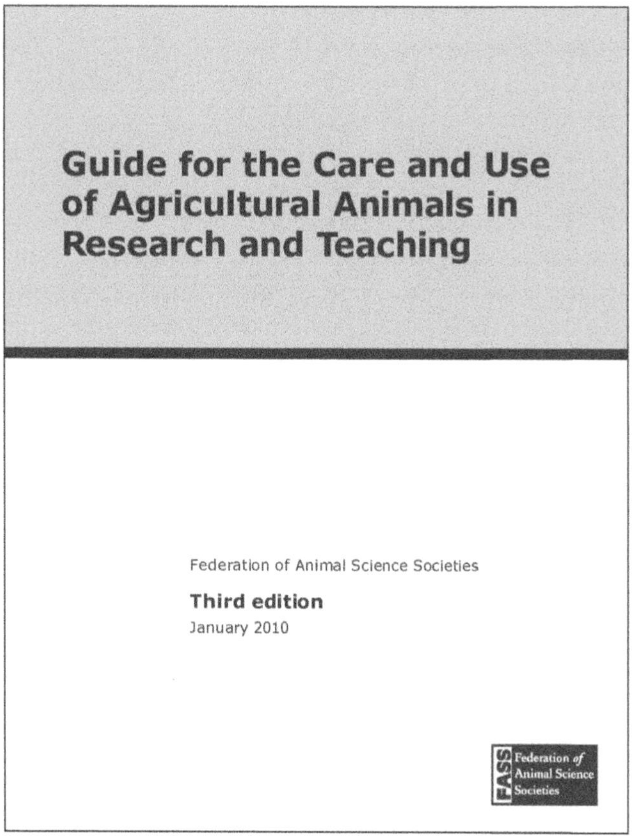

Guide for the Care and Use of Agricultural Animals in Research and Teaching

Federation of Animal Science Societies

Third edition

January 2010

FASS Federation of Animal Science Societies

Fig 2.3. *Ag Guide* book cover. (*Source:* Used by permission of American Dairy Science Association®, American Society of Animal Science, and Poultry Science Association. Use does not constitute endorsement by any of the rights holders.)

Good Laboratory Practice Regulations

Good Laboratory Practice (GLP) regulations provide the framework for performing high-quality, well-documented, and repeatable safety studies conducted under the oversight of responsible, designated individuals. The GLP regulations were first adopted in 1978 for nonclinical safety studies funded by the Food and Drug Administration (FDA) (21 CFR 58) and then in 1983 for studies funded by the Environmental Protection Agency (EPA) (40 CFR 160). These regulations specifically address and define standards for research facilities engaged in product safety testing designed for human and veterinary applications. Quality assurance and strict adherence to standard operating procedures are central components of the regulations. Each study must have an approved written protocol that defines the study title and purpose, the test article being studied, the testing facility, details about animal use, and study sponsorship. Laboratories must maintain extensive records of all aspects of the study and make them available to the FDA or the EPA, as needed. For animal studies, required records include those pertaining to animal acquisition, housing, and procedures; facility environmental monitoring; and sample collection and processing. The FDA and the EPA have the legal authority to inspect study records and the facilities where studies are conducted.

The Chimpanzee Health Improvement, Maintenance, and Protection Act

The Chimpanzee Health Improvement, Maintenance, and Protection (CHIMP) Act (PL 106-551) was signed into law in December 2000. It created a "sanctuary" retirement system for chimpanzees previously used, bred, or purchased for use in medical research supported by the agencies of the federal government. Chimp Haven, located near Shreveport, Louisiana, was selected to operate the National Chimpanzee Sanctuary System and is financially supported predominantly through federal funds. The CHIMP Act also mandated that standards of care for chimpanzees in the sanctuary be developed to ensure the well-being and the health and safety of the chimpanzees. The law originally contained a clause that allowed, under special circumstances, further use of the chimpanzees in research. However, passage of the Chimp Haven is Home Act (PL 110-170) in December 2007 repealed that portion of the original legislation and prohibited removal of chimpanzees from the sanctuary system for all research purposes, except for noninvasive behavioral studies.

The 21st Century Cures Act

The 21st Century Cures Act (PL 114–255) became law in December 2016. It is designed in part "to help accelerate medical product development and bring new innovations and advances to patients who need them faster and more efficiently," such as through the reduction of inconsistent, overlapping, or duplicative policies and regulations that hinder the conduct of animal research. It remains to be seen if the Act will achieve its intended purpose.

Animal Welfare Information Center

The AWIC is part of the USDA National Agricultural Library. It was established in 1986, as mandated by amendments to the Animal Welfare Act, to provide information on improved animal care and use in research, teaching, and testing. The AWIC combines personnel with subject expertise, state-of-the-art technology, and networking to assist those interested in learning more about methods for the humane care, use, and handling of animals in research, testing, and teaching. The AWIC provides the research community with specific information on employee training and identification of improved research methods that could reduce or replace animal use and minimize pain and distress to animals. It also assists researchers in conducting appropriate literature searches designed to identify animal alternatives and prevent unintended duplication of animal experimentation. In addition, the AWIC provides educational opportunities through workshops, publications, and public exhibits. See https://www.nal.usda.gov/awic for additional information.

State Regulations

In the United States, all 50 states and the District of Columbia have laws that protect animals. Most of these laws protect animals from cruel treatment and require that animals have access to food and water and be provided with shelter from extreme weather. Some states have public health and agriculture regulations that specifically cover animals used in research. Additionally, a number of states, cities, and towns regulate the release of impounded animals for research as well as the adoption of retired research animals.

AAALAC International

Initially organized by veterinarians and researchers in 1965, AAALAC International (AAALAC) is a private, nonprofit organization that promotes the humane treatment of animals in science by encouraging high standards of animal care, use, and well-being through voluntary accreditation and assessment programs (Figure 2.4). The name of the organization has changed over time from "American Association for Accreditation of Laboratory Animal Care" to "Association for the Assessment and Accreditation of Laboratory Animal Care, International," then finally to its current name (AAALAC International) to reflect its continued international expansion. AAALAC-accredited institutions are now present in over 47 countries worldwide.

It is important to note that AAALAC is not a regulatory entity and institutions are under no legal requirement to obtain or maintain AAALAC accreditation. Rather, institutions volunteer to participate in the AAALAC accreditation process to demonstrate their commitment to the highest quality of animal care and use (Box 2.5).

AAALAC exists due to the work of multiple groups. An administrative staff coordinates all organizational activities. Over 60 premier scientific, educational, and other organizations are AAALAC Member Organizations including American Heart Association, American Hospital Association, American Psychological Society, Association of Public and Land-Grant Universities, European Federation of Pharmaceutical Industries and Associations, Federation of American Societies for

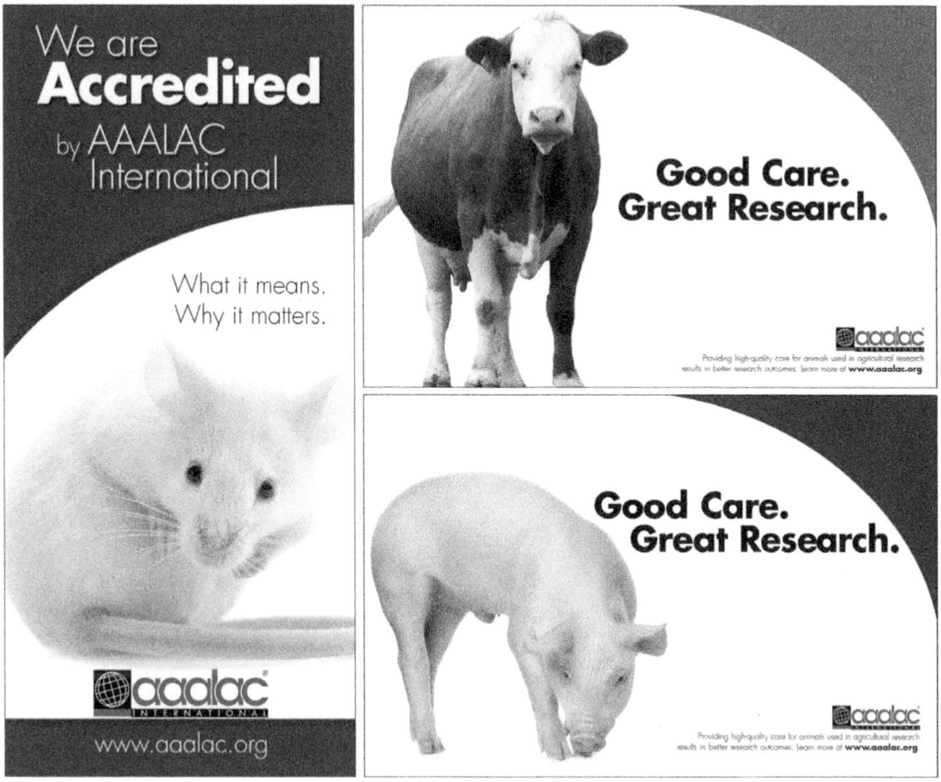

Fig 2.4. AAALAC brochures. (*Source*: Photo courtesy of AAALAC International.)

Box 2.5

Institutions volunteer to participate in the AAALAC accreditation process to demonstrate their commitment to the highest quality of animal care and use.

Experimental Biology, and the Society of Toxicology. Each Member Organization appoints one delegate to serve on AAALAC's International Board of Trustees. Delegates serve in an advisory role to AAALAC on behalf of their organizations. Delegates also attend and vote during AAALAC's annual business meeting.

AAALAC's Council on Accreditation performs the majority of institutional site visits and program evaluations. The Council is composed of professionals from around the world with expertise in the fields of veterinary medicine, laboratory animal science, and animal research. The Council is geographically and administratively divided into three regions: North American, European, and Pacific Rim.

Council members and designated ad hoc consultants conduct peer review evaluations of laboratory animal care facilities and programs. These site visits occur once every 3 years. The number of site visitors and the duration of the visit are based upon the size and complexity of a program. One of the most valuable aspects of the accreditation process is the writing of the program description, which requires institutions to carefully describe the details of their animal care and use program, and through this process to perform a self-assessment. The program description outline follows the chapters of the *Guide*, including animal care and use policies and responsibilities; animal environment, housing, and management; veterinary medical care; and physical plant.

AAALAC uses three primary standards in conducting evaluations of laboratory animal care and use programs: the *Guide for the Care and Use of Laboratory Animals* (ILAR, 2011); the *Guide for the Care and Use of Agricultural Animals in Research and Teaching* (FASS, 2010); and the European Convention for the Protection of Vertebrate Animals Used for Experimental and Other Scientific Purposes, Council of Europe (ETS 123). AAALAC also refers to other specialty publications and reference resources for supplemental information about procedures or techniques related to the care and use of laboratory animals. A list of these resources and AAALAC International policy statements can be found at www.aaalac.org.

REFERENCES

American Veterinary Medical Association (AVMA). 2013. *AVMA Guidelines for the Euthanasia of Animals*. Available at http://www.avma.org/KB/Policies/Documents/euthanasia.pdf [accessed March 15, 2013].

Animal and Plant Health Inspection Service (APHIS). 2017. *Animal Welfare Act and Animal Welfare Regulations as of January 1, 2017*. Washington, DC: US Department of Agriculture. Available at https://www.aphis.usda.gov/animal_welfare/downloads/AC_BlueBook_AWA_FINAL_2017_508comp.pdf [accessed October 7, 2018].

Congressional Research Service (CRS). 2016. *The Animal Welfare Act: Background and Selected Animal Welfare Legislation*. Available at http://nationalaglawcenter.org/wp-content/uploads/assets/crs/RS22493.pdf [accessed October 7, 2018].

Federation of Animal Science Societies (FASS). 2010. *Guide for the Care and Use of Agricultural Animals in Research and Teaching*, 3rd ed., J. McGlone and J. Swanson (eds.). Champaign, IL: FASS.

Institute of Laboratory Animal Resources (ILAR). 2011. *Guide for the Care and Use of Laboratory Animals*, 8th ed. ILAR, National Research Council. Washington, DC: National Academies Press.

Office of Laboratory Animal Welfare (OLAW). 2015. *Public Health Service Policy on Humane Care and Use of Laboratory Animals*, Available at https://olaw.nih.gov/policies-laws/phs-policy.htm [accessed October 22, 2018].

FURTHER READING

Bayne, K. and L. C. Anderson, 2015. Laws, regulations, and policies affecting the use of laboratory animals. In *Laboratory Animal Medicine*, 3rd ed., J. G. Fox, G. Otto, K. R. Pritchett-Corning, and M. T. Whary (eds.), pp. 23–42. San Diego, CA: Academic Press.

Office of Laboratory Animal Welfare (OLAW). Tutorial: PHS Policy on Humane Care and Use of Laboratory Animals. Available at https://olaw.nih.gov/resources/tutorial [accessed November 8, 2018].

CHAPTER 2 REVIEW

Match Up

Match the following with their respective descriptions:

A. 1
B. 2
C. 3
D. 5
E. Guide for the Care and Use of Agricultural Animals in Research and Teaching
F. Guide for the Care and Use of Laboratory Animals
G. IO
H. APHIS Animal Care
I. Health Research Extension Act of 1985
J. AWIC
K. Performance standards
L. Engineering standards
M. GLP
N. AWR
O. AAALAC
P. IACUC
Q. AVMA
R. OLAW
S. PHS

(Continued)

1. ____ Responsible for administration and enforcement of the AWA
2. ____ This organization publishes *Guidelines for Euthanasia*
3. ____ Governmental body responsible for interpreting and implementing the PHS Policy and evaluating institutional compliance with it
4. ____ Interprets the Animal Welfare Act into enforceable standards
5. ____ NIH, FDA, and CDC are part of this
6. ____ Provides the legislative mandate for the PHS Policy
7. ____ Individual who holds ultimate responsibility for an institution's animal care and use program
8. ____ Defines laboratory animals as "any vertebrate (e.g., traditional laboratory animals, farm animals, wildlife, and aquatic animals) used in research, testing, or education"
9. ____ According to the AWA, this is the minimum number of IACUC members.
10. ____ Minimum number of years that health records must be held after the final disposition or death of a USDA-regulated species
11. ____ This is part of the National Agriculture Library
12. ____ Direct the user to achieve a specific goal but does not specify the methods used to achieve the outcome
13. ____ Regulations used for preclinical safety studies funded by the FDA
14. ____ Must inspect animal facilities every 6 months
15. ____ Administers a voluntary accreditation program of laboratory animal care

Fill in the blank

Fill in the blank with one of the following regarding the AWA:
Yes = AWA regulations apply
No = AWA regulations do not apply

16. ____ BALB/c mouse
17. ____ Pig used in a dermatology study
18. ____ Guinea pig used in pregnancy toxemia study
19. ____ Rabbit used in gene therapy study
20. ____ Wild rat used in leptospirosis study
21. ____ Rhesus monkey used in vaccine study
22. ____ Sheep used in fetal human surgery study
23. ____ Dog used in cardiovascular study
24. ____ Cow used in milk production study
25. ____ Pigeon bred for research, used in behavioral study

3

Facility Design, Housing, Equipment, and Management

LABORATORY ANIMAL FACILITY DESIGN

The design, construction, and maintenance of an animal facility are key factors in an institution's ability to support both research animals and personnel and to minimize research variables due to environmental conditions. Anticipated research activities, the types and species of animals to be housed, and the available space and funds for construction are substantial factors in determining the overall design of a facility.

General Facility Design

Typically, institutions authorize the construction or renovation of animal research facilities to support a specific area of research (e.g., cancer research) or type of animal (e.g., transgenic or immunocompromised rodents). However, the research conducted within a facility frequently evolves over time with the arrival and departure of research groups, scientific advances, and changes in funding. Therefore, facilities should be designed to allow flexibility in their use over time without large-scale and expensive renovations. To this end, active involvement of a broad range of knowledgeable individuals, including architects, engineers, animal care personnel, veterinarians, biosafety professionals, and researchers is paramount in designing a well-functioning and efficient animal facility (Box 3.1). Furthermore, once a facility is constructed, specially trained building and facility maintenance engineers are instrumental in their maintenance as many contemporary facilities are composed of highly sophisticated and

Clinical Laboratory Animal Medicine: An Introduction, Fifth Edition.
Lesley A. Colby, Megan H. Nowland, and Lucy H. Kennedy.

Companion website: www.wiley.com/go/colby/clinical

Box 3.1

Active involvement of a broad range of knowledgeable individuals is paramount in designing a well-functioning and efficient animal facility.

Box 3.2

Construction of an interstitial area is highly recommended for most large facilities.

Table 3.1. Functional areas commonly present in animal research facilities

- Animal housing
- Animal procedure areas
- Receiving and storage for food, bedding, and supplies
- Cage wash and processing
- Waste material holding
- Containment facilities to support use of hazardous biological, physical, or chemical agents
- Specialized laboratories such as:
  - Surgery
  - Intensive care
  - Necropsy
  - Radiography
  - Clinical pathology
- Locker rooms and change areas
- Break rooms
- Administrative support

integrated resources that require continuous support and modifications. Involvement of maintenance engineers in the design process is the key to ensuring that a building and its systems can be properly maintained and supported throughout the building's anticipated lifespan.

Single-level facilities are preferable over multi-floor facilities as they avoid the need for elevators which can be costly to design, build, and maintain; can inhibit efficient movements within the facility; and can negatively affect building HVAC operations. Construction of an interstitial level is highly recommended for both single- and multi-level animal facilities (Box 3.2). Interstitial levels contain the wiring, ductwork, piping, and other system components that support adjacent levels. Because interstitial areas are physically separated from the animal facility, building support personnel can conduct regular and emergency systems maintenance without entering the facility and often without interrupting normal facility operations and activities.

Animal facilities are normally composed of several functional areas including those listed in Table 3.1. The relative location of each area within a facility should be carefully chosen to facilitate facility operations while also minimizing cross-contamination or disruptions. For instance, to minimize movement of large pallets within a facility, bulk feed and bedding storage areas are frequently located near the facility dock; cagewash rooms with noise- and vibration-generating equipment are normally isolated from rodent breeding rooms. For health protection and human comfort, personnel areas such as offices, conference rooms, and break rooms should be separated from other areas, but still easily accessible so as not to hinder their use. Table 3.2 is a useful resource when considering functional adjacencies, the purposeful positioning of areas based on their use or functions within a facility.

Corridors must be wide enough to allow movement of equipment and animals. In most animal facilities, 6- to 8-foot-wide corridors are adequate. In the past, it was common to include systems of "clean" and "dirty" corridors into the overall building design (Figure 3.1). In these systems, all movements of personnel, supplies, and animals are restricted to one direction: from clean to dirty areas. The return of personnel to a clean area during a single workday either is strictly prohibited or requires personnel to shower and/or change clothes. Although clean/dirty corridor systems can be highly effective in preventing cross-contamination between rooms, they are rarely incorporated into contemporary facilities due to the high proportion of overall building space required and the inefficiencies associated with their implementation. Common-use corridors have largely replaced clean/dirty corridor systems, with emphasis placed on operational practices to decontaminate or contain potentially contaminated items as well as the proper donning, doffing, and use of personal protective equipment (PPE).

Provision of adequate space is a challenge in every facility. In the past, many experimental procedures were conducted in animal housing rooms or in laboratories external to the animal facility. Both are now strongly discouraged. As a result of this and an increased use of large, expensive, and/or specialized equipment, the relative size and number of animal procedure rooms within facilities have markedly increased. Provision of adequate storage space is also challenging. Out of necessity, items are often stored in corridors, however this should be avoided whenever possible.

Critical building and animal support systems should be connected to emergency power sources such as gas generators, uninterrupted power sources (UPS), or batteries to ensure continuous operations without risks to personnel, animal health, and research integrity (Box 3.3).

As building systems and many items of research equipment are now internet-enabled, animal facilities require robust and reliable information technology (IT) systems. Both wired and Wi-Fi internet connections should exist, with sufficient bandwidth to support all users as well as robust cybersecurity features to protect systems and data.

Facility design must also incorporate equipment and systems to protect personnel health and safety. For instance, emergency eyewashes and safety showers must be positioned near chemical use areas. Active waste anesthetic gas (WAG) scavenging systems should be present in areas where gas anesthesia is frequently utilized. Oxygen monitors may be required in areas where a cryogen gas (e.g., liquid nitrogen) is stored or handled, including near MRI units with cryogen gas cooling systems. Seismic restraint devices can be used to stabilize equipment in earthquake-prone areas.

Walls, Ceilings, Doors, and Floors

There are several important considerations to address during the facility design process. Interior surfaces such as walls and ceilings need to be durable, impervious to moisture, fire-resistant, and as seamless as possible. Surfaces must be able to with-

Table 3.2. Communicating priorities for functional adjacencies in research animal facilities

	Main entrance	Administrative/office area	Conference/training area	Locker/dressing/shower/restrooms	Technician break area	Diagnostic laboratories	Necropsy	Surgery	Veterinary clinical support area	Imaging Laboratories	Animal procedures labs (multiple[a])	Cage sanitation area	Bedding storage	Feed storage	Supply storage	Bulk chemical storage	Animal carcass storage	Housekeeping storage	Janitorial service closets (Multiple[b])	Conventional small-animal housing	Conventional large-animal housing	Rodent barrier area	Biocontainment area	Chemical & nuclear containment	Rodent quarantine	Dock/receiving/shipping area
Main entrance		1	1	2	2	2	5	3	3	3	3	4	3	3	3	3	5	3	3	3	4	3	3	3	3	4
Administrative/office area	1		1	2	2	2	4	2	3	3	3	4	3	3	3	3	5	3	3	3	4	3	3	3	3	4
Conference/training area	1	1		2	2	2	4	2	3	3	3	4	3	3	3	3	5	3	3	3	4	3	3	3	3	4
Locker/dressing/shower/restrooms	2	2	2		1	3	4	3	3	3	3	4	3	3	3	3[c]	5	3	3	3	3	3	3	3	3	3
Technician break area	2	2	2	1		3	4	3	3	3	3	4	3	3	3	3	5	3	3	3	4	3	3	3	3	3
Diagnostic laboratories	2	2	2	3	3		2	3	2	3	3	4	3	3	3	3	5	3	3	3	3	3	3	3	3	3
Necropsy	5	4	4	4	4	2		3	3	3	3	3	3	3	3	3	2	3	3	3	3	3	3	3	3	2
Surgery	3	2	2	3	3	3	3		2	2	3	4	3	3	3	3	5	3	3	3	1	3	3	3	3	4
Veterinary clinical support area	3	3	3	3	3	2	3	2		2	3	4	3	3	3	3	4	3	3	3	1	3	3	3	3	3
Imaging Laboratories	3	3	3	3	3	3	3	2	2		3	3	3	3	3	3	4	3	3	3	1	1	3	3	3	3
Animal procedures labs (multiple)[a]	3	3	3	3	3	3	3	3	3	3		4	3	3	3	3	4	3	3	1	1	1	1	1	1	3
Cage sanitation area	4	4	4	4	4	4	3	4	4	3	4		1	1	3	3[c]	5	3	3	2	2	2	2	1[d]	2	3
Bedding storage	3	3	3	3	3	3	3	3	3	3	3	1		2	3	3	5	3	3	3	2	2	2	2	2	3
Feed storage	3	3	3	3	3	3	3	3	3	3	3	1	2		3	3	5	3	3	3	3	3	3	3	3	3
Supply storage	3	3	3	3	3	3	3	3	3	3	3	3	3	3		3	4	3	3	3	3	2	2	3	3	3
Bulk chemical storage	3	3	3	3	3	3	3	3	3	3	3	3*	3	3	3		3	3	3	3	3	3	3	3	3	1
Animal carcass storage	5	5	5	5	5	5	2	5	4	4	4	5	5	5	4	3		3	3	3	3	3	3	3	3	1
Housekeeping storage	3	3	3	3	3	3	3	3	3	3	3	3	3	3	3	3	3		3	3	3	3	3	3	3	3
Janitorial service closets (Multiple)[b]	3	3	3	3	3	3	3	3	3	3	3	3	3	3	3	3	3	3		3	3	3	3	3	3	3
Conventional small-animal housing	3	3	3	3	3	3	3	3	3	3	1	2	3	3	3	3	3	3	3		4	4	4	3	4	5
Conventional large-animal housing	4	4	4	3	4	3	3	1	1	2	1	2	2	3	3	3	3	3	3	4		3	3	3	3	2
Rodent barrier area	3	3	3	3	3	3	3	3	3	1	1	2	2	3	2	3	3	3	3	4	3		4	3	5	4
Biocontainment area	3	3	3	3	3	3	3	3	3	3	1	2	2	3	2	3	3	3	3	4	3	4		3	3	4
Chemical & nuclear containment	3	3	3	3	3	3	3	3	3	3	1	1[d]	2	3	3	3	3	3	3	3	3	3	3		4	3
Rodent quarantine	3	3	3	3	3	3	3	3	3	3	1	2	2	3	3	3	3	3	3	4	3	5	3	4		2
Dock/receiving/shipping area	4	4	4	3	3	3	2	4	3	3	3	3	3	3	3	1	1	3	3	5	2	4	4	3	2	

Source: Reprinted with permission: Hessler (2009).

Proximity priorities: 1 = close/high; 2 = close/medium; 3 = no priority; 4 = separation/medium; 5 = separation/high.

[a] Animal procedure labs are to be scattered throughout all the animal housing areas.

[b] Janitorial closets area to be scattered throughout the facility and within special areas such as surgery, biocontainment, barriers, etc.

[c] Bulk chemical storage is best located at the dock with chemicals piped to the cage-washers. If not, then the bulk chemical storage should be in a separate room in the cage sanitation area.

[d] The exit for cages from the Chemical and nuclear containment area should enter directly into the soiled side of the cage sanitation area so that the cage- and rack-washer can be used to decontaminate the cages when codes permit.

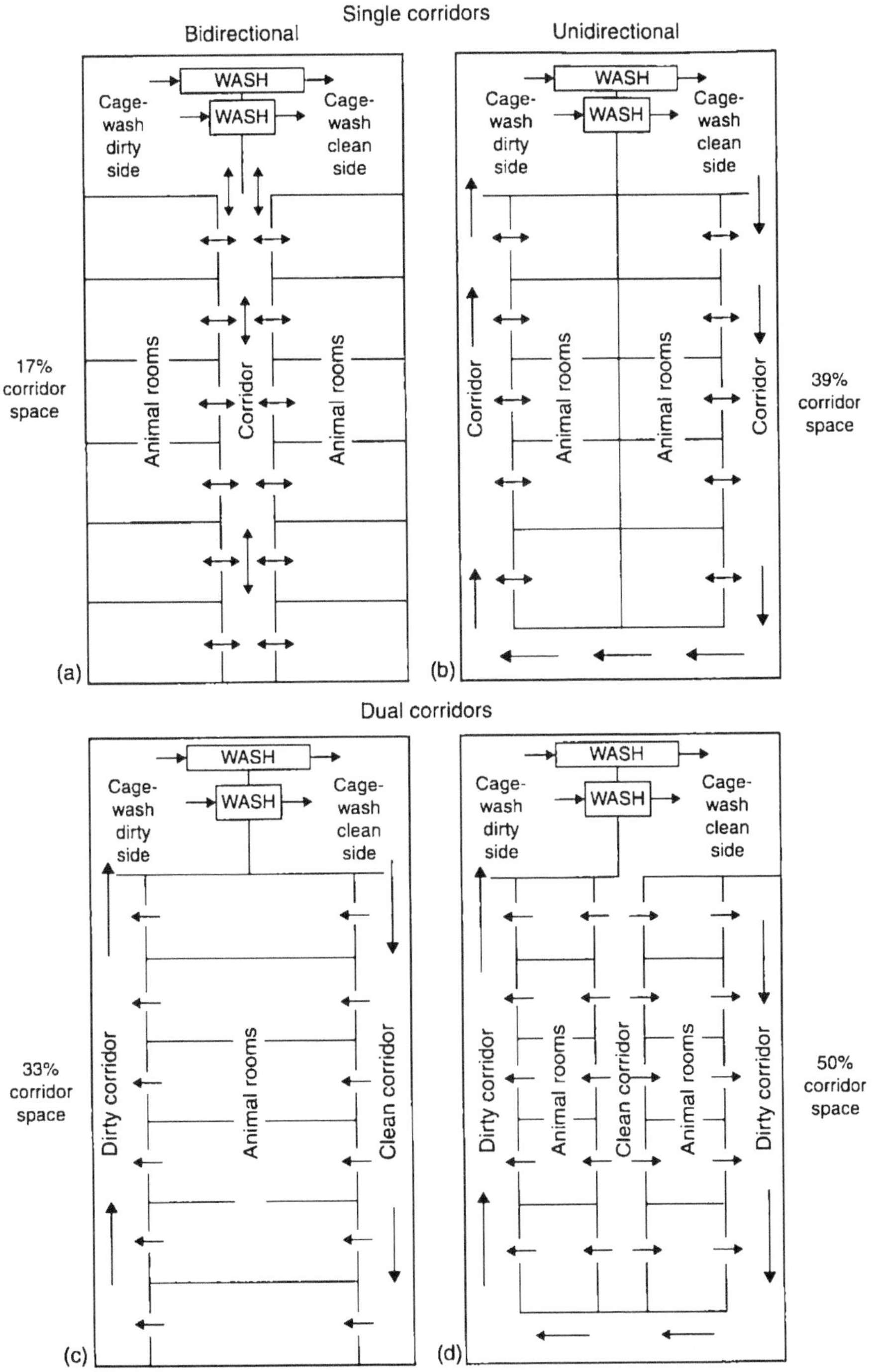

Fig 3.1. Four examples of circulation patterns within identical footprints are shown with arrows pointing in the direction(s) of traffic flow around the cage washing area: (a) a single-corridor bidirectional flow pattern; (b) a single-corridor unidirectional flow pattern; (c) a dual-corridor flow pattern with large animal rooms; and (d) a dual-corridor flow pattern with smaller animal rooms. The percentage of the footprint occupied by corridors is shown for each pattern. These percentages only serve to illustrate the impact of circulation pattern choices, and do not apply to any specific floor plan. (*Source:* Hessler and Lehner, 2009, *Planning and Designing Research Animal Facilities*, p. 102, figure 9.2.)

Box 3.3

Critical building and animal support systems should be connected to emergency power sources to ensure continuous operations without risks to personnel, animal health, and research integrity.

stand cleaning agents, high-pressure sprays, and impacts by carts and cage racks. Construction materials should be selected to minimize sound transmission. This is especially important in facilities with loud equipment (e.g., cage washers or MRIs) or housing multiple species as perception of some noises can be stressful to animals. For instance, dog barking is known to induce stress in sheep. When production of noise is unavoidable, its effects can be fully or partially mitigated through installation of sound-insulating walls, doors, and panels. Similarly, vibration-producing equipment should be avoided or isolated from animals as some animal's perception of vibrations can be distressful.

Walls within the facility are frequently constructed of reinforced, moisture-resistant wallboard or cement block. Where permissible, decoration of walls with colors or designs can be visually pleasing to personnel and help to improve their work environment. Metal or rubber wall guards and corner guards are valuable in minimizing wall damage from mobile equipment. Similarly, ceilings must be easily sanitizable. They should be sufficiently tight-fitting to prevent insect intrusions, but still allow access to underlying structures (e.g., ducts, pipes), if needed. Doors should open into the animal room and be sufficiently sized, minimally 42 by 84 inches, to easily accommodate passage of large equipment. Door hinges should allow the door to swing open to the maximum angle desired and not effectively obstruct the door frame opening. Recessed handles and kickplates add longevity to doors. Door windows allow personnel to evaluate a room's interior prior to entry, but corridor lighting must be considered and excluded during the night phase of the animal's photoperiod as even minute levels of light can disrupt the circadian rhythm of many species. Hatch-type ports or tinted glass that does not transmit specific wavelengths of visible light may be used. However, great care must be exercised when considering the use of tinted glass as the spectrum of visible light varies among different species and available window tinting materials may not adequately exclude unwanted wavelengths. Sweeps and flexible door gaskets may be required to block light from shining into rooms with controlled light cycles. Door sweeps should be present on key doors to help prevent entry of vermin (insects and wild animals) into the facility as well as escape of research animals (e.g., a mouse accidentally dropped on a housing room floor).

Floors should be durable, nonabsorbent, impact-resistant, and as seamless as possible. They should be relatively smooth to aid in sanitation, yet slip proof. Coving of the floor to create a continuous surface with the adjacent wall limits the accumulation of debris and facilitates cleaning. Floor drains are commonly installed in animal rooms in which animals are housed in pens or runs, but are frequently not necessary in other housing arrangements. When drains are present, floors should be sloped toward them and the drain should be of adequate size, at least 4 inches in diameter, for rapid removal

> **Box 3.4**
>
> *The spectrum and intensity of lighting has a direct effect on animal physiology.*

of water and excrement. Grates or baskets installed over drains can prevent small items, such as toys and bedding material, from clogging plumbing.

Lighting

The wavelength (spectrum) and intensity of lighting has a direct effect on animal physiology (Box 3.4). Recommended ranges of both exist for many species. For many years, fluorescent lighting has been routinely installed in animal use areas. In recent years, interest has risen in the use of light-emitting diodes (LEDs) due to potential energy and cost savings. However, the influence of LEDs on animal physiology has not yet been fully elucidated. Installation of lights in an animal housing room should be coordinated with the type and location of animal enclosures so that animals do not experience light of unacceptably high or low intensity. Light fixtures should be easily sanitizable and, at a minimum, water-resistant. An automated room lighting system is necessary to provide consistent and reliable day/night (lights on/lights off) cycles of room illumination. While mechanical light timers can be sufficient, fully programmable electronic lighting control systems are preferable as they are less prone to failure and can be modified only by authorized personnel. Regardless of type, lighting control systems should be monitored to ensure proper function. This can be accomplished by personnel observing room lighting during both the scheduled day and night cycle periods, through use of mobile light monitoring devices, or ideally as a component of the building environmental control system. Special lighting features are also available. These include red lights that are not (or only minimally) perceived by rodents to be used by personnel during the rodent dark cycle, high-intensity lighting ("task lighting") used by personnel during brief periods to facilitate in-room tasks, and "dawn-to-dusk" lighting that slowly increase or decrease light intensity to emulate sunrise and sunset.

Heating, Ventilation, and Air Conditioning (HVAC), Airflow, and Differential Pressures

The building heating, ventilation, and air conditioning (HVAC) system must be reliable and able to closely regulate temperature and humidity in all housing areas. The HVAC system should be capable of maintaining room temperatures within 2°F of the temperature set point and relative humidity within the range of 30%–70%, which is recommended for most common terrestrial laboratory animal species. While 10–15 room air changes per hour (ACH) are frequently recommended, optimal room ventilation rates are heavily influenced by a number of factors including animal numbers, animal species, and housing systems (e.g., individually ventilated versus static rodent caging). Refer to the *Guide for the Care and Use of Laboratory Animals* (the *Guide*) (ILAR, 2011) for more information on appropriate ventilation for animal housing rooms.

Consistent directional airflow and maintenance of differential air pressures between areas are recommended to control cross-contamination by airborne particles. For example, animal quarantine and nonhuman primate housing rooms should be kept under negative pressure relative to their adjacent corridor or anteroom, whereas surgery and specific pathogen-free animal housing rooms should be kept under positive pressure relative to adjacent areas. High-efficiency particulate air (HEPA) filtration of air exhausted from rooms or equipment (e.g., individually ventilated rodent cage racks) can also be useful for this purpose.

Monitoring and Alarms

Facilities should be equipped with a security access system, such as a card-key entry, to limit personnel access and alert authorities to attempts of unauthorized access. Facilities should also be equipped with environmental monitoring systems to monitor animal housing room parameters such as temperature, humidity, and airflow and alert personnel when parameters extend beyond predetermined limits (Box 3.5). It is critical that these alarms be reliably communicated to personnel 24 hours a day so that unacceptable environmental conditions can be quickly addressed. Local alarms may be sufficient for other monitored systems, including supply levels for central delivery systems of medical gases such as carbon dioxide or oxygen.

Fire alarm systems should be designed to minimally impact animals while still adequately alerting personnel to potential dangers. For instance, fire alarms are available that are audible to humans yet outside the hearing range of rodents. Similarly, red strobe lights are available that are imperceptible to rodents but visible to humans. However, federal and local fire safety ordinances must be followed. Alternative alarm systems should be approved by appropriate fire safety regulators.

COMMON FACILITY CLASSIFICATIONS

Biosecurity can be defined as the procedures or processes used to prevent the introduction or spread of harmful biological organisms within an area (Box 3.6). The overall design and operational procedures implemented at each animal facility are

Box 3.5

Facilities should be equipped with environmental monitoring systems to monitor animal housing room parameters and alert personnel when parameters extend beyond predetermined limits.

Box 3.6

Biosecurity can be defined as the procedures or processes used to prevent the introduction or spread of harmful biological organisms within an area.

driven by the level of biosecurity judged necessary to protect animals, humans, and the environment. Many factors contribute to this determination including animal immune status, the operational practices and facility design of animal sources (e.g., vendors, other institutions), frequency and methods of animal transportation into and within an institution, scientific needs, and the purposeful administration of infectious agents to animals.

Conventional and Barrier Facilities

The degree of biologic separation or isolation of animal colonies is a significant consideration when planning the movement of personnel, animals, and supplies into and within the facility. A combination of facility design and operational practices strongly influences these movement activities. Animal facilities are loosely categorized as either "conventional" or "barrier" facilities, however the precise definition of each varies across institutions. In general, *conventional facilities* are less restrictive in preventing the introduction or spread of unwanted microbial organisms. Relatively free movement of animals and supplies are allowed into and within the facility. Agents excluded from the facility may be limited only to highly pathogenic zoonotic agents. *Barrier facilities* are designed to exclude unintentional contamination of an area, adding a higher degree of protection to animals housed in them and helping to maintain animals in a disease-free condition. Barrier facilities were once used almost exclusively for specialized animal colonies such as immunocompromised animals and transgenic breeding lines. Now, recognizing the scientific and economic investment in animal research colonies, the majority of institutions favor the construction and operation of barrier facilities over conventional facilities for most of their animal colonies including rodents, fish, large animals, and nonhuman primates. Common design features and equipment associated with barrier facilities include equipment entry points with interlocked double doors allowing only one door to open at a time; connecting "rodent receiving" rooms separated by a pass-through biological safety cabinet for the clean transfer of rodents into the facility; equipment decontamination chambers or disinfectant misting tunnels; large capacity, pass-through autoclaves; and personnel entry areas (e.g., locker rooms) permitting multistage transition from one's original garb, possibly through a wet, chemical, or air shower, and into a uniform and required PPE. Items of PPE should be required only if they can reasonably be expected to provide a benefit to human or animal health, or to the environment. Institutions will vary in the intensity of the barriers that they choose to implement based on the associated financial and operational costs versus perceived benefits.

Gnotobiotic Facilities

Multiple areas of research now require that animals be either maintained completely free of all organisms (i.e., *germ-free* or *axenic*) or colonized only by a known or purposefully administered mixture of organisms (i.e., *defined flora*). Both germ-free and defined flora animals are considered gnotobiotic animals, animals in whom all forms of life are known. Gnotobiotic animals must be maintained in a strictly controlled environment to prevent inadvertent contamination of the animals. Gnotobiotic animals are most commonly housed in rigid or flexible-film isolators (Figure 3.2) maintained under positive pressure with respect to the surrounding room and supplied with HEPA-filtered air. Operators

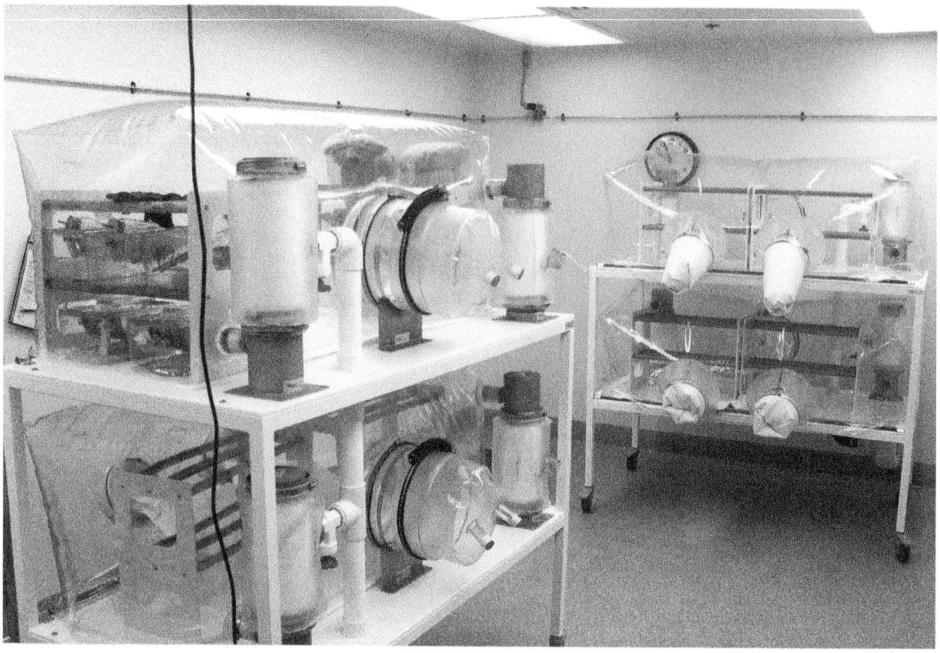

Fig 3.2. Isolator within a gnotobiotic facility containing rodent cages. (*Source*: Photo courtesy of University of Washington Gnotobiotic Core.)

work inside the isolator through gloves affixed to the unit. In some instances, gnotobiotic animals can be maintained in specially designed, air-tight shoebox-style cages with a HEPA-filtered air supply. For both housing types, special equipment and techniques are used to prevent the introduction of contaminants when handling the animals and introducing items into the isolators or cages.

Biohazard Facilities

Multiple types of hazardous organisms and substances are used in animal facilities, including infectious organisms, chemicals, x-rays, radioisotopes, and lasers. Many require special building features or operational practices for safety. Biohazard facilities are designed to prevent exposure of animal populations, humans, and the environment to infectious organisms. As described in the *Biosafety in Microbiological and Biomedical Laboratories* (*BMBL*) (CDC, 2009), the relative risk of an infectious organism is determined in part by its routes of transmission, severity of induced disease, susceptibility to treatments, and by its natural presence within the local environment. Biological safety levels (BSL) have been established that describe the recommended facility features, practices and techniques, and safety equipment appropriate for containing an organism within a laboratory. Similarly, animal biosafety levels (ABSL) outline recommended containment measures for housing and handling animals administered an infectious agent. For each, the lowest designation (BSL1, ABSL1) signifies the lowest level of risk and intensity of recommended containment measures, while the highest designation (BSL4, ABSL4) indicates the greatest level of risk and intensity of containment measures needed. ABSL1 and ABSL2 containment

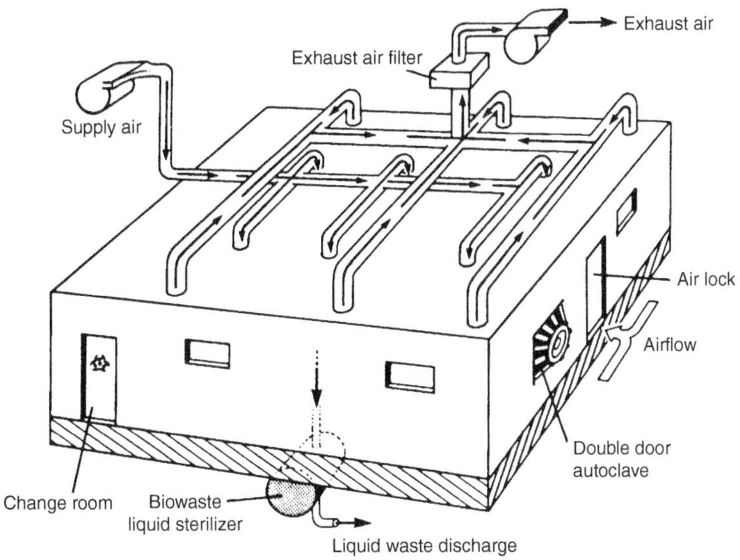

Fig 3.3. This containment facility provides treatment for all exiting air, fluids, equipment, and personnel. Ideally, building systems such as HVAC, lighting systems, electrical wiring, and plumbing are designed to permit servicing from outside the containment area. (*Source:* From AALAS, 2003, *Laboratory Animal Technician Training Manual*, p. 82, figure 7.10.)

facilities are common in animal research facilities. ABSL3 facilities are significantly more complex to build and operate and are uncommon. ABSL4 facilities are highly complex and expensive; they are rare with only approximately a dozen present in the United States and only a few dozen in existence worldwide. A formal process of risk assessment should be conducted to determine appropriate biosafety and animal biosafety levels necessary for containment.

Design features of biohazard facilities may include HVAC systems with high-efficiency particulate air (HEPA) filtration to capture and contain airborne organisms such as bacteria and viruses, airlocks to prevent unintended air movements between areas, autoclaves to sterilize contaminated materials, biological safety cabinets for material and animal handling, local handwashing sinks for hand hygiene, and self-closing doors to help maintain directional airflow and prevent accidental entry into containment areas. HEPA filters are constructed to capture at least 99.97% of all particles 0.3 microns in size, with a greater capture efficiency for both larger and smaller particles. Critical building systems are typically supported with redundant backup systems to maintain containment in the event of a system failure. For instance, emergency generators may automatically activate to provide power to biological safety cabinets when standard building power is interrupted. Figure 3.3 illustrates one potential design of a biocontainment facility.

Access into biohazard facilities is restricted to authorized and trained personnel. Personnel protection and environmental containment of biohazardous materials can be thought of in a three-tiered system. Primary containment of materials begins at the building and engineering level with airlocks, appropriate construction, and HVAC systems providing the first line of defense. Personnel practices and procedures provide the second layer and include entry and exit procedures and waste disposal practices. The final level of protection is PPE which is used to mitigate risks that cannot be controlled by the primary or the secondary methods. Personnel may be required to employ enhanced PPE as dictated by the ABSL designation of the room or area. For ABSL2 areas, this may include disposable gowns, multiple pairs of gloves, shoe covers, and masks and/or eyewear for mucous membrane protection. Additional or different PPE may be required in higher containment areas. For instance, ABSL3 may require full body coverage and full face protection with respirator use, while ABSL4 commonly requires use of a positive pressure ventilated suit with attached boots. Waste materials generated within a biohazard facility must be appropriately decontaminated or sterilized prior to disposal. Autoclaves, gas or vapor decontamination chambers, incinerators, and digesters can be useful for this purpose. Further guidelines and principles of biosafety can be found in the most recent edition of the *BMBL* (CDC, 2009).

HOUSING

A variety of housing systems may be used in a laboratory animal facility. The system used depends upon the animal species, the nature of the research, and the design of the facility. Space recommendations for group and individually housed animals are provided in multiple documents including the Animal Welfare Act (APHIS, 2017), the *Guide*, and the *Guide for the Care and Use of Agricultural Animals in Research and Teaching (Ag Guide)* (FASS, 2010). Space recommendations, adapted from the *Guide,* for housing mice, rats, hamsters, and guinea pigs of various sizes are shown in Table 3.3. Figure 3.4 illustrates calculations used to determine acceptable animal numbers per cage.

Rodent Housing

Shoebox-style cages are most commonly used to house rodents. The shoebox-style cage is a solid-bottomed cage usually made of a plastic material that has a stainless steel lid with a V-shaped trough to hold food and a water bottle or pouch. Caging materials must be durable and able to withstand repeated sanitation. Plastic cages are made of polystyrene, polypropylene, polycarbonate, polysulfone, or polyphenylsulfone. Each differs in its resistance to heat, steam, and chemicals, as manifested by ease of breakage and visible clouding of the plastic. With some plastic materials, there is potential for bisphenols to leach into the rodent's microenvironment when the plastic is repeatedly exposed to high temperatures, such as through autoclaving, and therefore should be avoided. Polystyrene cages are disposable and intended for single use, most often with biohazard or chemical hazard protocols. Polypropylene cages are opaque and occasionally used for rodents needing more seclusion, such as breeding animals. Polycarbonate cages are clear and have high-impact strength; an autoclavable version is used for protocols that require sterile caging. Both polypropylene cages and polycarbonate cages can withstand high temperatures. Polyphenylsulfone caging is produced in a variety of clear colors to allow a range of transparency and can withstand over 2000 autoclaving cycles.

Table 3.3. Recommended minimum space for commonly used group-housed laboratory rodents

Species	Weight (grams)	Floor Area per Animal (inches²)	Height (inches)[a]
Mice	<10	6	5
	Up to 15	8	5
	Up to 25	12	5
	>25	≥15	5
	Female housed with a litter	51[b]	5
Rats	<100	17	7
	Up to 200	23	7
	Up to 300	29	7
	Up to 400	40	7
	Up to 500	60	7
	>500	≥70	7
	Female housed with a litter	124[b]	7
Hamsters	<60	10	6
	Up to 80	13	6
	Up to 100	16	6
	>100	≥19	6
Guinea pigs	Up to 350	60	7
	>350	≥101	7

Source: Guide for the Care and Use of Laboratory Animals (ILAR, 2011).

[a] From cage floor to cage top.

[b] Recommended space for housing group.

Microisolation (MI) caging is an improvement of the shoebox-style cage system in that it includes a plastic cover with an integral air-permeable filter positioned over the shoebox-style cage bottom (Figure 3.5). Enclosing the cage with a filter-top lid helps to decrease the risk of a contaminant inadvertently entering the cage and release of organisms and allergens from the cage into room air. MI cages can be used as static (without forced ventilation) or as ventilated cages. Static cages are most frequently placed on or suspended from shelving units. Rarely, these shelving units are placed adjacent to mass horizontal air displacement devices designed to partially capture heat and odors emitted from the cage tops. Over the past decade, ventilated caging systems have become increasingly popular as they provide an improved environment for animals, decrease human allergen exposure, and permit a greater density of caging within a given space. Animals that must be fully separated from the room environment, such as severely immunocompromised animals or germ-free animals, can be housed in isolators (see Gnotobiotic Facilities section).

Individually ventilated cages (IVCs) (Figure 3.6) are a refinement to the static MI caging system. IVCs are constructed to fit onto ventilated cage racks (Figure 3.7) equipped with air delivery ports. When a cage docks with a rack port, a continuous flow of fresh air is delivered into the cage (Figure 3.8). IVC systems provide containment and

You measure your mouse cage and find it to be: 7.5 in. in width
11.5 in. in length
5.0 in. in height

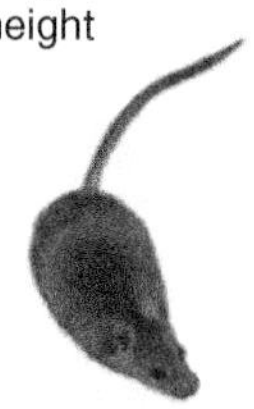

You weigh the mice to be housed and find they weigh 35 g.

From Table 3.1 you see the cage needs to be at least 5 in. in height and that each adult mouse (>25 g) needs minimally 15 in.^{2} of floor space.

Calculate the floor area by utilizing the formula: length x width.

$$7.5 \times 11.5 = 86.25 \text{ in.}^2$$

Then divide by 15 in.^{2} per mouse to determine the number of mice you can house.

86.25 in.^{2} divided by 15 in.^{2} = 5.75

You can house 5 mice in this cage.

Fig 3.4. Calculations used to determine acceptable occupant numbers per cage.

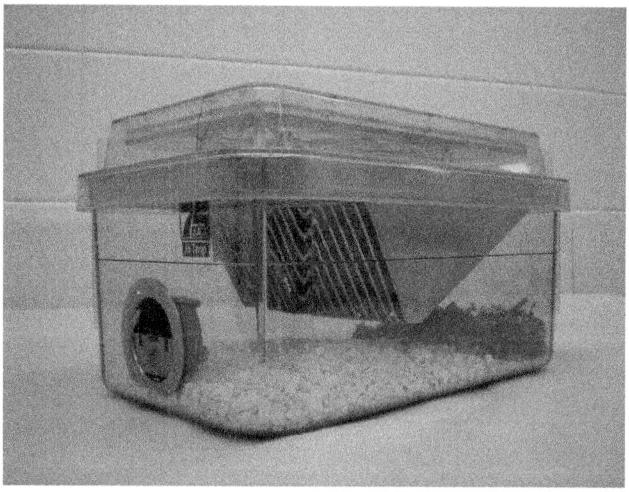

Fig 3.5. Static microisolation cage.

microbiological protection for the rodent while constant air exchange mitigates humidity, ammonia, and carbon dioxide levels that develop in an enclosed environment. As a result, IVC cages may not need to be cleaned as frequently as static MI cages. Depending on the rack design, air exhausted from each cage is captured either directly from the cage interior or from the area immediately surrounding the cage, such as near the cage-lid junction. To minimize personnel exposure to allergens, most facilities elect to discharge rack exhaust air either directly to the outdoors or through a HEPA filter.

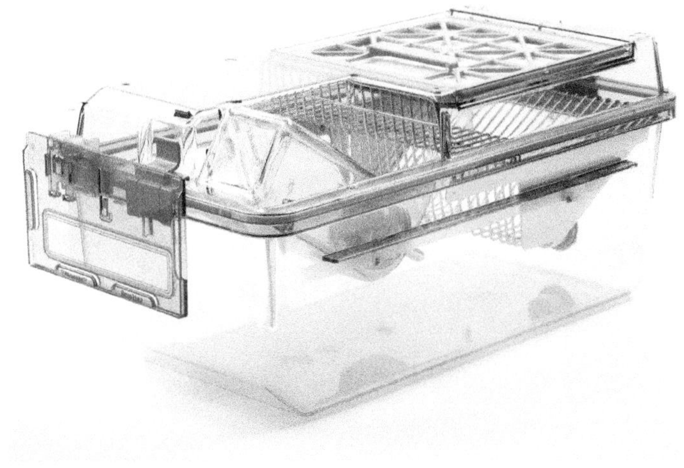

Fig 3.6. Individually ventilated cage for mice with wire bar feeder, water bottle, filter-top lid, and front-mounted cage card holder. (*Source:* Photo courtesy of Allentown Inc.)

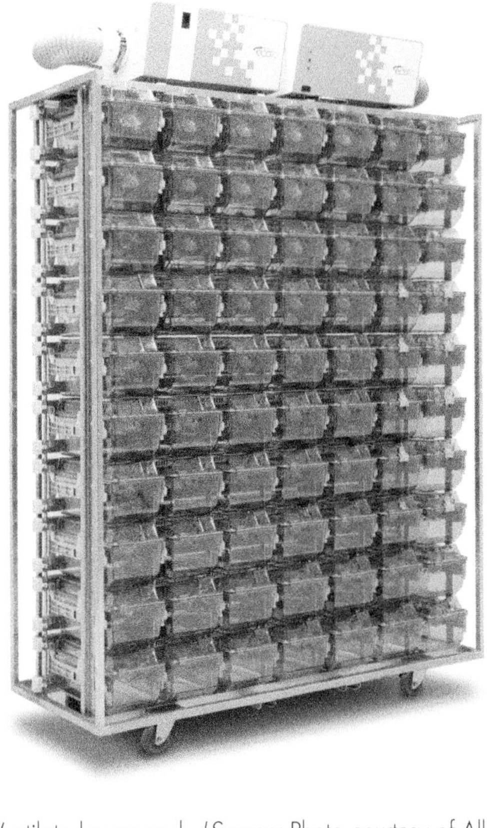

Fig 3.7. Ventilated cage rack. (*Source:* Photo courtesy of Allentown Inc.)

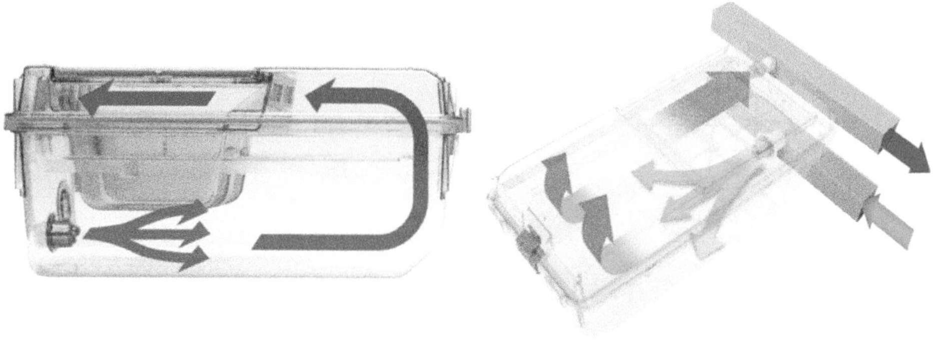

Side view Top view

Fig 3.8. Airflow pattern within a rodent individually ventilated cage (IVC) system. In this manufacturer's caging system, fresh air (blue arrows) travels through the rack supply air plenum and is introduced into the cage near the cage floor. Air is exhausted (red arrows) near the top of the cage before traveling through the rack exhaust air plenum. Different patterns of airflow exist in IVC systems produced by other manufacturers. (*Source:* Photos courtesy of Allentown Inc.)

Box 3.7

Rodents should be housed in solid-bottom caging whenever possible.

Rodents demonstrate a preference for solid-bottom caging with bedding substrate and should be housed in this manner whenever possible (Box 3.7). However, it is sometimes necessary to house rodents in suspended caging with perforated or wire-mesh flooring as this flooring allows animal wastes to drop through to a collection pan located beneath the cage. Perforated and wire flooring is discouraged for housing rodents because it may produce foot pathology in heavier animals housed for extended periods of time. When their use is unavoidable, use of solid resting platforms positioned within the cage is recommended when possible.

Housing for Other Small Mammals

Front-opening cages are commonly used to house rabbits, chinchillas, and ferrets. They are available as individual cages or as multiple-cage racks and, as the name suggests, provide front rather than top access to the animal. Front-opening cages can be made of stainless steel or plastic and have slotted bar or perforated flooring with trays under the flooring to collect excreta. Drawer-type rabbit cages offer the advantage of being able to examine the animal without fully removing it from the enclosure. Figure 3.9 shows front-opening, drawer-type caging. A J-type feeder is often used in this type of caging system. Group housing of social animals should be used whenever possible. Options include use of large enclosures designed specifically for this purpose, removable walls or installed openings between individual cages, and floor pens. For each option, animal and personnel safety as well as ease of husbandry and sanitation must be considered. Animal innate behavior and their past housing experiences may

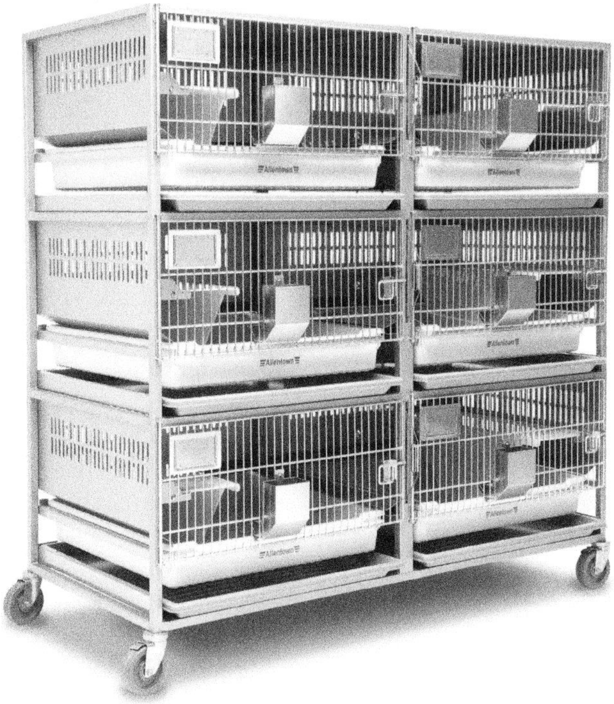

Fig 3.9. Front-opening drawer-type caging. (*Source:* Photo courtesy of Allentown Inc.)

strongly influence the success of group housing arrangements. For instance, severe fighting is likely to develop if group housing unfamiliar adult male rabbits. Two dominant or two submissive animals that are pair-housed may fight when establishing their social hierarchy. Furthermore, the influence of animal behaviors exhibited during group housing should be considered on research results. For instance, mounting activity exhibited by group-housed female rabbits may induce pseudopregnancy in some individuals which could significantly affect some research outcomes.

Housing for Large Animals

The regulations that apply to housing traditional agricultural species (e.g., sheep, goats, and swine) are dictated by the type of research in which they are employed. For example, the Animal Welfare Act Regulations apply to farm animals utilized in research, teaching, and testing, but not to animals "used or intended for use for improving animal nutrition, breeding, management, or fiber." Despite this, the AWA Regulations do not provide specific cage space requirements for some species, such as sheep, goats, and swine. For these, the *Guide* and *Ag Guide* recommendations are useful.

Housing animals in a traditional agricultural setting may be appropriate for the conduct of some biomedical research. When agricultural facilities are not locally available or when greater control of environmental parameters is required, then housing in indoor research facilities is necessary. Noise and odor levels common to large animal housing rooms heavily influence facility design and room construction. Engineered

> **Box 3.8**
>
> *Social species should be housed in compatible groups whenever possible.*

sound barriers (e.g., sound-insulating walls and ceilings) and robust room ventilation systems help contain noise and odors. Rooms may also be located distant from sensitive areas. Common large animal enclosures include freestanding, mobile cages; cages permanently installed within a room; and pens or runs with raised flooring or incorporating the room floor surface. Common types of raised flooring include reinforced fiberglass slatted panels and plastic-coated metal grate panels. Slat and grate openings should be appropriately sized for animal species and age to prevent entrapment of body parts (e.g., feet, hooves, teats) while still allowing passage of urine and feces. Flooring must be of sufficient texture to provide good footing without causing skin abrasions. Bedding such as straw or pine shavings may be used. Drinking water may be provided by automated watering systems with water valves or bowls positioned inside the enclosure. Alternatively, water pails may be suspended above the floor surface. Rooms and aisles should be sized not only to accommodate animal enclosures, but also to provide sufficient space for husbandry duties, limited supplies, and movement of carts and animals.

Social species should be housed in compatible groups whenever possible (Box 3.8). For flexibility of use with multiple co-housed animals, cages, pens, and runs should be designed with gates, removable walls, or other openings that can be selectively used to allow animals free movement between enclosures. When group housing is not possible due to research needs or animal medical or behavioral issues, animals should be provided visual, auditory, and/or olfactory contact with others of the same species. Animals should be provided opportunities to play and exercise. If properly equipped, hallways or room aisles may be suitable as temporary areas for these activities. Room features as well as animal enclosures and their contents such as shelving units, doors, gates, latches, and enrichment items (i.e., toys) should be regularly assessed for both human and animal safety. The integrity and cleanability of floor and wall surfaces are especially important when animals are housed in direct contact with them. Defects in floor and wall surfaces should be promptly identified and repaired as some species, such as swine, can be highly destructive in their rooting and chewing behavior and may quickly expand damage to the surrounding area. Water hoses and floor drains are essential for room cleaning. Drain size and placement within a room are dictated based on anticipated room use and can vary from small, centrally located drains to trench drains extending along entire walls. Sloping of floors can facilitate drainage. Drain grates or baskets should be designed to prevent bedding or enrichment from entering plumbing. Maintaining large animals within a research facility is physically demanding and labor intensive. All equipment and procedures should be regularly evaluated and refined to maximize personnel safety and minimize ergonomic injuries.

Housing for Nonhuman Primates

Similarly to some species of large animals, nonhuman primates may be housed in indoor or outdoor enclosures determined largely by research needs. Nonhuman primates should be socially housed whenever possible. Combining animals into stable social pairs or groups requires consideration of individual animals' health, reproductive status, and behavior and the involvement of personnel specially trained in the process.

Indoor enclosures vary from room-sized group housing pens to mobile or permanently installed cages designed for individual, pair, or group housing. Cages equipped with removable side, floor, or ceiling panels allow flexibility for co-housing one or more animals within multiple cages. Such an arrangement is especially useful when animals must be temporarily separated each day, such as for feeding or experimental observations. Specially designed *squeeze cages* are used to house some species of nonhuman primates and to safely restrain them. These cages have devices that move the false back of the cage forward to allow animal immobilization. Cages and pens may be equipped with perches, solid resting boards, or swings to increase cage complexity and improve animal comfort. Drinking water may be provided by automated watering systems with water valves positioned inside the enclosure or with externally mounted water bottles. Multiple forms of enrichment are regularly provided to nonhuman primates. Items used to mount or secure enrichment items, such as puzzle feeders or mirrors, on or within animal enclosures must not present entrapment or strangulation hazards.

Common outdoor housing enclosure types include "corncrib" pens, a roofed enclosure with metal mesh walls and gravel or concrete flooring and "corrals," large, open-air walled areas. Food and water are provided in multiple locations to avoid food hoarding by dominant animals. Cage complexities may be provided by ropes, swings, hammocks, and sturdy children's play structures. The design of each enclosure type must include means to capture individual animals when needed, such as for periodic health assessments.

Specialized Housing Systems

Metabolism cages are used in studies where urine or feces collection is required. The metabolism cage has a funnel-like apparatus to separate urine and feces, and a drinking valve or lixit located on the outside of the cage to avoid contamination of urine sample with drinking water. *Exercise cages* are used as a form of enrichment or for housing animals in specialized research studies such as those involving nutrition or exercise. *Transport cages* are used either to move animals from one part of the facility to another or for shipping. *Shipping containers* have design features to ensure the comfort and well-being of animals in transit. Live animal signage and arrows delineate the correct cage positioning. The container typically has screened windows with filters to reduce airborne contamination, and top or side offsets to prevent close positioning of cages and help ensure adequate air circulation.

Food and Bedding Materials

Food and bedding materials should be obtained from vendors and suppliers who ensure the quality of their products (Box 3.9). Areas in which laboratory animal diets and bedding materials are stored should be kept clean to minimize the introduction of disease, parasites, and potential disease vectors.

Animals should be fed a diet that is palatable, uncontaminated, and nutritionally adequate. Most dry, natural-ingredient diets should be stored below 70°F and 50% relative humidity to preserve nutritional content and can be fed up to 6 months after

Box 3.9

Food and bedding materials should be obtained from vendors and suppliers who ensure the quality of their product.

manufacture. Purified and chemically defined diets are less stable than natural-ingredient diets and should be stored at or below 39°F. The shelf life of these diets may be less than 6 months. Autoclavable and irradiated diets are adjusted in nutrient concentrations and ingredients to allow for degradation during sterilization or decontamination and ensure that adequate nutritional value is maintained. Autoclaved food should be labeled with the date of sterilization. Perishable foods should be refrigerated and used quickly to ensure freshness of product. Food milling, manufacture, and/or expiration date should be clearly visible when items are stacked in the storage area. Stock should be rotated to ensure animals are fed fresh food. Unopened bags of food should be stored off the floor on pallets, racks, or carts and positioned away from the wall to facilitate cleaning of the area and observing evidence of pests, such as rodent droppings. Opened bags of food should be stored in sealed, vermin-proof containers that also protect against moisture or other environmental contaminants.

Depending upon the species, housing method, and experimental conditions, the type of bedding material used varies. Bedding material should be selected based on its ability to provide animal comfort and its absorbency, availability, cost, low dust factor, and ease of disposal. In addition, bedding material should be nontoxic, nonnutritive, and nonpalatable. To minimize contamination and maintain quality, bedding materials should be stored off the floor on pallets, racks, or carts.

Environmental Enrichment

Over its successive editions, the *Guide* has placed an increased emphasis on the appropriate provision of environmental enrichment to help meet the psychological needs of all species. As stated in the *Guide* (ILAR, 2011), "The primary aim of environmental enrichment is to enhance animal well-being by providing animals with sensory and motor stimulation, through structures and resources that facilitate the expression of species-typical behaviors and promote psychological well-being through physical exercise, manipulative activities, and cognitive challenges according to species-specific characteristics (NRC 1998a; Young 2003)."

Environmental enrichment may include cage complexities that maximize use of existing space (e.g., shelves, perches, and swings) or increase an animal's interaction with its environment (e.g., water-filled children's pool, running wheels, puzzle feeders); shelters (e.g., plastic or disposable huts); nesting material; food treats; and manipulanda, items that animals can handle and manipulate (e.g., KONG®, Nylabone®, gnawing sticks). For animal health and safety, all enrichment items should be nontoxic and safe and reusable items should be sanitizable.

It must be noted that animals may interpret an object in a very different way than a human may predict. Enrichment items may induce unintended effects such as increased territoriality and aggression or physical trauma. For instance, a dominant

> **Box 3.10**
>
> *The physical and mental development of some animals can be directly affected by the absence or provision of enrichment items within their environment.*

nonhuman primate may attack its cagemate to protect a highly valued object. Cotton nesting material may traumatize the eyes of nude mice that do not possess eyelashes or may wrap around and strangulate their toes. Controversy exists regarding which enrichment items provide the greatest benefit and least risk to the animals. This is largely complicated by the difficulty of interpreting an animal's response to or desire for an object. Therefore, the use of all enrichment items must be critically evaluated.

In addition, scientific studies have shown that the physical and mental development of some animals can be directly affected by the absence or provision of enrichment items within their environment (Box 3.10). Both consistency and caution must be exercised in the provision of environmental enrichment when differences or changes in their use may impact research results. For these reasons, clear communication between the principal investigator, the IACUC, and the facility veterinarian regarding the introduction or standard use of any enrichment items is vital.

FACILITY EQUIPMENT

An animal facility requires the use of specialized equipment to provide high-quality care and sanitation in an efficient manner. Common pieces of equipment can be viewed on this book's accompanying website.

The level of cleanliness required of rooms and items within an animal facility varies based upon their use. It is important to critically determine the level of cleanliness that must be achieved for each situation as well as methods necessary to achieve the desired level. The *Guide* defines cleaning, sanitation, and disinfection as follows:

- "*Cleaning* removes excessive amounts of excrement, dirt, and debris"
- "*Sanitation* [is] the maintenance of environmental conditions conducive to health and well-being"
- "*[D]isinfection* reduces or eliminates unacceptable concentrations of microorganisms"

In addition, *sterilization* can be defined as follows:

- The "validated process used to render a product free of all forms of viable microorganisms" (Rutala and Weber, 2008).

The potential of all items and areas to introduce a contaminant to animal populations and/or to present an infectious health risk to personnel must be evaluated. The cleanliness of items in direct contact with animals (e.g., enclosures, caging, food bowls) and animal wastes are of greatest concern. Facility floor, walls, and ceiling should be cleaned and sanitized at a regular frequency. Mobile equipment and caging is commonly transported to a designated washroom for cleaning while items permanently affixed within a room (e.g., pens) must be cleaned in place. Brushes, wet and dry mops, water hoses, power washers, and detergent and chemical dispensers may facilitate in-room cleaning.

Personnel working in washroom areas must be advised of safety issues that are inherent in these types of facility operations such as noise, heat and chemical exposure, wet floors, performance of repetitive motions, and heavy equipment movement. Another potential health concern for cagewash personnel is the occupational exposure to laboratory animal allergens and other potential allergens (e.g., dust from clean bedding material). Procedures must be used to minimize exposure to aerosolized bedding material, animal dander, fur, and dust. Engineering controls such as negative pressure HEPA-filtered cage dumping systems, safe work practices, and appropriate PPE should be employed.

Cage Washers

Cage washers are used to clean and sanitize mobile equipment that can endure exposure to copious quantities of hot water. Three types of automated cage washers are commonly found in animal facilities: rack, cabinet, and tunnel washers. For each of these, personnel place items in the washer chamber and the machine then performs a series of washing and rinsing cycles, followed by a drying cycle. A rack washer (Figure 3.10) is sized to accommodate large pieces of equipment such as caging racks, shelving units, or portable kennels. A cabinet washer is a smaller version of a rack washer and resembles an oversized dishwasher. Tunnel washers (Figure 3.11) carry equipment on a conveyer belt from one end of the machine, through each step of the cleaning process, with clean and dry items exiting on the opposite side of the machine. All types of cage washers are designed to control wash water and dryer temperatures, addition of acids and/or detergent to wash water, and the overall sequence and duration of cycles. Specially designed lidded baskets or optional washer components are available for washing small cage components, such as environmental enrichment items, cage cardholders, water bottles, and sipper tubes.

Cage washers utilize a combination of water and heat, with or without the addition of chemical detergents, to sanitize items. It is generally recommended that when only heat is used, the temperature of the final rinse water be 180°F as measured at the item's surface. Visual indicators are commercially available for temperature monitoring. When a chemical detergent is added to the washing process, then sanitation may be achievable with rinse water of a lower temperature. Local government or water utility sewage regulations may require that waste water be conditioned (e.g., cooled or pH neutralized) prior to discharge into the sanitary sewage system.

The effectiveness of sanitation should be monitored at regular, established intervals through use of temperature test strips and biologic tests. Two commonly used methods include RODAC plate testing and ATP bioluminescent technology. RODAC is an acronym for "replicate organism detection and counting"—a system that measures bacterial colonies remaining on sanitized equipment. ATP bioluminescent technology measures the presence of adenosine triphosphate, a molecule present in all living organisms, to assess effectiveness of sanitization procedures. Equipment logs should be kept to document sanitation effectiveness as well as equipment failure and repairs.

Numerous potential safety hazards are specifically associated with cage washers,

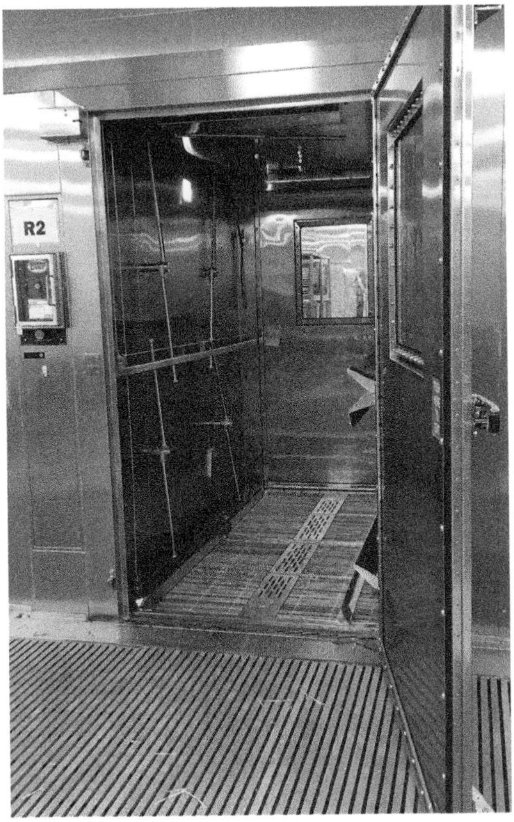

Fig 3.10. Rack washer.

including risks of thermal or chemical burns and personnel entrapment. Depending on the type and style of equipment, required safety features include emergency shutoff devices, easy-release door latches, and posted safety signage.

Autoclaves

Autoclaves are commonly used to sterilize a wide variety of items utilized in laboratory animal research. Small, single-door autoclaves similar to those used in medical clinics and laboratories are normally used to sterilize small items such as surgical materials and laboratory media and supplies. Large items and sizeable quantities of items, such as full carts of rodent caging materials, are more efficiently sterilized in oversized "bulk" autoclaves. Generally speaking, bulk autoclaves accommodate wheeled carts or equipment, thereby eliminating the need to manually lift and transfer items into the autoclave chamber. Bulk autoclaves equipped with doors on opposing ends of their sterilization chamber (pass-through autoclaves) can be positioned to traverse a wall between rooms containing non-sterile and sterile items. This design is frequently implemented in rodent cagewash facilities where clean cage components are loaded into the autoclave from the washroom, sterilized, and then removed into a sterile item storage room. Safety features and procedures are essential to protect personnel working with and near bulk autoclaves, including means to prevent personnel entrapment within the sterilization chamber and to easily and quickly stop machine operation.

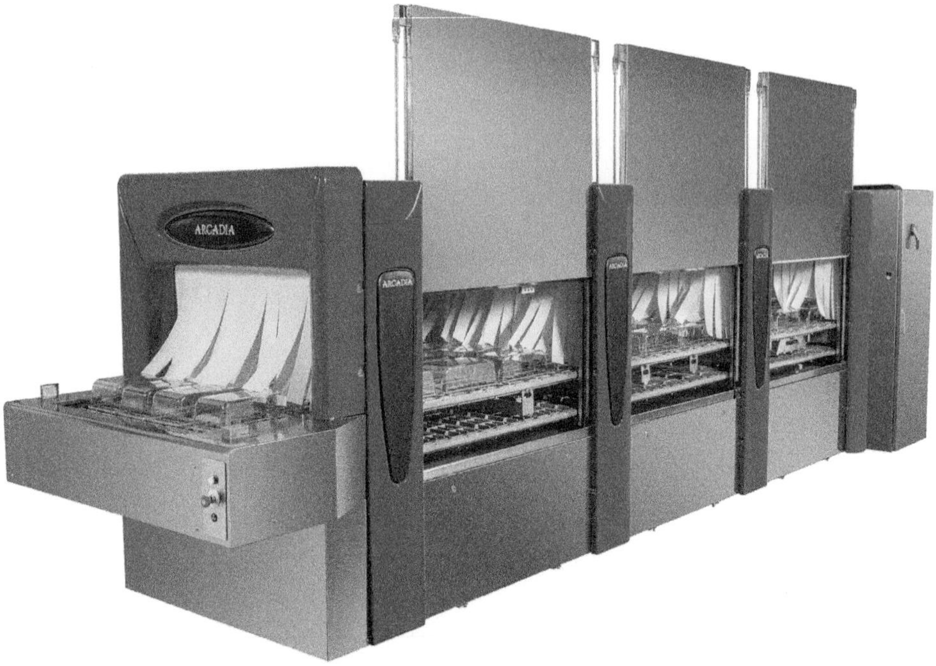

Fig 3.11. Tunnel washer. Side mechanical access panels raised to show three functional areas: the prewash, wash, and rinse sections of the unit through which items are carried on the tunnel's conveyor belt. (*Source:* Photo courtesy of Tecniplast.)

Watering Equipment

Drinking water provided to animals should be of high quality, without contaminants, and of consistent quality to help ensure animal health and minimize experimental variability across locations and over time. Multiple processes may be used to treat drinking water including filtration, exposure to ultraviolet lighting, hyperchlorination, acidification, reverse osmosis, and autoclaving. The degree of water quality control desired often varies by species or animal health status. For instance, for most agricultural animals, use of well or city tap water is sufficient whereas immunocompromised animals may require water purified by reverse osmosis and then slightly acidified (2.5–3.0 pH) or chlorinated (3–10 ppm of free chlorine) to inhibit bacterial growth. Regardless of the water source, automated watering systems have replaced use of water bottles and water bowls in many facilities as automated systems are less labor intensive and reduce ergonomic issues inherent in bottle handling. While more convenient, automated systems do require continual monitoring and maintenance. Water is delivered from the water source to rooms, usually through stainless steel piping affixed to walls or ceilings, and then through flexible water hoses to mobile cage racks or room pens. Water terminates at valves positioned within individual cages or pens. Animals can then physically activate these one-way valves to receive water (Figures 3.12 and 3.13). All system components should be checked regularly to ensure proper function and uninterrupted water delivery. To prevent water from becoming stagnant, systems are designed to automatically flush fresh water through all water lines at least daily (Figure 3.14). Despite this, a biofilm can eventually develop within the lines necessitating periodic sanitation of the system, such as with a bleach-based solution.

In some instances, other water delivery methods are preferable. Bottles with sipper tubes or water pouches (e.g., Hydropac®, Sipper Sack®) can be used with small animals when water consumption must be monitored or measured, or when specific medications or compounds are given. Packets of gelled water placed within the cage can be used for short periods of time and are particularly useful when transporting or shipping rodents.

Laminar Flow Rodent Change Stations

In most contemporary animal research facilities, rodent cage changes (movement of animals from soiled to clean cages) are performed within laminar flow hoods (LFHs) designed primarily to protect animals from potential airborne contaminants present in the room. When the laminar flow of air is vertically directed (from the top of the work area down to the work surface), LFHs also provide personnel some degree of protection from airborne particulates originating from the cage or the animals themselves as air passing over the work surface is partially captured and filtered before it is

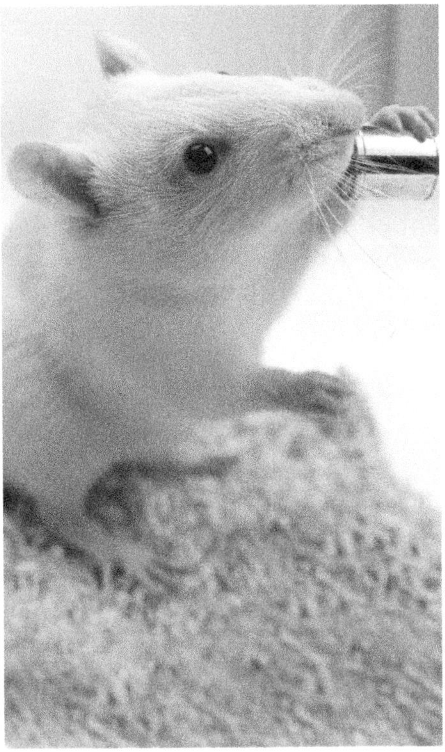

Fig 3.12. Rat drinking from a water valve supplied by an automated drinking system. (*Source:* Photo courtesy of Edstrom, a part of Avidity Science.)

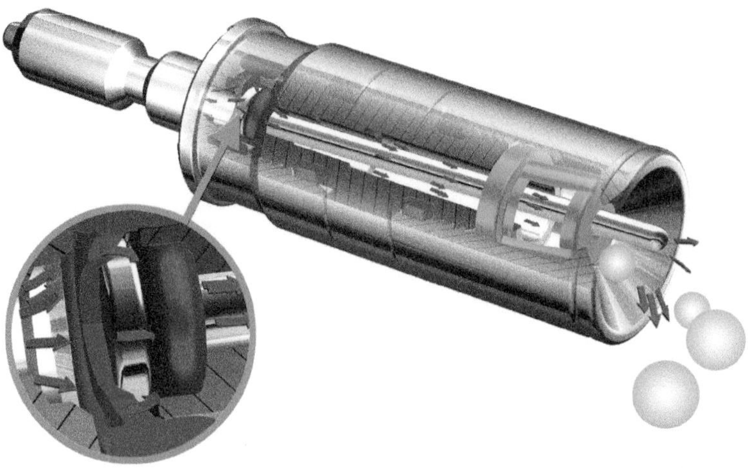

Fig 3.13. Automated drinking system water valve. Red arrows depict the flow of water. (*Source:* Photo courtesy of Edstrom, a part of Avidity Science.)

recirculated within the hood (Figure 3.15). LFHs are not comparable to biological safety cabinets (BSCs) in the level of protection they provide to animals or personnel. Only BSCs should be used to contain hazards or to provide a sterile work area. Most LFHs are mounted on wheels so that they can be easily moved between or within rooms.

Biological Safety Cabinets

When proper practices and procedures are followed, BSCs can provide protection to personnel, the environment, and items contained within the work area. Three types of BSCs exist (Class I, Class II, and Class III) based on the pattern of air circulation and HEPA filtration within the cabinet. Class II BSCs are used in most animal research facilities requiring ABSL2 or ABSL3 containment (Figure 3.16). Multiple types of Class II BSCs exist (e.g., A1, A2, B1, B2, C1). In all types, supply air is drawn from the room and HEPA filtered prior to delivery to the work area; air from the work area is again HEPA filtered prior to its recirculation within the cabinet or its exhaust to either the room or the building air exhaust system. Small quantities of volatile chemicals (e.g., isoflurane) can be safely used in some types of Class II BSCs and must be avoided in others due to the potential for explosion. Appendix A of the *BMBL* (CDC, 2009) provides a thorough overview of BSC design and function.

Imaging Techniques

Great advances have been made in rodent and small animal imaging over the last two decades. Many imaging modalities once used only in humans (e.g., digital x-ray imaging, magnetic resonance imaging (MRI), computed tomography (CT), positron emission tomography (PET), dual-energy x-ray absorptiometry (DEXA) scan, and ultrasound) have been adapted for use with these species, producing images of exquisitely fine detail. In addition, novel imaging techniques have been developed for use in animal research, including *in vivo* optical imaging. Some x-ray units (e.g., Faxitron animal imaging and

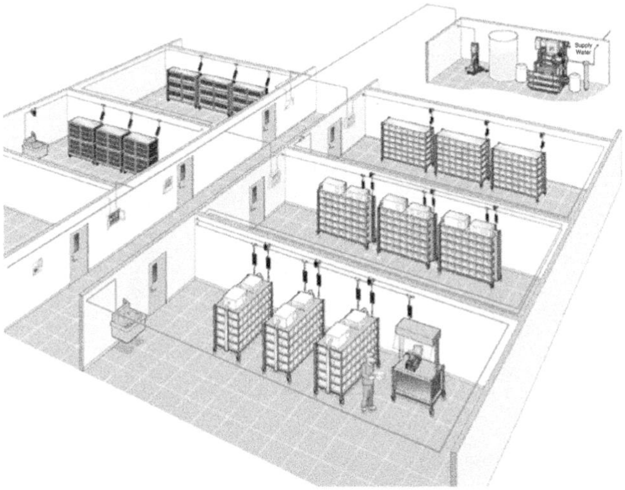

(a) Flushing system

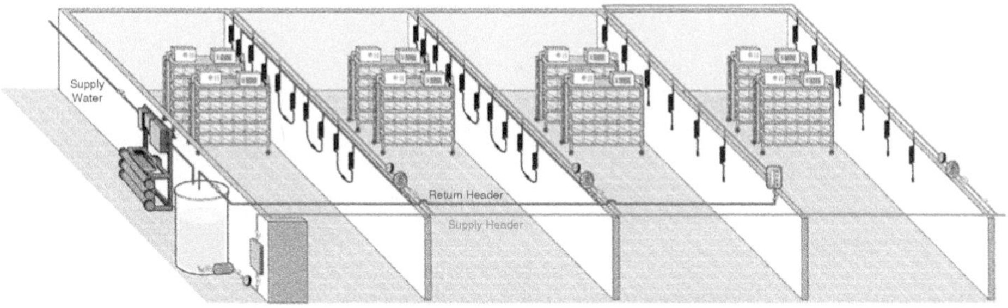

(b) Recirculating system

Fig 3.14. Automated drinking water system room design: (a) flushing system and (b) recirculating system. Water is rinsed through water piping at least daily to purge potentially stagnant water within the system. Flushing systems discharge the rinsed water into a drain. Recirculating systems capture and recycle the rinsed water within the system. (*Source:* Photos courtesy of Edstrom, a part of Avidity Science.)

irradiation systems) have been designed for use specifically with small rodents. These units produce a highly magnified and clear resolution image of the field of interest.

X-ray imaging equipment common in companion and large animal veterinary private practices is appropriate for use with ferrets, rabbits, most nonhuman primates, and agricultural animals. In contrast, with rodents and similarly sized animals, an x-ray machine with high milliamperage (e.g., 200- or 300-mA), low peak voltage (kVp), and the capability of small incremental changes can be ideal. High-detail film–screen combinations and short exposure times of 1/40 second or less should be used for high resolution and to decrease the chance of motion artifact. Alternatively, nonscreen film can be used with standard x-ray or dental units. Nonscreen film produces high-detail radiographs, but longer exposure times are needed. Digital imaging techniques offer substantial flexibility in image enhancement and delivery application and are now most commonly used for radiology. Animal restraint is best achieved through anesthesia or sedation coupled with use of adhesive tape for proper animal positioning.

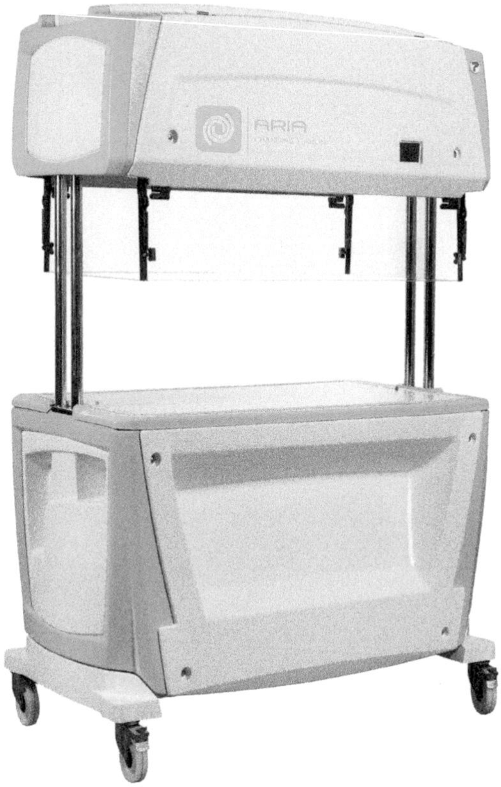

Fig 3.15. Mobile laminar flow hood. In this unit, used for handling rodent caging, HEPA filtered air is directed from the top of the unit, downward toward the work surface. (*Source:* Photo courtesy of Tecniplast.)

MANAGEMENT

A variety of administrative duties are required for the operation of an animal facility, including management of the budget and facility personnel, recordkeeping, preparation of standard operating procedures, executing the occupational health and safety program, and oversight of facility activities such as pest control and ordering of supplies and equipment. In most facilities, the researchers who use animals pay charges for animal housing that supports the majority of animal facility operating costs. The per diem, or per-day fee, is the cost to maintain one animal (or one cage of animals) for one day, calculated by determining the cost incurred for husbandry and for other services provided by the animal facility. Figure 3.17 shows a sample calculation of rabbit per diem charges.

Accurate, up-to-date records with sufficient detail must be kept to assure good animal care. Sophisticated computerized programs including, for example, radio-frequency identification systems now enable capture of most of the required information for an animal care and use program, including daily animal census, per diem charges, protocols, and animal health records.

Resources, including personnel, must be used efficiently for the facility to operate effectively. In large operations, use of bedding dispensers, automated watering, IVC

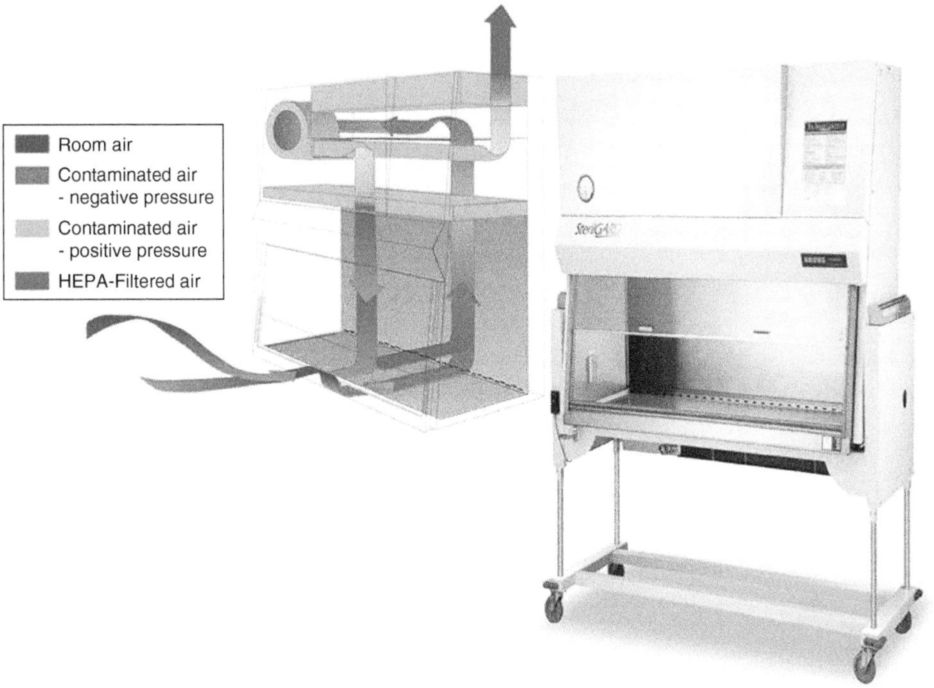

Fig 3.16. Class II – Type A2 Biological Safety Cabinet. Biological safety cabinets (BSCs) provide HEPA filtration of air exhausted from the unit. Class I, II, and III BSCs differ in their containment capabilities and performance features. Class II BSCs are most frequently utilized in laboratory animal facilities. (*Source:* Images courtesy of The Baker Company, www.bakerco.com.)

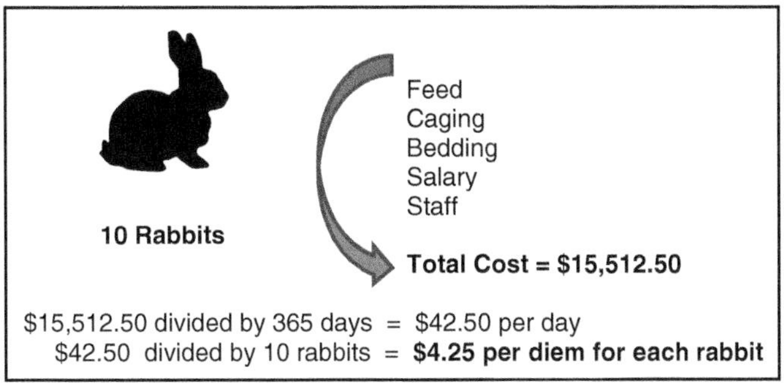

Fig 3.17. Calculation of per diems.

systems, and robots for cage handling may increase efficiency. Personnel must be trained in standard operating procedures and have basic knowledge of the species employed, including humane handling, restraint, and euthanasia techniques. They must understand the hazards and potential risks involved in carrying out their duties. Management must consider ergonomic issues to reduce personnel injury associated with tasks that are done repetitively. Although day-to-day responsibility for safety lies with the laboratory or facility supervisor, the institution's administration must be supportive of the occupational health and safety program as it relates to the use of animals in research.

Occupational Health and Safety Programs

Personnel in the course of their work with research animals may be exposed to hazards that could adversely affect their health. Physical hazards (e.g., animal bites, needle sticks), biological hazards (infectious agents and toxins), chemical hazards (e.g., carcinogens, cleaning chemicals), and radiation (e.g., x-rays, lasers, radionucleotides) all present potential hazards. Other hazards are inherent in animal use facilities such as laboratory animal allergens, zoonotic agents, use of cagewash equipment, wet floors, and lifting. The Occupational Safety and Health Standards (29 CFR Part 1910) requires employers to provide safe and healthy working conditions for their employees. In addition, the *Guide* states, "Each institution must establish and maintain an occupational health and safety program (OHSP) as a part of the overall program of animal care and use. The OHSP must be consistent with federal, state, and local regulations and should focus on maintaining a safe and healthy workplace. The nature of the OHSP will depend on the facility, research activities, hazards, and animal species involved." A risk assessment should be conducted to estimate the potential health risk of all who may enter the animal facility (e.g., visitors or vendors) or who may have contact with animals and equipment. Health questionnaires, physical exams, and self-reported changes in health status are commonly employed and are often invaluable in assessing personnel health risks. In addition to assessing individuals, the workplace should be periodically assessed for potential hazards and risks. Control and prevention are key to a successful program. Developing standard operating procedures, use of appropriate safety equipment, and provision of personal protective equipment are ways to manage hazards and risks. The National Research Council (NRC) offers two handbooks entitled *Occupational Health and Safety in the Care and Use of Research Animals* (NRC, 2003b) and *Occupational Health and Safety in the Care and Use of Nonhuman Primates* (NRC, 2003a). These books identify principles for building an effective safety program and discuss the accountability of institutional leaders, managers, and employees for a program's success.

Laboratory Animal Allergies

It must be noted that exposure to laboratory animal allergens is an occupational health concern for which each facility must establish a program of risk assessment and control. It is estimated that a third or more of laboratory animal handlers will develop laboratory animal allergies (LAAs) as a result of exposure to allergenic proteins found in the fur, dander, saliva, and urine of research animals. Factors in the work environment, such as the types of allergens and intensity and duration of exposure to the allergens, play a major role in the development of LAAs. Preventive measures include engineering controls, administrative policies, education and training of employees, and use of PPE. Engineering controls provide the most effective and practical measures to reduce allergen exposure. Numerous studies have demonstrated the effectiveness of housing mice in negatively pressurized IVCs and performing cage changes within a biological safety cabinet or laminar flow hood as all help to minimize release of allergens into the work environment. Personnel need to understand the importance of implementing preventative measures to reduce allergen exposure and recognizing and appropriately reporting development of allergy symptoms, if they occur. Visitors to animal research facilities should also receive training regarding laboratory animal allergens, including their potential risk of exposure. Further guidelines and principles regarding LAAs may be found in the latest editions of *Occupational Health and Safety in the Care and Use of Research Animals* (NRC, 2003b), the *BMBL* (CDC, 2009), and the *Guide* (ILAR, 2011).

BIBLIOGRAPHY

Animal and Plant Health Inspection Service (APHIS). 2017. *Animal Welfare Act and Animal Welfare Regulations as of January 1, 2017.* Washington, DC: US Department of Agriculture. Available at https://www.aphis.usda.gov/animal_welfare/downloads/AC_BlueBook_AWA_FINAL_2017_508comp.pdf [accessed October 7, 2018].

Centers for Disease Control and Prevention. 2009. *Biosafety in Microbiological and Biomedical Laboratories (BMBL)*, 5th ed. US Department of Health and Human Services, Washington, DC: US Government Printing Office.

Federation of Animal Science Societies (FASS). 2010. *Guide for the Care and Use of Agricultural Animals in Research and Teaching*, 3rd ed., J. McGlone and J. Swanson (eds.). Champaign, IL: FASS.

Hessler, J. R. 2009. Functional adjacencies, Table 10.1. In *Planning and Designing Research Animal Facilities*, J. R. Hessler and N. O. M. Lehner (eds.), pp. 107–108. San Diego, CA: Academic Press.

Institute for Laboratory Animal Research (ILAR). 2011. *Guide for the Care and Use of Laboratory Animals*, 8th ed. ILAR, National Research Council. Washington, DC: National Academies Press.

National Research Council (NRC). 2003a. *Occupational Health and Safety in the Care and Use of Nonhuman Primates.* Washington, DC: National Academies Press.

National Research Council (NRC). 2003b. *Occupational Health and Safety in the Care and Use of Research Animals.* National Research Council. Washington, DC: National Academies Press.

Rutala W. A., and D. J. Weber. 2008. *Guidelines for Disinfection and Sterilization in Healthcare Facilities*, Available at https://www.cdc.gov/infectioncontrol/pdf/guidelines/disinfection-guidelines.pdf [accessed November 15, 2018].

FURTHER READING

AAALAC International. 2018. *Safety Requirements for Walk-In Cage/Rack Washers and Bulk Sterilizers.* Available at https://www.aaalac.org/accreditation/positionstatements.cfm#walkin [accessed November 18, 2018].

Allen, E. D., E. F. Czarra, and L. DeTolla. 2018. Water quality and water delivery systems. In *Management of Animal Care and Use Programs in Research, Education, and Testing*, 2nd ed., Weichbrod, R. H., G. A. (Heidbrink) Thompson, and J. N. Norton (eds.), pp. 655–672. Boca Raton, FL: CRC Press.

Bush, R. K. 2001. Mechanism and epidemiology of laboratory animal allergy. ILAR 42(1): 4–11.

Corradi, M., E. Ferdenzi, and A. Mutti. 2012. The characteristics, treatment and prevention of laboratory animal allergy. Lab Anim (NY) 42(1): 26–33.

Dyson, M. C., C. B. Carpenter, and L. A. Colby. 2017. Institutional oversight of occupational health and safety for research programs involving biohazards. Comp Med 67(3):192–202.

Dyson, M. C., W. G. Greer, and L. A. Colby. 2018. Institutional responsibilities for the oversight of personnel safety in animal research. J Appl Biosaf 23(3):122–129.

Emmer, K. M., K. L. G. Russart, W. H. Walker, et al. 2018. Effects of light at night on laboratory animals and research outcomes. Behav Neurosci 132(4):302–314.

Hessler, J. R. 1999. The history of environmental improvements in laboratory animal science: Caging systems, equipment, and facility design. In *Fifty Years of Laboratory Animal Science*, C. W. McPherson and S. Mattingly (eds.), pp. 92–120. Memphis, TN: AALAS.

Hessler, J. R., and N. O. M. Lehner (eds.) 2009. *Planning and Designing Research Animal Facilities*. San Diego, CA: Academic Press.

Hildebrandt, I. J., H. Su, and W. A. Weber. 2008. Anesthesia and other considerations for *in vivo* imaging of small animals. ILAR 49(1):17–26.

Hogan, M. C., J. N. Norton, and R. P. Reynolds. 2018. Environmental factors: Macroenvironment versus microenvironment. In *Management of Animal Care and Use Programs in Research, Education, and Testing*, 2nd ed., Weichbrod, R. H., G. A. (Heidbrink) Thompson, and J. N. Norton (eds.), pp. 461–478. Boca Raton, FL: CRC Press.

Horn, M. J., S. V. Hudson, L. A. Bostrom, and D. M Cooper. 2012. Effects of cage density, sanitation frequency, and bedding type on animal wellbeing and health and cage environment in mice and rats. JAALAS 51(6):781–788.

Lipman, N. S., and S. L. Leary. 2015. Design and management of research facilities. In *Laboratory Animal Medicine*, 3rd ed., J. G. Fox, L. C. Anderson, G. Otto, K. R. Pritchett-Corning, and M. T. Whary (eds.), pp. 1543–1598. San Diego, CA: Academic Press.

Robert, K. B. and G. M. Stave. 2003. Laboratory animal allergy: An update. ILAR J 44(1):28–51.

Silverman, S., and L. A. Tell. 2005. *Radiology of Rodents, Rabbits, and Ferrets: An Atlas of Normal Anatomy and Positioning*. St. Louis, MO. Elsevier.

Stave, G. M. 2018. Occupational animal allergy. Curr Allergy Asthma Rep 18(2):11

Swearengen, J. R. (ed). 2012. *Biodefence Research Methodology and Animal Models*, 2nd ed. Boca Raton, FL: CRC Press.

Villano, J.S., J. M. Follo, M. G. Chappell, and M. T. Collins Jr. 2017. Personal protective equipment in animal research. Comp Med 7(3):203–214.

Zinn, K. R., T. R. Chaudhuri, A. A. Szafran, et al. 2008. Noninvasive bioluminescence imaging in small animals. ILAR 49(1):103–115.

CHAPTER 3 REVIEW

Multiple Choice

1. Interstitial areas
   A. allow building support personnel to access select building components without entering the animal facility.
   B. are recommended only for single-story facilities.
   C. are ideal locations for housing large animals.
   D. are necessary to support directional airflow within a facility.
2. Animal biosafety level designation that involves the highest level of risk is
   A. ABSL1.
   B. ABSL2.
   C. ABSL3.
   D. ABSL4.
3. Recommended relative humidity range for mouse housing rooms is
   A. 10%–40%.
   B. 20%–50%.
   C. 30%–70%.
   D. 40%–80%.
4. The guideline for ventilation in animal housing rooms is __________ air changes per hour.
   A. 4–8
   B. 8–10
   C. 10–15
   D. 15–20
5. For which of the following rooms should airflow be directed *into* the room from an adjacent hallway?
   A. personnel break room
   B. surgery room
   C. animal housing room with ABSL2 containment
   D. clean cagewash area
6. Most dry animal diets that are properly stored can be used up to _____ after milling.
   A. 3 months
   B. 6 months
   C. 9 months
   D. 1 year
7. A standard HEPA filter is 99.97% efficient in removing particles of 0.3 μm diameter. What is the efficiency of a standard HEPA filter in removing particles less than 0.3 μm in diameter?
   A. less than 99.97% efficiency
   B. 99.97% efficiency
   C. greater than 99.97% efficiency

(Continued)

8. Personnel protection and environmental containment of biohazardous materials can be achieved through use of a three-tiered system utilizing personal protective equipment (PPE), operational procedures and practices, and building and engineering controls. In what order should these systems be employed?
   A. PPE first, followed by building and engineering controls, and finally operational procedures and practices
   B. operational procedures and practices, followed by building and engineering controls, and finally PPE
   C. PPE first, followed by operational procedures and practices, and finally building and engineering controls
   D. building and engineering controls first, followed by operational procedures and practices, and finally PPE
9. A squeeze cage is routinely used for these animals.
   A. ferrets
   B. nonhuman primates
   C. rabbits
   D. chinchillas
10. The cage type used to separate and collect urine and feces is
    A. squeeze.
    B. gang.
    C. metabolism.
    D. microisolator.
11. Disinfection
    A. only removes excessive amounts of excrement, dirt, and debris.
    B. reduces or eliminates unacceptable concentrations of microorganisms.
    C. is the maintenance of environmental conditions conducive to health and well-being.
    D. is a validated process to render a product free of all forms of viable microorganisms.
12. ATP bioluminescent technology is used
    A. to determine facility airflow.
    B. to calculate room humidity levels.
    C. to balance room air pressure.
    D. to assess the efficacy of sanitation procedures.
13. Type of cage washing equipment designed to sanitize large pieces of equipment such as a cart is
    A. cabinet washer.
    B. rack washer.
    C. dish washer.
    D. tunnel washer.
14. Temperature suggested to achieve sanitation in an automated cage washer is
    A. 160°F.
    B. 180°F.
    C. 250°F.
    D. 280°F.

15. Potential risks to the health of cagewash personnel include
    A. noise, heat and chemical exposure.
    B. performance of repetitive motions and heavy equipment movement.
    C. exposure to laboratory animal allergens.
    D. all of the above.
16. True or False: Laminar change stations provide personnel a greater degree of protection against exposure to airborne particles than is provided by a biological safety cabinet.
17. The cost to maintain one animal (or one cage of animals) for one day is called
    A. per capita.
    B. perdu.
    C. per annum.
    D. per diem.
18. The ______ requires employers to provide safe and healthy working conditions for their employees.
    A. Occupational Protection Standards
    B. Occupational Safety and Health Standards
    C. Fair Employment Health Standards
    D. Safe Employee Health Standards
19. A ______ should be conducted to estimate the potential health risk of all who may enter an animal facility or who may have contact with animals and equipment.
    A. risk assessment
    B. physical exam
    C. health needs assessment
    D. job analysis
20. ________ provide(s) the most effective and practical measures to reduce personnel's exposure to laboratory animal allergens.
    A. Personal protective equipment
    B. Operational procedures and practices
    C. Engineering controls

Critical Thinking

21. A shipment of rats has arrived at the animal facility. You check the paperwork and notice the rats weigh between 150 and 175 g. The cages you have available are 8 inches high, 8.5 inches wide, and 17 inches long. How many rats can you place in each cage?

4

Mice

The laboratory mouse, *Mus musculus*, commonly known as the house mouse, belongs to the order Rodentia and the family Muridae. There are currently thousands of outbred stocks and inbred strains of mice in the world, with the number increasing almost daily. Although highly influenced by the stock or strain, adult mice usually weigh between 25 and 40 g and come in a variety of colors, including albino, black, brown, agouti, gray, and piebald (irregular patches of two colors).

GENETICS

Multiple genetic categories of mice are used in biomedical research: outbred stocks, inbred strains, F_1 hybrids, and transgenics. *Outbred stocks* are produced and maintained in large populations where the genetic composition of the population as a whole remains stable and matings are carefully planned to minimize unintended genetic changes such as inbreeding. Each outbred mouse should be unique, or heterogeneous, when compared with others in the population. To avoid genetic drift within a population, outbred stocks should not be subject to artificial selection for any characteristic (e.g., ease of handling, body conformation) other than possibly breeding efficiency. Common outbred stocks used in research include Swiss Webster, CD-1, and ICR.

In contrast to outbred stocks, all mice of an *inbred strain* are, by design, nearly genetically identical (Box 4.1). Strains are often produced to select for a specific trait that will be studied, such as diabetes mellitus or anemia. Following 20 generations of strategically planned brother × sister or parent × offspring matings, mice will exhibit at least 99% genetic homogeneity. With appropriate matings and genetic screening, established inbred strains can be maintained indefinitely. Three common

Clinical Laboratory Animal Medicine: An Introduction, Fifth Edition.
Lesley A. Colby, Megan H. Nowland, and Lucy H. Kennedy.

Companion website: www.wiley.com/go/colby/clinical

Box 4.1

Outbred mice are bred to maintain genetic heterogeneity. Inbred mice are bred to maintain maximum genetic homogeneity within a population.

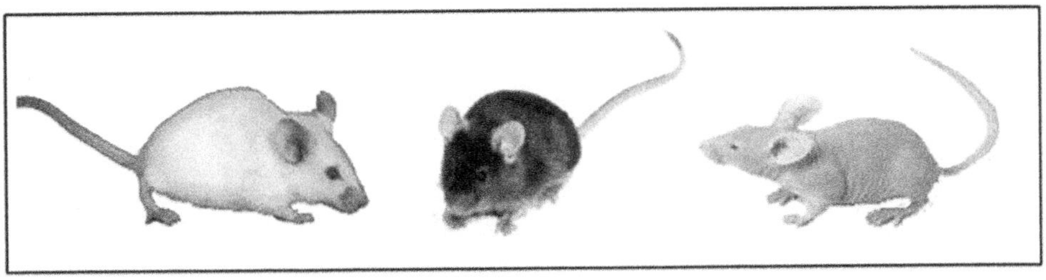

Fig 4.1. Strains of mice: BALB/c, C57BL/6J, and nude. (*Source*: Images courtesy of The Jackson Laboratory and Envigo.)

inbred strains are C57BL/6, BALB/c, and C3H mice. Two common inbred mutant strains used are the nude (nu/nu) and severe combined immunodeficient (SCID) mice. Figure 4.1 depicts common strains. Nude mice are deficient in T-cell lymphocytes but they have B cells and natural killer (NK) cell lymphocytes. As suggested by their name, nude mice lack normal coats; however, they are not truly nude and may, at times, exhibit some hair growth. SCID mice lack both T cells and B cells but have NK cells. Both of these strains are used most frequently in oncology research because they readily accept many transplanted human and murine tumors. This characteristic allows researchers to study tumor growth, metastasis, and chemotherapeutic efficacy.

F_1 hybrids are the first progeny of a mating between two different inbred strains and are genetically identical at all loci. All F_1 hybrids produced from mating two inbred strains are identical if and only if the parental sex from each strain is consistent (e.g., female of inbred strain 1 mated to male of inbred strain 2). F_1 hybrids produced from the reverse mating (e.g., male of inbred strain 1 mated to female of inbred strain 2) are similar but not identical. F_1 hybrids have the advantage of hybrid vigor, which means they are heartier than either of the parental strains. Inbred strains and F_1 hybrids are often chosen for research purposes because their genetic homogeneity eliminates an important variable in experimental work. Common F_1 hybrids used in research include B6D2F1 (C57BL/6 female mated with a DBA/2 male) and CD2F1 (BALB/c female mated with a DBA/2 male).

Transgenic technology is founded on the ability to alter the genetic makeup of an organism. Precisely ordered nucleotides (i.e., adenine, cytosine, guanine, and thymine) form the backbone of mammalian DNA. DNA is, in turn, ordered to comprise the functional unit of the gene and determines inherited characteristics. Through interactions with other cell components, DNA is responsible for protein synthesis and cellular metabolism and therefore orchestrates the function of the cell, an organ, an organ system, and the organism as a whole.

Although transgenic technologies have existed for over 50 years, the number of transgenic mice used in the study of gene functions and as models of human and animal disease has exploded since a draft of the mouse genome was published in 2002 (MGSC, 2002). Mice are referred to as *transgenic* if a foreign piece of DNA, a *transgene*, has been purposefully integrated in their genome. The DNA may originate from the mouse genome or from the genome of another organism. It may retain its original genetic sequence or be purposefully modified by the researcher.

Maintaining the genetic integrity of a strain or stock by controlling genetic drift and artificial selection of breeders is vitally important so that research results can be compared over the course of a study or between studies. The genetic composition of a strain or stock may vary between commercial animal vendors and between institutions. Therefore, to limit unintended genetic variability, all animals for a study should be obtained from only one source for the full duration of the study.

MICROBIOLOGIC CLASSIFICATIONS

In addition to being categorized by their genetic classification, mice are frequently classified by their microbiologic status: (1) germ-free or axenic, which are free of all detectable microflora; (2) gnotobiotic, which have associated known microflora; (3) specific pathogen–free, which are free of a defined list of pathogens; and (4) conventional, or animals with undefined microflora. While the number and prevalence of pathogens have declined considerably, many are still identified in laboratory animals and represent unwanted variables in research. Investigators using mice in biomedical experimentation should be aware of the profound effects that many of these agents can have on research. Animal care personnel and scientists must strive to ensure that research animals are free of disease to eliminate the unwanted variables that infections bring. Research institutions often institute a complex set of operational procedures designed to safeguard the microbiologic status of their existing mouse colonies. Of equal importance is the need for institutions to critically examine the microbiologic health status of animals obtained from other institutions or commercial vendors to ensure that the animals are suitable for their intended use and to minimize the health risk to the existing colonies.

Mice that either are infected with a known pathogenic agent or are of unknown health status may be bred and undergo cesarean rederivation or embryo transfer to obtain pathogen-free mouse pups. Cesarean rederivation is done near the time of parturition and involves surgical removal of full-term fetuses from the infected dam and fostering onto a specific pathogen-free dam with a litter of similar age. Embryo transfer is typically a surgical procedure in which early embryos are surgically removed from the infected pregnant dam and surgically implanted into a known pathogen-free foster dam. The embryos then develop and are born normally to the pathogen-free mouse. Recently, nonsurgical methods have also been developed to implant embryos into foster dams, which have some potential to reduce the level of surgical expertise needed for this technique. Another method to prevent transmission of select pathogens from dams to pups is through removal of the pups from the dam immediately postpartum. The pups are then cross-fostered to a lactating, specific pathogen–free female until weaning. The choice of which method to use is typically based on which pathogen is present, the strain, and the resources at the facility.

USES

More mice are used in research than any other mammal (Box 4.2). Mice have many attributes that make them valuable for research purposes, including a short life span, short gestation, large litter size, and wide genetic diversity. The short gestation and large litter size make them valuable in studies of reproduction, teratogenicity, and genetics. A short life span permits the study of several generations over a period of a few years. Furthermore, the anatomy, physiology, and genetics of mice have been studied extensively and are well characterized, providing a wealth of information for researchers to build upon. Common uses of mice in biomedical research include studies of infectious disease, oncology, autoimmune conditions, immunology, drug discovery, and product safety. Mice can be easily manipulated if handled gently; however, they do have a tendency to bite when they are startled or mishandled. Much of the complex equipment and imaging modalities (e.g., MRI, PET, ultrasound) originally developed for use in humans or larger animal species have been miniaturized to permit their use in mice. Mutant and genetically engineered strains of inbred mice provide investigators with a wide variety of animal models to study biologic processes and diseases.

The Food and Drug Administration requires the safety of a product to be proven prior to being marketed in the United States. Companies must use the most effective ways to test the safety of a product, which currently include animal testing. Relative to other species of research animals, mice are inexpensive to purchase and easy to maintain. Thus, they are frequently used for toxicity and carcinogenicity studies of various compounds for which large numbers of animals are required to provide statistically valid data.

BEHAVIOR

Mice are generally easy to handle and not aggressive toward humans. They are curious and social animals that normally sleep together in groups. They should be housed in same-sex groups unless they are part of a breeding pair or harem or are behaviorally incompatible. Although rodents are generally considered to be nocturnal animals, when housed indoors mice tend to have both active and resting periods throughout the day and night. Mice build nests in which to sleep and keep their litters.

Box 4.2

More mice are used in research than any other mammal.

Rodents are thigmotactic, possessing an innate preference for contact with the vertical perimeter of a bounded space (i.e., wall following, corner burrowing, or aggregating as a group) to avoid the perceived threat of open areas. Mice tend to be territorial. Adult males of many strains will fight when housed together unless they were cohoused at or soon after birth. Certain strains of mice (e.g., BALB/c, FVB, SJL/J) are more prone to aggression. Mice can inflict severe bite wounds that are not readily apparent around the genitals and tails and along the backs of their foes. Severe fight wounds can lead to morbidity and death. Female mice of most strains and stocks rarely fight unless defending their litters. Aggression may be reduced if mice are provided with enrichment objects, huts, or areas for hiding. Enrichment items must be carefully evaluated to insure they will not themselves promote territorial or aggressive behaviors. If aggression persists, population densities must be reduced until fighting ceases or animals must be individually housed. Incompatible animals may *not* remain together.

When group housed, one or more mice may remove the hair and whiskers from the faces, heads, and bodies of the other mice, a behavior known as barbering. This is an abnormal behavior and many factors may be involved in this idiosyncratic hair chewing. A distinct line of demarcation usually exists between the hairless and the haired areas, and the skin has no wounds. The "barber" mouse typically has no hair loss. Contrary to popular belief, barbering is not a dominance behavior, and both dominant and subordinate mice barber. Females are one-and-a-half times more likely than males to engage in this behavior. Barbering has been noted to increase during pregnancy. It appears to be strain dependent, with C57BL/6 mice showing a stronger likelihood to barber than do CD-1 mice. Barbering has been suggested as a model for the study of trichotillomania (compulsive hair pulling) in humans.

ANATOMIC AND PHYSIOLOGIC FEATURES

General biologic and reproductive data for the mouse are listed in Table 4.1. Mice have small bodies covered in soft, dense fur; short legs; and long, thin, hairless tails. Typical of other rodents, mice have a dental formula of 2(I 1/1, C 0/0, P 0/0, M 3/3). The incisors are open rooted, hypsodont (grow continuously throughout life), and are worn down by abrasion of the occlusal surface, whereas the molars have fixed roots.

Mice have a divided stomach consisting of a nonglandular forestomach and a glandular stomach. Their lungs consist of one large left lobe and four small right lobes. Brown fat tissue occurs in several places in the mouse, including between the scapulae. It is important in nonshivering thermogenesis during which the fat is metabolized to increase heat production in response to a cold environment.

Mice have five pairs of mammary glands: three thoracic and two abdominal. Mammary tissue is widely distributed in mice, with the glands extending well onto the sides and back. Both male and female mice have mammary glands, but the nipples are more prominent in females. Mice have open inguinal canals their entire life; therefore, to avoid herniation of abdominal organs, care should be taken to close the canals when castrating males. Males also have an os penis.

Table 4.1. Biologic and reproductive data for mice

Adult body weight: Male	20–40 g
Adult body weight: Female	25–40 g
Life span	1.5–3 y
Body temperature	36.5°–38 °C (97.7°–100.4 °F)
Heart rate	325–780 beats per minute
Respiratory rate	60–220 breaths per minute
Tidal volume	0.09–0.23 mL
Food consumption	12–18 g/100 g per day
Water consumption	15 mL/100 g per day
Breeding onset: Male	50 d
Breeding onset: Female	50–60 d
Estrous cycle length	4–5 d
Gestation period	19–21 d
Postpartum estrus	Fertile
Litter size	6–12
Weaning age	21–28 d
Breeding duration	7–9 mo
Chromosome number (diploid)	40

Source: Adapted from Harkness et al. (2010) and Harkness and Wagner (1995).

The most reliable criteria for differentiating the sexes are that the genital papilla is more prominent in the male, and that the distance between the anus and the genital papilla is about one-and-a-half to two times greater in the male (Figure 4.2). Sexing of neonatal mice requires practice but can be accomplished by comparing the anogenital distance; the size of the genital papillae; and in nonalbino mice, the presence of a pigmented spot on the perineum of the mouse pup between the genital papilla and the anus.

There are several distinctive characteristics of the hematologic and urinary profiles of mice. Lymphocytes are the predominant circulating leukocyte in mice.

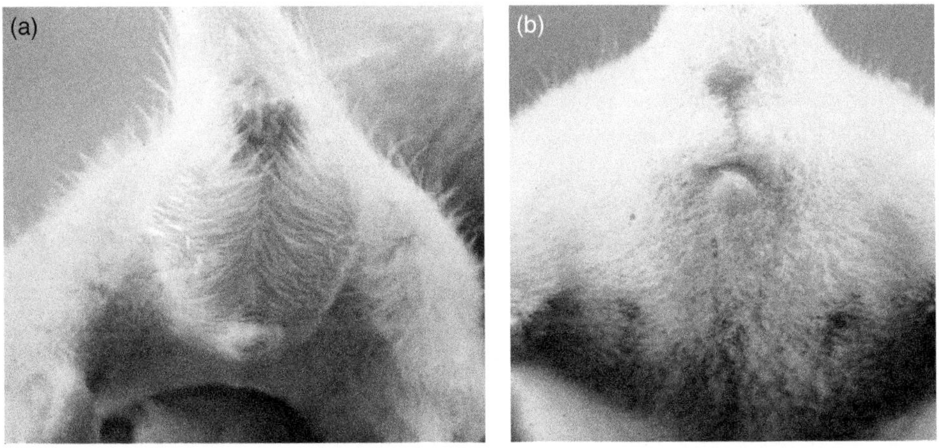

Fig 4.2. Sexing mice: (a) male and (b) female. (*Source*: Photo courtesy of Wayne State University.)

Basophils are rarely found in the circulating blood. Mature male mice have higher granulocyte counts than do female mice. Even such factors as site of collection and time of day can influence the number of leukocytes in peripheral blood. White blood cell counts, therefore, are of limited value in disease diagnosis. Mouse urine is excreted a drop at a time, is highly concentrated, and contains large amounts of protein. Taurine and creatinine are normal constituents of the urine while tryptophan is always absent. Urine pH is 7.3–8.5, with a mean specific gravity of 1.058. Hematologic and biochemical parameters for the mouse are listed in Appendix 1, "Normal Values."

BREEDING AND REPRODUCTION

Mice are continuously polyestrous without significant seasonal variations. The normal estrous cycle of mice is 4–5 days. Males and females can become reproductively active very soon after the recommended weaning age of 21 days. For this reason, sexes should be housed separately after weaning to prevent unintended pregnancies between littermates or parents and offspring. For maximum productivity, breeding should begin soon after animals reach sexual maturity (6–8 weeks, 20–30 g) and be continued throughout the breeding life of the female. It may be difficult to induce females to resume breeding if the breeding cycle is interrupted. Both monogamous (one male, one female) and polygamous (one male, multiple females) mating systems are routinely employed in mouse breeding. Monogamous systems may be preferentially selected when large numbers of offspring are not required and when defined mating pairs must be maintained. Polygamous mating systems may be selected to maximize breeding production and to maximize space utilization. The most commonly used polygamous breeding system is "trio breeding," in which two females are housed with one male. Depending on cage size, the adults and offspring may be cohoused until weaning or mice may need to be separated prior to parturition or when the offspring reach a designated body size or age, based on each institution's policies. Reproductive performance decreases with age, and many commercial suppliers suggest replacement of breeders at 8–10 months of age. Some females may be territorial, so if they are not cohoused, it is best to bring the female to the male's cage for breeding. Once bred, females will sometimes not accept another male for 21 days.

Pheromones play an important role in the reproductive behavior of mice. Pheromones are chemical substances secreted from the body that elicit a specific behavioral reaction in the recipient by activating the olfactory system. Large groups of females housed together without exposure to male pheromones tend to go into anestrus and do not cycle. If these females are introduced to males or their odor, they begin to cycle, and 40%–50% of the females will be in estrus within 72 hours. This synchronization of estrus is called the Whitten effect and can be attributed directly to pheromones. If a pregnant female mouse is exposed to the odor or presence of a strange male within 4 days of breeding, the existing pregnancy will often be aborted. This phenomenon is known as the Bruce effect and, like the Whitten effect, can be attributed to pheromones. Similarly, in what is known as the Lee–Boot effect, adult female mice housed in a group without exposure to a male will initially become synchronized in their estrus cycles.

Matings can usually be confirmed by the presence of sperm or a vaginal plug (firm whitish mass) in the female. Secretions from the vesicular and coagulating glands of the male form the plug. The plug may be deep in the vagina and difficult to observe. To look for a plug, lift the mouse by the base of the tail. If the plug is not obvious, a cotton-tipped swab may be used to gently spread the lips of the vulva. A blacklight can also assist in visualizing the plug. Vaginal plugs usually persist for 18–24 hours but may last up to 48 hours. Plugs do not guarantee pregnancy but do verify that mating occurred. Pregnant mice have an increased rate of weight gain by day 13 of gestation, marked mammary development, and a noticeably increased abdominal size by day 14. The fetuses can be palpated in mid- to late gestation.

The usual gestation period in mice is 19–21 days. In lactating mice, gestation is prolonged by 3–10 days because of a delay in uterine implantation of the blastocysts. Nonfertile matings result in a pseudopregnancy, which lasts for 14 days, during which estrus and ovulation do not occur. A fertile postpartum estrus may occur 14–28 hours after parturition; otherwise, mice will resume cycling 2–5 days postweaning.

Litter size is strain and age dependent but usually ranges between 6 and 12 pups. Smaller litter numbers are often noted with transgenic animals. To minimize cannibalism, dams and their litters should be left undisturbed for at least 2 days postpartum. Mice are altricial in that they are blind, naked, and deaf at birth. Pups are often called pinkies because of their color. The "milk spot" in their stomach can easily be observed through their thin skin to determine whether they are nursing. By day 10, mouse pups have a full covering of fine hair and their ears are open, and by day 12, their eyes are open. Mouse pups can begin eating solid food and drinking water by 2 weeks of age. Figure 4.3 depicts mice from 0 to 14 days of age. The usual weaning age is 21 days but may be as long as 28 days in some smaller inbred strains. Since thermoregulatory ability is not fully developed at weaning, pups should be cohoused with other weaned pups or adults or provided nesting materials to support body temperature maintenance (Figure 4.4). Cage size requirements for mice, including dams with litters, are outlined in the *Guide for the Care and Use of Laboratory Animals* (the *Guide*; ILAR, 2011) and further described in the housing section of Chapter 4.

HUSBANDRY

Housing and Environment

Mice are most frequently housed in shoebox-style cages constructed of a durable plastic, such as polycarbonate, polypropylene, or polysulfone. These plastics differ in their ability to withstand high temperatures and exposure to chemicals. Shoebox-style cages are comprised of a plastic housing component with a solid bottom and a fitted metal (usually stainless steel) lid consisting of parallel bars. A depression in the lid accommodates the pelleted food supply; a metal divider separates feed from the area designated for the water bottle. Solid-bottom caging with bedding is recommended. Mice may, when scientifically necessary, be housed in suspended cages with grid floors. Use of wire-bottom cages should be strongly avoided, however, as they are less

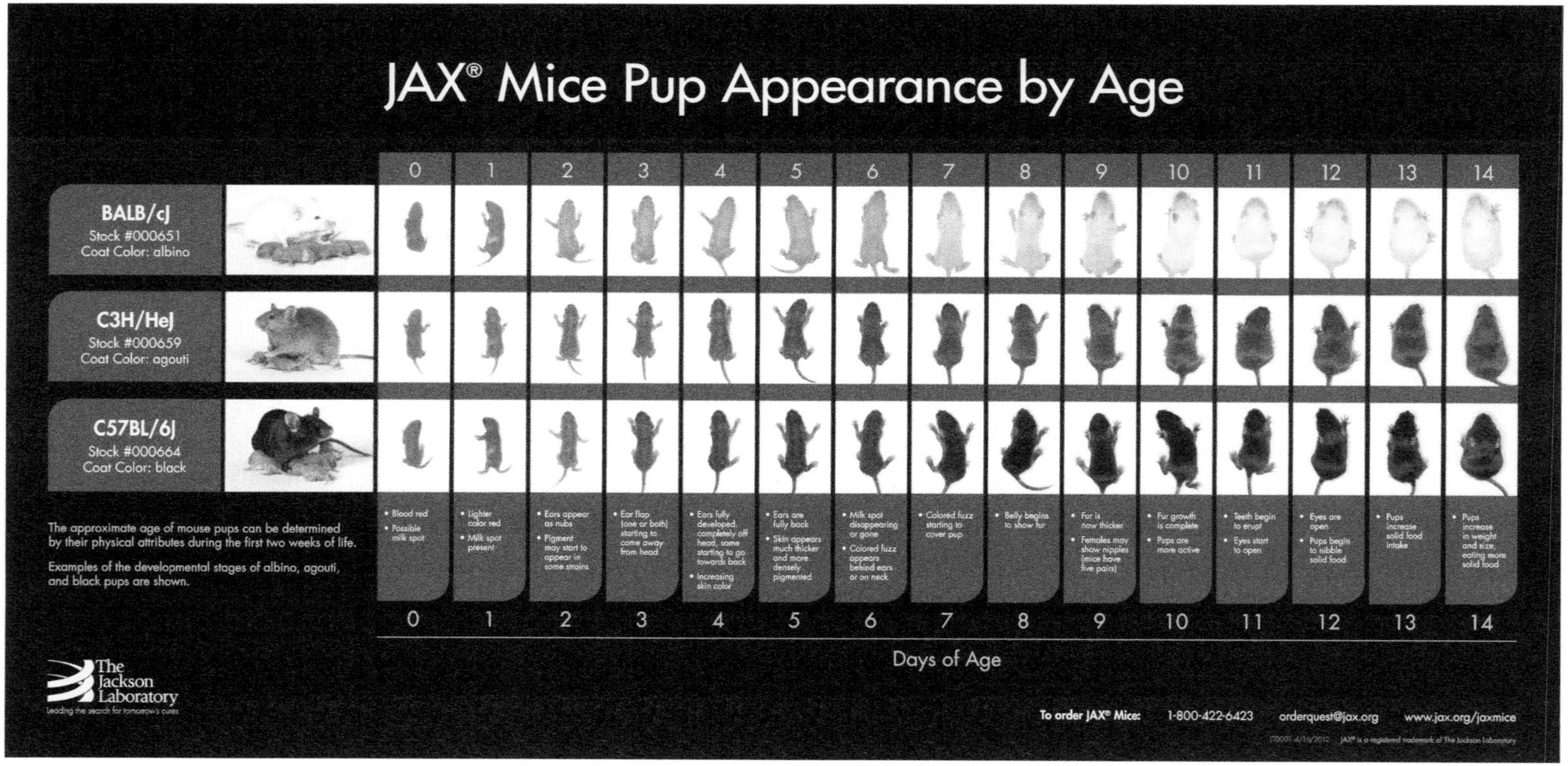

Fig 4.3. Mice pup appearance by age. (*Source*: Image courtesy of The Jackson Laboratory.)

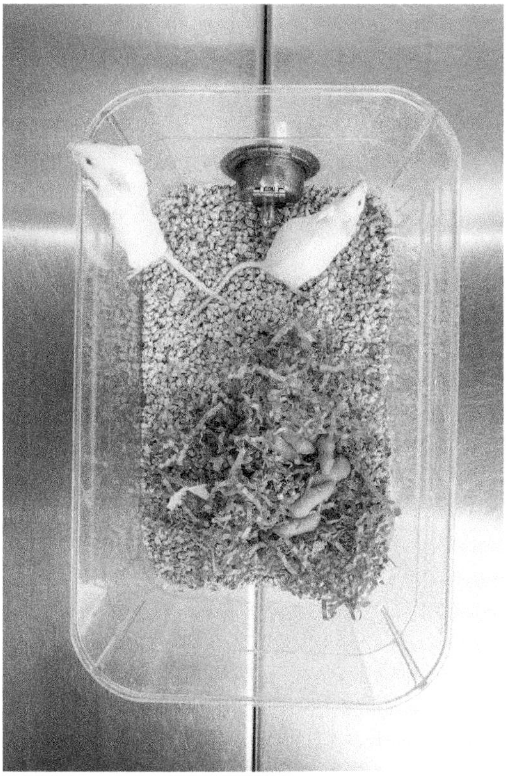

Fig 4.4. A breeding pair of mice with their litter in a nest. (*Source*: Courtesy of Austin Thomason, Michigan Photography—University of Michigan.)

comfortable for mice and are associated with increased incidence of limb injuries and lesions. Body temperature regulation is also hindered.

Microisolation (MI) cages are a refined type of shoebox-style cage commonly used to house laboratory mice. These cages are made of a durable plastic and have closed lids to reduce airborne disease transmission between cages. Microisolation cages are categorized as "static" or "ventilated" cages. Static cage lids incorporate filter material through which airflow into and out of the cage occurs through passive diffusion. One drawback of static caging is that humidity and ammonia levels increase with increasing numbers of mice. Ventilated caging systems are frequently used as an alternative to static MI caging. Ventilated caging systems consist of racks of shoebox-style cages designed with a ventilation port that attaches at the cage level to the ventilation system. The design allows individual cage ventilation and protection from airborne contaminants for the animals at the cage level. Additionally, the increased airflow inside the cage reduces buildup of humidity and ammonia to improve the microenvironment for the mice. Use of ventilated caging also benefits facility operations through a decreased frequency of necessary cage changes, the ability to house more animals in the same volume of room space (due to the denser arrangement of individual cages), and containment of allergens that would otherwise be released into the room. These caging systems must be evaluated to ensure that intracage airflow rates are not excessive and associated motor systems do not produce significant cage vibrations, each of which could disturb cage occupants. Single-use, disposable caging is also available. Its use can be especially beneficial in small or remote facilities with limited access to large cagewash systems and when animals are administered a substance hazardous to personnel (e.g., human pathogen, carcinogen, toxin).

As defined in the *Guide*, the minimal space requirements for group-housed adult mice larger than 25 g and without a litter are 96.7 cm^2 (15 $in.^2$) of floor space for each mouse and a cage height of 12.7 cm (5 in.). See Table 3.3 or the *Guide* for additional space requirements for smaller mice, females with litters, and larger mice. Mice tend to be proficient at escaping from their cages and do not return to them once they have escaped. To prevent escape, cages must have a secure cover such as a plastic lid or a metal grid that is fine enough to contain the animals. A contact bedding material, such as hardwood chips, composite recycled paper pellets, or corncob particles, is placed in the bottom of solid shoebox-style cages. Softwood bedding, such as pine or cedar chips, should not be used for laboratory mice because they produce aromatic hydrocarbons that induce hepatic microsomal enzymes. Nesting material is provided as a source of animal enrichment and to optimize animal comfort and thermoregulation.

In housing mice for research purposes, rigid control of room temperature, relative humidity, ventilation, and lighting is essential. A temperature range of 20°–26°C (68°–79°F) and a relative humidity range of 30%–70% are generally recommended. It is suggested that there should be 10–15 fresh air changes per hour in animal housing rooms to maintain adequate ventilation. This, however, is only a guideline, and determination of optimal ventilation should include careful consideration of the range of possible heat loads, number of animals involved, type of bedding and frequency of cage-changing, room dimensions, efficiency of air distribution from the secondary to the primary enclosure, and the design and function of the building ventilation system. A consistent cycle of darkness and light should be maintained in rooms housing mice. Typically, 12–14 hours of light per day should be provided and can be controlled through use of automatic timers. Fourteen hours is generally recommended for breeding mice although this may vary by strain or stock. Timer performance should be checked periodically to ensure proper lighting. During the dark portion of the light cycle, mice must experience complete darkness. Very short and/or low-intensity light exposure during the dark cycle can significantly alter their circadian rhythm and select physiological systems. Albino strains of mice should be housed under reduced lighting intensity as they are prone to retinal dysplasia. Consideration should be given to noise or vibration produced by surrounding rooms or buildings, as these can contribute significantly to stress and poor breeding performance in mice.

Environmental Enrichment and Social Housing

Mice are social animals and do best when housed in small, compatible groups. The provision of enrichment items may benefit mice. The types of enrichment items most frequently provided to mice are those that the animals can use for nesting materials (e.g., cotton nesting material, paper twists, facial tissues, soft paper towels), items that the animal can manually manipulate or gnaw on, and items that provide increased cage complexity (e.g., partially enclosed structures or huts, running wheels). It must be noted that mice may interpret an object in a very different way than a human may predict.

Enrichment items may also induce unintended effects such as increased territoriality and aggression or physical trauma. For instance, a dominant mouse may attack its cage-mates to protect a highly valued object. Cotton nesting material may traumatize the eyes of nude mice that do not possess eyelashes or may wrap around and strangulate their toes. Therefore, the use of all enrichment items must be critically evaluated before being routinely provided to a colony. In addition, scientific studies have shown that the physical and mental development of mice can be directly affected by social housing conditions (e.g., single- or group-housed) and the absence or provision of enrichment items within their environment. Both consistency and caution must be exercised in the use of environmental enrichment with study animals where the changes may impact research results. For these reasons, clear communication between the principal investigator, the IACUC, and the facility veterinarian regarding the introduction or standard use of any enrichment items is vital.

Feeding and Watering

Mice generally consume 4–5 g of solid food per day, although larger strains may consume more. Mice should be fed a nutritionally complete commercial rodent diet from a reputable company servicing the biomedical research community. There are a variety of diets available with a wide range in protein and fat composition depending on the needs of the animals. The diet should contain at least 16% protein and 4%–5% fat; higher fat levels may be indicated for breeding or nursing animals. Feed should be fed prior to the manufacturer's declared expiration date and stored in a cool (<70°F), dry location inaccessible to insects and vermin. Open bags of feed should be stored in a closed container. Feed is usually provided in the form of firm, dry pellets and fed *ad libitum* (free-choice). The food pellets should be placed in elevated hoppers (e.g., formed in the cage lid, attached to the cage wall) to protect it from contamination from the cage floor. Ill or very young mice may benefit from a container of moistened or gelatinous chow placed on the cage floor as they may not be able to access food or water near the cage top. Mice fed a powdered or soft diet are prone for incisor overgrowth since their teeth will not undergo normal wear from chewing. Provision of an object for chewing or occasional trimming may be needed to maintain the incisors at a normal length. Diet supplementation (e.g., fruits, seeds) is highly discouraged because mice may preferentially eat the supplements and not consume a well-balanced diet. Mice are coprophagic; consumption of their own feces serves as a significant source of B vitamins and other nutrients.

Adult mice drink 6–7 mL of water per day. Fresh, potable water should be available *ad libitum* through either water bottles with sipper tubes, sipper sacks (disposable, flexible plastic water containers), or automated watering systems. Mice must be carefully observed for dehydration after shipping. Additional forms of hydration, including gelatinous diets or moistened food pellets, on the cage floor will help to prevent dehydration. Weanling mice must be carefully observed for signs of dehydration for multiple days after separation from the nursing female as the weanlings may have initial difficulty learning to access the water source. Ill or impaired mice may have difficulty obtaining water from a cage's primary water source. In these situations, additional easily accessible water sources (e.g., lixit valves that extend closer to the cage floor) should be provided.

Sanitation

The required frequency of cage cleaning depends, to some extent, on the number and size of mice caged together and the amount of air movement in the room or cage. One to two times weekly is usually adequate for static MI cages housing up to five mice. More frequent cage changing may be required if the mice produce a large volume of urine (e.g., diabetic mice). Ventilated cages may require less frequent changes due to improved environmental conditions.

Cages, water bottles, and feed hoppers should be disinfected with chemicals, hot water 61.6°–82.2°C (143°–180°F), or a combination of both. Wardrip et al. (1994) showed that, when hot water is used alone, it is the combination of water temperature and time applied to the surface, known as the cumulative heat factor, that disinfects. Thus, a range of temperatures is acceptable as long as the water is applied to the surface for a long enough period of time to ensure destruction of common vegetative pathogenic organisms. Higher temperatures require less contact time than lower temperatures. Detergents and chemical disinfectants enhance the effectiveness of hot water, but they must be thoroughly rinsed from all caging surfaces with fresh water. Cage racks used with automated watering system manifolds (piping attached to cage racks) require special consideration. Before introducing the rack with attached manifolds into the cage washer, all residual water must be removed. Residual water within the pipes will adversely affect the rack washer's ability to achieve sanitization temperatures. It is recommended that both stainless steel and PVC types of manifolds be routinely treated with pressurized flushing and chemical agents or heat that are compatible with their chemical makeup. The pretreatment of the rack manifolds with chemical agents prior to introduction into the rack washer should also be considered. This process reduces the bioburden (biofilm) within the rack manifold prior to sanitization. In addition, before racks are placed in a rack washer, brushes or chemical agents should be used to clean the rack's air plenums, the small ductwork mounted to the rack through which air is distributed to each cage.

TECHNIQUES

Handling and Restraint

Exam gloves should always be worn when handling mice or the contents of their cages. To transfer a mouse from cage to cage, pick it up by the base of the tail with the fingers or with a pair of rubber-tipped forceps. Never grasp a mouse by the tip of its tail as this can result in a loss of skin and exposure of the caudal vertebrae. Alternatively, plastic tubes can be used to transfer mice from cage to cage (Figure 4.5).

To restrain a mouse, grasp the base of the tail with the thumb and forefinger of the dominant hand and place the mouse on a surface to which it will cling, such as a wire bar feeder. As the mouse attempts to move forward, quickly scruff the loose skin at the back of the neck between the thumb and the forefinger of the nondominant hand. When the skin is held properly, the mouse's head is immobilized so it cannot turn and bite. The mouse can be lifted and the tail secured between the pinky finger and the palm of the same hand. The dominant hand is then free to give injections (Figure 4.6)

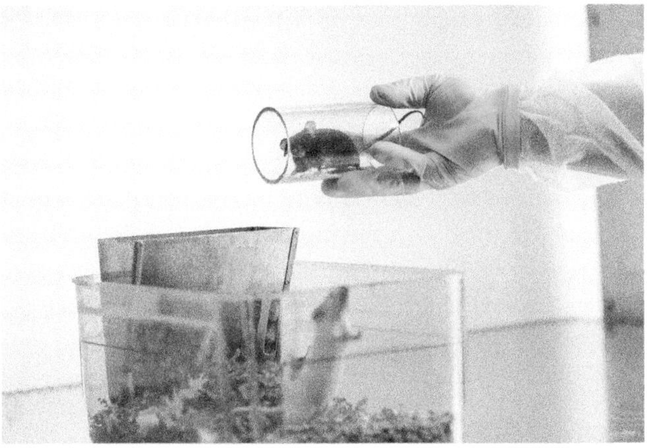

Fig 4.5. Use of a plastic tube for cage to cage transfer. (*Source*: Courtesy of Austin Thomason, Michigan Photography—University of Michigan.)

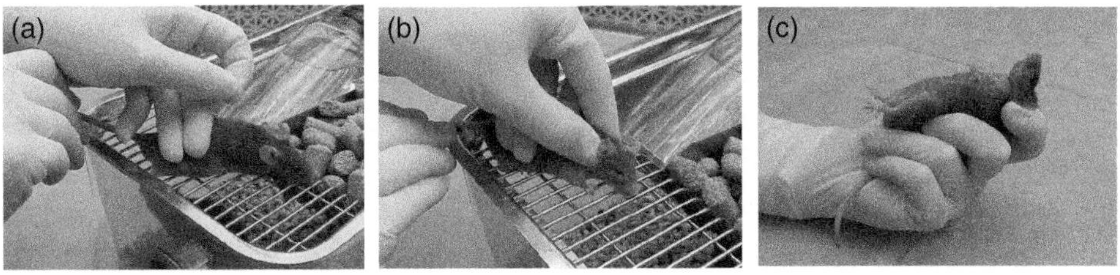

Fig 4.6. Restraint of the mouse. (*Source*: Photo courtesy of ULAM, University of Michigan.)

or dose the mouse by oral gavage. Mechanical restrainers made of rigid plastic are commercially available and allow access to blood collection and injection sites. Use of a soft towel to enfold the mouse can provide enough restraint for brief access to the tail or rear limbs. Alternatively, animals can be restrained within disposable, flexible, tapered plastic tubes for limited examination as well as for select injections or sample collections.

Identification

Cage cards may be used as a general means of identifying caged mice. Ear punching, ear tagging, ear or tail tattooing, or subcutaneous (SC) placement of a microchip (e.g., radio-frequency identification transponder) that allows electronic identification via a handheld scanner may be used for individual identification of mice. Temporary identification can be achieved by temporary ink tail markings and fur dyes. Toe amputation (toe clipping) is not allowed for identification alone at most institutions, as less invasive methods of animal identification are available.

Blood Collection

Assuming the animal is mature, healthy, and on an adequate plane of nutrition, the blood volume of most species averages 7% of the body weight in grams. A typical rule of thumb for blood withdrawal suggests that up to 10% of the circulating blood volume (or 1% of the body weight) can be withdrawn every 2–4 weeks from normal, healthy animals with minimal adverse effect. A larger volume or more frequent blood collection may be possible if fluid replacement is provided. Collecting blood from mice can be challenging because of their small size.

One of the most common sites used for large volume blood collection is the facial vein. The facial vein courses approximately from the lateral canthus of the eye to the point of the jaw before joining with the jugular vein. For the procedure, an unanesthetized mouse is restrained by grasping the skin over the neck and back, and the puncture site is identified at the point of the jaw. The puncture is made by fully inserting the point of an appropriately sized sterile lancet through the skin and vessel and up to 200 microliters (μL) of blood is allowed to drip freely into a collection tube. A 22- or 23-gauge hypodermic needle can sometimes be used in place of a lancet although this may be more difficult. Hemostasis is achieved by direct pressure on the site. Animals may die from blood loss if adequate hemostasis is not achieved. A video tutorial of the technique is available at www.medipoint.com. A similar technique has been recently described using the veins that are visible in the submental area of a mouse, which is the relatively unfurred area below the chin of the mouse. Submental blood collection is a simple technique that can be done in restrained mice and appears to have fewer side effects than facial blood collection.

Another site for blood collection is the retro-orbital sinus. As more techniques emerge that are considered less invasive, this method of blood collection is becoming less common. However, done properly and with appropriate training, it is still an acceptable and effective method of collecting blood. Individuals must be familiar with the anatomy of the retro-orbital sinus and receive training prior to attempting this blood collection technique. When performed correctly, multiple blood samples can be safely collected over time with no negative effect on vision. Mice must be anesthetized for this procedure and an ophthalmic anesthetic (e.g., proparacaine) can be applied. Sterile ophthalmic ointment should be used if the selected anesthetic will decrease the blink reflex for more than a brief period. Once the mouse is anesthetized, the forefinger and thumb of one hand are used to place pressure on the top and bottom lids of one eye to keep the eye open and slightly proptosed. Alternatively, the anesthetized mouse may be held by the scruff as described for general restraint. With the other hand, place the tip of a glass microcapillary tube in the medial or lateral canthus at approximately a 30°–45° angle toward the back of the eye. Using firm, steady forward pressure, rotate the tube between the thumb and the forefinger of the hand. This rotation will allow the tube to act as a cutting instrument through the conjunctiva at the back of the eye and enter the retro-orbital sinus. Once the conjunctiva has been bypassed, the tube will come up against bone; slightly withdraw the tube, and blood should flow into the tube by capillary action. A steady hand is required because additional movement of the tube tip can cause severe damage to the eye and the optic nerve, a clearly painful outcome. After collecting the blood sample, withdraw the tube, close the eyelids, and place slight pressure with a gauze square to stop the flow of blood. The eye will not be affected when proper technique is used because the capillary tube merely passes along the side and back of the globe. If mice show signs of ocular damage or pain, they should be promptly euthanized or provided analgesia with treatment to the eye injury. If mice will be bled over several days to weeks by this

Table 4.2. Adult mouse blood volumes and suggested sample size

	Volume (mL)
Total blood	1.6–3.2
Single sample	0.2–0.3
Exsanguination	1–1.5

Source: Adapted from Harkness et al. (2010).
Note: Values are approximate.

method, consideration should be given to alternating eyes and using sterile capillary tubes to minimize the chances for retro-orbital abscesses.

The lateral saphenous vein is an excellent site for blood collection from a conscious mouse. Restraint is accomplished by placing the mouse head first into a 50-mL tissue culture conical tube with perforations to allow air movement and then grasping the skin between the caudal aspect of the thigh and the tail to help extend the leg. The hair over the lateral aspect of the distal thigh is shaved with an electric clipper or scalpel blade. A sterile, oil-based ointment is applied topically to prevent blood from dispersing over the surface of the skin. Using a 23- or 25-gauge needle, a puncture is made into the vessel, and the drops of blood are collected into a microcapillary or other appropriate tube. Up to 100 µL can be collected. Multiple samples can be taken at a later date by removing the scab that forms over the collection site.

Small amounts of blood can also be collected by capillary tube collection from the hub of a needle placed in the dorsal tail artery or lateral tail veins or from a clipped toenail. Larger blood samples can be collected from a cardiac puncture. This procedure must be performed when the mouse is fully anesthetized and usually only when the animal will be euthanized prior to anesthetic recovery. The cardiac puncture technique is described in more detail in the rat chapter. To collect a terminal blood sample in euthanized mice, the axillary muscles and vessels of the front leg can be transected and a Pasteur pipette used to collect the blood as it pools. Approximate blood volumes for mice are listed in Table 4.2. It should be noted that hematological and blood chemistry values may be significantly influenced by the site of blood collection.

Urine Collection

On average, a healthy adult mouse produces 0.5–1.0 mL of urine per day. Mice may be stimulated to urinate upon handling or upon placement on a cold surface or in a cooled plastic bag. A urine sample is best collected with a specially designed metabolic cage, which separates fecal pellets from urine.

Drug Administration

Most drug administration techniques used in small animal practice can be used with rodents when modified to fit their small size. The tendency to overdose mice and other small rodents is attributable to overestimation of their body weight. Small digital laboratory scales are useful for obtaining accurate body weights. To increase dosing accuracy of small drug volumes, substances may be diluted to larger, more easily measured volumes and syringes designed for small volume administration (e.g., tuberculin syringe) used. Dosing volumes are most accurate when calculated on

Table 4.3. Maximum dosing volumes for a 30-g mouse.

Route	Amount (mL)
IP	2.0
SC	2.5
IM	0.05 per injection site [not recommended due to small muscle mass]
IV	0.125
PO	1.25

Source: Adapted from Harkness and Wagner (1995), Lukas (1999), and Diehl et al. (2001).

the basis of milliliters per kilogram (mL/kg) and not simply "per mouse." Table 4.3 lists the maximum recommended dosing volumes for an average, adult 30-g mouse.

Medication is frequently administered orally and is most easily accomplished by mixing the medication into the water or feed. Many factors may affect a mouse's willingness to drink or eat medicated water or food. Additionally, despite stability of medications in water and food, studies have shown that it is difficult to reach therapeutic levels in the blood. Therefore, administration of all substances, especially analgesics, in feed or drinking water is discouraged unless it can be shown that all animals will consume required amounts. Specialized gavage needles, available in metal as well as flexible plastic, are used to deliver a substance directly into the stomach for greater accuracy or for administering unpalatable liquids. Flexible gavage needles may be considered a refinement to the rigid type. In addition, use of ball-tipped gavage needles helps to prevent the needle passing into the trachea. The gavage technique can be rapidly accomplished in mice through proper restraint and extension of the head although the technique requires training and practice. A maximum volume of 1.25 mL is recommended for administration.

Smaller hypodermic needles, such as 25 or 23 gauge, should be used when giving injections. Medication can be administered through subcutaneous (SC) injections with a maximum volume of 2.5 mL administered under the loose skin over the shoulders or in the skin fold of the flank near the hind legs. Intramuscular (IM) injections are not recommended in mice due to their small muscle mass. The quadriceps muscle of the hind legs is the preferred site when IM injections are necessary. Volume should not exceed 0.05 mL per site with a maximum of two muscle sites. Certain drugs, such as ketamine, can cause muscle damage and nerve irritation that can lead to self-mutilation of the affected limb. As mice have such a small muscle mass, the intraperitoneal (IP) route is best for administration of ketamine and other irritating drugs (Box 4.3). The maximum injection volume for intraperitoneal injection is 2 mL. To administer an intraperitoneal injection, the mouse should be securely restrained to minimize movement with the head tilted slightly downward, and the injection administered in

Box 4.3

As mice have a small muscle mass, the intraperitoneal route is best for administration of ketamine and other irritating drugs.

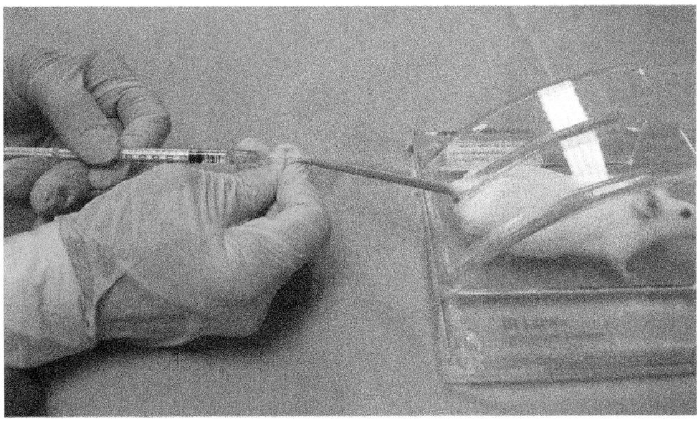

Fig 4.7. Lateral tail vein injection using a mouse restraint system. (*Source*: Photo courtesy of ULAM, University of Michigan.)

the lower abdominal quadrant just off of midline. Care should be used in male mice to avoid testicular injections. Before injection, the syringe should be aspirated to ensure that the needle has not entered the bladder or intestines of the mouse. Intravenous (IV) injections may be given into the lateral tail vein of mice using a 25-gauge or smaller needle at a maximum dose of 0.125 mL (Figure 4.7). IV injections can also be given into the retro-orbital sinus with appropriate anesthesia. Video tutorials for mouse injection techniques are available at www.procedureswithcare.org.uk.

Anesthesia, Surgery, and Postoperative Care

Preanesthetic fasting is not recommended in mice unless an empty stomach is inherent to the success of the procedure. A few common anesthetic and tranquilizing agents used in mice are listed in Table 4.4. Because of the small volumes of anesthetics required for mice, dilution of all injectable anesthetics is recommended. A dilution ratio of at least 1 part anesthetic to 10 parts either sterile distilled water or physiologic saline, based on manufacturer's recommendations works well. The age, sex, strain, health, and body condition of the animal influences the dose of anesthetic needed. Thus, a conservative dose is best given initially. The combination of ketamine and an α-2 adrenergic agonist such as xylazine or dexmedetomidine is frequently chosen as an injectable regimen for surgical procedures. When administered concurrently, they provide about 30–45 minutes of general anesthesia and can be mixed and given in one injection to minimize handling stress. Solutions should be mixed to the quantity required for short-term use. Mixed solutions have been reported to lose stability and effectiveness over time.

Tribromoethanol was once frequently used to induce a surgical plane of anesthesia in mice such as during embryo transfer procedures for transgenic production. However, its use is decreasing as more information is discovered regarding associated negative health effects (e.g., induced peritonitis with repeated administration) and unpredictable drug stability. If used, the drug must be freshly mixed, protected from light, and stored in a refrigerator.

Pentobarbital was commonly used in the past, but its use has significantly decreased due to its respiratory and cardiovascular depressant effects, variable anesthetic duration, and prolonged recovery partially due to induced hypothermia.

Table 4.4. Anesthetic agents and tranquilizers used in mice

Drug	Dosage	Route	Reference
Inhalants			
Isoflurane	1%–4% to effect	Inhalation	Markovic et al. (1993)
Sevoflurane	~5%	Inhalation	Cesarovic et al. (2010)
Injectables			
Acepromazine	2–5 mg/kg	IP	Flecknell (2016)
Alphaxalone	10 mg/kg	IV	Flecknell (2016)
Dexmedetomidine	15–50 μg/kg	SC	Flecknell (2016)
Diazepam	5 mg/kg	IP	Flecknell (2016)
Fentanyl	0.06 mg/kg	SC	Harkness et al. (2010)
+ metomidate	60 mg/kg	SC	
Fentanyl/fluanisone	0.3–0.6 mL/kg	IP	Redrobe (2001)
Fentanyl/fluanisone	0.4 mL/kg	IP	Flecknell (2016)
+ diazepam	5 mg/kg	IP	
Ketamine	100 mg/kg	IP	Flecknell (2016)
+ acepromazine	5 mg/kg	IP	
Ketamine	100 mg/kg	IP	Flecknell (2016)
+ diazepam	5 mg/kg	IP	
Ketamine	75 mg/kg	IP	Flecknell (2016)
+ dexmedetomidine	0.5 mg/kg	IP	
Ketamine	100 mg/kg	IP	Flecknell (2016)
+ midazolam	5 mg/kg	IP	
Ketamine	80–100 mg/kg	IP	Flecknell (2016)
+ xylazine	10 mg/kg	IP	
Ketamine	80–100 mg/kg	IP	Flecknell (2016)
+ xylazine	10 mg/kg	IP	
+ acepromazine	3 mg/kg	IP	
Midazolam	5 mg/kg	IP	Flecknell (2016)
Pentobarbital	40–50 mg/kg	IP	Flecknell (2016)
Propofol	26 mg/kg	IV	Flecknell (2016)

IM = intramuscular; IP = intraperitoneal; IV = intravenous; and SC = subcutaneous.

With the creation of anesthetic machines with multiple flow meters and nonrebreathing systems, use of inhalation anesthesia in rodents is common and often ideal in the research environment. Isoflurane and sevoflurane have high inherent vapor pressures and are best used in a precision vaporizer with a mask or nose cone apparatus in conjunction with a nonrebreathing anesthetic system. Several anesthetic and ventilation machines have been designed specifically for use in small mammals, which provide very precise anesthesia to the animal with minimal use and loss of the anesthetic agent. Alternatively, very brief (~1 minute) inhalant anesthesia can be induced independent of a precision vaporizer, through use of an anesthetic chamber. A simple anesthetic chamber can be fashioned by placing a cotton ball soaked with 300 μL of isoflurane in the bottom of a 500-mL glass beaker. A platform of hardware cloth or similar material should be placed over the cotton ball to separate the mouse from the anesthetic. Placing the mouse in the beaker and covering the beaker with a lid then induces anesthesia. When limb movement ceases and respiration is relatively slow and steady, the mouse is removed from the chamber. Use of volatile anesthetics should always be performed with appropriate scavenging systems or under a fume hood to avoid exposing personnel to the anesthetic vapors.

Contrary to some theories, rodents are no more resistant to infection than are other mammals, and surgeries should be performed using aseptic technique. Some research projects require multiple-rodent surgical procedures to be performed in 1 day. Sterilizing several small surgical packs is not always possible when surgical instruments are limited. In these situations, use of a hot bead sterilizer is ideal as it provides a rapid method to achieve sterilization of instruments, is easy to use, keeps the instruments dry and clean, and requires minimal bench space. Instruments must be cleaned of tissue and blood prior to placement in the bead sterilizer or the tissues will bake onto the instruments and potentially damage them. Instruments should be allowed to cool for several seconds prior to using on tissues. In situations where use of multiple surgical packs or a hot bead sterilizer is not possible, one sterilized pack can be used for a small number of animals (<5) with the instruments cleaned of gross debris with a cold sterilant and then rinsed between animals.

Likewise, adequate intraoperative and postoperative care is important for all animals. Rodents are particularly prone to hypothermia because of their small size (Box 4.4). A small circulating water blanket, a medical-grade heat pack or heating system is essential in maintaining the normal body temperature of a mouse during anesthesia. To help prevent drying of a rodent's eyes, sterile ophthalmic ointment must be used in animals that lose their blinking reflex for more than a momentary period such as with injectable anesthetics or continually administered inhalant anesthetics.

Because of the high ratio of evaporative surface area to body mass, mice have a greater sensitivity to water loss than do most mammals. Administering warmed saline or lactated Ringer's solution subcutaneously (1–2 mL) to mice that have undergone a prolonged anesthetic period or surgical procedure helps prevent hypothermia and dehydration and assists with recovery.

It is an ethical imperative that analgesics be administered to all animals, including mice, for control of surgical pain. Procedures that are known to cause pain in humans must be assumed to cause pain in other animals unless proven otherwise. Rodents are difficult to assess for signs of pain. Studies of postsurgical mice have shown that decreases in both water and food intake as well as decreases in activity and piloerection (involuntary erection of hair) are strong indicators of pain. A facial-expression-based pain coding system, similar to ones used with humans, has been developed and validated for use with mice. One reason clinical signs of pain may be overlooked is

Box 4.4

Mice are particularly prone to hypothermia because of their small size.

that the normal active phase of rodents is during the dark cycle, when personnel are usually not present. Analgesics should be provided sufficiently *prior to* the initiation of a painful procedure to allow the analgesic to reach effective levels at the time of the painful stimulus.

Nonsteroidal anti-inflammatory drugs (NSAIDs), such as meloxicam or carprofen, inhibit the production of the chemical mediators that activate peripheral pain receptors. Care must be taken when using NSAIDs because they may cause gastric ulceration, renal toxicity, and platelet inhibition. NSAIDs may be sufficiently potent to treat musculoskeletal, incisional, inflammatory, and acute, mild-to-moderate visceral pain.

The opioids are effective analgesics for moderate-to-severe pain. Opioids are controlled drugs, and careful documentation of use is required as directed by Drug Enforcement Administration (DEA) regulations. Buprenorphine works well to control severe acute or chronic visceral pain but also causes sedation. Sustained release formulations of buprenorphine are available, but data on length of efficacy in mice are inconsistent. Table 4.5 lists several analgesics that can be used in mice.

Anesthetized mice should be placed on a dry paper or cloth towel in a safe and enclosed area for recovery. An anesthetized mouse should not be placed back into a cage with animals that are not anesthetized as rodents may cannibalize animals that appear nonresponsive. Anesthetized mice should never be placed on small-particle bedding because it can be aspirated. Use of an incubator, circulating water blanket under half of the cage, or heat lamp directed at one corner of the cage is critical to preventing hypothermia in recovering mice. Nonambulatory mice should be turned approximately every 30 minutes to prevent hypostatic lung congestion. Provision of moistened chow or a critical care supplement can assist in the recovery phase.

Table 4.5. Analgesic agents used in mice

Drug	Dosage	Route	Reference
Buprenorphine	0.05–0.1 mg/kg q12h	SC	Flecknell (2016)
Buprenorphine sustained release	0.15–1.0 mg/kg(one 72-hour injection)	SC	Carbone et al. (2012)
Butorphanol	1–2 mg/kg q4h	SC	Flecknell (2016)
Carprofen	5 mg/kg q24h	SC	Flecknell (2016)
Diclofenac	8 mg/kg	PO	Flecknell (2016)
Flunixin meglumine	2.5 mg/kg q12–24h	SC	Heard (1993)
Ibuprofen	30 mg/kg	PO	Flecknell (2016)
Ketoprofen	5 mg/kg	SC	Flecknell (2016)
Meloxicam	5 mg/kg	PO,SC	Flecknell (2016)
Morphine	2.5 mg/kg q2–4h	SC	Flecknell (2016)
Nalbuphine	4–8 mg/kg q3h	IM	Heard (1993)
Oxymorphone	0.2–0.5 mg/kg q4–6h	SC	Flecknell (2016)
Piroxicam	3 mg/kg q24h	PO	Harkness et al. (2010)
Tramadol	5 mg/kg	SC, IP	Flecknell (2016)

IM = intramuscular; IP = intraperitoneal; PO = per os; and SC = subcutaneous.

Imaging Techniques

Great advances have been made in rodent and small animal imaging over the last decade. For a detailed description of current imaging modalities, see Chapter 3.

Euthanasia

The term euthanasia literally translates as "good" (*eu*) and "death" (*thanatos*). Euthanasia should provide a rapid death with little to no pain or distress. Individuals must be appropriately trained to use the various methods of euthanasia to minimize the chances of pain or distress if performed inappropriately. Methods must be consistent with the most current American Veterinary Medical Association (AVMA) *Guidelines for the Euthanasia of Animals* (AVMA, 2013), performed by trained personnel, detailed in the research protocol, and approved by the IACUC. Per AVMA Guidelines, "Carbon dioxide is acceptable with conditions for euthanasia in those species where aversion or distress can be minimized. Carbon dioxide exposure using a gradual fill method is less likely to cause pain due to nociceptor activation by carbonic acid prior to onset of unconsciousness; a displacement rate from 10% to 30% of the chamber volume/min is recommended. Whenever gradual displacement methods are used, CO_2 flow should be maintained for at least 1 minute after respiratory arrest. If animals need to be combined, they should be of the same species and, if needed, restrained so that they will not hurt themselves or others. Oxygen administered together with CO_2 appears to provide little advantage and is not recommended for euthanasia. The practice of immersion, where conscious animals are placed directly into a container prefilled with 100% CO_2, is unacceptable. Carbon dioxide and CO_2 gas mixtures must be supplied in a precisely regulated and purified form without contaminants or adulterants, typically from a commercially supplied cylinder or tank. The direct application of products of combustion or sublimation [author note: e.g., dry ice] is not acceptable due to unreliable or undesirable composition and/or displacement rate. As gas displacement rate is critical to the humane application of CO_2, an appropriate pressure-reducing regulator and flow meter or equivalent equipment with demonstrated capability for generating the recommended displacement rates for the size of the container being utilized is absolutely necessary."

The euthanasia of mouse fetuses and neonates requires special consideration. Neonates are resistant to hypoxia and require greater duration of exposure to CO_2 to effect euthanasia; for this reason, other methods may be preferred for this age group. Fetal mice under 15 days of gestation may be euthanized by allowing them to remain in utero following routine euthanasia of the dam. Alternatively, euthanasia can be induced by removal of the fetus from the uterus. However, fetuses removed from the uterus and allowed to breathe air must be promptly euthanized by a physical method of euthanasia (e.g., cervical dislocation or decapitation). Neonatal mice under 10 days of age may show marked resistance to CO_2. CO_2 euthanasia may still be used with these animals although prolonged exposure time may be required. Alternate methods of euthanasia of neonatal mice include injection of anesthetics, decapitation, or cervical dislocation. Death must always be verified prior to carcass disposal.

Other inhalant anesthetics may also be used for euthanasia, including isoflurane and sevoflurane. Anesthetic waste gas must be captured and diverted away from personnel. Another method that may be used to euthanize small numbers of mice is intraperitoneal administration of an overdose of an injectable barbiturate at three to four times the anesthetic dose or commercial euthanasia solution.

When anesthetics or tranquilizers have been documented to impact research results, it may be necessary to euthanize animals by physical means of euthanasia, such as by cervical dislocation or decapitation. Investigators must fully justify the need for using such a euthanasia method, personnel training must be insured, and the method must be approved by the IACUC. When guillotines are utilized for decapitation, a preventive maintenance program must be in place to ensure proper functioning and adequate sharpness of the blades.

Euthanasia of rodents inside an animal room should be carefully considered because under some conditions doing so may cause stress in the remaining animals. Per the AVMA Guidelines, "Distress vocalizations, fearful behavior, and release of certain odors or pheromones by a frightened animal may cause anxiety and apprehension in other animals. Therefore, for sensitive species, it is desirable that other animals not be present when individual animal euthanasia is performed."

There should always be a method to ensure death of animals, especially when noninvasive euthanasia procedures are used. Examples of assurance methods include performing a bilateral pneumothorax, cervical dislocation, removal of a vital organ, or exsanguination by transection of a major vessel. This step will ensure that death has occurred rather than just a deep plane of anesthesia from which the animal might later recover.

Humane Endpoints

To support humane animal treatment, an animal may require premature removal from a study due to its impaired physical condition or imminent death. The *humane endpoint* constitutes the discrete criteria used to determine when euthanasia should occur and is designed to occur prior to the time that an animal's potential suffering outweighs the value of the experimental data that may be acquired. The appropriate humane endpoint must be determined for each type of experiment performed and often for each strain of mouse utilized. Common criteria considered when determining a humane endpoint include loss of a percentage of body weight; inability to eat, drink, or ambulate; respiratory distress; loss of consciousness; severe or uncontrollable neurologic symptoms; large tumor mass; and hypothermia.

SPECIAL TECHNIQUES: TRANSGENIC PRODUCTION TECHNOLOGY

In recent years, multiple advances have been made in technologies to produce transgenic animals. Initially, two primary methods were commonly used to create transgenic mice: pronuclear injection (the injection of DNA into fertilized eggs) and gene targeting (the injection of genetically engineered embryonic stem cells into preimplantation embryos). With the advent of endonuclease systems, such as zinc-finger nucleases (ZFNs), transcription activator-like effector nucleases (TALENs), and most significantly, clustered regularly interspaced short palindromic repeats (CRISPR), the creation of transgenic mice has become more precise and efficient. That said, the basic techniques are still utilized and worth understanding.

Many health complications may arise in transgenic mice, including compromised immune function, decreased reproductive ability, altered growth patterns, and development of painful musculoskeletal conditions. Many of these can initially go unnoticed by researchers who depend on husbandry and veterinary staff to monitor animal health and development. Regardless of the method used to create a transgenic animal strain, the background mouse strains utilized can significantly influence phenotypic expression as well as the disease conditions and pathologic lesions that develop in the transgenic strain over time.

Pronuclear Injection

The first method of producing transgenic mice requires injection of foreign DNA into the egg- or sperm-derived pronuclei prior to their fusion within the fertilized egg. The basic steps for producing a transgenic animal through pronuclear injection are as follows:

1. Foreign DNA containing a gene of interest (the transgene) is injected into the male or female pronuclei of a fertilized egg. The injected DNA integrates at a random location and in variable numbers (up to hundreds of copies) in the chromosomes of the developing egg. However, since some cell division may have occurred prior to the DNA injection, *not all* cells present may carry the transgene.
2. Multiple fertilized eggs, each injected with the foreign DNA, are surgically implanted in a recipient, pseudopregnant female (female previously mated to a sterile male), where they develop normally into pups.
3. Following birth, a tissue sample from each pup is genetically tested to identify the pups whose genome has successfully incorporated the foreign DNA. Each of these pups is considered a genetic "founder." Each founder is genetically unique; founder animals produced even from the same litter are not genetically identical due to the random nature of DNA integration following pronuclear injection.
4. Each founder animal is then backcrossed to an inbred strain to produce a unique mouse strain that is homozygous for the transgene.

The FVB mouse strain are frequently used in pronuclear injection as their pronuclei tend to be larger and more well-defined than in other strains. Also, FVB females produce large numbers of embryos and are good mothers. The common complications of this technique are attributed to the random (i.e., nontargeted) insertion of an uncontrolled number of transgenes into an animal's genome. For instance, the random insertion of a transgene may disrupt a gene responsible for development, viability, or reproduction. Alternatively, transgene insertion may disrupt a necessary biochemical pathway or prevent production of a specific protein.

Gene Targeting

Gene targeting of mouse embryonic stem (ES) cells is most frequently used to alter the mouse genome at a specific location (Figure 4.8). The basic steps of gene targeting are as follows:

1. A preimplantation embryo is harvested from a donor female. At this stage, the embryo is composed of ES cells that possess the ability to differentiate into any cell type (e.g., skin, muscle, nervous tissue) and can be maintained and propagated in culture.

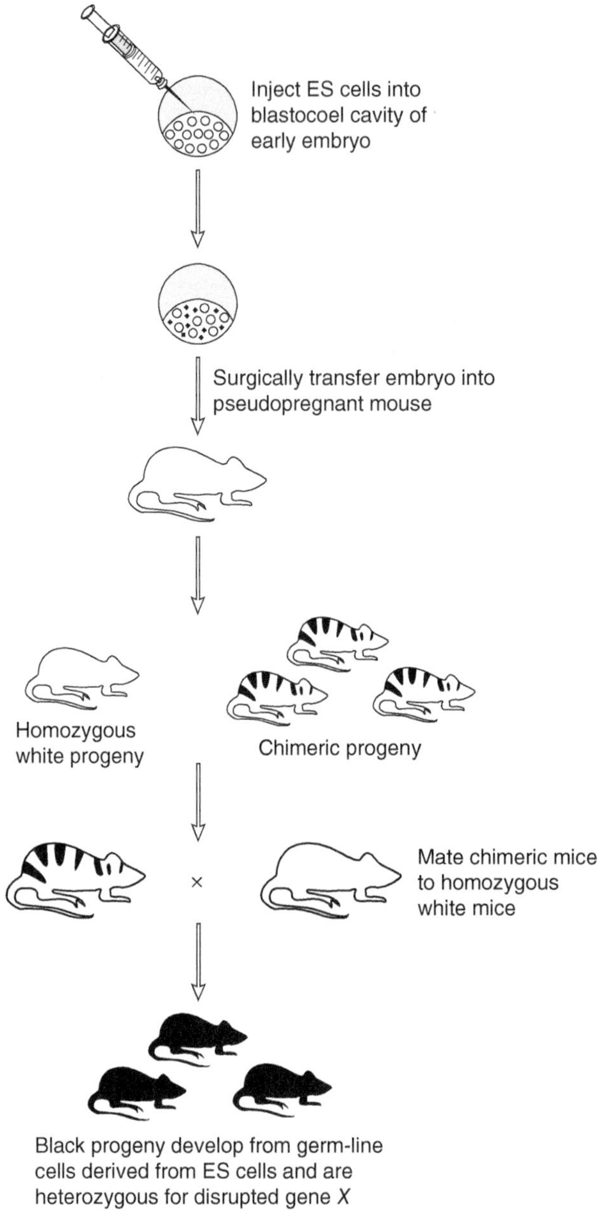

Fig 4.8. Gene targeting for the creation of transgenic mice. (*Source*: M. R. Capecchi, 1989, *Trends Genet* 5: 70. Reproduced with permission of Elsevier.)

2. The ES cells are mixed with DNA segments containing the transgene flanked on either side with a genetic sequence that is identical, or homologous, to the targeted gene in the ES cells. Through manipulation of the culture environment (e.g., passing an electric current through the cell thereby increasing the cell's membrane permeability), the DNA segments enter the ES cells and insert in the chromosome. A high proportion of insertions occur randomly, at unintended locations throughout the genome. A smaller number of targeted insertions occur

through homologous recombination where the genetic sequences flanking the transgene correspond with the genetic sequence of the ES cell.

3. The now genetically modified ES cells are screened in culture to select those in which the transgene was successfully inserted in the targeted location in the cell's genome. Genetically modified ES cells with nontargeted insertions are discarded.
4. The ES cells with the desired genetic mutation are injected into a host preimplantation embryo, where the modified ES cells and the host cells mix prior to their differentiation and proliferation during embryo development.
5. The embryo is surgically implanted in a surrogate, pseudopregnant dam (a female mouse previously mated to a sterile male), where it develops normally to a pup. The tissues of the pup will have derived either exclusively from the normal embryo (if ES cell injection was unsuccessful) or from a mixture of normal and modified ES cells. Animals with tissues derived from both ES cell lines are termed *chimeras*. If the coat color of the normal and modified ES cells' strains were different (e.g., normal ES cells from white strain and modified ES cells from black strain), then chimeras can be visually identified by altered coat color and pattern (e.g., white and black fur patches).
6. Chimeras are bred to select those with incorporation of the desired mutation in their germline (cells that give rise to eggs or sperm). These individuals are then bred to yield a population of animals each possessing the identical, targeted genetic mutation.

The two strains of mice frequently used in gene targeting are 129 and C57BL/6. Selection of these strains is useful as their coat colors allow ready differentiation of each strain and the resulting chimeras. The white strain 129 mice are used as a source of ES cells. The black strain C57BL/6 are used as a source of host embryos.

There are many practical applications to gene targeting. For instance, *knockout* (KO) mice can be engineered in which a specific gene is deleted or disrupted. By examining the abnormalities induced by the absence of the gene, scientists can infer the gene's normal function.

While this is simple in concept, many possible complications need to be considered. For instance, select strains of KO mice exhibit no observable change from their wild-type (natural genetic composition of the standard strain) counterparts due to compensatory replacement of the knocked-out gene's function by other unaltered genes or body systems. In these instances, a different strategy is required to determine gene function. Similarly, the function of a gene may change over time so that the primary function in young animals may differ from that in older animals. In other KO mice, high mortality rates or negative health complications may arise if gene expression is necessary for proper physiologic function during all or part of the animal's life. If the health complications manifest at an earlier age than the researcher wishes, the study may be compromised. Conditional gene modification systems (e.g., the loxP-Cre recombination system) can be used in these situations to effectively knock out the gene of interest in only select tissues or during a specific developmental stage or age.

Another application of gene targeting is the creation of *knock-in* (KI) mice, in which a transgene is inserted in a specific location in the genome without deletion or inactivation of the normal genetic sequence. This technique has been used to insert human genes into the mouse genome to create "humanized mice," which are used in studies to understand the impacts of specific human genes in disease models.

Endonuclease Gene Editing Systems

In recent years, several new gene editing technologies have been discovered. The ZFN and TALEN systems enjoyed a brief time in the spotlight, however, CRISPR is quickly becoming the primary gene editing technique used due to its relatively high success rate, low cost, and procedural ease. CRISPR are short repeated sections of DNA that many bacteria and archaea carry in their genomes. For the bacteria and archaea, these DNA portions are designed for defense; they allow for the recognition and removal of foreign DNA that might come from a virus or foreign plasmid. The Cas (CRISPR-associated) genes produce proteins that are essential for the function of the defense system. This technology has been taken and adapted from its natural origin to a powerful tool for cutting or snipping DNA efficiently and accurately.

The technique for using CRISPR/Cas to generate transgenic mice is very similar to the pronuclear injection procedure described previously. CRISPR/Cas mixtures containing the DNA of the gene of interest or the DNA sequence of interest are injected into the pronuclei or cytoplasm of a fertilized egg from a donor female. The eggs are then surgically transplanted into a recipient pseudopregnant female, where they complete their embryonic development and are born normally.

The power of this system lies in its ability to accurately and easily cut very specific sequences of DNA directly, with minimal off-target effects. It also takes fewer donor eggs and less time to produce the transgenic mouse of interest. It is very quickly becoming the top technique utilized to create transgenic animals, in multiple species. Outside of genome editing of research mammals such as mice, researchers are looking at this system to directly edit genes that produce human disease, such as the *CFTR* gene that causes cystic fibrosis.

Genotyping

To fully characterize the genetic makeup of breeding or genetically engineered rodents, a sample of DNA is usually collected from the tail tip. This involves removal of a few millimeters of the distal tip of the tail with sharp scissors or a scalpel blade. Minimal bleeding usually occurs, but if needed, hemostasis is achieved by applying pressure to the site. Anesthesia is used if mice over 21 days are biopsied; additional analgesia may be warranted and should be provided sufficiently *prior to* the initiation of a painful procedure to allow the analgesic to reach effective levels at the time of the painful stimulus. Alternative tissues that may also be collected include an ear punch, a swab of oral or rectal mucosa, feces, saliva, hair follicles, or an amputated toe. The use of ear punches as a genetic sample continues to increase in popularity, as it is minimally invasive, does not require anesthesia or analgesia, and commercial DNA extraction kits are now capable of generating the required amount of DNA from the tissue acquired. Toe amputation (toe clipping) is strongly discouraged but may be allowed on neonates less than 10 days of age with specific criteria that may include sampling not more than one toe per foot and amputation of only the distal-most phalange. The tissue collected from animal identification procedures (e.g., tail or ear punch) can and should be the tissue sample used for genetic testing.

Prior to performing any tissue collection method, investigators should contact the genetic testing laboratory to make sure they collect an appropriate amount of tissue and ship it in optimal conditions for maximum testing accuracy.

THERAPEUTIC AGENTS

Suggested mouse antimicrobial and antifungal drug dosages are listed in Table 4.6. Antiparasitic agents are listed in Table 4.7, and miscellaneous drugs are listed in Table 4.8.

INTRODUCTION TO DISEASES OF MICE

In the past 50 years, research and improved environmental controls and husbandry have led to the identification and eradication of a large number of infectious agents in laboratory rodents. Most laboratory rodent colonies today are relatively free of the viruses, bacteria, parasites, and fungi that cause clinical disease. However, these agents

Table 4.6. Antimicrobial and antifungal agents used in mice

Drug	Dosage	Route	Reference
Ampicillin	20–100 mg/kg q12h	PO, SC, IM	Anderson (1994)
Cephalexin	15 mg/kg q12h	IM	Flecknell (2016)
Cephalosporin	30 mg/kg q12h	SC	Harkness et al. (2010)
Chloramphenicol	30–50 mg/kg q8–12h	SC	Burgmann and Percy (1993)
Chlortetracycline	25 mg/kg q12h	PO, SC	Morrisey and Carpenter (2011)
Ciprofloxacin	7–20 mg/kg q12h	PO	Harkness et al. (2010)
Doxycycline	2.5–5 mg/kg q12h	PO	Harkness et al. (2010)
Enrofloxacin	5–10 mg/kg q12h	PO, SC	Harkness et al. (2010)
Erythromycin	20 mg/kg q12h	PO	Morrisey and Carpenter (2011)
Gentamicin	2–4 mg/kg q8–12h	SC	Harkness et al. (2010)
Griseofulvin	25–50 mg/kg q12h for 14–60 d	PO	Harkness et al. (2010)
	1.5% in DMSO for 5–7 d	Topical	Harkness et al. (2010)
Ketoconazole	10–40 mg/kg q24h for 14 d	PO	Harkness et al. (2010)
Metronidazole	20–60 mg/kg q8–12h	PO	Harkness et al. (2010)
Oxytetracycline	10–20 mg/kg q8h	PO	Burgmann and Percy (1993)
Sulfadimethoxine	10–15 mg/kg q12h	PO	Harkness et al. (2010)
Tetracycline	10–20 mg/kg q8–12h	PO	Burgmann and Percy (1993)
Trimethoprim/sulfa	30 mg/kg q12h	PO, SC	Harkness et al. (2010)
Tylosin	10 mg/kg q24h	PO, SC	Harkness et al. (2010)

DMSO = dimethyl sulfoxide; IM = intramuscular; PO = per os; and SC = subcutaneous.

Table 4.7. Antiparasitic agents used in mice

Drug	Dosage	Route	Reference
Carbamate (5%)	Twice weekly	Topical	Harkness et al. (2010)
Fenbendazole	20 mg/kg q24h for 5 d	PO	Allen et al. (1993)
	150 mg/kg in feed; provide for 7 d on, 7 d off for 3 treatments		Boivin et al. (1996)
Fipronil	7.5 mg/kg q30–60d	Topical	Richardson (1997)
Ivermectin	8 mg/L drinking water for 4 d on, 3 d off, for 5 wk		Klement et al. (1996)
	0.2–0.5 mg/kg q7d for 3 wk	PO, SC	Harkness et al. (2010)
Mebendazole	40 mg/kg q7d for 21 d	PO	Adamcak and Otten (2000)
Metronidazole	30–40 mg/kg q8–12h	PO	Harkness et al. (2010)
Moxidectin	0.5 mg/kg of 0.5% pour-on solution applied to the dorsum	Topical	Pullium et al. (2005)
	2 mg/kg repeated once in 15 d	PO	Harkness et al. (2010)
Permethrin	4 g of 0.25% dust once weekly in bedding for 4 wk		Bean-Knudsen et al. (1986)
	Cotton balls with 5%–7.4%		Mather and Lausen (1990)
	In bedding (w/w) active permethrin, used as nesting material for 4–5 wk		Hill et al. (2005)
Praziquantel	6–10 mg/kg	PO	Harkness et al. (2010)
	140 ppm in feed for 5 d		Harkness et al. (2010)
Pyrethrin powder	3 times a week for 3 wk	Topical	Harkness et al. (2010)
Thiabendazole	100–200 mg/kg	PO	Harkness et al. (2010)
	0.3% in feed for 7–10 d, use repeated treatments		Sebesteny (1979)

PO = per os and SC = subcutaneous.

still cause sporadic outbreaks of disease in the laboratory setting. The evaluation of clinical signs in mice is difficult because of their small size and their tendency, as a prey species, to hide signs of weakness or illness. In many cases, serology, histopathology, microbiology, and polymerase chain reaction (PCR) are required for a definitive diagnosis. The introduction of a pathogen into a facility may stem from many sources. For instance, infectious organisms may arrive in association with personnel, contaminated equipment, infected animals, or biologic materials. To improve biosecurity, some laboratory animal programs have prohibited employees from owning pet rodents, although the value of such a policy is in question. Facilities routinely prohibit sharing of equipment among institutions, facilities, and areas within a facility. Biologic material (e.g., cell cultures, serum) are screened for contamination. There is also a recognized threat of spreading infectious agents via the transportation and sharing of rodents and their tissues both nationally and internationally. Some infectious agents, notably those causing a gradual cumulative or subtle disease, may be present in an enzootic (constantly present) state in many research colonies. Finally, the use of immunocompromised and genetically engineered strains of mice is on the rise.

Table 4.8. Miscellaneous agents used in mice

Drug	Dosage	Route	Reference
Atipamezole	0.1–1 mg/kg	SC, IP, IM, IV	Flecknell (2016)
Atropine	0.05–0.1 mg/kg	SC	Harkness and Wagner (1995)
Cimetidine	5–10 mg/kg q6–12h	PO, SC	Allen et al. (1993)
Dexamethasone	0.5–2 mg/kg then decreasing dose q12h for 3–14d	PO, SC	Harkness and Wagner (1995)
Diphenhydramine	1–2 mg/kg q12h	PO, SC	Morrisey and Carpenter (2011)
Doxapram	5–10 mg/kg	IP, IV	Flecknell (2016)
Flumazenil	0.1–10 mg/kg	IP, SC	Flecknell (2016)
Furosemide	1–4 mg/kg q4–6h	IM	Harrenstien (1994)
Glycopyrrolate	0.01–0.02 mg/kg	SC	Huerkamp (1995)
Naloxone	0.01–0.1 mg/kg	IV, IP	Harkness et al. (2010)
Oxytocin	0.2–3 IU/kg	SC, IV	Anderson (1994)
Prednisone	0.5–2.2 mg/kg	SC, PO	Anderson (1994)
Sucralfate	25–50 mg/kg	PO	Morrisey and Carpenter (2011)
Vitamin B complex	0.02–0.2 mL/kg	SC	Anderson (1994)
Vitamin K	1–10 mg/kg q24h for 4–6d	IM	Harkness and Wagner (1995)
Yohimbine	0.2 mg/kg	IV	Flecknell (2016)
	0.5 mg/kg	IM	

IM = intramuscular; IP = intraperitoneal; IV = intravenous; PO = per os; and SC = subcutaneous.

These animals are more susceptible to disease, and this population increases the likelihood of outbreaks from a variety of adventitious agents (Box 4.5). Depending on the competency of their immune systems, identifying infected but subclinically infected immunocompromised mice can be especially challenging. Basic knowledge of the variety of infectious agents that may infect a rodent population is imperative to being able to quickly and appropriately respond to a disease outbreak. Presented here is a general overview of common bacterial, viral, fungal, and parasitic agents of mice and some standard diagnostic and treatment modalities.

Bacterial Diseases

Pneumonia and Respiratory Diseases

Primary bacterial pneumonia is uncommon in mice unless the animals are immunologically deficient or stressed. Infection with *Mycoplasma pulmonis*, a bacterium that lacks a cell wall, is one causal organism, but it is a much more serious disease issue in rats. Refer to Chapter 5 for a more detailed description of mycoplasmosis.

Box 4.5

Immunocompromised and genetically engineered strains of mice are generally more susceptible to disease, increasing the likelihood of outbreaks from a variety of adventitious agents.

Concurrent infection with Sendai virus or the cilia-associated respiratory (CAR) bacillus may result in a fatal pneumonia. Bacteria are often cultured from pneumonic lungs of mice with primary viral or mycoplasmal infections.

CAR bacillus is a Gram-negative bacillus that has been found between the cilia lining the respiratory tract of mice and other laboratory and domestic species. In mice, it appears to be opportunistic, as it has only been found in association with other respiratory pathogens. A histologic change noted in mice is peribronchitis. Sulfamerazine or ampicillin, administered at a dose of 500 mg/L of drinking water, has been reported to eliminate colonization of the organism as well as reduce the severity of the peribronchitis. Other bacteria occasionally associated with respiratory disease in mice include *Klebsiella pneumoniae*, *Corynebacterium kutscheri*, *Bordetella bronchiseptica*, and *Pasteurella pneumotropica*.

Clinical signs associated with pneumonia in mice include teeth chattering, labored respiration, weight loss, and conjunctivitis. Treatment with antibiotics is frequently not practical in a research colony; however, antimicrobials such as ampicillin, oxytetracycline, or trimethoprim sulfa may be effective when circumstances justify their use.

Helicobacter spp. Infection

Helicobacter spp. are small spiral- to rod-shaped, Gram-negative, motile bacteria that inhabit the gastrointestinal tract from the stomach to the colon in a variety of species, including mice, rats, hamsters, ferrets, cats, dogs, and humans. They are generally, but not always, host-specific. To date, at least 12 different *Helicobacter* species have been identified in mice, but this list will likely expand as the ability to recognize these agents improves. Transmission occurs by the fecal–oral route, and infections are persistent. Mouse strains vary greatly in their susceptibility to infection, with A/JCr mice being highly susceptible and C57BL/6 mice being resistant to *Helicobacter hepaticus* infection. In addition to the differences in strain susceptibility, the different rodent helicobacters vary in pathogenicity. Infection with *Helicobacter* spp. cannot be equated with disease.

Helicobacter bilis and *H. hepaticus* have been documented as pathogens in a wide range of mouse strains and should therefore be regarded as pathogens of susceptible hosts. They have been associated with disease syndromes, including chronic active hepatitis, hepatic neoplasia, inflammatory bowel disease, proliferative colitis, and rectal prolapse. Mice infected with these pathogens should not be used in long-term studies or housed near immunodeficient animals. Although the organism can be readily transmitted between animals in physical or close contact, the organism is sensitive to desiccation. Thus it is not readily transmitted between rooms or facilities employing routine biosecurity practices. Clinical signs are usually not seen until the liver disease is nearing end stage. Immunodeficient mice and aged mice have demonstrated a higher frequency of intestinal and hepatic lesions as well as an increased incidence of hepatocellular tumors, which may confound interpretation of experimental results. Gross lesions include multiple white foci in the liver, sites of hepatic necrosis. *H. hepaticus* serves as a model for *H. pylori*–induced chronic gastritis, gastric ulcers, and gastric adenocarcinoma in humans.

Helicobacter rappini, *H. muridarum*, and *H. rodentium* have rarely been associated with disease and should probably be regarded as undesirable contaminants of mice.

Their presence might be considered conditionally acceptable for some programs. Programs with substantial populations of susceptible immunodeficient, inbred, or transgenic mouse strains should consider excluding all *Helicobacter* spp. from the facility.

Sentinel mice exposed to soiled bedding can be used to screen for the presence of *Helicobacter* spp. Diagnosis of *Helicobacter* spp. is possible in several ways, including culture, histology, and PCR. No serologic assays are commercially available due to difficulties with assay specificity. PCR testing of fecal pellets or intestinal tissue samples is currently the most accurate and sensitive diagnostic tool available.

Eradication of *Helicobacter* spp. from a colony can be achievable by transferring neonates to *Helicobacter*-negative foster dams on the first day of life. Additionally, use of good microisolation technique can effectively prevent the horizontal transmission of *Helicobacter* spp. to other cages in the same room. Infection may be treated with a multi-antibiotic regimen although complete elimination of the organism is not always successful.

Tyzzer's Disease

Mice, rats, hamsters, gerbils, guinea pigs, rabbits, dogs, cats, several nonhuman primate species, and other animals are susceptible to Tyzzer's disease caused by *Clostridium piliforme*. *C. piliforme* is a long, thin, Gram-negative spore-forming bacterium. Tyzzer's disease occurs more frequently and is usually more severe in recently weaned animals, immunosuppressed animals, and those housed in unfavorable conditions. Different strains of mice have varied susceptibility to this organism. Clinical signs may include diarrhea, dehydration, and anorexia. Animals may be found dead in the absence of obvious signs of illness. Gross lesions seen at necropsy include miliary, pale foci throughout the liver, and at times a slightly reddened lower intestinal tract. Spores can remain stable up to 1 year at room temperature and are a likely means of transmission, especially through contaminated food or bedding. Diagnosis is made by histologic detection of intracellular organisms in the liver or intestine, by enzyme-linked immunosorbent assay (ELISA) or, ideally, by PCR. Treatment with antibiotics is frequently not effective because of spore formation; however, favorable results have been reported using high doses of tetracycline in the drinking water for 4–5 days. Barrier housing, good husbandry practices, and strict quarantine help to prevent outbreaks or control spread of infection.

Colonic Hyperplasia Disease

Citrobacter rodentium causes a disease syndrome in mice called transmissible murine colonic hyperplasia. Infection induces enterocolitis that leads to clinical signs of diarrhea, retarded growth, ruffled fur, soft feces, and occasionally rectal prolapse. The mortality rate is variable and depends on age and strain susceptibilities with recently weaned mice having a higher mortality. The characteristic gross finding at necropsy is thickening of the distal half of the colon. Microscopically, mucosal hyperplasia, infiltration of inflammatory cells, and mucosal erosions may be evident in the affected portion of the colon. Diagnosis can be made by culture, but PCR offers a more sensitive diagnostic assay. Recommended treatments include neomycin, tetracycline, and sulfamethazine.

Hyperkeratosis-Associated Coryneform (HAC)

Corynebacterium bovis has been associated with a severe hyperkeratotic dermatitis in nude mice of all ages and in neonatal SCID mice. The infection is often referred to as scaly skin disease. Transmission is by direct contact, fomites, and cell lines. People can serve as the source of infection for mice. The disease may cause high mortality in suckling nude and SCID mice. Clinical signs include dry, white flaky skin, dehydration, and pruritus that typically last 1 week. Mice that recover from the clinical signs may be persistently infected. Definitive diagnosis requires culturing the organism on select media or by PCR identification. There is no known treatment, and affected animals should be euthanized to prevent spread of the organism within a clean colony. Strict adherence to microisolation technique is necessary to limit spread of disease in immunodeficient mice.

Miscellaneous Bacterial Diseases

Staphylococcus aureus is a Gram-positive coccus that commonly infects the skin and mucous membranes of animals. Staphylococci are prevalent and can be found on the skin and in the nasopharynx and gastrointestinal tract. *S. aureus* is a pathogen that is most frequently associated with abscesses, conjunctivitis, and superficial pyoderma, particularly around the head and face. Bite wounds are often secondarily infected with *S. aureus*. Suppurative dermatitis or furunculosis caused by *S. aureus* is a particularly troublesome condition in nude mice and treatment is rarely successful. Diagnosis is usually by culture.

Staphylococcus xylosus is a Gram-positive coccus that is ubiquitous in nature and a common commensal of the skin and mucous membranes of many species, including immunocompetent rodents and humans. The organism has been identified as the causative agent for morbidity and mortality in select strains of transgenic mice. Mice with clinical infections frequently exhibit abscesses or other skin lesions. Modified husbandry procedures may decrease the rate of clinical disease in susceptible strains.

Streptococcus spp. infections are associated with dermatitis, pharyngitis, cervical lymphadenitis, bacteremia, and a variety of other disease processes. Immunodeficient mice are more susceptible to infection. Systemic antibiotics and improved sanitation may be beneficial in treatment.

Pseudomonas aeruginosa is frequently found in association with water and is not part of the mouse's normal microflora. In animal facilities, contaminated, untreated drinking water is the most common source of *P. aeruginosa* and has been shown to be a source of infection in animals. As an opportunist, this organism, once established, may be found chronically in the oropharynx, nasopharynx, and gastrointestinal tract and is frequently isolated from preputial gland abscesses. Mice that are irradiated or otherwise immunologically compromised are susceptible to developing a *P. aeruginosa* septicemia. The septicemia is usually rapid, and clinical signs may include listlessness, equilibrium disturbances, conjunctivitis, serosanguinous nasal discharge, edema of the head, skin lesions, anorexia, and death. Diagnosis is usually by culture of the nasal mucosa or water sipper tubes. Decontamination of water prior to presentation to animals can be accomplished by a number of techniques, including reverse osmosis, deionization, microfiltration, reverse osmosis–deionization–ultrafiltration, autoclaving, hyperchlorination, and acidification. Infections can be avoided but not eliminated by chlorinating the drinking water with sodium hypochlorite to achieve 10–13 ppm of free chlorine or by acidifying to a pH of 2.5–3.0 with hydrochloric acid. Acidity of the water should be tested before use.

Corynebacterium kutscheri is a Gram-positive organism that is usually inapparent in mice, but it produces a disease in stressed or immunosuppressed mice termed pseudotuberculosis. Transmission occurs by multiple routes from asymptomatic carriers. The disease is characterized by septicemia with high mortality and produces disseminated abscesses, especially in the kidneys and liver, in surviving mice. Treatment is usually not successful, but prevention can be achieved by barrier housing and good husbandry practices.

Salmonella spp. infections were extremely common in research colonies at one time but are now rare as a result of the institution of proper management practices. Mice can be intermittent shedders for several months without showing clinical signs of disease. Salmonella infection is significant due to its ability to infect and cause disease in humans.

Streptobacillus moniliformis infections are not common in mice. Epizootics are most likely to occur in mice that are housed near rats that may harbor the organism in the nasopharynx. The importance of this organism is that it has been identified as one of the causes of rat-bite fever, which is a zoonotic influenza-like disease in humans.

VIRAL DISEASES

Parvoviruses

Parvoviruses are small and nonenveloped DNA viruses; thus they are resistant to heat, lipid solvents, and acidic environments and can persist in the environment for months to years. Mouse parvovirus (MPV) and mouse minute virus (MMV) are the two parvoviruses known to naturally infect laboratory mice and are among the most prevalent infectious agents found in contemporary laboratory mouse colonies. Both viruses target rapidly dividing cells including those of the intestinal tract and lymphoid tissue. However, the intestinal tract is not usually significantly affected in infected animals. Neither of these viruses typically causes clinical disease in adult mice although runting and cerebral hypoplasia may be noted in neonates infected with MMV. MPV is a greater concern because of its known effects on the immune system of mice. There are differences in strain sensitivities to these infections. C57BL/6 mice are known to have increased resistance to infection. Transmission of MPV is relatively slow and is thought to be primarily fecal–oral although transmission can also occur through administration of contaminated biologic materials (e.g., cell lines, tumor cells, and serum). It appears to require direct contact with contagious mice or contaminated fomites. MPV is different from MMV in at least three ways: adult mice are as susceptible as neonates to infection, MPV causes immune dysfunction because of its tropism for lymphocytes, and MPV can infect and persist in immunocompetent mice but no one knows for how long. Diagnosis is usually made by serological screening of sentinel mice. PCR testing can also be used to confirm diagnosis by screening infected tissues such as mesenteric lymph nodes. PCR assays have been developed to detect the virus' genetic material in the environment. Knowledge of MPV's influence on physiologic systems and biologic pathways is continually expanding. Due to the virus' known persistence in lymphoid tissue and effects on the immune system, institutions devote significant efforts to excluding the virus from their colonies. Control of infection generally includes depopulation of infected mice and/or cesarean rederivation or embryo transfer for valuable mice. Environmental decontamination is considered important by some, and the use of a chemical disinfectant such as chlorine dioxide or hydrogen peroxide that can be vaporized to reach all surfaces should be considered.

Mouse Hepatitis Virus

Mouse hepatitis virus (MHV) is a coronavirus that is ubiquitous and highly contagious. Mice shed the virus in their feces and respiratory secretions. Transmission occurs through direct contact, fomites, and airborne particles. Although it is much less common in research colonies today, it remains one of the more common viral contaminants of conventionally housed mice due to its ease of transmission. There are many related strains of MHV that generally fall into two disease patterns: the enteric pattern and the respiratory pattern. Enterotropic strains are much more common.

Mouse hepatitis virus infections are usually enzootic and subclinical, with epizootics occurring in naive suckling mice. Clinical signs in nursing mice may include severe diarrhea, runting, an empty stomach, or disappearance of the milk spot (milk outwardly visible within the stomach), encephalitis with tremors, and high mortality. Infection of immunodeficient mice is associated with a severe wasting syndrome. Gross signs in adult mice include multifocal miliary white foci throughout the liver due to the necrotizing hepatitis that occurs with some strains of MHV. The most distinctive histologic finding is syncytial cells in the small intestinal mucosa and liver parenchyma. Diagnosis of MHV is most often achieved by use of ELISA with diagnosis confirmation through use of immunofluorescent assays (IFA) or PCR testing. MHV does not persist in immunocompetent mice and can be eliminated from a colony by cessation of breeding and no introduction of susceptible mice for at least 4 weeks to allow all infected mice to clear the infection. This eradication method may fail in transgenic mice if the genetic modification has altered immune function—an unintended and often unrecognized effect of genetic modification.

Epizootic Diarrhea of Infant Mice

Epizootic diarrhea of infant mice (EDIM) is a rotavirus that causes disease in suckling mice less than 2 weeks of age. It is characterized by the presence of soft, yellow feces or an accumulation of dried feces around the anus. Unlike in MHV infection, affected mice usually continue to nurse, as evidenced by the milk spot, but their growth is often stunted. Diagnosis is usually by ELISA serology. No treatment exists other than supportive care.

Murine Norovirus

Noroviruses are important human pathogens worldwide and cause more than 90% of all cases of nonbacterial epidemic gastroenteritis. Currently, over 40 strains of MNV have been detected worldwide; none are known to be zoonotic. MNV is a common viral infection in laboratory mice although a growing number of research institutions have eliminated the virus from their animal colonies by rederivation and cross-fostering very young neonates with uninfected dams. Transmission is primarily via the fecal–oral route. Certain infected immunodeficient strains of mice have high mortality with encephalitis, pneumonia, and hepatitis and may remain persistently infected. Immunocompetent mice frequently exhibit no clinical signs and are only transiently infected. Further studies are required to fully determine the consequences of infection; the virus has been shown to frequently affect the immune system although the effects of MNV infection varies significantly across mouse strains and with each MNV strain. Tests used to detect animal infection include ELISA, IFA, and PCR. Growth of many strains in cell culture has been challenging. A 1:10 dilution of bleach is the only disinfectant currently known to kill the virus.

Sendai Virus

Sendai virus (SV) is closely related to human parainfluenza I virus. While once very common, the virus is rarely detected in modern laboratory colonies. Viral infection can cause clinical respiratory disease in adult immunocompetent mice. Rats, hamsters, and guinea pigs are also susceptible to infection. It usually exists as an inapparent infection. It may, however, produce acute disease that is sometimes fatal, particularly in suckling or weanling mice. There is a distinct strain variation in susceptibility to infection. Immunosuppressed mice are highly susceptible and develop a wasting disease. Transmission is by aerosol, and the virus is highly contagious. Modern outbreaks have been associated with the administration of biologic agents (e.g., blood, serum, tissue, cell cultures) contaminated with the virus. Sendai virus infection suppresses the normal antibacterial activity of the lungs, thereby predisposing infected mice to secondary bacterial pneumonia. Clinical signs include a hunched posture, ruffled or erect hair coat, rapid weight loss, dyspnea, crusty eyes, and chattering sounds. Sendai virus has also been associated with otitis media and interna as well as exacerbations of pneumonia due to *M. pulmonis*. Gross lesions include consolidated, plum-colored lungs. The severity of disease is intensified by secondary bacterial infection. Diagnosis is generally made by ELISA serology, but reverse transcriptase–PCR can also be used to detect virus in the lungs. Sendai virus infections are self-limiting in immunocompetent mice. Susceptible animals must not be introduced into a colony for 4–6 weeks to allow "burnout" of the organism. Barrier housing will easily prevent spread of infection. Antibiotics may be beneficial in preventing or eliminating secondary bacterial infection.

Murine Retroviral Infection

All mice harbor both endogenous murine leukemia virus (MuLV) and endogenous murine mammary tumor virus (MuMTV) in their genome. Expression of disease is mouse strain-, age-, and cell-type-specific. The proviruses are transmitted genetically as inherited Mendelian characteristics and, as such, cannot be eradicated by traditional methods (e.g., test-and-cull, rederivation, cross-fostering of pups).

Lymphocytic Choriomeningitis Virus

Lymphocytic choriomeningitis virus (LCMV) is an arenavirus and is the only latent virus of mice that naturally infects humans, causing an influenza-like disease. The natural reservoir of LCMV is wild mice although many other rodent species can be infected. Mice may serve as long-term asymptomatic carriers of the virus, so care should be taken when contacting tissue, feces, or urine of suspect animals.

Ectromelia (Mousepox)

Ectromelia is caused by a poxvirus and is very uncommon in the United States yet still persists in other countries. It is significant when it occurs in research mice because it may be associated with high morbidity and mortality without additional clinical signs. Mice that survive the initial infection may have clinical signs, including conjunctivitis and a poxlike rash that can develop anywhere on the body. Severe infection of the feet and tail can lead to amputation, hence the name infectious ectromelia (*ectro* =loss of; *melia* =limbs). The disease is usually introduced through imported mice, tumor transplants, or other biologic materials. This underscores the need to screen all imported biologic materials by PCR or other methods prior to using them in animal studies.

Pneumonia Virus of Mice

Pneumonia virus of mice (PVM) is a pneumovirus that naturally infects mice, rats, guinea pigs, hamsters, and probably other rodents. Infections are asymptomatic, but may cause dyspnea, listlessness, and a wasting disease in immunodeficient mice. PVM has a worldwide distribution and may be prevalent in conventional colonies. It replicates only in the respiratory tract epithelium. Diagnosis is usually by ELISA screening of sentinel mice. Infections are acute and self-limiting in immunocompetent mice, thus control and elimination are similar to those described for SV.

Miscellaneous Viral Infections

Mice are susceptible to a vast number of other viral infections, including K virus, mouse polyoma virus, reovirus type 3, Theiler's encephalomyelitis virus, mouse adenovirus, and lactic dehydrogenase elevating virus. These rarely cause disease in immunocompetent mice and are primarily of concern in immunodeficient mice and as potential variables in biomedical research. They are most often introduced into colonies as contaminants of cell cultures or in subclinically infected mice being transported from a noncommercial source. Clinical signs are rarely seen in animals beyond the age of weaning. Quarantine of incoming mice with serologic and/or PCR screening should routinely be performed to ensure that only animals of appropriate health status are used for research.

Parasitic Diseases

Mites

Mites are sporadically detected in research colonies. The more common species of pelage-inhabiting mites are *Myobia musculi*, *Radfordia affinis*, and *Myocoptes musculinus*. The degree of pathogenicity is highly variable, but *Myobia musculi* is considered the most pathogenic because it feeds on skin secretions and interstitial fluid.

Light infestations are usually inapparent, whereas heavy infestations cause dermatitis, alopecia, greasy-appearing hair, and self-inflicted trauma. Some transgenic strains are especially sensitive to infection presumably due to often-unrecognized alterations of their immune systems. An allergic component may also be involved. Mite infestations can induce immunologic changes with marked systemic consequences that act as a variable in research. Mite lesions must be differentiated from fight wounds, ringworm, and other skin disorders.

Premortem diagnosis can be accomplished by several methods, including skin scrapings, fur plucks, and applying cellophane tape to the fur and examining the tape under the microscope for nits (eggs) or mites. The body site with the heaviest infestation, and therefore the highest chance of detection, varies with mite species and most frequently includes the dorsal neck and shoulder regions, the dorsal caudal thoracic or cranial pelvic region, the ventral abdomen, and the axilla regions. In addition, PCR assays have been developed as a diagnostic method. Each diagnostic method has varying degrees of sensitivity. All three stages of the life cycle—the egg, nymph, and adult—attach to the hairs on the host. Euthanizing the mouse and either collecting the mites as they leave the cold carcass or removing the mouse skin, placing it in a petri dish, and examining the bottom of the dish under low magnification after several hours usually achieve more conclusive results than antemortem assays. If mites are present, they should be transferred to a glass slide for identification.

Psorergates simplex is a follicle-inhabiting mite that produces dermal pouches that appear as small white nodules on the visceral surface of the reflected skin. These mites are rarely seen today.

Acaricides can reduce and even eliminate the mite population. Complete eradication of mites in a large mouse population, however, is difficult and requires an intensive treatment regimen. Ivermectin given by a number of routes, and to a lesser extent permethrin dusts, have been shown to be effective in eliminating mites. Cotton balls impregnated with permethrin have been successfully used to eliminate infestations after 4–8 weeks. Caution should be used when treating suckling mice because they may be more sensitive to topical applications of acaricides.

The most reliable means to eradicate mites from a colony is surgical rederivation. This method is more technically demanding and costly but highly effective. Cross-fostering within 36 hours in combination with topical ivermectin therapy has also been used to effectively eradicate murine fur mites. Extreme caution must be used with ivermectin administration as death or neurologic disease can be induced if the drug passes into the central nervous system through an incomplete or damaged blood–brain barrier. Ivermectin treatments should be administered to representative animals (e.g., varying age and sex) to evaluate safety prior to colony-wide administration.

Pinworms

Syphacia obvelata and *Aspiculuris tetraptera* inhabit the cecum and colon and are the most common nematode parasites that affect mice. A high proportion of conventional colonies are estimated to house mice infected with these parasites. In most cases, clinical signs are absent; however, heavy infestations may be associated with poor hair coat, mucoid enteritis, anal pruritus, rectal prolapse, and intestinal impaction or intussusceptions. Pinworm infection can alter the humoral immune response. Mice strains differ in their susceptibility to infection with pinworms, and this difference may be partially related to differences in immune function. Neither species of pinworms is transmissible to humans.

Premortem diagnosis of infection can be challenging, especially given the intermittent shedding of eggs in an infected mouse's feces, the need to have a mixed-sex infection to induce egg production, and the reduction in parasite load with age. The banana-shaped ova of *S. obvelata* can occasionally be detected by pressing a strip of cellophane tape to the perianal area, applying the tape to a glass slide, and examining the tape under a microscope. The more oval eggs of *A. tetraptera* may be detected by fecal examination. The most definitive diagnostic procedure involves examining the cecal contents for adults under a dissecting microscope. PCR assays are also available to detect infection.

Anthelmintics effective in treating pinworms include fenbendazole, ivermectin, piperazine citrate, thiabendazole, and mebendazole, many of which can be formulated in the feed or drinking water. Caution must be used with the administration of each medication as many may induce severe adverse effects in some strains of mice or may alter experimental results. The eggs may remain infectious in the environment for prolonged periods. Complete elimination of *S. obvelata* without repopulation and strict sanitation is difficult to achieve.

Lice

Polyplax serrata, the house mouse louse, is a bloodsucking louse that causes skin irritation, anemia, and debilitation. It is highly uncommon in laboratory mice. Ivermectin has been effectively used to eliminate lice. Dusts, such as permethrin dust, applied to the animals and the bedding are also reported to be effective against lice.

Tapeworms

Mice may harbor *Rodentolepis nana*, the dwarf tapeworm, and *Hymenolepis diminuta*, the rat tapeworm. Both species are transmissible to humans. Only *R. nana*, however, presents a practical public health concern because *H. diminuta* requires an intermediate host such as a grain beetle, whereas *R. nana* can directly infect its definitive host. Tapeworms are uncommon in modern mouse colonies.

Diarrhea and retarded growth may occur with heavy infestations, but most cases are clinically silent. Infestations can be detected by the presence of ova upon fecal flotation or by observing the adults in the small intestine at necropsy. Treatments may include thiabendazole or praziquantel, but treatments are generally not recommended because of the zoonotic hazard. Eradication by means other than repopulation is extremely difficult.

Flagellates

Spironucleus muris and *Giardia muris* are flagellates that occur in the small intestine and cecum. In young animals, the parasites may cause diarrhea and occasionally death, but older animals are generally asymptomatic. Giardia may be treated with metronidazole that controls outbreaks, but does not eliminate the parasite. There are no available treatments for spironucleosis.

Neoplasms

The incidence and types of tumors occurring in mice are highly strain- and age-related. Retroviral infections play a key role in the development of most neoplasms of the lymphoreticular and hematopoietic systems as well as of the mammary gland. Most mammary tumors are adenocarcinomas, which can produce large, firm masses on the abdomen, sides, or back of a mouse because of the wide distribution of mammary tissue. The C3H strain has a high incidence of mammary tumors; AKR mice have a high incidence of lymphoma.

Miscellaneous Conditions

Bite Wounds

Some strains of mice, including BALB/c, SCID, SJL, and FVB, are prone to aggression and can inflict severe bite wounds to their cagemates. Aggression is seen most often in males. In general, cohousing of multiple adult males not raised and maintained in the same litter is not possible. Housing males together prior to weaning can sometimes decrease aggressive behavior, but this is challenging when research requires randomization of mice. Wounds are seen primarily around the tail and perineum but also along the back, shoulders, and head. These wounds may become secondarily infected with *S. aureus*, which can lead to an ulcerative dermatitis with moist eczematous lesions. The stress from fighting likely impacts the physiology of the mice, and infection with *S. aureus* has been shown to alter immune responses.

Treatment of severe bite wounds is usually ineffective, and euthanasia is indicated. For animal welfare and scientific reasons, aggressive mice should be identified and removed from cages to decrease wounding and stress (Box 4.6). Removing the aggressor may resolve the problem, but a new dominant animal may emerge and fighting may continue. Addition of enrichment, such as nesting material, huts, and chewing objects, may result in decreased fighting by promoting other natural behaviors and providing an escape for subordinate mice.

Ulcerative Dermatitis

Ulcerative dermatitis (UD) is a genetically linked skin syndrome found most frequently in C57BL/6 mice and strains of mice on the C57BL/6 background. Clinical signs include severe pruritus with excoriation, ulceration, and loss of skin segments. Lesions are most common over the dorsal cervical and scapular regions, although lesions may occur over any aspect of the body. Histologically, mice with UD frequently have splenomegaly and peripheral lymphadenopathy secondary to ulceration and inflammation. A diagnosis of UD should be made only after eliminating other etiologies (e.g., ectoparasite infestation, fighting wounds). Treatment options have included antibiotics, corticosteroids, antihistamines, antifungal and antibacte-

Box 4.6

For animal welfare and scientific reasons, aggressive mice should be identified and removed from cages to decrease wounding and stress.

rial ointments (e.g., zinc oxide, silver sulfadiazine), and dietary vitamin (e.g., vitamin E) supplementation all with limited therapeutic efficacy. Success has been reported with trimming an affected animal's nails early in the disease process. Left untreated, UD may lead to such severe lesions that euthanasia is required for animal welfare reasons.

Dehydration

Dehydration should not be overlooked as a possible cause of acute death in mice. Water may be unavailable because of an air lock in the sipper tube even when a water bottle is full. Malfunction of drinking valves in automated watering systems can also result in a lack of water. In addition, mice may be slow in learning how to use a novel watering system when moved to a new environment. Mice undergoing surgical procedures should routinely be provided an IP or SC injection of warm saline or lactated Ringer's solution at 1–2 mL per adult mouse to offset the decrease in water consumption that often occurs postoperatively.

Hair Loss

Mice frequently develop bilaterally symmetrical areas of alopecia on the muzzle, which can be caused by friction from bars on the feeder. A more common cause of hair loss is barbering by a cagemate and most frequently involves hair chewing of the vibrissae or head region. Although long believed to be a show of dominance, studies have revealed that both dominant and submissive mice exhibit this behavior, and its causes are multifactorial. Additional information on barbering is provided in the behavior section of this chapter.

Malocclusion

Overgrowth of the incisors can occur when the jaw is malformed, there are missing opposing teeth, or the diet is too soft. If severe and undetected, overgrown incisors can lead to emaciation and death due to an inability to eat. A common clinical sign in later stages is excessive drooling of saliva with matting of the fur around the chin and neck. Incisors can be trimmed with suture removal scissors or toenail clippers, but this practice may lead to fractures of the teeth. A dental bur is a better tool to trim teeth without causing fractures. The use of a mouth speculum will protect the animal and the handler during examination and trimming. Some malocclusions have a genetic basis. Variable incidences are seen between strains, with some transgenic strains being severely affected. In these cases, it is recommended that affected animals be culled (removed) from the breeding population to decrease the incidence of malocclusion in future generations.

REFERENCES

Adamcak, A., and B. Otten. 2000. Rodent therapeutics. *Vet Clin North Am: Exotic Anim Pract* 3: 221–237.

Allen, D. G., J. K. Pringle, and D. A. Smith. 1993. *Handbook of Veterinary Drugs*. Philadelphia: JB Lippincott.

American Veterinary Medical Association (AVMA). 2013. *AVMA Guidelines for the Euthanasia of Animals.* Available at http://www.avma.org/KB/Policies/Documents/euthanasia.pdf [accessed November 8, 2018].

Anderson, N. L. 1994. Basic husbandry and medicine of pocket pets. In *Saunders Manual of Small Animal Practice*, S. J. Birchard and R. G. Sherding (eds.), pp. 1363–1389. Philadelphia: WB Saunders.

Arras, M., P. Autenried, A. Rettich, D. Spaeni, and T. Rulicke. 2001. Optimization of intraperitoneal injection anesthesia in mice: Drugs, dosages, adverse effects, and anesthesia depth. *Comp Med* 51(5): 443–456.

Atanasov, N.A., J.L. Sargent, J.P. Parmigiani, R. Palme, and H.E. Diggs 2015. Characterization of train-induced vibration and its effect on fecal corticosterone metabolites in mice. *JAALAS* 54(6): 737–744.

Bean-Knudsen, D. E., J. E. Wagner, and R. D. Hall. 1986. Evaluation of the control of *Myobia musculi* infestations on laboratory mice with permethrin. *Lab Anim Sci* 36(3): 268–270.

Boivin, G. P., I. Ormsby, and J. E. Hall. 1996. Eradication of *Aspiculuris tetraptera*, using fenbendazole-medicated food. *Contemp Topics* 35(2): 69–70.

Burdette, E. C., R. A. Heckmann, and R. Ochoa. 1997. Evaluation of five treatment regimens and five diagnostic methods for murine mites (*Mycoptes musculinus* and *Myobia musculi*). *Contemp Topics* 36(2): 73–76.

Burgmann, P., and D. H. Percy. 1993. Antimicrobial drug use in rodents and rabbits. In *Antimicrobial Therapy in Veterinary Medicine*, 2nd ed., J. F. Prescott and J. D. Baggot (eds.), pp. 524–541. Ames, IA: Iowa State University Press.

Carbone, E. T., K. E. Lindstrom, S. Diep, and L. Carbone. 2012. Duration of action of sustained-release buprenorphine in 2 strains of mice. *Lab Anim Sci* 51(6): 815–819.

Cesarovic, N., F. Nicholls, A. Rettich, et al. 2010. Isoflurane and sevoflurane provide equally effective anaesthesia in laboratory mice. *Lab Anim* 44: 329–336.

Clark T. S., D. D. Clark, and R. F. Hoyt Jr. 2014. Pharmacokinetic comparison of sustained-release and standard buprenorphine in mice. *JAALAS* 53(4): 387–391.

Cole, J. S., M. Sabol-Jones, B. Karolewski, and T. Byford. 2005. *Ornithonyssus bacotic* infestation and elimination from a mouse colony. *Contemp Top Lab Anim Sci* 44(5): 27–30.

Collins, B. R. 1995. Antimicrobial drug use in rabbits, rodents, and other small mammals. In *Antimicrobial Therapy in Caged Birds and Exotic Pets*, pp. 3–10. Trenton, NJ: Veterinary Learning Systems.

Cruz, J. I., J. M. Loste, and O. H. Burzaco. 1998. Observations on the use of medetomidine/ketamine and its reversal with atipamezole for chemical restraint in the mouse. *Lab Anim* 32: 18–22.

Cui L., Zhang Z., Sun F., et al. 2014. Transcervical embryo transfer in mice. *JAALAS* 53(3): 228–231.

Diehl, K. H., R. Hull, D. Morton, et al. 2001. A good practice guide to the administration of substances and removal of blood, including routes and volumes. *J Appl Toxicol* 21: 15–23.

Dole, V. S., J. Zaias, D. M. Kyricopoulos-Cleasby, et al. 2011. Comparison of traditional and PCR methods during screening for and confirmation of *Aspiculuris tetraptera* in a mouse facility. *JAALAS* 50(6): 904–909.

Flecknell, P. A. 1997. Medetomidine and atipamezole: Potential uses in laboratory animals. *Lab Anim (NY)* 26(2): 21–25.

Flecknell, P. A. 2009. *Laboratory Animal Anaesthesia*, 3rd ed. London, UK: Academic Press.

Flecknell, P. A. 2012. Personnel communication. Ketamine/medetomidine subcutaneous dose.

Flecknell, P. A. 2016. *Laboratory Animal Anaesthesia*, 4th ed. Oxford, UK: Academic Press.

Foltz, C. J., J. G. Fox, L. Yan, and B. Shames. 1996. Evaluation of various oral antimicrobial formulations for eradication of *Helicobacter hepaticus*. *Lab Anim Sci* 46(2): 193–197.

Fried, J. H., D. B. Worth, A. K. Brice, and F. C. Hankenson. 2015. Type, duration, and incidence of pathologic findings after retroorbital bleeding of mice by experienced and novice personnel. *JAALAS* 54(3): 317–327.

Garner, J. P., S. M. Weisker, B. Dufour, and J. A. Mench. 2004. Barbering (fur and whisker trimming) by laboratory mice as a model of human trichotillomania and obsessive–compulsive spectrum disorders. *Comp Med* 54(2): 216–224.

Gozalo, A. S., V. J. Hoffmann, L. R. Brinster, W. R. Elkins, L. Ding, and S. M. Holland. 2010. Spontaneous *Staphylococcus xylosus* infection in mice deficient in NADPH oxidase and comparison with other laboratory mouse strains. *JAALAS* 49(4): 480–486.

Harkness, J. E., and J. E. Wagner. 1995. *Biology and Medicine of Rabbits and Rodents*, 4th ed. Philadelphia: Williams & Wilkins.

Harkness, J. E., P. V. Turner, S. VandeWoude, and C. L. Wheler. 2010. *Harkness and Wagner's Biology and Medicine of Rabbits and Rodents*, 5th ed. Ames, IA: Wiley-Blackwell.

Harms D. W., R. M. Quadros, D. Seruggia, et al. 2015. Mouse genome editing using CRISPR/Cas system. *Curr Protoc Hum Genet* 83: 15.7.1–15.7.27.

Harrenstien, L. 1994. Critical care of ferrets, rabbits, and rodents. *Semin Avian Exotic Pet Med* 3: 217–228.

Heard, D. J. 1993. Principles and techniques of anesthesia and analgesia for exotic practice. *Vet Clin North Am Small Anim Pract* 23(6): 1301–1327.

Heyne G. W., E. H. Plisch, C. G. Melberg, E. P. Sandgren, J. A. Peter, and R. J. Lipinski. 2015. A simple and reliable method for early pregnancy detection in inbred mice. *JAALAS* 54(4): 368–371.

Hill, W. A., M. M. Randolph, K. L. Boyd, and T. D. Mandrell. 2005. Use of permethrin eradicated the tropical rat mite (*Ornithonyssus bacoti*) from a colony of mutagenized and transgenic mice. *Contemp Top Lab Anim Sci* 44(5): 31–34.

Hill, W. A., M. M. Randolph, and T. D. Mandrell. 2009. Sensitivity of perianal tape impressions to diagnose pinworm (*Syphacia* spp.) infections in rats (*Rattus norvegicus*) and mice (*Mus musculus*). *JAALAS* 48(4): 378–380.

Hoff, J. 2000. Methods of blood collection in the mouse. *Lab Anim (NY)* 29(10): 4753.

Holson, R. R. 1992. Euthanasia by decapitation: Evidence that this technique produces prompt, painless unconsciousness in laboratory rodents. *Neurotoxicol Teratol* 14: 253–257.

Huerkamp, M. J. 1995. Anesthesia and postoperative management of rabbits and pocket pets. In *Kirk's Current Therapy XII—Small Animal Practice*, J. D. Bonagura (ed.), pp. 1322–1327. Philadelphia: WB Saunders.

Hughes, H. C. 1981. Anesthesia of laboratory animals. *Lab Anim (NY)* 10(5): 40–56.

Institute for Laboratory Animal Research (ILAR). 2011. Environment, housing and management. In *Guide for the Care and Use of Laboratory Animals*, 8th ed. ILAR, National Research Council. Washington, DC: National Academies Press.

Karst, S. M., C. E. Wobus, M. Lay, J. Davidson, and H. W. Virgin IV. 2003. STAT1-dependent innate immunity to a Norwalk-like virus. *Science* 299(5612): 1575–1578.

Kelmenson, J. A., D. P. Pomerleau, S. Griffey, W. Zhang, M. J. Karolak, and J. R. Fahey. 2009. Kinetics of transmission, infectivity, and genome stability of two novel mouse norovirus isolates in breeding mice. *Comp Med* 59(1): 27–36.

Kendall L. V., R. J. Hansen, K. Dorsey, S. Kang, P. J. Lunghofer, and D. L. Gustafson. 2014. Pharmocokinetics of sustained-release analgesics in mice. *JAALAS* 53(5): 478–484.

Klement, P., J. M. Augustine, K. H. Delaney, G. Klement, and J. I. Weitz. 1996. An oral ivermectin regimen that eradicates pinworms (*Syphacia* spp.) in laboratory rats and mice. *Lab Anim Sci* 46(3): 286–290.

Lawson, G. W., A. Sato, L. A. Fairbanks, and P. T. Lawson. 2005. Vitamin E as a treatment for ulcerative dermatitis in C57BL/6 mice and strains with a C57BL/6 background. *Contemp Top Lab Anim Sci* 44(3): 18–21.

Le Blanc, S. A., R. E. Faith, and C. A. Montgomery. 1993. Use of topical ivermectin treatment for *Syphacia obvelata* in mice. *Lab Anim Sci* 43(5): 526–528.

Lipman, N. S., S. D. Dalton, A. R. Stuart, and K. Arruda. 1994. Eradication of pinworms (*Syphacia obvelata*) from a large mouse breeding colony by combination oral anthelmintic therapy. *Lab Anim Sci* 44(5): 517–520.

Livingston, R. S., L. K. Riley, C. L. Besch-Williford, R. R. Hook, and C. L. Franklin. 1998. Transmission of *Helicobacter hepaticus* infection to sentinel mice by contaminated bedding. *Comp Med* 48(3): 291–293.

Lodish, H., A. Berk, C. A. Kaiser, et al. 2008. *Molecular Cell Biology*, 6th ed. New York: W. H. Freeman.

Lukas, V. 1999. Volume guidelines for compound administration. In *The Care and Feeding of an IACUC*, M. L. Podolsky and V. S. Lukas (eds.), p. 187. Boca Raton, FL: CRC Press.

Markovic, S. N., P. R. Night, and D. M. Murasko. 1993. Inhibition of interferon stimulation of natural killer cell activity in mice anesthetized with halothane or isoflurane. *Anesthesiology* 78(4): 700–706.

Marx J. O., D. Vudathala, L. Murphy, S. Rankin, and F. C. Hankenson. 2014. Antibiotic administration in the drinking water of mice. *JAALAS* 53(3): 301–306.

Mather, T. N., and N. C. G. Lausen. 1990. A new insecticide delivery method for control of fur mite infestations in laboratory mice. *Lab Anim (NY)* 19: 25–29.

Matsushita, S., and E. Suzuki. 1995. Prevention and treatment of cilia-associated respiratory bacillus in mice by use of antibiotics. *Lab Anim Sci* 45(5): 503–507.

McKeel, R., N. Douris, P. L. Foley, and S. H. Feldman. 2002. Comparison of an espB gene fecal polymerase chain reaction assay with bacteriologic isolation for detection of *Citrobacter rodentium* infection in mice. *Comp Med* 52(5): 439–444.

Metcalf Pate, K. A., K. A. Rice, R. Wrighten, and J. Watson. 2011. Effect of sampling strategy on the detection of fur mites within a naturally infested colony of mice (*Mus musculus*). *JAALAS* 50(3): 337–343.

Morrisey, J. K., and J. W. Carpenter. 2011. Drug formulary. In *Ferrets, Rabbits, and Rodents: Clinical Medicine and Surgery*, K. E. Quesenberry and J. W. Carpenter (eds.), pp. 566–575. St. Louis, MO: WB Saunders.

Mouse Genome Sequencing Consortium (MGSC). 2002. Initial sequencing and comparative analysis of the mouse genome. *Nature* 420(6915): 520–562.

O'Rourke, C. M., G. K. Peter, and P. L. Junken. 1994. Evaluation of ketamine–xylazine–acepromazine as a combination anesthetic regimen in mice. *Contemp Topics* 33: A–25.

Pullium, J. K., W. J. Brooks, A. D. Langley, and M. J. Huerkamp. 2005. A single dose of topical moxidectin as an effective treatment for murine acariasis due to *Myocoptes musculinus*. *Contemp Top Lab Anim Sci* 44(1): 26–28. Erratum: *Contemp Top Lab Anim Sci*, 2005 May, 44(3): 56.

Redrobe, S. 2001. Imaging techniques in small animals. *Semin Avian Exotic Pet Med* 10: 187–197.

Regan, R. D., J. E. Fenyk-Melody, S. M. Tran, G. Chen, and K. L. Stocking. 2016. Comparison of submental blood collection with the retroorbital and submandibular methods in mice (*Mus musculus*). *JAALAS* 55(5): 570–576.

Richardson, V. C. G. 1997. *Diseases of Small Domestic Rodents.* Oxford, UK: Blackwell Scientific.

Scanziani, E., A. Gobbi, L. Crippa, A. M. Giusti, E. Pesenti, E. Cavalletti, and M. Luini. 1998. Hyperkeratosis-associated coryneform infection in severe combined immunodeficient mice. *Lab Anim* 32(3): 330–336.

Sebesteny, A. 1979. Syrian hamsters. In *Handbook of Diseases of Laboratory Animals*, J. M. Hime and P. O'Donoghue (eds.), pp. 111–136. London, UK: Heinemann.

Shek, W. R., F. X. Paturzo, E. A. Johnson, G. M. Hansen, and A. L. Smith. 1998. Characterization of mouse parvovirus infection among Balb/c mice from an enzootically infected colony. *Comp Med* 48(3): 294–297.

Smith, D. A., and P. M. Burgmann. 1997. Formulary. In *Ferrets, Rabbits, and Rodents: Clinical Medicine and Surgery*, E. V. Hillyer and K. E. Quesenberry (eds.), pp. 392–404. Philadelphia: WB Saunders.

Urbanski, H. F., and S. T. Kelley. 1991. Sedation by exposure to a gaseous carbon dioxide–oxygen mixture: Application to studies involving small laboratory animal species. *Lab Anim Sci* 41(1): 80–82.

Waddington, S. M., R. Privolizzi, R. Karda, and H. C. O'Neill. 2016. A broad overview and review of CRISPR-Cas technology and stem cells. *Curr Stem Cell Rep* 2: 9–20.

Wardrip, C. L., J. E. Artwohl, and B. T. Bennett. 1994. A review of the role of temperature versus time in an effective cage sanitation program. *Contemp Topics* 33(5): 66–68.

West, W. L., J. C. Schofield, and B. T. Bennett. 1992. Efficacy of the micro-dot technique for administering topical 1% ivermectin for the control of pinworms and fur mites in mice. *Contemp Topics* 31(6): 7–10.

Whary, M. T., J. H. Cline, A. E. King, et al. 2000. Containment of *Helicobacter hepaticus* by use of husbandry practices. *Comp Med* 50(1): 78–81.

Whary, M.T., N. Baumgarth, J.G. Fox, and S.W. Barthold. 2015. Biology and diseases of mice. In *Laboratory Animal Medicine*, 3rd ed. J.G. Fox, L. Anderson, G. Otto, K. Pritchett-Corning, and M. Whary (eds.), pp. 43–149. Amsterdam: Academic Press

White, W. J., and K. J. Field. 1987. Anesthesia and surgery of laboratory animals. *Vet Clin North Am Small Anim Pract* 17(5): 989–1017.

FURTHER READING

Animal Research Advisory Committee (ARAC). 2016a. Guidelines for endpoints in animal study proposals. ARAC, National Institutes of Health. Available at oacu.od.nih.gov/ARAC/index.htm [accessed April 25, 2018].

Animal Research Advisory Committee (ARAC). 2016b. Guidelines for the euthanasia of rodent fetuses and neonates. ARAC, National Institutes of Health. Available at oacu.od.nih.gov/ARAC/index.htm [accessed April 25, 2018].

Baker, D. G. 1998. Natural pathogens of laboratory mice, rats, and rabbits and their effects on research. *Clin Microbiol Rev* 11(2): 231–266.

Barthold, S. W. 2002. "Muromics": Genomics from the perspective of the laboratory mouse. *Comp Med* 52(3): 206–223.

Chichlowski, M., and L. P. Hale. 2009. Effects of *Helicobacter* infection on research: The case for eradication of *Helicobacter* from rodent research colonies. *Comp Med* 59(1): 10–17.

Code of Federal Regulations (CFR). 1986. Title 16 (Federal Hazardous Substances Act Regulations), Secs. 1400.40, 1400.41, and 1400.42. Washington, DC: Office of the Federal Register.

Croy, B. A., K. E. Linder, and J. A. Yager. 2001. Primer for non-immunologists on immune-deficient mice and their applications in research. *Comp Med* 51(4): 300–313.

Dauchy, R. T., L. M. Dupepe, T. G. Ooms, et al. 2011. Eliminating animal facility light-at-night contamination and its effect on circadian regulation of rodent physiology, tumor growth, and metabolism: A challenge in the relocation of a cancer research laboratory. *JAALAS* 50(3): 326–336.

Dobromylskyj, P., P. A. Flecknell, B. D. Lascelles, P. J. Pascoe, P. Taylor, and A. Waterman-Pearson. 2000. Management of postoperative and other acute pain. In *Pain Management in Animals*, P. Flecknell and A. Waterman-Pearson (eds.). London, UK: WB Saunders.

Eaton, G. J. 1976. Hair growth cycles and wave patterns in "nude" mice. *Transplantation* 22(3): 217–222.

Edmond, M., S. Faubert, and M. Perkins. 2003. Social conflict reduction program for male mice. *Contemp Top Lab Anim Sci* 42(5): 24–26.

Festing, M. F. W., and E. M. C. Fisher. 2000. Mighty mice. *Nature* 404: 815.

Fish, R., P. J. Danneman, M. Brown, and A. Karas. 2008. *Anesthesia and Analgesia in Laboratory Animals*, 2nd ed. San Diego, CA: Academic Press.

Flecknell, P. A. 2001. Analgesia of small mammals. *Vet Clin North Am: Exotic Anim Pract* 4: 47–56.

Foley, P. L. 2005. Common surgical procedures in rodents. In *Laboratory Animal Medicine and Management*, J. D. Reuter and M. A. Suckow (eds.), doc no. B2515.0605. Ithaca, NY: International Veterinary Information Service. Available at www.ivis.org.

Forbes, N., C. Brayton, S. Grindle, S. Shepherd, B. Tyler, and M. Guarnieri. 2010. Morbidity and mortality rates associated with serial bleeding from the superficial temporal vein in mice. *Lab Anim (NY)* 39(8): 236–240.

Fox, J. G., L. C. Anderson, F. M. Loew, and F. W. Quimby. 2002. *Laboratory Animal Medicine*, 2nd ed. San Diego, CA: Academic Press.

Fox, J. G., X. Li, L. Yan, et al. 1996. Chronic proliferative hepatitis in A/JCr mice associated with persistent *Helicobacter hepaticus* infection: A model of *Helicobacter*-induced carcinogenesis. *Infect Immun* 64: 1548–1558.

Gadad, B. S., J. P. L. Daher, E. K. Hutchinson, et al. 2010. Effect of fenbendazole on three behavioral tests in male C57BL/6N mice. *JAALAS* 49(6): 821–825.

Gaertner, D. J., T. M. Hallman, F. C. Hankenson, and M. A. Batchelder. 2008. Anesthesia and analgesia for laboratory rodents. In *Anesthesia and Analgesia in Laboratory Animals*, 2nd ed., R. Fish, P. J. Danneman, M. Brown, and A. Karas (eds.), pp. 239–297. San Diego, CA: Academic Press.

Hickman-Davis, J. M., and I. C. Davis. 2006. Transgenic mice. *Paediatr Respir Rev* 7: 49–53.

Hoyt, R. F., J. V. Hawkins, M. B. St Clair, and M. J. Kennett. 2006. Mouse physiology. In *The Mouse in Biomedical Research*, 2nd ed., Volume 3, *Normative Biology, Husbandry, and Models*, J. G. Fox, S. W. Barthold, M. T. Davisson, C. E. Newcomer, F. W. Quimby, and A. Smith (eds.), pp. 23–90. San Diego, CA: Academic Press.

Hubrecht, R., and J. Kirkwood. 2010. *The UFAW Handbook on the Care and Management of Laboratory and Other Research Animals*, 8th ed. Ames, IA: Wiley-Blackwell.

Huerkamp, M. J., L. A. Zitzow, S. Webb, and J. K. Pullium. 2005. Cross-fostering in combination with ivermectin therapy: A method to eradicate murine fur mites. *Contemp Top Lab Anim Sci* 44(4): 12–16.

Institute for Laboratory Animal Research (ILAR) homepage. Available at http://dels.nas.edu/ilar [accessed April 25, 2018].

Institute of Laboratory Animal Resources (ILAR). 1991. *Infectious Diseases of Mice and Rats.* Committee on Infectious Diseases of Mice and Rats, ILAR, Commission on Life Sciences, National Research Council. Washington, DC: National Academies Press.

Isogenic.info. Isogenic strains & design of laboratory animal experiments. Available at http://www.isogenic.info [accessed April 25, 2018].

Jackson Laboratory Mouse Genome Informatics. Available at http://www.informatics.jax.org [accessed April 25, 2018].

Jacoby, R. O., and A. L. Smith. 2003. Mouse parvovirus: Survival of the fittest [Editorial]. *Comp Med* 53(5): 470–471.

Langford, D. J., A. L. Bailey, M. L. Chanda, et al. 2010. Coding of facial expressions of pain in the laboratory mouse. *Nat Methods* 7(6): 447–449.

Lavin, L. M. 2007. Avian and exotic radiography. In *Radiography in Veterinary Technology*, 4th ed., pp. 294–301. St. Louis, MO: WB Saunders.

Marx J. O., A. K. Brice, R. C. Boston, and A. L. Smith. 2013. Incidence rates of spontaneous disease in laboratory mice used at a large biomedical research institution. *JAALAS* 52(6): 782–791.

Marx J. O, D. J. Gaertner, and A. L. Smith. 2017. Results of survey regarding prevalence of adventitial infections in mice and rats at biomedical research facilities. *JAALAS* 56(5): 527–533.

MEDIpoint, Inc. Facial vein bleeding technique. Available at http://www.medipoint.com/html/animal_lancets.html [accessed April 25, 2018].

Memarzadeh, F., P. C. Harrison, G. L. Riskowski, and T. Henze. 2004. Comparison of environment and mice in static and mechanically ventilated isolator cages with different air velocities and ventilation designs. *Contemp Top Lab Anim Sci* 43(1): 14–20.

Militzer, K. 2001. Hair growth pattern in nude mice. *Cells Tissues Organs* 168(4): 285–294.

Monastersky, G. M., and J. G. Geitsfeld. 2002. Transgenic and knockout mice. In *Laboratory Animal Medicine*, 2nd ed., J. G. Fox, L. C. Anderson, F. M. Loew, and F. W. Quimby (eds.), pp. 1129–1141. San Diego, CA: Academic Press.

Nagy, A., M. Gertsenstein, K. Vintersten, and R. Behringer. 2003. *Manipulating the Mouse Embryo: A Laboratory Manual*, 3rd ed. New York: Cold Spring Harbor Laboratory Press.

Neimark, H., W. Peters, B. L. Robinson, and L. B. Stewart. 2005. Phylogenetic analysis and description of *Eperythrozoon coccoides*, proposal to transfer to the genus *Mycoplasma* as *Mycoplasma coccoides* comb. nov. and request for an opinion. *Int J Syst Evol Microbiol* 55(3): 1385–1391.

Pacheco, K. A., C. McCammon, P. S. Thorne, et al. 2006. Characterization of endotoxin and mouse allergen exposures in mouse facilities and research laboratories. *Ann Occup Hyg* 50(6): 563–572.

Pecaut, M. J., A. L. Smith, T. A. Jones, and D. S. Gridley. 2000. Modification of immunologic and hematologic variables by method of CO_2 euthanasia. *Comp Med* 50(6): 595–602.

Percy, D. H., and S. W. Barthold. 2007. *Pathology of Laboratory Rodents and Rabbits*, 3rd ed. Ames, IA: Wiley-Blackwell.

Pritchett, K., D. Corrow, J. Stockwell, and A. Smith. 2005. Euthanasia of neonatal mice with carbon dioxide. *Comp Med* 55(3): 275–281.

Ray, M. A., N. A. Johnston, S. Verhulst, R. A. Trammell, and L. A. Toth. 2010 Identification of markers for imminent death in mice used in longevity and aging research. *JAALAS* 49(3): 282–288.

Redrobe, S. 2002. Soft tissue surgery of rabbits and rodents. *Semin Avian Exotic Pet Med* 11: 231–245.

Smith, A., and D. J. Corrow. 2005. Modifications to husbandry and housing conditions of laboratory rodents for improved well-being. *ILAR* 46(2): 140–147.

Smith, A. L., S. L. Mabus, and Y. Woo. 2005. Effects of housing density and cage floor space on three strains of young adult inbred mice. *Comp Med* 55(4): 368–376.

Suckow, M. A., P. Danneman, and C. Brayton. 2012. *The Laboratory Mouse*, 2nd ed. Boca Raton, FL: CRC Press.

Taylor, B., S. A. Orr, J. L. Chapman, and D. E. Fisher. 2009. Beyond-use dating of extemporaneously compounded ketamine, acepromazine, and xylazine: Safety, stability, and efficacy over time. *Lab Anim Sci* 48(6): 718–726.

Weisbroth, S. H., R. Peters, L. K. Riley, and W. Shek. 1998. Microbiological assessment of laboratory rats and mice. *ILAR* 39(4): 272–290.

Wiles, S., B. D. Robertson, G. Frankel, and A. Kerton. 2009. Bioluminescent monitoring of *in vivo* colonization and clearance by light-emitting bacteria. *Bio Biolum* 574(5): 137–153.

Wixson, S. K., and K. L. Smiler. 1997. Anesthesia and analgesia in rodents. In *Anesthesia and Analgesia in Laboratory Animals*, D. F. Kohn, S. K. Wixson, W. J. White, and G. J. Benson (eds.), pp. 183. San Diego, CA: Academic Press.

Wolfer, D., and M. Stagljar-Bozicevic. 1998. Spatial memory and learning in transgenic mice: Fact or artifact? *Physiology* 13: 118–123.

CHAPTER 4 REVIEW

Short Answer

1. Define outbred stocks and inbred strains.
2. What type of mice would you order if you needed mice free of all detectable microflora? What about free of a defined list of pathogens?
3. What federal organization requires the safety of a product to be proven in animal models prior to being marketed for humans?
4. True or False: Mammary tissue is only found on the abdomen of mice.
5. Which pheromone effect are you taking advantage of if group-housed female mice are exposed to male mouse urine to synchronize estrous?
6. Which type of nesting material should be avoided in nude mice, and why?
7. True or False: Mice must be anesthetized for retro-orbital blood collection or injections.
8. What is a chimera?
9. What does CRISPR stand for?
10. What is a minimally invasive tissue collection technique for genotyping that does not require anesthesia or analgesia?

Match up

A. Ectromelia virus
B. Mouse hepatitis virus
C. mites
D. tapeworms
E. pinworms
F. *Pseudomonas aeruginosa*
G. ulcerative dermatitis
H. Murine norovirus
I. *Corynebacterium bovis*
J. Pneumonia virus of mice
K. Mouse minute virus
L. Sendai virus
M. barbering
N. *Helicobacter hepaticus*

11. ____ bacteria associated with chronic active hepatitis
12. ____ parvovirus that targets intestinal and lymphoid tissue
13. ____ hair chewing of vibrissae on head region
14. ____ *Syphacia* and *Aspicularis*
15. ____ poxvirus that can lead to amputation of feet and tail
16. ____ *Myobia* and *Mycoptes*
17. ____ coronavirus that is highly contagious; enteric and respiratory patterns
18. ____ genetically linked skin syndrome found frequently in C57BL/6 mice
19. ____ cause of scaly skin disease in nudes
20. ____ found in association with water, not part of normal flora

5

Rats

The laboratory rat strains most commonly used in research are believed to be domesticated albino strains of the Norway rat (*Rattus norvegicus*) that originated in Asia and migrated to Europe and then North America. Rats, like mice, belong to the order Rodentia and the family Muridae. Rats generally weigh between 250 and 500 g when they reach adulthood, with males being significantly larger than females by 9 weeks of age. Most laboratory rats are albino with white coats and pink eyes. There are several other color varieties, including brown, black, and hooded.

GENETICS

Like mice, rats are genetically classified as outbred stocks, inbred strains, or genetically engineered. Refer to Chapter 4, for a brief description of each. Outbred stocks are valuable in modeling natural populations that inherently possess genetic diversity. Three of the most common outbred stocks of rats used in research are the Sprague-Dawley, Wistar, and Long-Evans (Figure 5.1). Sprague-Dawley and Wistar rats are albinos, in contrast to the Long-Evans which is hooded (color on the head and shoulders with a pigmented dorsal stripe).

Inbred rats are commonly utilized to limit experimental variability and to capitalize on a desired characteristic, often arising through a spontaneous mutation, for which the strain has been selectively bred. Examples of inbred strains of rats include the Fischer 344 (F344), the Spontaneously Hypertensive (SHR), Wistar-Kyoto (WKY), and the Buffalo (BUF). Each of these is selected for use due to its unique desirable characteristics. However, each also has characteristics that can conflict with or complicate experimental interpretation, thereby necessitating careful strain

Clinical Laboratory Animal Medicine: An Introduction, Fifth Edition.
Lesley A. Colby, Megan H. Nowland, and Lucy H. Kennedy.

Companion website: www.wiley.com/go/colby/clinical

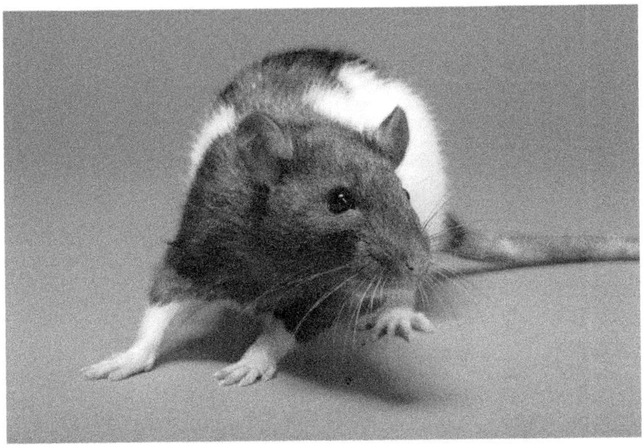

Fig 5.1. Long-Evans, outbred hooded rat. (*Source*: Photo courtesy of Taconic.)

selection when designing experimental studies. For example, F344 rats have a high incidence of testicular tumors, large granular lymphocytic leukemia, and retinal degeneration. They are commonly used in gerontology and long-term toxicity studies. SHR rats develop hypertension and are used to study therapies for this disease; the WKY has normal blood pressure and functions as the control for the SHR. Buffalo rats have a high incidence of autoimmune thyroiditis, also known as Hashimoto's disease. Other popular rat strains that have been developed following a spontaneous mutation event include the nude rat and the Zucker Diabetic Fatty (ZDF) rat. The nude rat, similar to the nude mouse, lacks a thymus and thus is deficient in T cells; they are used in oncology studies because they readily accept xenografts of human tumors. "Nude" is somewhat of a misnomer in this case as it frequently possesses a sparse but noticeable coat. The ZDF, with a body weight of 400–600 g at 15 weeks of age, develops hyperlipidemia and hyperglycemia at 8 weeks and diabetes at 12 weeks when fed a high-fat diet.

Genetically engineered strains are useful in elucidating gene functions and the modeling of human conditions not represented in existing inbred strains. The number of specifically designed, genetically modified strains continues to increase, although it is still significantly less than that of mice. Two genetically modified strains are the p53 knockout used in oncology research and the RIP-HAT developed for use in diabetes research. Mutant strains of inbred rats provide investigators a large variety of animal models with which to study biologic processes and diseases.

MICROBIOLOGIC CLASSIFICATIONS

In addition to being categorized by their genetic classification, rats, like mice, are frequently classified by their microbiologic status. These are (1) germ-free or axenic, which are free of all detectable microflora; (2) gnotobiotic, which are colonized only with a known population of microflora; (3) specific pathogen–free, which are free of a defined list of pathogens; and (4) conventional, or animals with undefined microflora. The majority of rodents used for research are specific pathogen–free and are maintained within barrier facilities, specifically designed and operated to exclude the unintentional introduction of organisms to an animal colony.

USES

Rats rank second only to mice in the number of mammals used in biomedical research (Box 5.1). Rats and mice combined account for more than 95% of all mammals used. Rats share most of the attributes of mice that make them valuable for research purposes, including a short lifespan, a short gestation length, a large litter size, abundant genetic diversity, and ease of maintenance. Hypertension, neoplasia, teratology, toxicology, embryology, and aging are just a few of the research areas for which these animals are used.

BEHAVIOR

Rats are generally quiet, gentle animals that are intelligent and easily trained. They seldom bite unless provoked and do not have the distinct musty odor that is characteristic of mice. Rats appear to tolerate single housing but social housing in pairs or small groups is recommended whenever possible; single housing should be employed only when scientifically justified. Unlike mice, rats rarely fight, and younger males can be housed together with few problems. Older males may be aggressive toward other males and therefore group housing of males after weaning age should be done with caution. Females with litters may not tolerate the company of other females. Most strains are docile and curious, and easily adapt to various environments. Rats are thigmotaxic, with an innate preference for contact with the vertical perimeter of bounded spaces. They display this behavior by wall-following, corner-burrowing, group aggregation, and the strong avoidance of open areas. This behavioral preference can be used in acclimating animals to handling by holding them securely with as much surface contact as possible. Some strains (e.g., Long-Evans and F344) can be more difficult to handle than others. Docile behavior can be markedly improved by frequent and gentle handling, especially when initiated with young animals. Rats may bite out of fear if they are handled roughly.

Rats are nocturnal, sleeping much of the day. They like to burrow and, although variability exists across strains, females may build nests if pups are present and they are provided with appropriate nesting material. Rats may escape from their cages if

Box 5.1

Rats rank second only to mice in the number of mammals used in biomedical research.

not securely closed, but will often return to them after a brief exploration period. Pups left alone by the dam emit high-frequency (22–80 kHz) vocalizations. Adults routinely vocalize under a variety of circumstances although nearly all vocalizations are beyond the range of human hearing.

ANATOMIC AND PHYSIOLOGIC FEATURES

Biologic and reproductive data for the rat are listed in Table 5.1. Rats are much larger than mice. They have conical heads; cylindrical bodies covered in thick, short fur; and short legs. Their tails are sparsely haired and slightly shorter than the length of the body.

The rat gastrointestinal system is anatomically similar to that of the mouse with a few notable exceptions. Both mice and rats have a dental formula of 2(I 1/1, C 0/0, P 0/0, M 3/3) and continuously growing incisors. Rat lungs are similar to those in mice, consisting of one left lobe and four small right lobes. The cecum is large, thin-walled, and populated with a high concentration of organisms that contribute to the fermentation of nondigestible food components. The stomachs of both mice and rats are divided into two compartments: a nonglandular forestomach and the glandular corpus. It is believed that neither species can vomit, but their stomach anatomy differs in that the mucosa that separates the nonglandular and glandular portions of the rat stomach is raised in a structure called the "limiting ridge." The rat's inability to vomit is partially attributed to the ridge's physical interaction with the esophageal opening

Table 5.1. Biologic and reproductive data for rats

Early adult body weight: Male	450–520 g
Early adult body weight: Female	250–300 g
Life span	2.5–3.5 y
Body temperature	35.9°–37.5°C (96.6°–99.5°F)
Heart rate	250–450 beats per minute
Respiratory rate	70–115 breaths per minute
Tidal volume	0.6–2 mL
Food consumption	5–6 g/100 g per day
Water consumption	10–12 mL/100 g per day
Breeding onset: Male	65–110 d
Breeding onset: Female	65–110d
Estrous cycle length	4–5d
Gestation period	21–23d
Postpartum estrus	Fertile
Litter size	6–12
Weaning age	21d
Breeding duration	350–440 d
Chromosome number (diploid)	42

Source: Adapted from Harkness et al. (2010).

to the stomach. However, other physical and neurologic factors likely play more significant roles in the rat's inability to vomit. Other unique features of the rat digestive system include the absence of a gallbladder and tonsils, a diffuse and lobulated pancreas, and prominent salivary glands in the anterior neck between the submandibular lymph nodes and the sternum. The liver has four lobes: median, left lateral, right lateral, and caudate.

Behind each eye lies a large, horseshoe-shaped lacrimal structure called the Harderian gland. Although the full function of the gland is unknown, it is known to secrete lipids that provide lubrication to the eye. During periods of animal stress or illness, the gland also secretes the red pigment porphyrin in tears (termed chromodacryorrhea or "red tears") that may stain fur around the eyes. After passing down the nasolacrimal duct, the pigment may also be seen on the fur around the nose. The red discoloration may be mistaken for blood but an ultraviolet light can be used to detect the fluorescence characteristic of porphyrin.

Zymbal's glands, specialized sebaceous glands, are located anterior and ventral to the base of the external ear canal with the gland's ducts opening into the external ear canal near the tympanic membrane. Occasionally, tumors develop in the glands of older rats. Zymbal's gland tumors are rarely metastatic, but are frequently locally invasive and present as masses near the ear base that may ulcerate. As with other rodents, brown fat is important in thermogenesis and is found between the scapulae and in the ventral cervical region. Due to its location and coloration, brown fat may initially be confused on necropsy with salivary glands or lymph nodes.

Identifying the sex of neonates is accomplished by observing the anogenital distance and the size of the genital papillae. A greater anogenital distance and a larger genital papilla are present in males as compared to females (Figure 5.2). The sex of adult rats is readily determined as the testes are obvious in the scrotum of males. Testes descend into the scrotum at about 15 days of age and remain retractable throughout life due to open inguinal canals. Males have paired bulbourethral glands, seminal vesicles, and a large prostate gland, as well as an os penis.

Females have a bicornuate (double-horned) uterus with two distinct uterine horns and associated cervices that communicate with the vagina. At birth, the vaginal opening

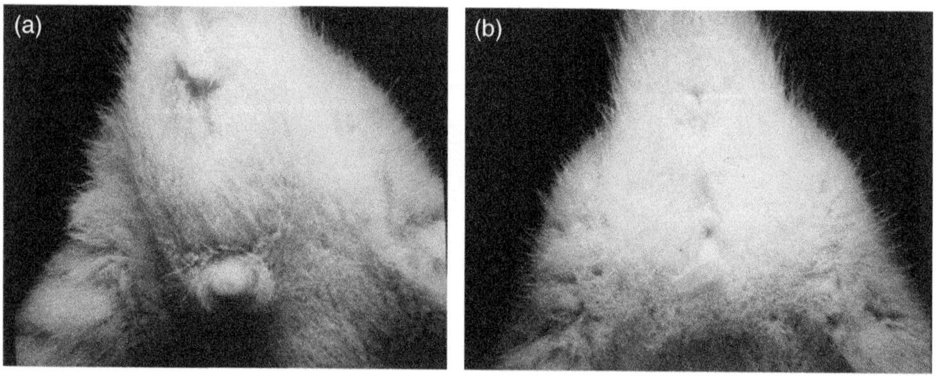

Fig 5.2. Anogenital distance in (a) male and (b) female rats. (*Source:* Photo courtesy of ACLAM.)

is closed by the vaginal plate composed of compact epithelium. This structure begins to degenerate at 3–5 weeks of age, and the vagina is completely open between 40 and 80 days. Rats, like mice, have extensive mammary tissue, ranging ventrally from the neck to the inguinal region and onto the sides and back. They have six pairs of mammary glands: three thoracic and three abdominal.

The hematologic and urinary profiles of rats have several distinctive characteristics. Lymphocytes comprise about 80% of the peripheral blood leukocyte population and basophils are rarely seen in circulation. Males generally have higher granulocyte and lymphocyte counts than do females. Rats have the ability to concentrate urine twice that of humans. While values differ between strains and stocks and across ages, rat urine normally has a pH of approximately 6.5–8.5 and a specific gravity in the range 1.015–1.070. Hematologic and biochemical parameters for the rat are listed in Appendix 1.

BREEDING AND REPRODUCTION

Both monogamous and polygamous breeding systems can be successfully used with rats. In a monogamous mating system, one male and one female are paired and the offspring are removed when they reach weaning age. A polygamous mating system typically entails cohousing one male and two or more females. Pregnant females are removed a few days prior to parturition to minimize cannibalism and abandonment of litters. Females are then returned to the breeding cage after their litters are weaned.

The age at puberty varies across sex, stock, and strain. In general, rats reach puberty between 2 and 3 months of age, and are normally not bred until about 3 months of age. Females are continuously polyestrous, spontaneous ovulators with an estrous cycle length of 4–5 days. Vaginal plugs, formed by coagulated seminal vesicle and coagulating gland secretions, may persist in the vagina for 12–24 hours after coitus and are useful to confirm mating. Outbred stocks regularly achieve conception rates greater than 85%, while a lower rate is common in inbred strains. Nonfertile matings and cervical stimulation can induce a pseudopregnancy of 12–14 days duration.

When compared with mice, pheromones appear to play a muted role in the reproductive behavior of rats. The Whitten effect (pheromone-mediated synchronization of estrus) and the Bruce effect (the spontaneous abortion or absorption of embryos by dams exposed to pheromones of novel males) do occur in rats but are less pronounced than in the mouse.

The usual gestation period of a rat is 21–23 days but may extend an additional 8–22 days in lactating rats due to a period of blastocyst dormancy and delayed implantation. Developing fetuses are most easily detected by manual palpation after 12 days of gestation. Abdominal enlargement and mammary development may be noted by approximately 13 and 14 days of gestation, respectively. Pregnant females should be isolated from disturbances for a few days before and after parturition as stress may induce dams to cannibalize their pups (Box 5.2). Dams do experience a fertile postpartum estrus, however they are not normally intentionally bred during this time due to potential complications with the young litter. Estrous cycles then resume 2–4 days postweaning.

Box 5.2

Pregnant females should be isolated from disturbances for a few days before and after parturition as stress may induce dams to cannibalize their pups.

Rat litter sizes average between 6 and 12 pups but varies with strain and age. Rat pups are altricial (hairless, blind, deaf, and completely dependent on the dam at birth). Developmental milestones include the following:

- 2.5–3.5 days—external ears open
- 6–8 days—incisors erupt
- 7–10 days—fully haired
- 14–17 days—eyes open
- Approximately 2 weeks—eat solid food

In a laboratory setting, most pups are weaned from their dams at 20–21 days of age.

HUSBANDRY

Housing and Environment

The *Guide for the Care and Use of Laboratory Animals* (the *Guide*; ILAR, 2011) provides recommended minimum cage sizes for rats based on animal body weights, with special consideration of the housing of females with litters. At a minimum, rat cages should be 7 inches (17.8 cm) in height. Rats are most commonly housed in microisolation cages composed of a durable plastic, solid-bottom shoebox-style cage; contact bedding; a wire bar feeder; and a plastic cagetop with integral filter. In special circumstances such as toxicology studies, stainless steel cages with wire-mesh bottoms may be used. However, wire-mesh flooring should be avoided whenever possible as rats prefer solid-flooring with bedding (Box 5.3). Also, larger animals housed on wire-mesh are at increased risk of developing foot lesions. See Chapter 3 for additional information regarding caging types and considerations.

A contact bedding material such as corncob particles, composite recycled paper pellets, or select hardwood chips should be placed in the bottom of solid shoebox-style cages. Cedar wood chips or shavings should not be used due to the adverse physiologic effects (e.g., increased tumor incidence, liver disease) induced by volatile compounds emitted from this type of wood.

Box 5.3

Wire-mesh flooring should be avoided whenever possible as rats prefer solid-flooring with bedding.

As recommended in the *Guide*, rat housing rooms should be maintained within a temperature range of 20°–26°C (68°–79°F) and a relative humidity range of 30% and 70%. Ten to fifteen air changes per hour are suggested to maintain adequate ventilation. This airflow exchange rate, however, is only a guideline. Determination of optimal ventilation should include careful consideration of the heat, humidity, and volatile compounds present in the housing room. Each is influenced by the number of animals present, bedding type, cage change frequency, and room size. The rate of air exchange between the cage and the room is a key factor in this consideration. For instance, a room air exchange rate below 10 ACH may be sufficient when all animals are housed in individually ventilated cages receiving 30–60 air changes per hour and air exhausted from cages is directed exclusively into the building heating, ventilation, and air conditioning (HVAC) system. Rats are nocturnal and must be provided with regular light–dark cycles for normal behavior and physiologic processes. Light–dark cycles providing 12 hours of light and 12 hours of darkness (12L:12D) and 14L:10D are common. If regular light cycles are not maintained, circadian rhythm will be disrupted, possibly resulting in inconsistent responses to experimental manipulation. The position of animals relative to light sources should be carefully selected to reduce potential experimental variability induced by differing light exposure levels. For instance, depending on the caging type, animals housed on the top row of cage racks may have significantly more light exposure than those housed nearer to the floor. In addition, albino strains of rats should be housed under reduced lighting intensity as they are prone to light-induced retinal damage.

Social Housing and Environmental Enrichment

Over its successive editions, the *Guide* has placed an increased emphasis on the use of social housing and the appropriate provision of environmental enrichment and to help meet the psychological and social needs of all species. The *Guide* states that social animals should be housed in physical contact with conspecifics when it is appropriate and compatible with the protocol. Rats are social animals and do best when housed in pairs or small, compatible groups (Box 5.4). The provision of enrichment items may benefit rats; objects should be nontoxic, nondigestible, sanitizable, and safe. The type of enrichment items most frequently provided to rats are those that the animal can manually manipulate or gnaw, such as tissues, shredded papers, or Nylabones. Additional items that provide increased cage complexity include elevated shelves to increase usable floor space (Figure 5.3), resting platforms, tunnels, and huts. Each is commercially available for laboratory animal use. Additional information regarding environmental enrichment can be found in Chapter 3.

> **Box 5.4**
>
> *Rats are social animals and do best when housed in pairs or small, compatible groups.*

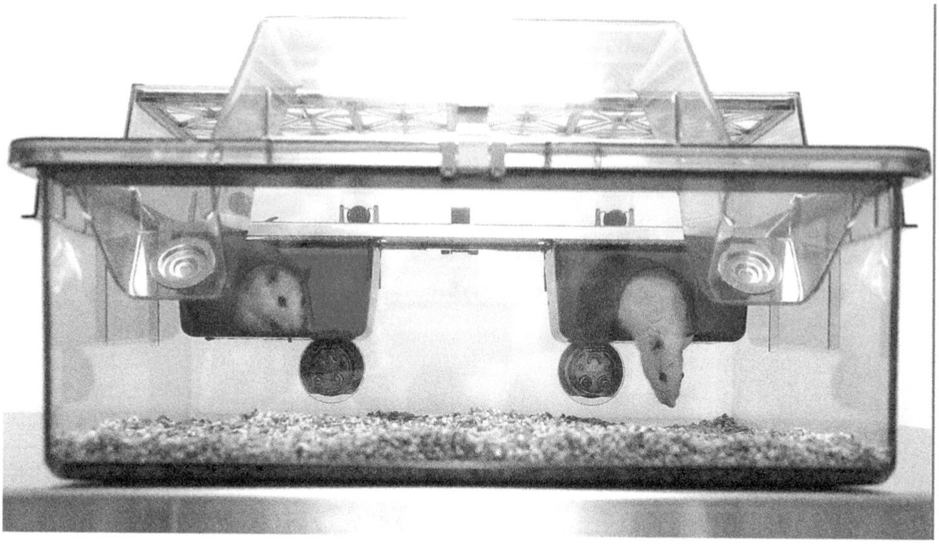

Fig 5.3. Red cage enrichment item that increases usable floor space. (*Source:* Photo courtesy of Allentown Inc.)

Feeding and Watering

Most rats grow and reproduce well when maintained on a standard commercial rodent diet containing at least 20%–25% protein and 4% fat. Rodent chow is usually provided in the form of firm, dry blocks or pellets. Rats eat an average of 5–6 g of chow per 100 g of body weight per day. They tend to become obese if fed *ad libitum* (free choice); restricted feeding is recommended for animals used in long-term studies. Restriction of caloric protein and fat, as well as feeding soy protein rather than casein (present in high levels in dairy products), extends the life span of some rat strains. Food pellets are provided within the cage either in a wire bar feeder or in a specially designed food hopper attached to one wall of the cage. Food should not be placed directly on the cage floor unless animals are debilitated or too young to otherwise reach the food. Supplemental feeding is not necessary or indicated for research animals except in a limited amount as an approved form of enrichment or prescribed supportive care. Like most other rodents, rats are coprophagic, consuming their own feces to conserve important nutrients. Adult rats drink an average of 10–12 mL of water per 100 g of body weight per day. Fresh, potable water should be made available *ad libitum*, from either an automated drinking water system, water bottles, or water pouches.

Sanitation

Caging should be cleaned as frequently as necessary to limit accumulated feces, moisture, and ammonia levels. The required frequency can vary (most commonly once or twice weekly for up to five group-housed rats in a static MI cage) and is heavily influenced by the number and size of rats, the type of caging (static versus ventilated), and study requirements (e.g., select surgical models, conditions inducing polyuria). As stated in the *Guide*, cages, water bottles, and feeders should be disinfected with chemicals, hot water

61.6°–82.2°C (143°–180°F), or a combination of both. Detergents and chemical disinfectants enhance the effectiveness of hot water, but they must be thoroughly rinsed from all caging surfaces with fresh water. Cage racks used with automated watering system manifolds (piping attached to cage racks) require special consideration. Before introducing the rack with attached manifolds into the cage washer, residual water should be removed. Manifolds should be routinely treated with pressurized flushing and chemicals or heat, as is compatible with the manifold materials, to reduce the accumulation of bioburden (biofilm) on the manifold interior. In addition, before racks are placed in a rack washer, brushes or chemical agents should be used to clean the rack's air plenums, the small ductwork mounted to the rack through which air is distributed to each cage. Additional information regarding sanitation is presented in Chapter 3.

TECHNIQUES

Handling and Restraint

If young rats are handled gently and frequently, they become quite docile (Box 5.5). Older rats that have not been handled often may be nervous or fractious. Transferring rats from one cage to another is easily accomplished by picking them up by the base of the tail. Rats should never be picked up by the middle or tip of the tail because the skin may be stripped off, creating a painful degloving injury. For routine handling, place a hand under the body and cradle the rat in the crook of the handler's elbow. By placing the opposite hand to cover or secure the animal's body, the rat's preference for physical contact is accommodated.

Rats can be restrained by a number of methods. One method includes placing the index and middle fingers behind each ear as shown in Figure 5.4. The ring finger and thumb encircle the thorax caudal to the front limbs, while a second hand supports the rat's body weight. Another method involves holding the rat with one hand by the base of the tail and placing the other hand firmly over the back and ribcage. The thumb and forefinger of this hand are then placed directly behind the rat's elbows to push the legs forward so that they cross under the chin. Care must be taken to avoid placing too much pressure on the thorax as doing so will impede respiration.

Docile rats can be safely handled while wearing only exam gloves. Properly trained personnel eliminate the need for protective gloves that are difficult to sanitize, often awkward to manipulate, and can make rats more fearful and difficult to handle. When administering compounds or with select other procedures, a hand towel can be wrapped around the body of the rat to facilitate restraint.

Alternatively, clear plastic restraint bags are commercially available and formed in the shape of a cone with an opening at the tapered end. They are especially helpful for individuals working alone with large or fractious rats. The bag is held open in one

Box 5.5

If young rats are handled gently and frequently, they become quite docile.

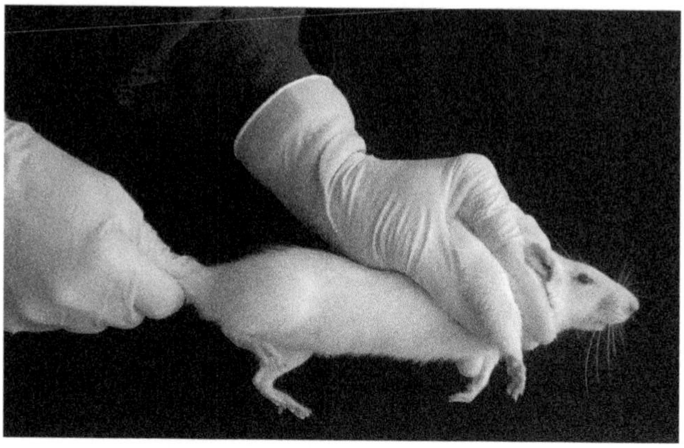

Fig 5.4. Rat manual restraint.

hand with the tapered end pointing down. The rat is picked up by the base of the tail and quickly lowered, head first, into the bag. As the animal enters the bag, the bag is quickly tilted upward to encourage the rat to advance toward the open end. The individual then rapidly gathers the rear of the bag until the animal's nose projects from the end and its body is fully restrained. Injections can be given directly through the bag. Animals should be restrained only for short periods in this manner because they can quickly overheat and may become stressed. Rigid plastic restrainers that have openings to permit injections, blood collection, and other manipulations are also commercially available.

Identification

Cage cards are most often used to identify groups of animals. There are several permanent methods to identify rats individually, including ear tagging; ear, tail, and toe tattooing; subcutaneous placement of a microchip for electronic identification; and ear punching. Dyes, permanent markers, or clipped fur can be used as temporary identification methods.

Blood Collection

Table 5.2 lists approximate adult rat blood volumes. Assuming the animal is mature, healthy, and on an adequate plane of nutrition, the blood volume of most terrestrial mammals averages approximately 7% of lean body weight in grams. A typical rule of

Table 5.2. Adult rat blood volumes and suggested sample size

	Volume (mL)
Total blood	20–40
Single sample	2–3
Exsanguination	8–12

Source: Adapted from Harkness et al. (2010).

Note: Values are approximate.

Box 5.6

In general, up to 10% of the circulating blood volume can be withdrawn from normal, healthy animals every 2–3 weeks with minimal adverse effect.

thumb for blood withdrawal suggests that up to 10% of the circulating blood volume (or 1% of the lean body weight) can be withdrawn from normal, healthy animals every 2–3 weeks with minimal adverse effect (Box 5.6).

The lateral tail veins are good sites for collecting small-to-moderate amounts of blood. A clear plastic rigid or flexible restrainer can be used to restrain the rat's body while allowing free access to the tail. Dipping the tail in warm water (40°C) for approximately 10 seconds allows vasodilation of the tail veins. An alarming thermometer should be used to ensure that the water temperature does not exceed 40°C because hotter temperatures can cause scalding. A 23-gauge butterfly needle with all but a short (~1″) section of tubing cut off can be used to enter the vein and allow the blood to drip into a collection tube. Hemostasis is achieved by applying direct pressure to the site. A needle and syringe can also be used to collect blood from the tail veins. Alternatively, capillary tube collection from the hub of a needle placed in the lateral tail veins is an effective method. Multiple successive blood samples can be taken by entering the same site or moving toward the tail base. The ventral tail artery can also be used to obtain a small amount of blood.

Up to approximately 1 mL of blood can be collected from the lateral saphenous vein (Figure 5.5). For this commonly used technique, the cranial portion of the conscious rat is restrained. Firm but gentle manual pressure is applied slightly proximal and lateral to the knee to extend the leg and dilate the vessel. Fur over the caudolateral

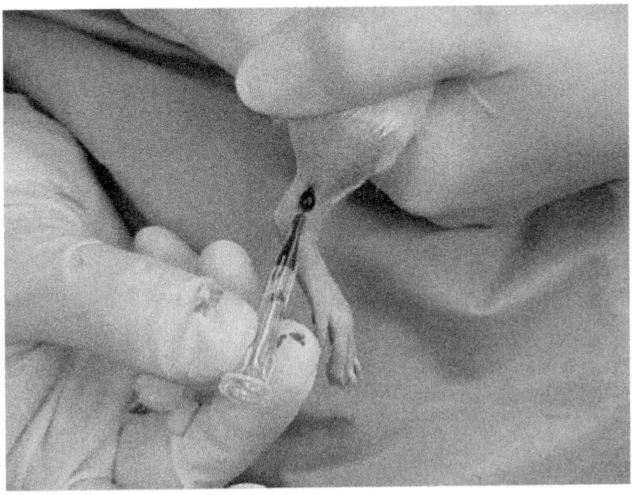

Fig 5.5. Blood collection from the saphenous vein. (*Source:* Photo courtesy of ULAM, University of Michigan.)

aspect of and slightly proximal to the hock joint is removed by shaving or with use of a depilatory agent. A sterile ointment is applied to the skin to prevent blood from dispersing over the skin surface and seeping into the adjacent fur. A 20-gauge needle is used to puncture the vessel and the blood is collected. Hemostasis is achieved by applying pressure to the collection site. Smaller volumes of blood can be similarly collected from the dorsal pedal vein.

Larger volumes of blood may be obtained from the jugular veins of a conscious or (preferably) anesthetized rat. Special restraining boards are available to restrain a rat in dorsal recumbency and expose the neck for jugular access. In a conscious rat, two people are required for collection: one to restrain the rat and turn its head to the side and the second to collect the sample. The cranial vena cava can also be used to collect larger samples from an anesthetized rat. In this technique, the needle is directed through the thoracic inlet on the right side of the neck and slowly advanced caudally and medially toward the rat's opposite elbow. Slight negative pressure is maintained on the syringe so that when a flash of blood is seen in the needle hub, advancement ceases and the sample is collected. These procedures must be performed with a steady hand because unintended movement of the needle may lacerate the vessels or thoracic tissues and be fatal.

The retro-orbital plexus is a site from which moderate amounts of blood can be collected in rats, although less invasive alternatives are available and may be preferred. This procedure requires anesthesia and the use of a microhematocrit tube to penetrate the venous plexus behind the eye. Individuals must be familiar with the anatomy of the retro-orbital plexus and receive training prior to attempting this blood collection technique. Following anesthetic induction, an ophthalmic anesthetic (e.g., proparacaine) can be applied. Sterile ophthalmic ointment should then be used if the selected anesthetic will decrease the blink reflex for more than a brief period. With the rat in lateral recumbency, the forefinger and thumb of one hand are used to place pressure on the top and bottom lids of one eye to keep the eye open and slightly proptosed. Alternatively, the rat may be held by the scruff with the length of the body partially resting on the handler's forearm. The other hand is used to place the tip of a glass microcapillary tube just dorsal to the medial canthus at approximately a 30°–45° angle toward the back of the eye. Using firm, steady forward pressure, the tube is rotated between the thumb and the forefinger allowing the tube to act as a cutting instrument through the conjunctiva at the back of the eye and entering the retro-orbital sinus. If bone is felt, slight withdrawing of the tube should result in the flow of blood into the tube by capillary action. A steady hand is required because additional movement of the tube tip can cause severe damage to the eye and the optic nerve, a clearly painful outcome. After collecting the blood sample, withdraw the tube, close the eyelids, and place slight pressure with a gauze square to promote hemostasis. The eye will not be affected when proper technique is used as the capillary tube passes along the side and back of the globe. If rats show signs of ocular damage or pain, they should be promptly euthanized or provided analgesia with treatment for the injury. The retro-orbital blood collection method should be avoided when possible, and especially when collection of multiple samples is required.

Surgically placed jugular vein, femoral vein, or carotid artery catheters may be used for studies that require multiple blood collections. Catheterization is a refined blood collection method as it avoids the stress and discomfort caused by multiple periods of restraint and needle penetrations although it is both costly and time consuming.

Automated technology advancements continue to produce options that can be of great benefit to both personnel and animals in the research setting. Commercial, automated blood samplers are now available and offer several advantages over standard dosing and blood collection methods. Surgically catheterized rats are placed into a jacket that allows the catheter(s) to exit through a swivel port, and permits free movement of the rats inside their cages while remaining connected to the computerized unit. Using a series of peristaltic pumps, a computer program simultaneously schedules and controls dosing and blood sample collection for multiple rats. In addition, volumes withdrawn can be automatically replaced with fluids to help maintain physiologic stability. This technology not only reduces handling stress, but also makes research more efficient because it reduces personnel required for both dosing and blood collection. It should be noted, however, that catheters must be handled with strict aseptic technique, regularly flushed, filled with a catheter locking solution when not actively used, and inspected to maintain their patency throughout their anticipated functional time period (commonly 1–5 weeks).

Cardiac puncture can be performed on anesthetized rats for a terminal blood collection. The heart is approached from the abdomen just left of the xiphoid process with the needle directed at an approximately 30°–35° angle from the thoracic midline. Alternatively, cardiac puncture can be performed by passing a needle through the lateral thoracic wall, just caudal to the rat's elbow. A terminal sample can also be collected from the blood that pools after laceration of the axillary vessels.

Urine Collection

Specially designed metabolism cages facilitate collection of urine and feces over an extended period (hours to weeks). These cages are designed with feed and water containers positioned to prevent contamination of the urine and feces separating units located below the cage floor. Alternatively, the natural tendency of rodents to urinate and defecate when handled can provide a small sample to be collected from the table.

Drug Administration

Medications are routinely added to the water or feed for ease of administration to large groups. However, it is important to note that this method relies on each animal consuming its expected quantity of food or water each day, which may not occur if it is unpalatable or unfamiliar to the animal, or if the animal's appetite is decreased. A gavage needle can be used for dosing individuals with liquid medication. Gavage needles, available in both metal and flexible plastic, have large blunted ends (balls) on their tips to help minimize the risk of esophageal perforation or accidental entry into the trachea. Maximum dosing volumes for multiple routes of administration are listed in Table 5.3.

Smaller gauge needles, such as 23- or 25-gauge needles, should be used for injections. Subcutaneous (SC) injections can be given in the loose skin over the back. Rats have such a small muscle mass that intramuscular (IM) injections should be used only when absolutely necessary (Box 5.7). Irritation of the sciatic nerve from a misplaced injection or from certain drugs, such as ketamine, will often lead to self-mutilation of

Table 5.3. Maximum dosing volumes in rats

Route	Amount (mL/100 g)
IP	2.0
SC	2.0
IM	0.1–0.3/site
IV	0.5
PO	2.0 (5 mL max)

Source: Adapted from Harkness and Wagner (1995) and Lukas (1999).

Box 5.7

Rats have such a small muscle mass that intramuscular injections should be used only when absolutely necessary.

the limb. Intraperitoneal (IP) injections are preferred over IM injections and should be placed in a rat's lower right abdominal quadrant, just off the midline. This location is recommended to help decrease the likelihood of penetrating the liver, bladder, or cecum. Before injection, the syringe should be aspirated to ensure that the needle has not entered the bladder or intestines of the mouse. Video tutorials for rat injection techniques are available at www.procedureswithcare.org.uk.

Although continuous or repeated intravenous (IV) administration of drugs can be challenging, it is often accomplished for research purposes by surgical placement of a vascular access port or an indwelling catheter in the jugular or femoral veins. The free end of the catheter is tunneled through subcutaneous tissues and exteriorized in the dorsal cervical or interscapular region. Alternatively, the tail vein can be used for intravenous administration in rats. Mini-osmotic pumps are designed to deliver a constant infusion of drugs via the SC, IP, or IV route. Their function is based on differences in osmotic pressure between the compartment within the pump and the tissue space in which the pump is implanted. The pumps are aseptically prepared with the drug of choice and then surgically implanted. Drug delivery rates and durations can be selected from a wide range, for example 0.11–10.0 μL/h and 1 day to 6 weeks, respectively. Pumps can be surgically accessed, refilled, and reimplanted in an individual animal. Use of mini-osmotic pumps is considered a refinement in dosing because it avoids the stress of daily handling; however, it does require surgical intervention.

Anesthesia, Analgesia, Surgery, and Postoperative Care

Agents commonly used for anesthesia and tranquilization of rats and recommended dosages are listed in Table 5.4. Preanesthetic fasting is not recommended in rodents unless an empty stomach is inherent to the success of the procedure. Injectable anesthetic regimens are used mainly for shorter procedures when administration of inhalant anesthesia is difficult due to equipment availability or its use is not compatible with research needs. A combination of ketamine and xylazine is frequently used to induce a

Table 5.4. Anesthetic agents and tranquilizers used in rats

Drug	Dosage	Route	Reference
Inhalants			
Carbon dioxide	50%–80% CO_2 mixed with 20%–50% O_2	inhalation	Fenwick and Blackshaw (1989)
Isoflurane	1.5%–3%	inhalation	Flecknell (2016)
Sevoflurane	3.5%–4%	inhalation	Flecknell (2016)
Injectables			
Diazepam	2.5–5 mg/kg	IP, IM	Flecknell (2016)
Fentanyl	0.3 mg/kg	IP	Flecknell (2016)
+ medetomidine	0.3 mg/kg	IP	
Ketamine	75 mg/kg	IP	Flecknell (2016)
+ acepromazine	2.5 mg/kg	IP	
Ketamine	75 mg/kg	IP	Wellington et al. (2013)
+ dexmedetomidine	1 mg/kg	IP	
Ketamine	40–80 mg/kg	IP	Wixson et al. (1987)
+ diazepam	5–10 mg/kg	IP	
Ketamine	75 mg/kg	IP	Flecknell (2016)
+ medetomidine	0.5 mg/kg	IP	
Ketamine	75 mg/kg	SC	Harkness et al. (2010)
+ medetomidine	0.5 mg/kg	SC	
Ketamine	75 mg/kg	IP	Flecknell (2016)
+ midazolam	5 mg/kg	IP	
Ketamine	40–80 mg/kg	IP	Wixson et al. (1987)
+ xylazine	5–10 mg/kg	IP	
Midazolam	2.5–5 mg/kg	IM, IP	Flecknell (2016)
Pentobarbital	30–40 mg/kg	IP	Wixson et al. (1987)
Propofol	10 mg/kg	IV	Flecknell (2016)
Tiletamine-zolazepam	40 mg/kg	IP	Flecknell (2016)
Tiletamine-zolazepam	20–40 mg/kg	IP	Wilson et al. (1992)
+ butorphanol	1.25–5 mg/kg	IP	
Tiletamine-zolazepam	20–40 mg/kg	IP	Wilson et al. (1992)
+ xylazine	5–10 mg/kg	IP	

IM = intramuscular; IP = intraperitoneal; and IV = intravenous; SC = subcutaneous.

surgical plane of anesthesia to facilitate relatively short-term procedures (e.g., less than 45 minutes). The appropriate dose of this combination may vary between ages and strains of rats. Once mixed, the drug combination will degrade over time and may lose its sterility; therefore, institutions routinely recommend that a new mixture be made at a predetermined interval (e.g., daily or weekly). The acid pH of ketamine has been associated with muscle damage and nerve irritation and should be given preferentially by the intraperitoneal route. A bland ophthalmic ointment should be placed in each eye of the animal to prevent corneal drying during the anesthetic period as the blinking reflex is reduced or absent. Pentobarbital was once the most frequently used injectable anesthetic, but it has been found to have a narrow safety margin and significant depressant effects on the cardiovascular systems causing hypothermia and prolonged anesthetic recovery times. Occasionally, it is still used when the newly obtained experimental results must be compared with historical results.

Inhalant anesthetics are safe and convenient for the induction and maintenance of brief periods of anesthesia in rats. With the use of appropriate anesthetic and monitoring equipment, inhalation anesthesia can be maintained successfully for prolonged periods (i.e., hours). Intubation and positive pressure ventilation systems are available for use in rats and other small rodents. Of the inhalant anesthetic agents, isoflurane and sevoflurane are preferable and must be used with a precision vaporizer. Volatile anesthetics should always be used with appropriate waste gas scavenging systems or in a fume hood.

Common surgical procedures of rats include castrations and mammary tumor excisions. To prevent intestinal entrapment, care should be taken to close the open inguinal canals during castration. Mammary tumors are usually well encapsulated and easy to remove; however, they frequently reoccur. Other surgical procedures commonly performed on research rats including hypophysectomy, adrenalectomy, thymectomy, and jugular and femoral vein or carotid artery catheterization.

Surgeries should be performed in an aseptic manner. Although a misconception may exist that rodents are inherently resistant to surgical infections, studies have shown that rats do develop significant physiological abnormalities when poor aseptic technique is employed. Care should be taken to avoid hypothermia, blood loss, and dehydration, which can lead to slow anesthetic recoveries and death (Box 5.8).

Postanesthetic recovery includes, at a minimum, placing the animal on a clean paper towel or dry cloth as an interface between the rat and small-particle bedding which might otherwise be aspirated. A circulating-water heating blanket, self-regulating heating pad, or other method of providing heat should be used to promote euthermia. Use of drugstore-quality heating blankets must be avoided as they can cause thermal burns. Subcutaneous administration of warmed saline or lactated Ringer's solution (up to 2 mL/100 g) following a prolonged anesthetic period or surgical procedure helps to prevent hypothermia and dehydration and assists with recovery. To prevent hypostatic lung congestion, the rat should be turned approximately every 30 minutes until it is ambulatory. To avoid cannibalism, an anesthetized rat should not be placed back in a cage with conscious cagemates until it is fully ambulatory. Provision of moistened chow or critical care supplements can assist in the recovery phase.

Analgesics should be provided to rats as a standard of care for alleviating pain associated with surgical or other painful procedures. If a procedure is known to cause pain in humans, it must be assumed to also cause pain in rats unless proven otherwise (Box 5.9). Scientific justification must be provided and approved by the IACUC if

Box 5.8

Hypothermia, blood loss, and dehydration can lead to slow anesthetic recoveries and death.

Box 5.9

If a procedure is known to cause pain in humans, it must be assumed to also cause pain in rats unless proven otherwise.

there is a need to withhold analgesics for research animals. Research rodents present some unique challenges for pain control, including the need to dose many rodents at a time and determining the potential confounding effects of analgesic administration on research results. Detection of pain in rats can be extremely challenging and requires careful observation of their movement, behavior, and physiologic functions.

Animal care and research staff have an ethical responsibility to continue to look for better ways to reduce pain and distress in their research subjects. Pain assessment scales have been developed based on visual observation of animals' facial expressions. These scales are referred to as "grimace scales." Each scale is unique to one species and has been validated for use with specifically defined pain conditions (e.g., acute inflammation-induced pain). Use of the scales can be labor- and time-intensive. However, automation is being employed to facilitate their use. Liposome-encapsulated opioids have been developed to provide a slow-release, long-acting analgesic for moderate-to-severe pain in rats; their efficacy is still being assessed. The use of such drugs could provide consistent and reliable pain relief without the need for frequent and repeated animal handling and injection. Also, significant efforts had been devoted to incorporating analgesics in drinking water or food items (e.g., flavored gelatin) that a rat would freely consume. However, these methods have not been successful for multiple reasons, including an instinctual avoidance of novel food items (neophobia), poor palatability, and limited consumption of drug-supplemented food or water.

The provision of analgesics prior to pain induction (preemptive analgesia) affords better pain control than administration after the painful procedure and may decrease required anesthetic dosages. Buprenorphine is commonly used both for mild postoperative discomfort and to control acute or chronic visceral pain. When administered at high doses (0.05–0.3 mg/kg), buprenorphine may induce pica (consumption of non-food items such as fur or bedding). A sustained-release formulation of buprenorphine (Buprenorphine SR-LAB) has been developed, but currently is not commercially available in all states. Both carprofen and meloxicam are good choices for mild-to-moderate musculoskeletal and visceral pain and have longer duration of action (24 hours) than opioids without sustained-release formulation. Meloxicam comes in an injectable and oral liquid form that is very palatable. Multimodal analgesia, administration of two or more drugs that act by different mechanisms, may provide a superior level of analgesia than can be achieved by administration of a single drug class. For example nonsteroidal anti-inflammatory agents, such as carprofen and meloxicam, used in combination with opioids may provide better analgesia than either could provide independently. Table 5.5 lists several analgesics commonly administered to rats.

Table 5.5. Analgesic agents used in rats

Drug	Dosage	Route	Reference
Buprenorphine	0.01–0.05 mg/kg q8-12h	SC, IV	Flecknell (2016)
Buprenorphine sustained release	1–1.2 mg/kg (one 72-h injection)	SC	Foley et al. (2011)
Butorphanol	1–2 mg/kg q4h	SC	Flecknell (2016)
Carprofen	5 mg/kg	SC	Flecknell (2016)
Flunixin meglumine	2.5 mg/kg q12-24h	SC	Heard (1993)
Ketoprofen	5 mg/kg	SC	Flecknell (2016)
Meloxicam	1 mg/kg q24h	PO, SC	Harkness et al. (2010)
Morphine	2.5 mg/kg q2-4h	SC	Flecknell (2016)
Oxymorphone	0.2–0.5 mg/kg q6-12h	SC	Harkness et al. (2010)
Tramadol	5 mg/kg	SC, IP	Flecknell (2016)

IP = intraperitoneal; IV = intravenous; PO = per os; and SC = subcutaneous.

Imaging Techniques

Many imaging modalities once used only in humans [e.g., digital x-ray imaging, magnetic resonance imaging (MRI), computed tomography (CT), positron emission tomography (PET), dual-energy x-ray absorptiometry (DEXA) scan, and ultrasound] have been adapted for use with laboratory animal species. See Chapter 3 for more detailed information regarding imaging in laboratory animals.

Euthanasia

The term euthanasia literally translates as "good" (*eu*) and "death" (*thanatos*). Euthanasia should provide a rapid death with little to no pain or distress. Individuals must be appropriately trained to use the various methods of euthanasia to minimize the chances of pain or distress if performed inappropriately. Methods must be consistent with the most current American Veterinary Medical Association (AVMA) *Guidelines for the Euthanasia of Animals* (AVMA, 2013), performed by trained personnel, detailed in the research protocol, and approved by the IACUC. Per AVMA Guidelines, "Carbon dioxide is acceptable with conditions for euthanasia in those species where aversion or distress can be minimized. Carbon dioxide exposure using a gradual fill method is less likely to cause pain due to nociceptor activation by carbonic acid prior to onset of unconsciousness; a displacement rate from 10% to 30% of the chamber volume/min is recommended.... CO_2 flow should be maintained for at least 1 minute after respiratory arrest." Conscious animals should never be placed in an area prefilled with 100% CO_2 as this can cause pain of the mucous membranes. Furthermore, only a pure form of CO_2 must be used, such as from a commercially supplied cylinder.

The euthanasia of rat fetuses and neonates requires special consideration. Neonates are resistant to hypoxia and require greater duration of exposure; for this reason, other methods may be preferred for this age group. Fetal rats (unborn

Table 5.6. Antimicrobial agents used in rats

Drug	Dosage	Route	Reference
Amikacin	10 mg/kg q12h	SC	Morrisey and Carpenter (2004)
Ampicillin	20–50 mg/kg q12h	PO, SC	Morrisey and Carpenter (2004)
Cephalexin	15 mg/kg q12h	SC	Flecknell (2016)
Doxycycline	5 mg/kg q12h	PO	Harkness et al. (2010)
Enrofloxacin	0.05–0.2 mg/mL drinking water for 14 d		Harkness et al. (2010)
	5–10 mg/kg q12h	PO, SC	Harkness et al. (2010)
Erythromycin	20 mg/kg q12h	PO	Morrisey and Carpenter (2004)
Gentamicin	5–10 mg/kg divided q8-12h	SC	Morrisey and Carpenter (2004)
Metronidazole	10–40 mg/kg q24h	PO	Burgmann and Percy (1993)
Pencillin G	22,000 IU/kg q24h	SC	Morrisey and Carpenter (2004)
Trimethoprim-sulfa	15–30 mg/kg q12h	PO, SC	Morrisey and Carpenter (2004)

PO = per os; and SC = subcutaneous.

animals who have not breathed) under 15 days of gestation may be euthanized by allowing them to remain in utero following routine euthanasia of the dam. Alternatively, euthanasia can be induced by removal of the fetus from the uterus. However, fetuses removed from the uterus and allowed to breathe air must be promptly euthanized by a physical method of euthanasia (e.g., cervical dislocation or decapitation). Neonatal rats under 10 days of age may show marked resistance to CO_2. Carbon dioxide euthanasia may still be used with these animals although prolonged exposure time may be required. Alternate methods of euthanasia of neonatal rats include injection of anesthetics, decapitation, or cervical dislocation. Death must always be verified prior to carcass disposal.

Other acceptable methods of euthanasia include overdose of an inhalant anesthetic and IP administration of a barbiturate anesthetic at three to four times the anesthetic dose.

Many other euthanasia methods are acceptable when performed only on a fully anesthetized animal, including exsanguination and the use of potassium chloride (KCl) administered intravenously to induce cardiac arrest. Occasionally, it is necessary to euthanize animals without the use of anesthetics or tranquilizers (e.g., decapitation with a guillotine) that have been documented to complicate research results. Investigators must fully justify the need for using such a euthanasia method and the method must be approved by the IACUC.

THERAPEUTIC AGENTS

Suggested rat antimicrobial drug dosages are listed in Table 5.6. Antiparasitic agents are listed in Table 5.7, and miscellaneous drugs are listed in Table 5.8.

Table 5.7. Antiparasitic agents used in rats

Drug	Dosage	Route	Reference
Fenbendazole	20 mg/kg q24h for 5 d	PO	Allen et al. (1993)
	150 mg/kg of feed; provide for 7 d on, 7 d off for 3 treatments		Boivin et al. (1996)
Fipronil	7.5 mg/kg q30–60 d	Topical	Morrisey and Carpenter (2004)
Ivermectin	0.2–0.4 mg/kg every 7–10 d for 3 treatments	PO, SC	Harkness et al. (2010)
	25 mg/L drinking water for 4d on, 3d off for 5wk		Klement et al. (1996)
Mebendazole	40 mg/kg q7d for 21 d	PO	Adamcak (2000)
Metronidazole	10–40 mg/animal	PO	Morrisey and Carpenter (2004)
	2.5 mg/mL drinking water for 5 d		Adamcak (2000)
Moxidectin	0.2 mg/kg for 4 d	PO	Oge et al. (2000)
Piperazine citrate	2–5 mg/mL drinking water for 7 d, off 7 d, repeat		Anderson (1994)
Praziquantel	6–10 mg/kg	PO	Harkness et al. (2010)

PO = per os and SC = subcutaneous.

chapter 5

INTRODUCTION TO DISEASES OF RATS

Most contemporary laboratory rodent colonies in the United States are relatively free of bacteria, viruses, parasites, and fungi that cause clinical disease. However, sporadic outbreaks of disease still occur, in part due to the transfer of rodents between institutions, both within the United States and internationally. Laboratory personnel who own pet rodents may serve as a possible source of contamination to research animals although the associated degree of risk has not been fully quantified. Gaertner (2004) postulated three reasons infectious agents continue to occur in otherwise clean facilities: some agents are extremely contagious (mouse hepatitis virus, MHV), some are highly resistant to environmental inactivation (parvoviruses), and some are difficult to diagnose or eradicate (pinworms). Basic knowledge of the variety of infectious agents that may infect rats ensures a quick and appropriate response to a disease outbreak if it does occur. Presented here is a general overview of common bacterial, viral, parasitic, and fungal pathogens of rats as well as some general diagnostic and treatment modalities. Readers who are faced with managing a disease outbreak are encouraged to review the current scientific literature for the most up-to-date information.

Bacterial Diseases

Pneumonia and Respiratory Diseases

Mycoplasma pulmonis is a Gram-negative bacterium that is uncommon in barrier-maintained laboratory rats but remains an important pathogen for conventional

Table 5.8. Miscellaneous agents used in rats

Drug	Dosage	Route	Reference
Atipamezole	0.1–1 mg/kg	SC, IM, IP, IV	Flecknell (2016)
Atropine	0.05–0.1 mg/kg	SC	Harkness and Wagner (1995)
Cimetidine	5–10 mg/kg q6-12h	PO	Allen et al. (1993)
Dexamethasone	0.5–2 mg/kg then decreasing dose q12h for 3–14 d	PO, SC	Harkness and Wagner (1995)
Diphenhydramine	1–2 mg/kg q12h	PO, SC	Morrisey and Carpenter (2004)
Doxapram	5–10 mg/kg	IP, IV	Morrisey and Carpenter (2011)
Furosemide	2–10 mg/kg q12h	SC, PO	Morrisey and Carpenter (2004)
Glycopyrrolate	0.01–0.02 mg/kg	SC	Huerkamp (1995)
	0.5 mg/kg	IM	Flecknell (2016)
Naloxone	0.01–0.1 mg/kg	SC, IP	Huerkamp (1995)
Oxytocin	0.2–3 IU/kg	SC, IV	Anderson (1994)
Prednisone	0.5–2.2 mg/kg	SC, PO	Anderson (1994)
Sucralfate	25–50 mg/kg	PO	Morrisey and Carpenter (2004)
Vitamin B complex	0.02–0.2 mL/kg	SC	Anderson (1994)
Yohimbine	0.5–1 mg/kg	IV	Harkness and Wagner (1995)

IM = intramuscular; IP = intraperitoneal; IV = intravenous; PO = per os; and SC = subcutaneous.

colonies and pet rats. Susceptibility to infection varies across strains and stocks. It can induce a chronic respiratory disease syndrome called murine respiratory mycoplasmosis (MRM) or chronic respiratory disease, and has also been associated with infections of the genital tract. Although *M. pulmonis* is the etiologic agent of MRM, other viruses (e.g., Sendai, sialodacryoadenitis) and bacteria [e.g., cilia-associated respiratory (CAR) bacillus, *Streptococcus pneumoniae*, *Bordetella bronchiseptica*] are often recovered from the lungs of infected animals.

Mycoplasma pulmonis can be transmitted by direct contact between an infected dam and her offspring, by intrauterine or sexual transfer, and by aerosol. The organism has an affinity for the epithelial cells of the respiratory tract, middle ear, and endometrium. The disease is usually subclinical, especially in young animals, and slowly progressive, with clinical signs becoming evident only when an advanced stage of disease is reached. Factors such as high ammonia levels, other respiratory pathogens, and various forms of stress have a profound effect on the clinical course and severity of the disease.

A serous or catarrhal nasal and ocular discharge may occur, but the sound of snuffling is usually more obvious than other early clinical signs. Animals with extensive pulmonary involvement may exhibit labored breathing, weight loss, lethargy, a hunched posture, and a rough hair coat. Sudden deaths are usually the result of secondary bacterial infections. Unilateral or bilateral otitis interna, characterized by the presence of a head tilt, is part of the chronic respiratory disease syndrome. The infection frequently extends up the eustachian tube into the middle ear and then to the inner ear, causing a labyrinthitis. When rats with labyrinthitis are held by the tail in a vertical position, they typically spin, rotating their bodies rapidly.

In the earliest stage, pulmonary lesions are limited to peribronchiolar lymphoid hyperplasia, visible only on microscopic examination of the lung. As the disease progresses, well-demarcated foci of firm, red–gray consolidation appear. Accumulation of inflammatory debris and mucus may result in bronchial distention, which can give the surface of the lung a "cobblestone" appearance. Genital disease may be characterized by purulent endometritis, salpingitis, and perioophoritis. Additionally, pregnant rats infected with *M. pulmonis* have had a variety of adverse outcomes, including low birth weight, small litter size, stillbirths, and fetal resorption.

Diagnosis is based on history, clinical findings, gross and microscopic lesions, and isolation of *M. pulmonis* from the nasopharynx, tympanic bullae, trachea, or lungs. A serum enzyme-linked immunosorbent assay (ELISA) is the most rapid tool for screening colonies for the presence of *M. pulmonis* infection although additional tests are often required to differentiate *M. pulmonis* from the nonpathogenic *M. arthritidis*. A polymerase chain reaction (PCR) test offers a rapid way to screen cell lines, biological agents, and tissues of animals; for initial diagnostic testing of individual animals; and for confirmatory testing following serologic screening.

Bacterial culture and sensitivity testing are necessary to determine the most appropriate choice of antibiotics. Antimicrobials added to the drinking water for periods of a week or more will suppress *M. pulmonis* infection but will not eliminate the disease. Parenteral antibiotic administration may rarely be effective for treatment of individual animals; rather treatment may only prolong survival until an acceptable experimental endpoint can be reached. Elimination of this disease requires cesarean rederivation of breeding stock and maintenance of animals under a barrier system. Areas of research most affected by MRM include respiratory, reproductive, and immune system studies.

Evidence exists for *M. pulmonis* infection in pet owners and individuals in contact with laboratory rats (Piasecki et al., 2017). The clinical significance of human infection has not yet been determined.

Streptococcus pneumoniae, once a common cause of respiratory disease in young rats, is rarely found in contemporary research facilities. Infected rats harbor the organism in the upper respiratory tract, often without clinical signs. Aerosol transmission is most common, although transmission via contaminated fomites may be possible. Disease outbreaks can occur following stress. The disease tends to be acute to subacute and primarily affects younger animals. Affected animals exhibit depression, a serosanguinous to mucopurulent nasal discharge, a snuffling respiratory sound, dyspnea, ocular discharge, and ruffled fur. Gross lesions often found at necropsy include seropurulent and fibrinopurulent pleuritis, pericarditis, epicarditis, peritonitis, meningitis, otitis media and interna, metritis, and bronchopneumonia. Fibrinopurulent peritonitis and pleuritis are common with minimal involvement of lung parenchyma. Antibiotic treatment of individual animals can be effective, but depopulation of infected colonies is recommended.

Naturally occurring infections of CAR bacillus have been reported in rats, mice, rabbits, cattle, swine, and other species. The organism is a Gram-negative bacterium, although its taxonomic classification is controversial. In most species, it appears to be an opportunistic invader of the respiratory tract. Infection in rats is usually asymptomatic or induces nonspecific signs of illness and is lifelong. Transmission is predominantly by direct contact; animal colony surveillance by sentinels exposed to soiled bedding is not effective. On histology, CAR bacillus is found between and parallel to the cilia of the respiratory epithelium. Silver stains can be used to visualize the organism in respiratory tract scrapings or lung sections of infected animals. An ELISA test can be used to quickly screen colonies. PCR can also be used to confirm the presence of CAR bacillus in a colony. No effective treatment has been described, and elimination or rederivation may be necessary to rid a colony of the organism.

Pasteurella pneumotropica is a Gram-negative coccobacillus that is generally latent in rats, but is considered an opportunistic pathogen secondary to other agents such as Sendai virus and *M. pulmonis*. It is most often associated with the nasopharynx, cecum, vagina, uterus, and conjunctiva. Transmission is by direct contact. Most animals are asymptomatic, although clinical infections of the conjunctiva, endometrium, or mammary gland have rarely been reported. Selective antibiotic administration may be beneficial in controlling clinical manifestations of infection but will not eliminate the carrier state. Cesarean rederivation or embryo transfer can eliminate the organism from infected colonies.

Tyzzer's Disease

Clostridium piliforme is the causative agent of Tyzzer's disease. Infected adults are usually subclinically affected while overt disease is most likely to occur in weanlings. Transmission is by fecal–oral spread of spores, which are highly resistant in the environment and to some disinfectants. Disease occasionally manifests as an acute epizootic when stressors such as poor environmental conditions or concurrent infections lead to immunosuppression. Clinical signs may include diarrhea, dehydration, and anorexia. Animals may be found dead in the absence of obvious signs of illness. Gross lesions include miliary, pale foci throughout the liver, abdominal distention, megaloileitis (distended and hyperemic ileum), and hemorrhagic and ulcerated areas of the lower intestinal tract. The heart may also be affected with pale circumscribed areas or streaks. A definitive diagnosis may be difficult to establish and requires identification of the filamentous bacilli in affected tissues with silver, Giemsa, or methylene blue stain. Due to the organism's complexity, serology screens may yield false-positive results and require further investigations with alternate diagnostic methods. PCR of feces or tissue sections may be useful in detecting active infections. Infected colonies should be depopulated and rederived following effective disinfection of the environment to ensure that spores do not persist.

Helicobacter spp.

Multiple species of Gram-negative *Helicobacter* have been identified in rats including *H. muridarum, H. trogontum, H. bilis,* and *H. pullorum*. Fecal–oral transmission is suspected and animals remain persistently infected throughout life. It is uncertain if infection induces any clinical disease in immunocompetent rats. PCR is the optimal diagnostic method. Antibiotic treatment of individual animals might be effective, however colony rederivation is more reliable.

Staphylococcus

Staphylococcus aureus, a common environmental contaminant of human origin, may induce a variety of lesions in rats, including ulcerative dermatitis and pododermatitis. In immunocompetent animals, clinical infections require an inciting injury or event (e.g., skin or foot trauma). Trimming the toenails of rats affected with ulcerative dermatitis can help to reduce the self-trauma associated with scratching. Good sanitation procedures and, in some cases, parenteral antibiotics should be used to treat staphylococcal infections. Treatment with topical antibiotics is often impractical, as rats will frequently lick the medication from their skin.

Miscellaneous Bacterial Infections

Corynebacterium kutscheri, a Gram-positive rod, usually exists as a latent or subclinical infection but can persist and cause disease in older animals. The organism may be cultured from the submandibular lymph nodes, oropharynx, nasopharynx, middle ears, and preputial glands. Stressful situations often elicit a subacute respiratory disease with abscesses in the lungs. Abscesses may also be found in the liver, kidney, skin, and joints. In chronic cases, abscesses frequently contain caseous material, hence the term commonly used for this infection, pseudotuberculosis. Transmission appears to be by direct contact. Diagnosis is by culture or PCR detection of the organism (preferably from the submandibular lymph nodes) or through serology screens. Positive ELISA tests should always be confirmed by PCR or culture.

Pseudomonas aeruginosa, a Gram-negative bacillus, is usually not pathogenic in immunologically competent animals as it is a common commensal organism of rodents. Animals may, however, become septicemic following experimental manipulations that compromise their immune function, such as radiation exposure. Strict control of the animals' microbial environment is required to exclude the organism from colonies. Sterilization of all cage components, and possibly use of isolator housing, is necessary. Rederivation is required to eliminate the organism from infected colonies.

Salmonella spp. infections are uncommon in contemporary research animal facilities. With the possibility of introduction by wild rodents or infected feed or water, it should remain on the differential list for diseases of unknown etiology. Infections may exist in a subclinical form, elicit nonspecific clinical signs such as lethargy or weight loss, or cause acute disease with a high mortality; diarrhea is uncommon. Diagnosis is by culture or PCR of feces, blood, mesenteric lymph nodes, liver, or spleen. Salmonellosis is a concern because of its zoonotic disease potential and ready interspecies transmission. Rats can be asymptomatic carriers and shed the organism in the feces for many months. As a result, treatment of infected animals is not recommended. Rather, infected colonies should be depopulated and rederived.

Another zoonotic agent of concern is the Gram-negative pleomorphic bacterium, *Streptobacillus moniliformis*, an etiologic agent of rat-bite fever. The organism has been effectively eliminated from contemporary animal research facilities, but is still occasionally found in both wild and pet rats. Infected rats remain asymptomatic throughout infection. Fatal infections have been described in humans; clinical signs may include fevers, vomiting, arthralgia, and rashes. Infected animal colonies should be immediately depopulated to protect human health.

Viral Diseases

Rat Coronavirus (RCV)

A number of coronaviruses have been isolated from rats. Two prototype coronaviruses are sialodacryoadenitis virus (RCV-SDA) and Parker's rat coronavirus (RCV-P). Although the two viruses were once thought to cause distinctly different diseases, clinical signs and pathology cannot differentiate infection with either virus. These viruses are common in both pet and conventionally housed rat populations but are uncommon in barrier-maintained colonies. The coronaviruses of rats are highly contagious and cause inflammation of the salivary and lacrimal glands. Transmission is by direct contact, aerosol, fomites, or administration of contaminated biologics. Rat coronaviruses may induce asymptomatic infections. Alternatively, infections may lead to transient clinical disease. Overt disease occurs in preweanling, nonimmune rats within endemically infected breeding colonies as well as when postweaned animals from naïve colonies are first exposed to the virus. The later may result in explosive outbreaks. Tissue tropisms include salivary glands, lacrimal glands including the Harderian gland, and respiratory epithelium. Infections may exacerbate respiratory disease attributable to *M. pulmonis*.

Common signs of infection are eye squinting, swelling of the ventral cervical region and jaw, and exophthalmia (protrusion of the eye). Generally, clinical signs resolve within approximately 2 weeks. Keratoconjunctivitis is the only clinical sign of infection in some outbreaks. Affected rats usually remain active and continue to eat. Viral shedding lasts about one week. Persistent infection occurs only in severely immunodeficient animals. Although coronaviruses may spread rapidly in a susceptible colony, mortality is usually very low. Treatment is not indicated unless exophthalmia leads to corneal ulceration or keratitis, for which a topical ophthalmic preparation is indicated. Rats that are reinfected may show no clinical signs yet shed the virus for several weeks. Infected animals can be detected through serologic testing for the presence of antibodies, and PCR and histologic examination of tissues from acutely infected rats. Control of infection may entail colony depopulation or rederivation, especially with immunocompromised animals. Alternatively, the "burnout" technique can be used with fully immunocompetent rat colonies whereby breeding and the introduction to the colony of newly susceptible animals are halted for 6–8 weeks. Current colony animals are allowed to contract and then recover from the virus.

Parvoviruses

Parvoviruses are small, non-enveloped DNA viruses that are resistant to heat, lipid solvents, and acidic environments. There are several parvoviruses that naturally infect rats, including the prototypic (Kilham's) rat virus (RV), rat parvovirus (RPV), rat minute virus (RMV), and (Toolan's) H-1 virus. These viruses are among the most prevalent infectious agents found in contemporary laboratory rat colonies. Parvoviruses have predilection for actively dividing cells and neonates are typically more susceptible than adults to active disease. RV infections are sporadic and usually produce subclinical signs. Young adult rats may have clinical signs, including scrotal cyanosis, dehydration, and abdominal swelling. Pregnant rats with RV may have reduced litter size, runted litters, and neonatal death. Clinical disease is not normally observed with RPV, RMV, or H-1 infections in rats. Transmission is by aerosol, through direct contact, fomites, transplacental, and administration of infected biologics. Some infections are persistent for prolonged periods, but persistence is viral-strain dependent. Rat strain and immune status influence the susceptibility to infection as well as the severity and persistence of infection.

Polymerase chain reaction, ELISA, immunofluorescent assays (IFA), and other serologic methods can be used to diagnose parvovirus. PCR can also be used to screen infected tissues such as mesenteric lymph nodes or the spleen. The exact impact of parvoviruses on research is not fully known, but they are generally unwelcome because of their known effects on the immune system, tumor development, fetal development, and the actively dividing cells of the hematopoietic, neurologic, and gastrointestinal systems. Control of infection generally includes depopulation of infected rats and/or cesarean rederivation or embryo transfer for valuable rats. Parvoviruses can persist in the environment for months to years. Environmental decontamination of areas previously occupied by infected animals is vital.

Hantaviruses

Wild rodents serve as the primary reservoir hosts for hantaviruses worldwide. Wild rodents infected with hantaviruses have been identified in multiple regions of the United States, including in numerous cities. Multiple species of hantaviruses exist and present serious zoonotic health risks to people. In general and based on the infecting viral strain, infected humans develop one of two disease syndromes: Hantavirus pulmonary syndrome or hemorrhagic fever with renal syndrome. Each can be fatal.

Hantavirus infection of laboratory rats is exceedingly rare, but may occur through multiple means including the intrusion of wild rodents into a facility, housing and handling of animals not known to be infected (e.g., captured wildlife or international animal transfers), or use of contaminated biologics (e.g., cell cultures). Transmission of hantavirus from laboratory rats to people has been reported in Japan, Belgium, and the United Kingdom.

The virus is persistently shed in the urine and feces of infected rodents. Transmission may occur through bites, aerosols, direct contact with contaminated fomites, or ingestion of contaminated food and water. To help prevent introduction of the virus into research facilities, wild-caught rats and rats transferred from untrusted or untested sources should be carefully screened for hantaviruses. Furthermore, facilities should have robust pest management and exclusion programs.

Group B Rotavirus (Infectious Diarrhea of Infant Rats)

A Group B rotavirus, previously known as infectious diarrhea of infant rats (IDIR), causes a diarrheal disease in suckling rats. It usually occurs in animals less than 2 weeks of age and is characterized by the presence of soft yellow feces or an accumulation of dried feces or hemorrhage around the anus. Affected rats usually continue to nurse, as evidenced by a milk spot (milk in the stomach visible through the abdominal wall), but their growth is often stunted. Pathology findings include small intestinal villous atrophy and syncytial cells. The virus can persist in the environment for prolonged periods and is resistant to some disinfectants. Group B rotaviruses can also cause diarrheal disease in humans. Although most Group B rotaviruses are believed to be species-specific, human isolates have been shown to induce diarrhea in infant rats and an identical or very similar virus to IDIR has been associated with a small-scale human outbreak of diarrhea. Thus, the potential for cross-infectivity exists. No treatment exists other than supportive care. Methods to eliminate the virus from rat colonies include depopulation or rederivation.

Miscellaneous Viral Infections

A number of viruses, including cytomegalovirus, adenovirus, pneumonia virus of mice, and Sendai virus, produce naturally occurring infections in rats. Most infections are subclinical and rarely occur in contemporary US research facilities. However, latent or indigenous viruses that may be activated by stress or may alter the response of animals to experimental procedures are nevertheless of concern in the research laboratory. Emphasis must be placed on quarantine and screening of incoming rats of unknown origin. Additionally, PCR screening or other testing of transplantable tumors, cell lines, and other biological materials are important aspects of preventing viral contaminants from entering a research colony.

Parasitic Diseases

With the exception of pinworms, parasitic infections are extremely rare in colonies of laboratory rats. When they do occur, their source can most commonly be traced to wild rodents that have either been purposefully brought into the facility or entered as pests. When parasitic infections do occur, management personnel should critically examine the facility's integrated pest management program as well as animal transfer and quarantine practices. With parasites capable of harboring zoonotic diseases, personnel health evaluations may also be warranted.

Mites

Several mites can cause disease in rats. *Radfordia ensifera*, the fur mite of rats, can cause pruritus, hair loss, and debilitation with heavy infestations. *Notoedres muris*, a rare mange mite that burrows into the deeper layers of the epidermis, can produce red papules or reddened and thickened skin. *Ornithonyssus bacoti*, the tropical rat mite, is a bloodsucking mite that can cause pruritus and skin irritation. *O. bacoti* drops off of the rat after each feeding and has been associated with pruritus and skin lesions in humans, including animal caretakers. *O. bacoti* presents an additional human health risk as it can transmit multiple, serious diseases to humans, including Q fever, plague, Hantaan viruses, and western equine encephalitis. O. *bacoti* infections in barrier-maintained rat colonies are very rare, but they are possible if infected rats enter a facility either through purposeful animal transport or on infested, wild rodents. Select anthelmintics (e.g., ivermectin, moxidectin), administered topically, parentally, or mixed with food or water have been effective in treating mite infestations. Caution should be used when treating suckling rats or other rats with incomplete or damaged blood–brain barriers as they are sensitive to the neurotoxic effects of avermectins.

Pinworms

Syphacia muris, *S. obvelata*, and *Aspiculuris tetraptera* are pinworms that infect rats, with *S. muris* infections being most common. Each species of nematode is also capable of infecting other animal species, including mice. While horizontal transmission occurs with both, *Syphacia* and *Aspiculuris* differ in their lifecycles. *Syphacia* spp. have a direct life cycle of 11–15 days. Females deposit their eggs near the animal's anus. Eggs are then ingested, hatch in the small intestine, and mature in the cecum. In contrast, *Aspicularis* has a direct life cycle of 23–25 days. Eggs are passed in the feces and do not adhere to the perineum.

Infected animals are frequently asymptomatic, although an increased incidence of rectal prolapse may be observed. Infections may alter hematologic values and immunological responses, as well as cause reduced weight gain and growth rate of young rats. Diagnostic methods include observation of adult worms in intestinal sections collected during necropsy, identification of *Syphacia* eggs obtained from the perianal region through the use of cellophane tape pressed to the perianal region, and identification of *Aspiculuris* eggs through fecal flotation. All three methods are laborious and time consuming and perianal tape tests and fecal examinations can easily yield false-negative results. More recently, fecal PCR diagnostic tests have been developed. Unfortunately, these also can be laborious and expensive. Use of a combination of tests may yield the most accurate results.

Sound management practices are required to prevent the introduction of pinworms into a colony. Fenbendazole, ivermectin, and levamisole are among the anthelmintics used to treat pinworm infections in rats. When possible, administration of the drug in specially formulated feed can be ideal. Although pinworm eggs can be persistent in the environment, eradication can be achieved without environmental decontamination through multiple weeks of treatment with medicated feed. Anthelmintics have been shown to affect animal behavior and may negatively affect reproduction. The influence of these effects on animal welfare and research findings must be considered. If decontamination is necessary, dry heat (100°C for 30 minutes), ethylene oxide gas, vaporized hydrogen peroxide, and choline dioxide gas are reportedly effective at eliminating infectious eggs from contaminated equipment and areas.

Lice

Polyplax spinulosa, the spined rat louse, is a bloodsucking louse commonly seen in wild rats. Affected rats may exhibit no clinical signs, but heavy infestations may cause skin irritation, anemia, and debilitation. *P. spinulosa* can transmit the blood parasite *Mycoplasma haemomuris* among rats. Ivermectin has been effectively used to eliminate this louse. Permethrin dust applied to the animals and to the bedding is also reported to be effective.

Tapeworms

The rat is a definitive host for *Rodentolepis nana*, the dwarf tapeworm, and *Hymenolepis diminuta*, the rat tapeworm. These worms are pathogenic only with heavy infestations. Diagnosis of infection is usually by fecal flotation, fecal smear, or identification of the adult worms in the small intestine. Typical morphologic features used to differentiate *R. nana* from *H. diminuta* include adult worm size as well as the shape and characteristics of the scolex, eggs, and embryos.

Rodentolepis nana is of particular concern because of its direct life cycle, interspecies transmission, and zoonotic potential. Prevention of hymenolepid infections requires strict sanitation practices and elimination of vectors. Praziquantel and thiabendazole are reported to be effective in treating rat tapeworms. However, treatment is generally not recommended for *R. nana* infections because of the zoonotic potential. Total eradication in large rat populations is difficult to achieve without repopulation.

Mycotic Diseases

Pneumocystis Carinii

Pneumocystis carinii is a single-celled, airborne fungal pathogen transmitted by aerosol exposure and possibly through contact with contaminated fomites. The course of disease induced by the organism differs in immunocompetent and in immunocompromised animals. Infected immunocompetent animals develop an infectious interstitial pneumonia, a condition previously and erroneously attributed to rat respiratory virus, prior to clearing the infection. In contrast, the organism proliferates in the lungs of immunocompromised animals, causing a chronic progressive pneumonia, obstruction of alveolar spaces with fungal cysts, and eventual death. Disease is most commonly diagnosed postmortem through histologic identification of organisms in lung tissue with silver staining. Few organisms may be found in immunocompetent animals; suspected infections should be confirmed through PCR. Organisms are readily detected in infected immunocompromised animals. Antibiotic administration may suppress disease severity, but no treatment has been shown effective in completely eliminating the organism from infected animals. Rederivation is required to eliminate the infection from infected colonies.

Dermatophytosis (Ringworm)

Ringworm in rats is usually caused by *Trichophyton mentagrophytes*. Infection may cause widespread skin lesions in a colony or may produce asymptomatic carriers. Systemic mycoses are extremely rare in rats. Human ringworm infections have been associated with rats infected with this organism.

Neoplasia

Spontaneous neoplasms involving essentially every organ have been reported. The incidence depends to a large extent on the particular stock or strain and age of animals examined. Environmental influences and the presence or absence of pathogenic infections also play an important role, as does diet. Long-term dietary restriction (e.g., 20% reduction of *ad libitum* food consumption) has been associated with a significant reduction in overall incidence of tumors in Wistar rats.

Mammary Tumors

Mammary tumors are very common in most stocks of laboratory rats (Box 5.10). Up to 50% of aged female Sprague-Dawley rats develop mammary tumors. Tumors do, although rarely, occur in males. Because of the distribution of mammary tissue,

> **Box 5.10**
>
> *Mammary tumors are very common in most stocks of laboratory rats.*

tumors may occur over a wide area of the body and may reach enormous sizes. Mammary tumors are usually classified as benign fibroadenomas, are well encapsulated, and do not metastasize. They are usually freely mobile under the skin. Surgical removal is feasible, and prospects of recovery are favorable. Tumors frequently, however, reoccur.

Testicular Tumors

Interstitial cell tumors of the testes are extremely common (~80% incidence) in F344 rats, an inbred strain commonly used in toxicologic studies. Grossly, the tumors are yellow-brown with areas of hemorrhage. They are frequently soft and discrete and may occur unilaterally or bilaterally. Incidence in other rat stocks or strains is quite low, with Wistars having an 11% incidence.

Keratoacanthoma

Keratoacanthomas are benign tumors of the skin that can become quite large. They appear as proliferations of keratin or horny growths with craterlike centers and may occur anywhere on the skin. No treatment is required unless the tumor becomes large and/or inhibits mobility or normal body functions.

Large Granular Lymphocytic Leukemia

Large granular lymphocytic leukemia is a major cause of death in aging F344 rats, with up to a 50% incidence of tumor development in 2-year studies. This neoplasia is not associated with a retrovirus as it is in mice. A leukocytosis of up to 180,000/μL may occur. Clinical signs include weight loss, anemia, jaundice, and depression. Gross findings include marked splenomegaly with moderate hepatomegaly and lymphadenopathy. Histologically, a diffuse infiltration of large malignant lymphocytes in seen throughout many organs, including the spleen, liver, lymph nodes, and lungs.

Pituitary Adenomas

Pituitary adenomas occur frequently in aged rats, particularly in Sprague-Dawley and Wistar rats. They are histologically classified as chromophobe adenomas. These tumors are frequently slow-growing but can be large (up to 0.5 cm) and cause compression of adjacent central nervous system tissues. Grossly, the tumors are often hemorrhagic and appear dark red and soft. Clinical signs include severe depression, incoordination, torticollis, and death.

Zymbal's Gland Tumors

Tumors of Zymbal's gland, which is located at the base of the ear, occur with some frequency in rats. The tumor tends to be locally invasive but not metastatic.

Miscellaneous Conditions

Chromodacryorrhea

Aged, clinically ill, or stressed rats may have obvious signs of chromodacryorrhea; *chromo* meaning "colored," *dacryo* "tears," and *rrhea* "many") (Box 5.11). The Harderian gland, located posterior to the orbit, is a lacrimal gland that secretes porphyrins. When secretion becomes excessive, tears containing porphyrin form a red

Box 5.11

Aged, clinically ill, or stressed rats may display chromodacryorrhea.

crust around the eyes and may run down the nasolacrimal duct to form crusts around the nose (Figure 5.6). This dark, reddish-brown material resembles blood. The amount of secretion increases with age and during stressful conditions such as shipping. Treatment specifically for chromodacryorrhea is not indicated, although cleaning away the crusts may keep the rat more comfortable. The presence of excess secretions suggests the possibility of an underlying condition that should be further explored.

Chronic Progressive Glomerulonephropathy

Chronic progressive glomerulonephropathy (CPN) is a significant kidney disease of aged rats. In long-term rat studies, CPN is one of the most common causes of death. Several factors may play a role in the development of CPN, including age, sex, strain, and diet. Males have a higher incidence, earlier onset, and more severe lesions than females. Moderate diet restriction (80% of *ad libitum*–fed body weight) greatly reduces the incidence and severity of CPN. Clinical signs may include weight loss, unkempt hair coat, and sudden death from renal failure. There is marked proteinuria, and secondary hyperparathyroidism may develop with resultant widespread tissue mineralization. Grossly, the renal cortices are pitted and irregular.

Chronic Myocardial Disease

Some strains of rats, such as Sprague-Dawley, have a high incidence of chronic heart disease. Similar to CPN, this is more common in the aged male and in *ad libitum*–fed animals. Grossly, the heart is enlarged.

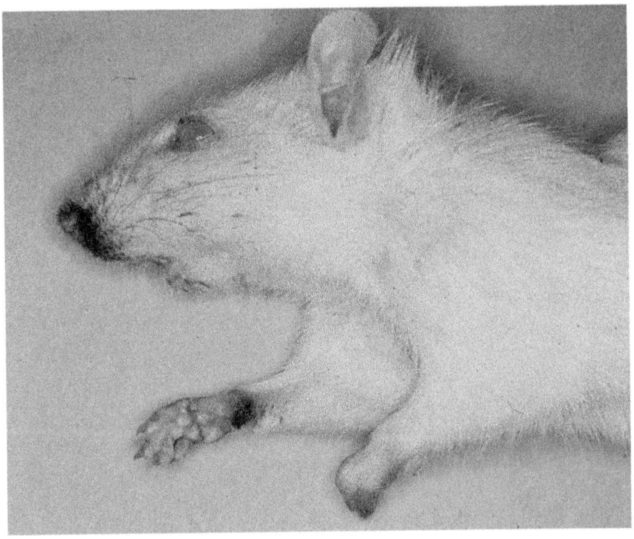

Fig 5.6. Chromodacryorrhea. (*Source*: Photo courtesy of ACLAM.)

Dehydration

Dehydration should not be overlooked as a possible cause of sudden death in rats. Water may be unavailable because of an air lock in the sipper tube even when a water bottle is full. Malfunction of drinking valves in automated watering systems can also result in a lack of water. Pain often results in a decrease in both food and water consumption. To check for dehydration, simply lift the skin over the interscapular region. The skin of a hydrated animal slides quickly and smoothly back into place, whereas the skin of a dehydrated animal will tent with a slow return to normal position. If tenting is observed, the rat is at least 10% dehydrated and requires fluid supplementation. Sunken eyes are a further sign of severe dehydration.

Malocclusion

Rat incisors grow continuously throughout their lives. Without proper alignment or wear from gnawing activities, the incisors will overgrow and may cause hard or soft tissue damage and inhibit or totally prevent food or water consumption. Underlying causes of malocclusion include congenital, traumatic, or research-induced disruption of normal tooth root activity, tooth loss, jaw deformity, and a lack of hard materials or surfaces for gnawing (Figure 5.7). If severe and undetected, overgrown incisors can lead to emaciation and death due to an inability to eat. Rodent incisors can be trimmed with a dental bur or sharp suture removal scissors, with the bur less likely to fracture the teeth. Affected animals should not be bred if malocclusion may be congenital in origin.

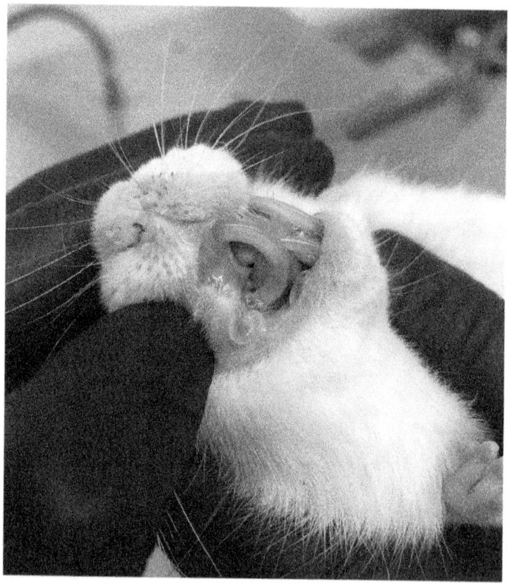

Fig 5.7. Malocclusion.

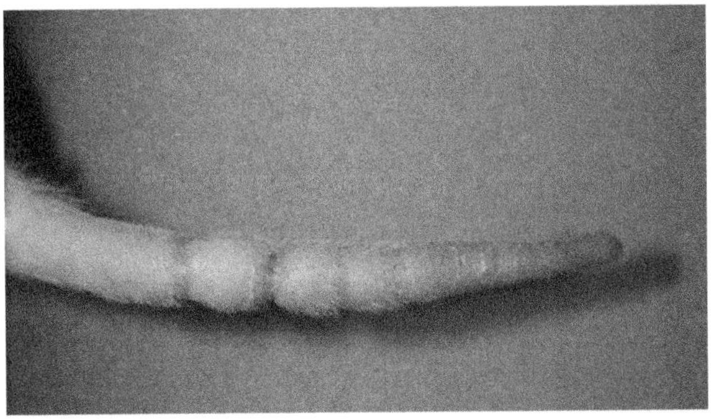

Fig 5.8. Ringtail. (*Source*: Photo courtesy of Wayne State University.)

Polyarteritis Nodosa

Polyarteritis nodosa is a chronic degenerative disease of aging rats, especially Sprague-Dawley and Spontaneously Hypertensive rats. At necropsy, gross findings include segmental thickening and marked tortuosity of the medium-sized arteries of the mesentery, testes, and pancreas, as well as of the pancreaticoduodenal artery. The cause of these lesions has not been determined but may be an immunologically mediated response.

Ringtail

Ringtail is a syndrome associated with suckling or preweaned rats housed in low (<20%) ambient relative humidity (Figure 5.8). It is usually seen in the winter months when heating systems are in use. However, lesions can develop in higher humidity levels. Ringtail appears as one or more annular constrictions of the tail. Distal to the constriction, the tail may become edematous or necrotic. The process is assumed to be painful and should not be ignored. Providing solid-bottomed cages with adequate bedding and maintaining relative humidity at approximately 50% can help to prevent ringtail.

Spontaneous Radiculoneuropathy

Radiculoneuropathy is a spontaneous aging disease of rats that involves degeneration of the spinal roots and concurrent atrophy of the skeletal muscles of the lumbar region and hind limbs. Affected animals exhibit posterior weakness or paresis.

BIBLIOGRAPHY

Adamcak, A. 2000. Rodent therapeutics. *Vet Clin North Am: Exotic Anim Pract* 3: 221–237.

Allen, D. G., J. K. Pringle, and D. A. Smith. 1993. *Handbook of Veterinary Drugs*. Philadelphia: JB Lippincott.

American Veterinary Medical Association (AVMA). 2013. *AVMA Guidelines for the Euthanasia of Animals*. Available at http://www.avma.org/KB/Policies/Documents/euthanasia.pdf [accessed December 4, 2018].

Anderson, N. L. 1994. Basic husbandry and medicine of pocket pets. In *Saunders Manual of Small Animal Practice*, S. J. Birchard and R. G. Sherding (eds.), pp. 1363–1389. Philadelphia: WB Saunders.

Baker, D. G. 1998. Natural pathogens of laboratory mice, rats, and rabbits and their effects on research. *Clin Microbiol Rev* 11(2): 231–266.

Barlow, S. C., M. M. Brown, and H. V. Price. 2005. Eradication of *Syphacia muris* from food-restricted rats without environmental decontamination. *Contemp Top Lab Anim Sci* 44(1): 23–25.

Barthold, S. W., S. M. Griffey, and D. H. Percy. 2016. *Pathology of Laboratory Rodents and Rabbits*, 4th ed. Ames, IA: Wiley-Blackwell.

Besselsen, D. G., A. M. Wagner, and J. K. Loganbill. 2002. Detection of rodent coronaviruses by use of fluorogenic reverse transcriptase–polymerase chain reaction analysis. *Comp Med* 52(2): 111–116.

Boivin, G. P., I. Ormsby, and J. E. Hall. 1996. Eradication of *Aspiculuris tetraptera* using fenbendazole-medicated food. *Contemp Top Lab Anim Sci* 35(2): 69–70.

Brown, C. 2006. Blood collection from the tail of a rat. *Lab Animal (NY)* 35(8): 24–5.

Burgmann, P., and D. H. Percy. 1993. Antimicrobial drug use in rodents and rabbits. In *Antimicrobial Therapy in Veterinary Medicine*, 2nd ed., J. F. Prescott and J. D. Baggot (eds.), pp. 524–541. Ames, IA: Iowa State University Press.

Chung, S. L., S. J. Hwang, S. B. Kwon, et al. 1998. Outbreak of rat mite dermatitis in medical students. *Int J Derm* 37(8): 591.

Clark, J. A., P. H. Myers, M. F. Goelz, et al. 1997. Pica behavior associated with buprenorphine administration in the rat. *Lab Anim Sci* 47(3): 300–303.

Cooper, D. M., D. DeLong, and C. S. Gillette. 1997. Analgesic efficacy of acetaminophen and buprenorphine administered in the drinking water of rats. *Contemp Top Lab Anim Sci* 36(3): 58–62.

De Vera Mudry M. C., S. Kronenberg, S. Komatsu, and G. D. Aguirre. 2013. Blinded by the light: Retinal phototoxicity in the context of safety studies. *Toxicol Path* 41(6): 813–25.

Dix, J., J. Astill, and G. Whelan. 2004. Assessment of methods of destruction of *Syphacia muris* eggs. *Lab Anim* 38(1): 11–6.

Dontas, I. A., A. I. Tsolakis., L. Khaldi, et al. 2010. Malocclusion in aging Wistar rats. *J Am Assoc Lab Anim Sci* 49(1): 22–26.

Esfandiani, A., T. Loya, and J. L. Lee. 2002. Skin tumors in aging Long-Evans rats. *J Natl Med Assoc* 94(6): 506–510.

Fenwick, D. C., and J. K. Blackshaw. 1989. Carbon dioxide as a short-term restraint anaesthetic in rats with subclinical respiratory disease. *Lab Anim* 23(3): 220–228.

Flecknell, P. A. 1991. Postoperative analgesia in rabbits and rodents. *Lab Anim (NY)* 20(9): 34–37.

Flecknell, P. A. 1997. Medetomidine and atipamezole: Potential uses in laboratory animals. *Lab Anim* 26(2): 21–25.

Flecknell, P. A. 2009. *Laboratory Animal Anaesthesia*, 3rd ed. London: Academic Press.

Flecknell, P. A. 2016. *Laboratory Animal Anaesthesia*, 4th ed. Oxford: Academic Press.

Foley, P. L., H. Liang, and A. R. Crichlow. 2011. Evaluation of a sustained release formulation of buprenorphine for analgesia in rats. *Lab Anim Sci* 50(2): 198–204.

Gaertner, D. J. 2004. Speculations on why some lab rodent pathogens continue to be prevalent [editorial]. *Contemp Top Lab Anim Sci* 43(3): 8.

Goodroe, A. E., V. K. Baxter, and J. Watson. 2016. Guidance regarding sample collection and refinement of fecal flotation exam for the isolation of *Aspiculuris tetraptera*. *J Am Assoc Lab Anim Sci* 55(5): 541–547.

Graham, J. E. and T. R. Schoeb. 2011. *Mycoplasma pulmonis* in rats. *J Exotic Pet Med* 20(4): 270–276.

Harkness, J. E., and J. E. Wagner. 1995. *Biology and Medicine of Rabbits and Rodents*, 4th ed. Philadelphia: Williams & Wilkins.

Harkness, J. E., P. V. Turner, S. VandeWoude, and C. L. Wheler. 2010. *Harkness and Wagner's Biology and Medicine of Rabbits and Rodents*, 5th ed. Ames, IA: Wiley-Blackwell.

Harrenstien, L. 1994. Critical care of ferrets, rabbits, and rodents. *Semin Avian Exotic Pet Med* 3: 217–228.

Heard, D. J. 1993. Principles and techniques of anesthesia and analgesia for exotic practice. *Vet Clin North Am Small Anim Pract* 23(6): 1301–1327.

Hedrich, H. J. 2000. History, strains and models. In *The Laboratory Rat*, G. Krinke (ed.), pp. 3–16. London: Academic Press.

Henderson, K. S., V. Dole, N. J. Parker, P. Momtsios, et al. 2012. *Pneumocystis carinii* causes a distinctive interstitial pneumonia in immunocompetent laboratory rats that had been attributed to "Rat Respiratory Virus." *Vet Pathol* 49(3): 440–452.

Hill, W. A., M. M. Randolph, and T. D. Mandrell. 2009. Sensitivity of perianal tape impressions to diagnose pinworm (*Syphacia* spp.) infections in rats (*Rattus norvegicus*) and mice (*Mus musculus*). *J Am Assoc Lab Anim Sci* 48(4): 378–380.

Hironaga, M., T. Fujigaki, and S. Watanabe. 1981. *Trichophyton mentagrophytes* skin infections in laboratory animals as a cause of zoonosis. *Mycopathologia* 73(2): 101–104.

Huber, A. C., R. H. Yolken, L. C. Mader, et al. 1989. Pathology of infectious diarrhea of infant rats (IDIR) induced by an antigenically distinct rotavirus. *Vet Pathol* 26(5): 376–385.

Huerkamp, M. J. 1995. Anesthesia and postoperative management of rabbits and pocket pets. In *Kirk's Current Veterinary Therapy XII: Small Animal Practice*, J. D. Bonagura (ed.), pp. 1322–1327. Philadelphia: WB Saunders.

Huerkamp, M. J., K. A. Benjamin, S. K. Webb, and J. K. Pullium. 2004. Long-term results of dietary fenbendazole to eradicate *Syphacia muris* from rat colonies. *Contemp Top Lab Anim Sci* 43(2): 35–36.

Ike F., M. Sakamoto, M. Ohkum, et al. 2016. Filobacterium rodentium gen. nov., sp. nov., a member of Filobacteriaceae fam. nov. within the phylum Bacteroidetes; includes a microaerobic filamentous bacterium isolated from specimens from diseased rodent respiratory tracts. *Int J Syst Evol Microbiol* 66(1): 150–157.

Institute of Laboratory Animal Resources (ILAR). 2011. *Guide for the Care and Use of Laboratory Animals*, 8th ed. ILAR, National Research Council. Washington, DC: National Academies Press.

Iwasaki, K., C. A. Gleiser, E. J. Masoro, et al. 1988. The influence of dietary protein source on longevity and age-related disease processes of Fischer rats. *J Gerontol* 43(1): B5–B12.

Jacoby, R. O., J. G. Fox, and M. Davisson. 2002. Biology and diseases of rats. In *Laboratory Animal Medicine*, J. G. Fox, L. C. Anderson, F. Loew, and F. Quimby (eds.), pp. 121–167. San Diego, CA: Academic Press.

Jekl, V., K. Hauptman, E. Jeklová, and Z. Knotek. 2005. Blood sampling from the cranial vena cava in the Norway rat (*Rattus norvegicus*). *Lab Animal* 39(2): 236–239.

Keen, R., M. Macinnis, P. Guilhardi, et al. 2005. The lack of behavioral effects of fenbendazole: A medication for pinworm infection. *Contemp Top Lab Anim Sci* 44(2): 17–23.

Kelaher, J., R. Jogi, and R. Katta. 2005. An outbreak of rat mite dermatitis in an animal research facility. *Cutis* 75: 282–286.

Klement, P., J. M. Augustine, K. H. Delaney, et al. 1996. An oral ivermectin regimen that eradicates pinworms (*Syphacia* spp.) in laboratory rats and mice. *Lab Anim Sci* 46(3): 286–290.

Kondo, S. Y., A. D. Taylor, and S. S. C. Chun. 1998. Elimination of an infestation of rat fur mites (*Radfordia ensifera*) from a colony of Long-Evans rats, using the micro-dot technique for topical administration of 1% ivermectin. *Contemp Top Lab Anim Sci* 37(1): 21–24.

Livingston, R. S., C. L. Besch-Williford, M. H. Myles, et al. 2011. *Pneumocystis carinii* infection causes lung lesions historically attributed to rat respiratory virus. *Comp Med* 61(1): 45–52.

Lukas, V. 1999. Volume guidelines for compound administration. In *The Care and Feeding of an IACUC*, M. L. Podolsky and V. S. Lukas (eds.), p. 187. Boca Raton, FL: CRC Press.

Marashi, V. and T. Rülicke. 2012. The Bruce effect in Norway rats. *Biol Reprod* 86(1): 1–5.

Martin, L. B. E., A. C. Thompson, T. Martin, and M. B. Kristal. 2001. Analgesic efficacy of orally administered buprenorphine in rats. *Comp Med* 51(1): 43–48.

Morrisey, J. K., and J. W. Carpenter. 2004. Formulary. In *Ferrets, Rabbits and Rodents: Clinical Medicine and Surgery*, K. E. Quesenberry and J. W. Carpenter (eds.), pp. 436–444. St. Louis, MO: Saunders.

Morrisey, J. K., and J. W. Carpenter. 2011. Drug formulary. In *Ferrets, Rabbits, and Rodents: Clinical Medicine and Surgery*, K. E. Quesenberry and J. W. Carpenter (eds.), pp. 566–575. St. Louis, MO: WB Saunders.

National Association for Biomedical Research. 2018 Laboratory animals: Species in research. Available at https://www.nabr.org/biomedical-research [accessed December 4, 2018].

Oge, H., E. Ayaz, T. Ide, and S. Dalgic. 2000. The effects of doramectin, moxidectin, and netobimin against natural infections of *Syphacia muris* in rats. *Vet Parasitol* 88(3–4): 299–303.

Olson, M. E., D. Vizzutti, D. W. Morck, and A. K. Cox. 1994. The parasympatholytic effects of atropine sulfate and glycopyrrolate in rats and rabbits. *Can J Vet Res* 58(4): 254–258.

Otto, G. M., C. L. Franklin, and C. B. Clifford, 2015. Biology and diseases of rats. In *Laboratory Animal Medicine*, 3rd ed., J. G. Fox, G. Otto, K. R. Pritchett-Corning, and M. T. Whary (eds.), pp.151–207. San Diego, CA: Academic Press.

Piasecki T., K. Chrzastek, and U. Kasprzykowska. 2017. *Mycoplasma pulmonis* of rodents as a possible human pathogen. *Vector Borne Zoonotic Dis* 17(7): 475–477.

Poul, J. M. 1988. Effects of perinatal ivermectin exposure on behavioral development of rats. *Neurotoxicol Teratol* 10(3): 267–272.

Pritchett, K. R., and N. A. Johnston. 2002. A review of treatments for the eradication of pinworm infections from laboratory rodent colonies. *Contemp Top Lab Anim Sci* 41(2): 36–46.

Reyes, L., D. A. Steiner, J. Hutchison, et al. 2000. *Mycoplasma pulmonis* genital disease: Effect of rat strain on pregnancy. *Comp Med* 50(6): 622–627.

Silverman, J., M. Huhndorf, M. Balk, and G. Slater. 1983. Evaluation of a combination of tiletamine and zolazepam as an anesthetic for laboratory rodents. *Lab Anim Sci* 33(5): 457–460.

Smith, A., and D. J. Corrow. 2005. Modifications to husbandry and housing conditions of laboratory rodents for improved well-being. *ILAR J* 46(2): 140–147.

Smith, L. J., L. Krugner-Higby, M. Clark, A. Wendland, and T. D. Heath. 2003. A single dose of liposome-encapsulated oxymorphone or morphine provides long-term analgesia in an animal model of neuropathic pain. *Comp Med* 53(3): 280–287.

Susana, G. S., R. E. Sorge, A. Zaloum, et al. 2011. The Rat Grimace Scale: A partially automated method for quantifying pain in the laboratory rat via facial expressions. *Mol Pain* 7: 55.

Thomas J, J. K. Haseman, J. I. Goodman, et al. 2007. A review of large granular lymphocytic leukemia in Fischer 344 rats as an initial step toward evaluating the implication of the endpoint to human cancer risk assessment. *Toxicol Sci* 99(1): 3–19.

Thompson, A. C., M. B. Kristal, A. Sallaj, et al. 2004. Analgesic efficacy of orally administered buprenorphine in rats: Methodologic considerations. *Comp Med* 54(3): 293–300.

Van Loo, P. L. and V. Baumans. 2004. The importance of learning young: The use of nesting material in laboratory rats. *Lab Animal* 38(1): 17–24.

Vorherr H. and U. F. Vorherr. 1984. Suckling-induced delay of implantation and increased fecundity in rats. *Gynecol Obstet Invest* 17(2): 106–110.

Waite, M. E., A. Tomkovich, T. L. Quinn, et al. 2015. Efficacy of common analgesics for postsurgical pain in rats. *J Am Assoc Lab Anim Sci* 54(4): 420–425.

Walling, B. E. and G. B. Marit. 2016. The eye and harderian gland. In *Atlas of Histology of the Juvenile Rat*, G. A. Parker and C. A. Picut (eds.), pp. 373–394. San Diego, CA: Academic Press.

Wellington, D., I. Mikaelian, and L. Singer. 2013. Comparison of ketamine–xylazine and ketamine–dexmedetomidine anesthesia and intraperitoneal tolerance in rats. *J Am Assoc Lab Anim Sci* 52(4): 481–487.

Wilson, R. P., I. S. Zagon, D. R. Larach, and C. M. Lang. 1992. Antinociceptive properties of tiletamine–zolazepam improved by addition of xylazine or butorphanol. *Pharmacol Biochem Behav* 43(4): 1129–1133.

Wixson, S. K., W. J. White, H. C. Hughes Jr., C. M. Lang, and W. K. Marshall. 1987. A comparison of pentobarbital, fentanyl–droperidol, ketamine–xylazine and ketamine–diazepam anesthesia in adult male rats. *Lab Anim Sci* 37(6): 726–730.

Yang, J., J. M. I. Maarek, and D. P. Holschneider. 2005. In vivo quantitative assessment of catheter patency in rats. *Lab Anim* 39(3): 259–268.

Yoshizwa, K. 2018. Specialized sebaceous glands—Zymbal's gland, preputial gland, clitoral gland, and perianal gland. In *Boorman's Pathology of the Rat: Reference and Atlas*, 2nd ed., A. W. Suttie (ed.), pp 347–365. San Diego, CA: Academic Press.

FURTHER READING

Meek, S., T. Mashimo, and T. Burdon. 2017. From engineering to editing the rat genome. *Mamm Genome* 28(7): 302–314.

National Centre for the Replacement, Refinement, and Reduction of Animals in Research. 2018. Grimace scales. Available at www.nc3rs.org.uk/grimacescales [accessed December 6, 2018].

Newcastle University. 2018. Procedures with Care. Available at www.procedureswithcare.org.uk [accessed November 30, 2018].

Sharp, J., T. Zammit, T. Azar, and D. Lawson. 2002. Does witnessing experimental procedures produce stress in male rats? *Contemp Top Lab Anim Sci* 41(5): 8–12.

Sylvie C., K. Wahl, C. Baker, and R. C. Newberry. 2014. The social buffering effect of playful handling on responses to repeated intraperitoneal injections in laboratory rats. *J Am Assoc Lab Anim Sci* 53(2): 168–173.

Vandamme, T. F. 2014. Use of rodents as models of human diseases. *J Pharm Bioallied Sci* 6(1): 2–9.

CHAPTER 5 REVIEW

Multiple Choice

1. Which of the following are outbred stocks of rats (more than one answer may be correct)
   A. Sprague–Dawley
   B. Buffalo
   C. Wistar
   D. Long-Evans
   E. F344
2. Which genetic classification is useful for modeling natural population diversity?
   A. genetically engineered
   B. inbred strain
   C. outbred stock

3. ____ animals colonized only with a known population of microflora.
   A. Germ-free
   B. Gnotobiotic
   C. Axenic
   D. Specific pathogen–free
4. Which is NOT an acceptable reason to singly house animals of a social species?
   A. cost
   B. scientific necessity
   C. observed social incompatibility (e.g., fighting)
   D. veterinary concerns regarding animal well-being
5. What is the usual gestation period of a rat?
   A. 17–19 days
   B. 19–21 days
   C. 21–23 days
   D. 23–25 days
6. Which of the following is INCORRECT regarding rat nutrition?
   A. Rats are copraphagic.
   B. Rats drink an average of 10–12 mL of water per day.
   C. Rats eat an average of 5–6 g of rodent chow per 100 g of body weight per day.
   D. Rats tend to become obese if fed ad libitum throughout adulthood.
7. As a general guideline, up to ______% of the circulating blood volume can be withdrawn every 2–3 weeks from normal, healthy animals with minimal effect.
   A. 5
   B. 7
   C. 10
   D. 12
8. If a procedure is known to cause pain in humans, it must be assumed to also cause pain in rats unless ___________.
   A. it is clinically insignificant
   B. it negatively affects research outcomes
   C. it is of short duration
   D. proven otherwise
9. Recommended site for administration of intraperitoneal injections in rats is
   A. upper right abdominal quadrant.
   B. lower left abdominal quadrant.
   C. upper left abdominal quadrant.
   D. lower right abdominal quadrant.
10. Recommended methods for the individual identification of adult rats include all but which of the following:
    A. toe clipping
    B. ear tagging

(Continued)

C. tattooing
D. microchip implantation

11. What is the name of the AVMA guidance document for members of the veterinary profession who carry out or oversee the euthanasia of animals?
A. Guidelines for the Euthanasia of Research Animals
B. Guidelines for the Euthanasia of Animals
C. Guidelines for the Practice of Euthanasia
D. Guidelines for Laboratory Animal Euthanasia for Research

Match Up

Match the following with their respective descriptions:

A. Clostridium piliforme
B. Radfordia ensifera
C. Sialodacryoadenitis
D. Parvoviruses
E. Mycoplasma pulmonis
F. Trichophyton mentagrophytes
G. Hantavirus
H. CAR bacillus
I. Rodentolepis nana
J. Ringtail
K. Pituitary adenoma
L. Syphacia
M. Streptobacillus moniliformis
N. Chromodacryorrhea

12. ____ Ringworm
13. ____ Fur mite of rat
14. ____ Gross lesions include miliary pale foci of the liver, abdominal distention, and megaloilietis
15. ____ Zoonotic agent endemic in some wild rodent populations
16. ____ "Red tears"
17. ____ Associated with low housing humidity
18. ____ Pinworm species for which the perianal tape test may be diagnostic
19. ____ Bacteria histologically visible between and parallel to the cilia of respiratory epithelium
20. ____ Etiologic agent of rat-bite fever
21. ____ Rat Coronavirus
22. ____ Bacteria that induces chronic respiratory disease and a "cobblestone" appearance of the lungs
23. ____ Predilection for actively dividing cells
24. ____ Zoonotic tapeworm
25. ____ Common tumor of aged rats

6

Gerbils

The Mongolian gerbil is a rodent of the family Muridae, which also includes the majority of rat and mouse species seen in research. Its scientific name is *Meriones unguiculatus*, which translates into "mammal having claws." The Mongolian gerbil is also known as the clawed jird. It is native to desert regions of China and Mongolia. Gerbils are intermediate in size between mice and hamsters. Adults typically weigh 50–100 g, with males slightly larger than females. The most common coat color is agouti, which has a light buff to white ventrum and mixed white, yellow, and black hairs dorsally, giving it an overall brown color. Gerbils may also be black, gray, white, cinnamon, dove, or piebald (patches of two or more colors, often including white).

USES

Gerbils have many attributes that contribute to their usefulness as a research animal. They are clean, friendly, easy to handle, and tame; they rarely bite and are nearly odor free. In addition, they tend to be very curious and quite active.

Gerbils are useful in a number of research areas, including stroke, behavior, parasitology, epilepsy, radiobiology, hearing, lipid metabolism, and infectious disease research. They are an important animal model for stroke research because they have an incomplete circle of Willis, which is the major arterial vascular supply to the base of the brain. This unique anatomic feature makes it possible to create ipsilateral cerebral ischemia by unilateral carotid ligation. Gerbils can be infected with a wide variety of parasites. They are particularly useful in studying diseases caused by filarial nematodes. Gerbils are also an important model for the study of epilepsy because they have a high incidence of spontaneous epileptiform seizures.

Clinical Laboratory Animal Medicine: An Introduction, Fifth Edition.
Lesley A. Colby, Megan H. Nowland, and Lucy H. Kennedy.

Companion website: www.wiley.com/go/colby/clinical

BEHAVIOR

Gerbils are social animals and, under normal circumstances, live peacefully in same-sex or mixed-sex groups formed prior to puberty. They may fight if crowded or if grouped as adults. Gerbils are active burrowers and, in their natural desert environment, construct elaborate tunnels with multiple entrances, nesting rooms, and food chambers. Food hoarding is common and primarily seen with females. Gerbils tend to be most active in the evening, with short periods of activity during the day. They frequently sit upright on their hind limbs in an inquisitive stance. When caged, they may commonly scratch a bottom corner repeatedly with their front paws while pushing bedding behind them with their hind limbs. Gerbils attract attention or express aggression by thumping their hind limbs to create a drumming sound. They generally mate for life, forming stable breeding pairs. Both sexes participate in nest building and take an active role in parenting.

ANATOMIC AND PHYSIOLOGIC FEATURES

Biologic and reproductive data for the gerbils are listed in Table 6.1. The gerbil has a longer and more slender body conformation than that of the hamster. Gerbils are characterized by a long tail that is fully furred with a tuft of longer hairs on the end. They have prominent furred ears; large, slightly protruding eyes; furred foot pads and strong claws for burrowing; and elongated hind limbs used for jumping or maintaining a semierect posture. Gerbils have a Harderian gland located poste-

Table 6.1. Biologic and reproductive data for gerbils

Adult body weight: Male	80–130 g
Adult body weight: Female	55–85 g
Life span	3–4 y
Body temperature	37°–38.5°C (98.6°–101.3°F)
Heart rate	360 beats per minute
Respiratory rate	90 breaths per minute
Food consumption	5–8 g/100 g per day
Water consumption	4–7 mL/100 g per day
Breeding onset: Male	70–85 d
Breeding onset: Female	65–85 d
Estrous cycle length	4–6 d
Gestation period	24–26 d
Postpartum estrus	Fertile
Litter size	3–7
Weaning age	20–26 d
Breeding duration	12–17 mo
Chromosome number (diploid)	44

Source: Adapted from Harkness et al. (2010).

rior to each globe within the ocular orbit. These exocrine glands secrete lipid- and porphyrin-rich material that lubricates the eyes and conjunctival space. The secretions drain through an opening in the nictitating membrane, down the nasolacrimal duct, to the external nares. Harderian gland secretions appear to play a role in pheromone-mediated behavior, temperature regulation, and protection and lubrication of the eye, and they may influence the retinal–pineal axis. Both sexes have an elliptical, midventral abdominal sebaceous gland covered with coarse hair. The ventral sebaceous gland, used in territorial marking, is nearly twice as large in the male and produces an orange, oily, and musky-scented secretion. The gerbil's dental formula is typical of rodents: 2(I 1/1, C 0/0, P 0/0, M 3/3). Only the incisors continuously grow. The stomach consists of a nonglandular forestomach and a glandular stomach. The adrenal glands are very large relative to the total body weight and are approximately three times larger than those of the rat. The thymus persists into adulthood. Gerbils have a great capacity for temperature regulation and for water and electrolyte conservation.

Sexing gerbils is fairly easy because the male has a prominent, darkly pigmented scrotum and a substantially greater anogenital distance than the female. The female has three body openings in the anogenital region: the urinary papilla, vagina, and anus. Newborn gerbils can be sexed by anogenital distance and by noting the male's larger genital papilla. Both females and males have four pairs of mammary glands, although nipples are only observable in females.

There are several distinctive characteristics of the hematologic and urinary profiles of gerbils. Gerbils frequently exhibit lipemia and hypercholesterolemia even when fed standard rodent diets. The lipemia can be accentuated by feeding high-fat chows or sunflower seeds. The life span of their red blood cells is relatively short, approximately 9–10 days. It is common to see large numbers of reticulocytes and erythrocytes with basophilic stippling in the peripheral blood, especially in young animals. Lymphocytes are the predominant leukocyte. Influenced by their desert ecology, gerbils produce small quantities of highly concentrated urine. Selected hematologic and biochemical values are listed in Appendix 1, "Normal Values."

BREEDING AND REPRODUCTION

Gerbils breed readily throughout the year, but they are not as prolific as mice. They are inclined to periods of nonbreeding, especially during the winter. Controlling light cycles to supply 14 hours of light per day, providing tunnels or huts for hideaways, changing the bedding type, or housing in an opaque cage may encourage nonbreeding gerbils to resume breeding. Pairs should be formed at 8 weeks of age or earlier and should not be separated unless they are incompatible. Breeding pairs are usually monogamous; if one mate is lost, the survivor generally will not accept another (Box 6.1). Compared with other rodents, puberty occurs later in gerbils. They should be bred when they are 10–12 weeks of age. Gerbils are polyestrous, spontaneous ovulators with an estrous cycle length of 4–6 days. They have a fertile postpartum estrus. A female in estrus acts restless and may have a congested vulva.

Box 6.1

Breeding pairs are monogamous; if one mate is lost, the survivor generally will not accept another.

Observation of both male and female behavior is a better guide to the presence of estrus than vaginal smears because the changes in the vaginal epithelium are not obvious as in the mouse or rat. Breeding usually occurs in the late evening. The female is actively pursued by the excited male until she stands to allow mounting. Copulation is characterized by multiple intromissions. A vaginal plug is formed during mating, but it is not readily detectable as it is small and lies deep in the vagina. Duration of gestation is 24–26 days in a nonlactating gerbil. If the female is bred while nursing a large litter or during periods of stress, implantation may be delayed and gestation may be as long as 42 days. The birthing process takes approximately 1 hour and the average litter size is five. Neonates are altricial, born hairless and blind. Their ears open at 3–7 days, hair grows at 7–10 days, and eyes open at 14–20 days of age. Newborns are rarely abandoned or cannibalized, although it is more common with small litters. Both males and females participate in nest building and care of the young. Development of young is somewhat slower in gerbils than in mice or rats. Young gerbils start eating solid foods around 2 weeks of age. Care should be taken to ensure that they can reach the food hopper and water supply. Food pellets can be placed on the cage floor or moistened and placed in a container on the cage floor. Gerbils are typically weaned at 20–26 days of age.

HUSBANDRY

Housing and Environment

Gerbils are best housed in rigid plastic rodent cages with a solid floor and deep bedding. The enclosure should be at least 15 cm (6 in.) in height to provide the animals adequate space to sit upright. Each adult gerbil should be provided with 230 cm^2 (36 $in.^2$) floor area while breeding pairs with litters should be provided 1300 cm^2 (180 $in.^2$). The cage needs to have a secure lid and be designed to prevent escape. Gerbils are active gnawers and burrowers and, although they do not climb well, they can jump. An escaped gerbil will generally return to its cage or move to the middle of a room rather than hide. Ground corncob, hardwood chips, composite recycled paper pellets, and sand are satisfactory for bedding. Cedar and pine shavings are not recommended as they are irritating to the skin and mucous membranes (Box 6.2) and may

Box 6.2

Cedar and pine shavings are not recommended bedding materials because they are irritating to the skin and mucous membranes.

induce hepatic enzymes that may alter normal drug metabolism. Bedding depth should be at least 2 cm (1 in.) to facilitate nest building and burrowing activity. The recommended temperature range for gerbils in a research facility is 20°–26°C (68°–79°F) with a relative humidity between 30% and 50%. Humidity in excess of 50% causes the gerbil's hair coat to become matted and wet. Providing a container of sand in the cage has been reported to be helpful in preventing oily coats. Ventilation should provide 10–15 air changes per hour. The light cycle is usually controlled by a timing device to provide 12 hours of light per day although 14 hours of daylight may improve breeding. Noise should be minimized in gerbil housing areas to decrease incidence of spontaneous seizure activity. Housing gerbils with other species should be avoided because interspecies transmission of diseases (e.g., *Salmonella* spp., *Bordetella bronchiseptica*, and *Syphacia*) can occur.

Sanitation

Gerbil caging requires less frequent cleaning than do the cages of other rodents because gerbils produce only a few drops of urine daily and their fecal pellets are small, dry, and hard. Ammonia levels have been shown to remain within acceptable limits for up to 6 weeks in pair-housed breeding gerbils housed in individually ventilated cages. The *Guide for the Care and Use of Laboratory Animals* (ILAR, 2011) recommends cages and cage accessories be sanitized at least once every 2 weeks. Cages, bottles, and feed hoppers can be disinfected with chemicals, hot water 61.6°–82.2°C (143°–180°F), or a combination of both. Detergents and chemical disinfectants enhance the effectiveness of hot water, but they must be thoroughly rinsed from the surfaces of the item. Refer to Chapter 4 for a more detailed description of disinfection methods.

Environmental Enrichment and Social Housing

An animal's social needs should be carefully considered when housing animals in the laboratory environment. Ideally, enrichment should increase the normal behavior for the species and decrease abnormal or stereotypic behaviors. Exercise wheels, items for hiding (e.g., PVC piping, huts, and tunnels), sufficient bedding for burrowing, and materials that can be shredded for nesting can be used to provide environmental enrichment (Figure 6.1). Clear communication between the principal investigator, the IACUC, and the facility veterinarian regarding the introduction or standard use of any enrichment item is vital to minimize introducing research variability.

Feeding and Watering

Gerbils should be fed a pelleted rodent chow that contains 16%–22% protein. They will consume an average of 5–8 g/100 g of body weight per day. Diet should be provided *ad libitum* in a food hopper. Food provided in wire bar feeders may lead to lower body weights in weanling and adult gerbils in comparison to animals fed with food in food hoppers (J feeders). Although gerbils prefer sunflower seeds to pelleted chows, these are not satisfactory as a balanced food source. Sunflower seeds are low in calcium and high in fat and do not meet the nutritional needs of the species.

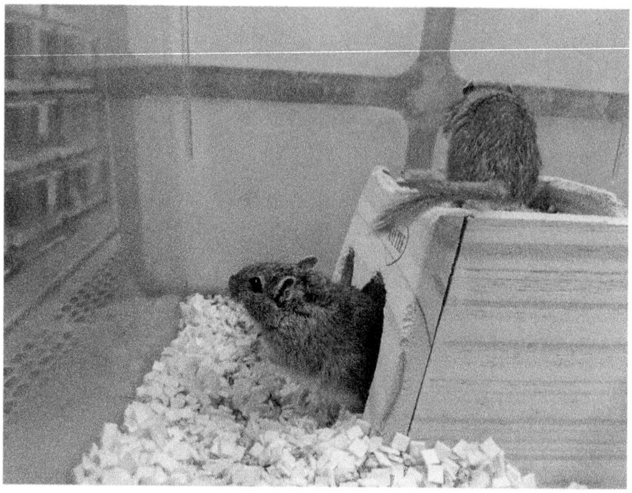

Fig 6.1. A hut used as enrichment for pair-housed gerbils. (*Source:* Photo courtesy of C. Thurman, New York University—Washington Square.)

Feeding excessive amounts of seeds can cause obesity, which can shorten a gerbil's life span. Gerbils, especially females, typically hoard food. Fresh, potable water should be supplied *ad libitum* by bottles, water pouches, or an automated watering system. Adults drink an average of 4–7 mL/100 g of body weight per day.

TECHNIQUES

Handling and Restraint

Although not inclined to bite, gerbils are quick and can leap great distances in an effort to escape. A gerbil may be lifted from its cage by grasping the base of the tail. Care must be taken not to grasp the tip of the tail as a degloving injury may result, in which the tail skin is pulled off to expose the underlying vertebrae (Box 6.3). A gerbil can also be scooped up in the palm of the hand; however, it should be held firmly. To restrain for examination or manipulation, first hold the base of the tail with one hand, then grasp the scruff of the neck with the other hand, as shown in Figure 6.2. Alternatively, the gerbil may be grasped by placing a hand over the gerbil's back to enclose the body firmly, as shown in Figure 6.3. Gerbils resist being placed on their back and tend to struggle. Injections or manipulations are more readily accomplished when animals are held in an upright position.

Box 6.3

Care must be taken not to grasp the tip of the tail as a degloving injury may result, in which the tail skin is pulled off to expose the underlying vertebrae.

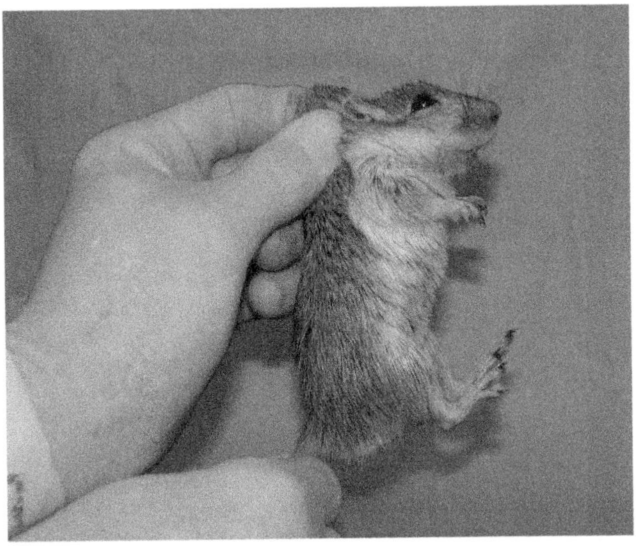

Fig 6.2. Two-hand method of gerbil restraint. (*Source:* Photo courtesy of M. Tear.)

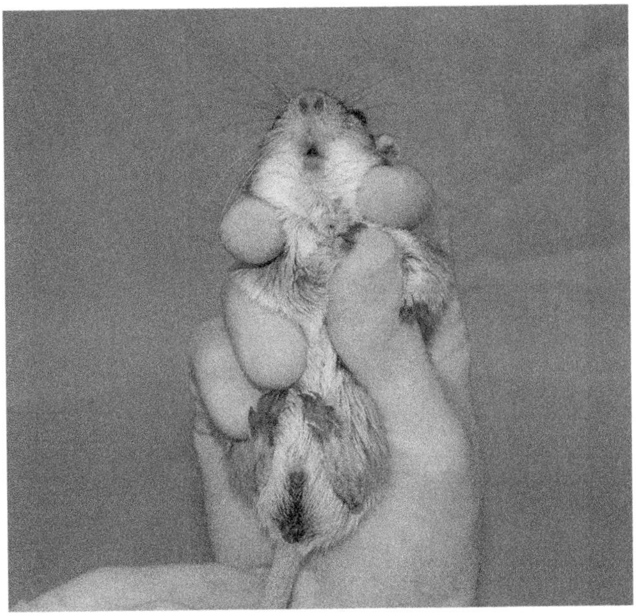

Fig 6.3. One-hand method of gerbil restraint. (*Source:* Photo courtesy of M. Tear.)

Identification

In the research setting, cage cards are most often used for general identification. Methods to permanently identify individual gerbils include ear punching, ear tagging, or subcutaneous (SC) placement of a microchip for quick electronic identification. Dyes, permanent markers, and fur clipping can be used as temporary identification methods.

Blood Collection

Assuming the animal is mature, healthy, and on an adequate plane of nutrition, the blood volume of most species averages 7% of the body weight in grams. Table 6.2 lists approximate adult gerbil blood volumes. A typical rule of thumb for blood withdrawal suggests that up to 10% of the circulating blood volume can be withdrawn from normal, healthy animals every 2–3 weeks with minimal adverse effect. If greater than 10% total blood volume is removed during a single collection, the blood volume should be replaced with lactated Ringer's or other physiologic solution. Small amounts of blood (0.1–0.3 mL) are best obtained from the lateral saphenous vein. Other sites for small blood volume collection are the lateral tail vein and the submandibular vein. Larger blood samples can be obtained from an anesthetized animal by retro-orbital puncture, jugular venous puncture, or cardiac puncture. Cardiac puncture is risky and normally is performed only if the animal will be euthanized prior to anesthetic recovery.

Urine Collection

Collecting urine from a gerbil can be a challenge because of the small quantities that are produced daily. Handling stress commonly causes gerbils to urinate. Metabolic cages can be useful for urine collection when necessary.

Drug Administration

Small scales are useful for obtaining accurate body weights to calculate a medication dose. Most drug administration techniques used in small animal practice can be used with gerbils when modified to fit their small size. Dosage accuracy is increased through dilution of drugs to create a more manageable volume and by use of a tuberculin syringe. Medication can be administered orally by mixing the medication in the water or feed. This method should only be used if the animal's consumption of the medicated food or water can be assured. If more accurate dosing is necessary, a syringe may be used to place the medication in the oral cavity or a small, ball-tipped gavage needle can be used to administer the medication directly into the stomach. Small-gauge hypodermic needles, such as 23 or 25 gauge, should be used for parenteral injections. Medication can be administered by subcutaneous (SC) injection using the skin over the shoulders, provided that the administered agent is not excessively irritating. A maximum volume of 3–4 mL is suggested. Because of the risk of accidental sciatic nerve injury, small muscle mass, and stress of restraint from extending the leg, the intraperitoneal (IP) route of drug administration is recommended over the intramuscular route. If intramuscular injections are required, volumes should be no

Table 6.2. Adult gerbil blood volumes and suggested sample size

	Volume (mL)
Total blood	4.4–8.0
Single sample	0.5–1.0
Exsanguination	2–4

Source: Adapted from Harkness et al. (2010).
Note: Values are approximate.

Table 6.3. Maximum adult gerbil dosing volumes

Route	Volume (mL)
IP	2–3
SC	3–4
IM	0.1
IV	0.3
PO	1.5

Source: Adapted from Harkness and Wagner (1995) and Lukas (1999).

greater than 0.1 mL. For the gerbil, the IP procedure is modified slightly from that of the mouse or rat as gerbils detest being placed on their backs. The gerbil should be restrained and held vertically to prevent it from struggling during the injection. Intraperitoneal injections, with a maximum volume of 2–3 mL, should be given in the lower quadrant of the abdomen, lateral to the midline. The lateral tail vein is a common site for intravenous injections. Although technically challenging, the lateral saphenous vein can also be used for intravenous injections. The maximum dosing volumes are summarized in Table 6.3.

Anesthesia, Surgery, and Postoperative Care

A variety of agents that can be used to tranquilize and anesthetize gerbils are listed in Table 6.4. Preanesthetic fasting is not recommended because the gerbil has a high metabolic rate and there is potential for inducing hypoglycemia and hypothermia. The use of acepromazine in this species is not recommended because it lowers the seizure threshold. Single-injection anesthesia techniques are generally used to minimize handling stress. Mixtures of ketamine with xylazine administered by the IP route produce fairly consistent anesthesia. Gerbils can be anesthetized through the use of an induction chamber or masked down with an inhalation agent delivered from a precision vaporizer. When using inhalation agents, care must be used to scavenge anesthetic gases to ensure the safety of personnel working with the animal or in the general area. Isoflurane and sevoflurane should be administered via a precision vaporizer with a mask or nose-cone apparatus in conjunction with a nonrebreathing system. Alternatively, very brief (~1–2 minutes) anesthesia can be produced through the use of a simple anesthetic chamber. See Chapter 4 for additional information.

Gerbils may show an idiosyncratic writhing before entering a surgical plane of anesthesia. This should not be confused with light anesthesia. The depth of anesthesia can be determined by using a combination of reflexes such as the righting reflex, pedal withdrawal reflex, and the abdominal pinch reflex. Muscle tone and purposeful movement in response to painful stimuli may also be used as indicators of anesthetic depth. Ocular position and the palpebral reflex are inconsistent and unreliable indicators of anesthetic depth in the gerbil.

While anesthetized, gerbils should have a sterile, bland ophthalmic ointment placed in their normally protruding eyes to prevent exposure keratitis. Use of a circulating water heating blanket or other suitable heating source designed for use with animals promotes euthermia and is recommended. Generic, electric heating pads should never be placed in direct contact with the animal as they may cause thermal burns.

Table 6.4. Anesthetic agents and tranquilizers used in gerbils

Drug	Dosage	Route	Reference
Inhalants			
Isoflurane	1%–4% to effect	Inhalation	Wixson (1994)
Sevoflurane	To effect	Inhalation	Morrisey and Carpenter (2004)
Injectables			
Acepromazine	Not recommended, lowers seizure threshold		
Alphaxalone/alphadolone	80–120 mg/kg	IP	Flecknell (2016)
Dexmedetomidine	0.05–0.1 mg/kg	IP	Flecknell (2016)
Diazepam	5 mg/kg	IP	Flecknell (2016)
Fentanyl-fluanisone	0.5–1 mg/kg	IP	Flecknell (2016)
Fentanyl-fluanisone	0.3 mL/kg	IP	Flecknell (2016)
+ diazepam	5 mg/kg	IP	
Fentanyl	0.05 mg/kg	SC	Flecknell (2016)
+ metomidate	50 mg/kg	SC	
Ketamine	50 mg/kg	IP	Flecknell (2016)
+ diazepam	5–10 mg/kg	IP	
Ketamine	75 mg/kg	IP	Flecknell (2016)
+ dexmedetomidine	0.25 mg/kg	IP	
Ketamine	50 mg/kg	IP	Flecknell (2016)
+ xylazine	2 mg/kg	IP	
Medetomidine	0.1–0.2 mg/kg	IP	Flecknell (2016)
Midazolam	5 mg/kg	IP	Flecknell (2016)
Pentobarbital	60–80 mg/kg	IP	Flecknell (2016)
Tiletamine-zolazepam	20 mg/kg	IP	Huerkamp (1995)
+ xylazine	10 mg/kg	IP	

IP = intraperitoneal and SC = subcutaneous.

Common clinical surgeries in gerbils include simple castration, tail amputation, or growth removal. Care should be taken to close the inguinal canals during castration to prevent intestinal entrapment. In research, one of the most common surgical procedures is to produce stroke by ligating one of the carotid arteries to cause cerebral infarction. Surgeries should be performed in an aseptic manner. Prevention of blood loss is an important consideration.

The anesthetized gerbil should be placed on a clean, dry paper or cloth towel and recovered in an escape-proof incubator. Small-particle bedding materials are contraindicated in recovery cages because they can stick to the eyes, nose, and mouth of the recovering animal and may be aspirated. Postoperative care should include hydration of the anesthetized animal (e.g., SC or IP injection of a warmed solution such as saline, saline–dextrose, lactated Ringer's), and support of normal body temperature. Hypostatic pulmonary congestion should be prevented by turning the animal at least every 30 minutes. It is important to maintain hydration and nutrition levels in the postoperative period to support normal metabolic processes and gut physiology.

Table 6.5. Analgesic agents used in gerbils

Drug	Dosage	Route	Reference
Acetylsalicylic acid	100–150 mg/kg q4h	PO	Heard (1993)
Buprenorphine	0.01–0.05 mg/kg q8h	SC, IP	Flecknell (2009)
Butorphanol	1–5 mg/kg q4h	SC	Heard (1993)
Carprofen	5 mg/kg q24h	SC	Pollack (2002)
Flunixin meglumine	2.5 mg/kg q12–24h	SC	Heard (1993)
Ketoprofen	5 mg/kg	SC	Pollack (2002)
Meperidine	20 mg/kg q2–3h	SC	Heard (1993)
Meloxicam	1 mg/kg q24h	SC	Flecknell (2009)
Morphine	2–5 mg/kg q2–4h	SC	Heard (1993)
Nalbuphine	4–8 mg/kg	SC	Mason (1997)
Oxymorphone	0.2–0.5 mg/kg q6–12h	SC	Heard (1993)
Pentazocine	10 mg/kg q2–4h	SC	Heard (1993)
Piroxicam	3 mg/kg q24h	PO	Harkness et al. (2010)
Tramadol	5–10 mg/kg q12–24h	PO	Morrisey and Carpenter (2011)

IP = intraperitoneal; PO = per os; and SC = subcutaneous.

Select commercially available supportive and critical care products for laboratory animals are provided in Appendix 3.

Table 6.5 lists analgesics than can be used. Gerbils that are in pain may have piloerection, a hunched posture, a reluctance to move, and may exhibit decreased interactions with their cagemates. Carprofen is recommended for mild postoperative discomfort. Buprenorphine works well to control acute or chronic visceral pain but causes more sedation.

Imaging Techniques

Great advances have been made in rodent and small animal imaging over the last decade. For a detailed description of current imaging modalities, see Chapter 3.

Euthanasia

Methods of euthanasia must be consistent with the most current American Veterinary Medical Association (AVMA) *Guidelines for the Euthanasia of Animals* (AVMA, 2013) and performed by trained personnel. Per AVMA Guidelines, "Carbon dioxide is acceptable with conditions for euthanasia in those species where aversion or distress can be minimized. Carbon dioxide exposure using a gradual fill method is less likely to cause pain due to nociceptor activation by carbonic acid prior to onset of unconsciousness; a displacement rate from 10% to 30% of the chamber volume/min is recommended.... CO_2 flow should be maintained for at least 1 minute after respiratory arrest." Conscious animals should never be placed in an area prefilled with 100% CO_2 as this can cause pain of the mucous membranes. Furthermore, only a pure form of CO_2 must be used, such as from a commercially supplied cylinder. Neonates are resistant to hypoxia and require greater duration of exposure. For this reason, other methods may be preferred for this age group. Studies have shown that the method of

CO_2 euthanasia can result in significant differences in immunologic and hematologic variables; thus consistency of method may be important in accurate interpretation of research data. Other acceptable methods of euthanasia include overdose of an inhalant anesthetic and IP administration of a barbiturate anesthetic at three to four times the anesthetic dose.

THERAPEUTIC AGENTS

Suggested gerbil antimicrobial and antifungal drug doses are listed in Table 6.6. Antiparasitic agents are listed in Table 6.7 and miscellaneous drugs are listed in Table 6.8.

INTRODUCTION TO DISEASES OF GERBILS

Most laboratory rodent colonies today are relatively free of the viruses, bacteria, parasites, and fungi that cause clinical disease. However, sporadic outbreaks may still occur, and it is important for individuals to have a basic knowledge of the most

Table 6.6. Antimicrobial and antifungal agents used in gerbils

Drug	Dosage	Route	Reference
Amikacin	2–5 mg/kg q8–12h	SC	Harkness et al. (2010)
Ampicillin	6–30 mg/kg q8h	PO	Anderson (1994)
Cephalexin	25 mg/kg q24h	SC	Flecknell (2016)
Chloramphenicol	50–200 mg/kg q8h	PO	Burgmann and Percy (1993)
	30–50 mg/kg q12h	SC	Burgmann and Percy (1993)
Ciprofloxacin	7–20 mg/kg q12h	PO	Harkness et al. (2010)
Doxycycline	2.5 mg/kg q12h	PO	Allen et al. (1993)
Enrofloxacin	5–10 mg/kg q12h	PO, SC	Harkness et al. (2010)
Gentamicin	2–4 mg/kg q8h	SC	Harkness et al. (2010)
Griseofulvin	25–50 mg/kg q12h for 14–60d	PO	Harkness et al. (2010)
	1.5% in DMSO for 5–7d	Topical	Harkness et al. (2010)
Ketoconazole	10–40 mg/kg q24h for 14d	PO	Rollin and Kesel (1995)
Metronidazole	7.5 mg/70–90 g animal q8h	PO	Collins (1995)
Neomycin	100 mg/kg q24h	PO	Burgmann and Percy (1993)
Oxytetracycline	10 mg/kg q8h	PO	Burgmann and Percy (1993)
	20 mg/kg q24h	SC	McKellar (1989)
Sulfadimethoxine	10–15 mg/kg q12h	PO	Harkness et al. (2010)
	10–20 mg/kg q8–12h	PO	Burgmann and Percy (1993)
Trimethoprim/sulfa	30 mg/kg q12–24h	PO, SC	Harkness et al. (2010)
Tylosin	10 mg/kg q24h	PO, SC	Collins (1995)

DMSO = dimethyl sulfoxide; PO = per os; and SC = subcutaneous.

Table 6.7. Antiparasitic agents used in gerbils

Drug	Dosage	Route	Reference
Amitraz	1.4 mL/L water using cotton-ball application q14d for 3–6 treatments	Topical	Harkness et al. (2010)
Fenbendazole	20 mg/kg q24h for 5 d	PO	Harkness et al. (2010)
Ivermectin	0.2 mg/kg q7d for 3 wk	PO, SC	Anderson (1994)
Pyrantel pamoate	50 mg/kg	PO	Rollin and Kesel (1995)
Praziquantel	30 mg/kg q14d for 3 treatments	PO	Burke (1995)
Pyrethrin powder	3 times per week for 3 wk	Topical	Anderson (1994)
Thiabendazole	100 mg/kg q24h for 5 d	PO	Allen et al. (1993)

PO = per os; and SC = subcutaneous.

Table 6.8. Miscellaneous agents used in gerbils

Drug	Dosage	Route	Reference
Atipamezole	0.1–1 mg/kg	SC, IP, IV	Flecknell (2016)
Atropine	0.05–0.1 mg/kg	SC	Harkness and Wagner (1995)
Cimetidine	5–10 mg/kg q6–12h	PO	Allen et al. (1993)
Dexamethasone	0.5–2 mg/kg then decreasing dose q12h for 3–14 d	PO, SC	Harkness and Wagner (1995)
Doxapram	5–10 mg/kg	IV, IP	Harkness (1993)
Furosemide	5–10 mg/kg q12h	SC	Allen et al. (1993)
Glycopyrrolate	0.01–0.02 mg/kg	SC	Huerkamp (1995)
Naloxone	0.01–0.1 mg/kg	SC, IP	Huerkamp (1995)
Oxytocin	0.2–3 IU/kg	SC	Anderson (1994)
Vitamin K	1–10 mg/kg q24h for 4–6 d	IM	Harkness and Wagner (1995)
Yohimbine	0.5–1 mg/kg	IV	Harkness and Wagner (1995)

IM = intramuscular; IP = intraperitoneal; IV = intravenous; PO = per os; and SC = subcutaneous.

common infectious agents and how to respond to them. Presented here is a general overview of common bacterial, viral, fungal, and parasitic agents of gerbils and some standard diagnostic and treatment modalities.

A sick gerbil typically presents with similar clinical signs regardless of the cause. General signs of illness include weight loss, porphyrin staining of the eyes or nose, loss of body and coat condition, and reduced activity. Hypothermia, anorexia, and dehydration are common and need to be treated aggressively. Supportive care in the form of warmed fluids given IP or SC and dietary supplementation are important. Unlike the hamster, guinea pig, and rabbit, whose normal intestinal microflora is highly susceptible to antibiotics with a Gram-positive spectrum, the gerbil can be safely treated with a wide variety of antibiotics. However, fatal cases of *Clostridium difficile* overgrowth subsequent to amoxicillin administration as well as ascending paralysis and death from dihydrostreptomycin administration have been reported, so careful monitoring of gerbils on any antibiotic regimen is recommended.

Bacterial Diseases

Tyzzer's Disease

Gerbils are highly susceptible to *Clostridium piliforme*, the causative agent of Tyzzer's disease. The disease is most frequently seen at weaning age, but adults can be affected. Mortality is high in young animals 3–7 weeks of age. Poor sanitation and stress are important contributing factors of disease. Affected animals typically have a rough hair coat, are lethargic and anorexic, and die within 1–3 days of infection. Diarrhea may be absent or mild in gerbils, in contrast to other species which show a profuse watery diarrhea. Transmission is thought to be fecal–oral. Characteristically, infected animals have hepatomegaly with numerous gray, white, or yellow foci measuring 1–2 mm in diameter. Edema and hemorrhage of the intestines, particularly in the ileocecal area, may also be present. Oxytetracycline or tetracycline can be used to suppress, but not eliminate, infection. Supplemental fluid therapy can be provided if indicated. In an outbreak, it is best to cull ill animals. Infectious spores can remain in the environment for prolonged periods of time and are resistant to numerous disinfectants. Therefore, all cages and feeding and watering equipment should be sterilized. Microisolation cages can be used to prevent cage-to-cage transmission.

Salmonellosis

Adult gerbils are fairly resistant to *Salmonella* spp.; however, disease has been observed in young gerbils. Clinical signs are generally nonspecific and include dehydration, depression, emaciation, and rough hair coat. The abdomen is frequently distended and diarrhea may or may not be present. Testicular enlargement may be observed in males. Sudden death may occur. Animals that recover may become asymptomatic carriers and transmit infection to other animals or humans. Therefore, animals that are positive on bacteriological culture should be culled from the colony. Treatment is contraindicated due to the zoonotic potential of the organism.

Staphylococcal and Streptococcal Infections

Beta-hemolytic *Staphylococcus aureus* has been associated with a diffuse dermatitis in young gerbils, with the face, feet, legs, and ventral body surface affected. In addition, bite wounds, nose abrasions secondary to burrowing, and the ventral sebaceous gland can become infected with *Staphylococcus* spp., *Streptococcus* spp., and other bacteria. Daily treatment with a topical antibacterial preparation is often beneficial. Tetracycline, sulfonamides, or chloramphenicol can be used for parenteral treatment.

Viral Diseases

No clinically significant and naturally occurring viral infections of gerbils have yet been identified.

Parasitic Diseases

Demodex

Alopecia and dermatitis associated with *Demodex* spp. have been reported in gerbils. Demodex mite infestations are not noted to be a problem in clinically healthy animals. Old age and debilitation are important predisposing factors to disease development. Gerbils can be treated similarly to hamsters, with a dilute solution of amitraz applied topically with a cotton ball.

Pinworms

Gerbils are susceptible to infection with several species of oxyurids, including *Syphacia muris* and *S. obvelata*. *Syphacia* spp. live in the distal region of the intestinal tract and can occasionally be diagnosed by applying clear adhesive tape to the perineum and then examining it microscopically for the presence of ova. Both *S. muris* and *S. obvelata* can be transmitted between gerbils as well as between other species (*S. muris*: mice, rats, hamsters; *S. obvelata*: mice). In contrast, gerbils are the primary natural host of *Dentostomella translucida*, which resides in the proximal small intestine. *Dentostomella* infection is detected by the fecal flotation method. Clinical disease is not observed in infected animals. Ivermectin, fenbendazole, or thiabendazole are effective treatments.

Tapeworms

Cestodiasis in gerbils is normally subclinical; however, severe infections with the dwarf tapeworm, *Rodentolepis nana*, have been reported. Infections have been associated with debilitation and diarrhea. *R. nana* is a concern because of its direct life cycle, transmission to other rodents, and zoonotic potential. Infected animals should be culled to eliminate the public health risk.

Neoplasia

The incidence of spontaneous tumors is relatively low in the gerbil. Neoplasms occur primarily in aged gerbils over 2 years of age. The most commonly recognized neoplasms in gerbils are squamous cell carcinoma of the ventral marking gland in males, ovarian granulosa cell tumors in females, adrenocortical tumors, cutaneous tumors such as squamous cell carcinoma and melanoma of the ear and foot, and renal and splenic hemangiomas.

Miscellaneous Conditions

Nasal Dermatitis (Sore Nose)

Nasal dermatitis, also known as facial eczema or sore nose, is most commonly encountered in recently weaned and adult gerbils. Affected animals initially exhibit alopecia around the external nares and upper labial region with a varying degree of red-brown, moist dermatitis and ulceration that may extend over the head, forelimbs, and torso. Chemical irritation of the skin by porphyrin-containing Harderian gland secretions is thought to be the primary cause. Mechanical trauma due to excessive burrowing may be an important contributing factor. Secondary infections with *Staphylococcus* spp. are common. Using sand as bedding material, providing access to a sand bath, cleaning the face, application of a topical antibacterial ointment, and removing stress factors may be helpful in treating the condition.

Tail Degloving (Tail Slip)

The gerbil tail is especially sensitive to degloving wounds (Figure 6.4), particularly if it is handled roughly or by the tip. During a traumatic degloving event, the skin of the distal tail is pulled off, exposing the underlying vertebral tissue. If a tail degloving injury occurs, the tail should be amputated at the level of the skin break and the remaining skin closed over the tail tip.

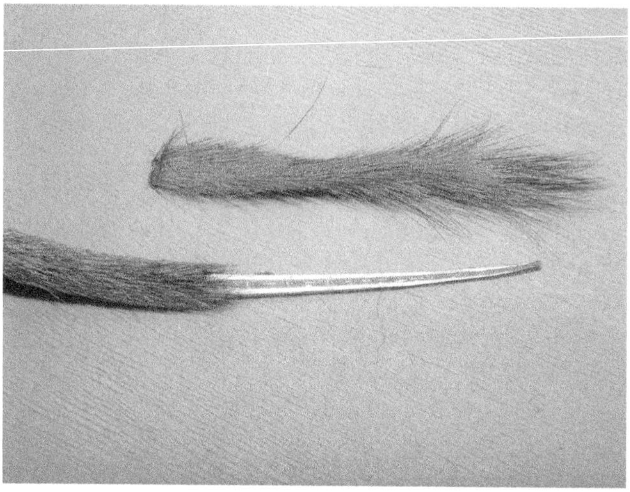

Fig 6.4. Degloved tail. (*Source:* Photo courtesy of M. Tear.)

Hair Loss (Barbering and Bald Nose)

Gerbils may barber each other if housed in overcrowded conditions or as a stereotypy. The hair around the base of the tail or along the tail is most frequently affected.

Bald nose can occur in gerbils housed in cages with wire bar feeders, through which gerbils may aggressively push their noses to obtain food. Selecting an alternative feeding method resolves the problem. A similar condition can occur in gerbils that have vigorous burrowing habits. Providing cage enrichment in the form of tunnels or nesting materials usually diminishes the behavior.

Epileptiform Seizures

Gerbils exhibit spontaneous epileptiform seizures that vary from hypnotic and cataleptic to grand mal. The seizures may be initiated by handling, stress, loud noises, or novel environment. Typically, the episodes are brief, lasting up to a few minutes. Animals resume normal activity soon afterward and show no ill effects. Frequent handling of young animals has been reported to decrease episodes. Treatment is generally not recommended.

Chromodacryorrhea

The Harderian gland in the orbit produces porphyrin-rich secretions. The porphyrins are normally removed by grooming; however, when there is excessive secretion, a red crust appears in the medial canthus of the eye or on the end of the nose. Animals that are stressed or ill commonly exhibit these "red tears."

Malocclusion

Malocclusion is rarely a problem in the gerbil but may occur as a result of upper incisor loss with overgrowth of the lower teeth. Trimming the teeth with a dental bur may be necessary to prevent overgrowth.

Cystic Ovaries

Cystic ovaries are very common in females over 2 years of age and can be associated with reduced litter size, infertility, symmetrical alopecia, abdominal swelling, dyspnea, lethargy, and anorexia.

Chronic Interstitial Nephritis

Aged gerbils are susceptible to chronic interstitial nephritis. Clinical signs include polyuria, polydipsia, and weight loss.

Aural Cholesteatoma

Spontaneous aural cholesteatomas frequently occur in gerbils over 2 years of age. Clinical signs include head tilt and keratin mass accumulation in the external ear canal.

Ocular Proptosis

Aged gerbils can develop ocular proptosis, including protrusion of the nictitating membrane.

BIBLIOGRAPHY

Allen, D. G., J. K. Pringle, and D. A. Smith. 1993. *Handbook of Veterinary Drugs*. Philadelphia, PA: JB Lippincott.

American Veterinary Medical Association (AVMA). 2013. *AVMA Guidelines for the Euthanasia of Animals*. Available at http://www.avma.org/KB/Policies/Documents/euthanasia.pdf [accessed August 9, 2018].

Anderson, N. L. 1994. Basic husbandry and medicine of pocket pets. In *Saunders Manual of Small Animal Practice*, S. J. Birchard and R. G. Sherding (eds.), pp. 1363–1389. Philadelphia, PA: WB Saunders.

Bergin, I. L., N. S. Taylor, P. R. Nambiar, and J. G. Fox. 2005. Eradication of enteric helicobacters in Mongolian gerbils is complicated by the occurrence of *Clostridium difficile* enterotoxemia. Comp Med 55(3): 265–268.

Burgmann, P., and D. H. Percy. 1993. Antimicrobial drug use in rodents and rabbits. In *Antimicrobial Therapy in Veterinary Medicine*, 2nd ed., J. F. Prescott and J. D. Baggot (eds.), pp. 524–541. Ames, IA: Iowa State University Press.

Burke, T. J. 1995. "Wet tail" in hamsters and other diarrheas of small rodents. In *Kirk's Current Veterinary Therapy XII—Small Animal Practice*, J. D. Bonagura (ed.), pp. 1336–1339. Philadelphia, PA: WB Saunders.

Collins, B. R. 1995. Antimicrobial drug use in rabbits, rodents, and other small mammals. In *Antimicrobial Therapy in Caged Birds and Exotic Pets*, pp. 3–10. Trenton, NJ: Veterinary Learning Systems.

Donnelly, T. M., I. Bergin, and M. Ihrig. 2015. Biology and diseases of other rodents. In *Laboratory Animal Medicine*, 3rd ed. J.G. Fox, L. Anderson, G. Otto, K. Pritchett-Corning, and M. Whary (eds), pp. 285–349. Amsterdam: Academic Press.

Flecknell, P. A. 1997. Medetomidine and atipamezole: Potential uses in laboratory animals. Lab Anim (NY) 26(2): 21–25.

Flecknell, P. A. 2009. *Laboratory Animal Anaesthesia*, 3rd ed. London: Academic Press.

Flecknell, P. A. 2016. *Laboratory Animal Anaesthesia*, 4th ed. Oxford: Academic Press.

Harkness, J. E. 1993. *A Practitioner's Guide to Domestic Rodents*. Lakewood, CO: American Animal Hospital Association.

Harkness, J. E., P. V. Turner, S. VandeWoude, and C. L. Wheler. 2010. *Harkness and Wagner's Biology and Medicine of Rabbits and Rodents*, 5th ed. Ames, IA: Wiley-Blackwell.

Harkness, J. E., and J. E. Wagner. 1995. *Biology and Medicine of Rabbits and Rodents*, 4th ed. Philadelphia, PA: Williams & Wilkins.

Heard, D. J. 1993. Principles and techniques of anesthesia and analgesia for exotic practice. Vet Clin North Am Small Anim Pract 23: 1301–1327.

Huerkamp, M. J. 1995. Anesthesia and postoperative management of rabbits and pocket pets. In *Kirk's Current Veterinary Therapy XII—Small Animal Practice*, J. D. Bonagura (ed.), pp. 1322–1327. Philadelphia, PA: WB Saunders.

Institute of Laboratory Animal Resources (ILAR). 2011. *Guide for the Care and Use of Laboratory Animals*, 8th ed. ILAR, National Research Council. Washington, DC: National Academies Press.

Johnson-Delaney, C. 1999. Postoperative management of small mammals. Exotic DVM 1(5): 19–21.

Lukas, V. 1999. Volume guidelines for compound administration. In *The Care and Feeding of an IACUC*, M. L. Podolsky and V. S. Lukas (eds.), p. 187. Boca Raton, FL: CRC Press.

Mason, D. E. 1997. Anesthesia, analgesia, and sedation for small mammals. In *Ferrets, Rabbits, and Rodents: Clinical Medicine and Surgery*, E. V. Hillyer and K. E. Quesenberry (eds.), pp. 378–397. Philadelphia, PA: WB Saunders.

McKellar, Q. A. 1989. Drug dosages for small mammals. Practice (March): 57–61.

Morrisey, J. K., and J. W. Carpenter. 2004. Formulary. In *Ferrets, Rabbits, and Rodents: Clinical Medicine and Surgery*, K. E. Quesenberry and J. W. Carpenter (eds.), pp. 436–444. St. Louis, MO: WB Saunders.

Morrisey, J. K., and J. W. Carpenter. 2011. Drug formulary. In *Ferrets, Rabbits, and Rodents: Clinical Medicine and Surgery*, K. E. Quesenberry and J. W. Carpenter (eds.), pp. 566–575. St. Louis, MO: WB Saunders.

Mulder G.B., K.R. Pritchett-Corning, M.A. Gramlich, and A.E. Crocker. 2010. Method of feed presentation affects the growth of Mongolian gerbils (*Meriones unguiculatus*). JAALAS 49(1): 36–39.

Pollack, C. 2002. Postoperative management of the exotic animal patient. Vet Clin North Am Small Anim Pract 5: 183–212.

Rollin, B. E., and M. L. Kesel. 1995. *The Experimental Animal in Biomedical Research. Volume II: Care, Husbandry, and Wellbeing. An Overview by Species*. Boca Raton, FL: CRC Press.

Wixson, S. K. 1994. Rabbits and rodents: Anesthesia and analgesia. In *Research Animal Anesthesia, Analgesia and Surgery*, A. C. Smith and M. M. Swindle (eds.), pp. 59–92. Greenbelt, MD: Scientists Center for Animal Welfare.

FURTHER READING

Barthold S.W., S.M. Griffey, and D.H. Percy. 2016. *Pathology of Laboratory Rodents and Rabbits*, 4th ed. Ames, IA: Wiley-Blackwell.

Batchelder, M., L. S. Keller, M. B. Sauer, and W. L. West. 2012. Gerbils. In *The Laboratory Rabbit, Guinea Pig, Hamster, and Other Rodents*, M. A. Suckow, K. A. Stevens, and R. P. Wilson (eds.), pp. 275–279. San Diego, CA: Academic Press.

Bauck, L. 1989. Ophthalmic conditions in pet rabbits and rodents. Compend Contin Educ Pract Vet 11(3): 258–268.

Bresnahan, J. F., G. D. Smith, R. H. Lentsch, W. G. Barnes, and J. E. Wagner. 1983. Nasal dermatitis in the Mongolian gerbil. Lab Anim Sci 33(3): 258–263.

Donnelly, T. M., and F. W. Quimby. 2002. Biology and disease of other rodents. In *Laboratory Animal Medicine*, 2nd ed., J. G. Fox, L. C. Anderson, F. M. Loew, and F. W. Quimby (eds.), pp. 275–279. San Diego, CA: Academic Press.

Lavin, L. M. 2007. Avian and exotic radiography. In *Radiography in Veterinary Technology*, 4th ed., pp. 294–301. St. Louis, MO: WB Saunders.

Lussier G., and F. M. Loew. 1970. Natural *Hymenolepis nana* infection in Mongolian gerbils (*Meriones unguiculatus*). Can Vet J 11(5): 105–107.

Moore, D. M. 1995. Hamsters and gerbils. In *The Experimental Animal in Biomedical Research*, B. E. Rollin and M. L. Kesel (eds.), pp. 309–333. Boca Raton, FL: CRC Press.

Norris, M. L., and C. E. Adams. 1972. Incidence of cystic ovaries and reproductive performance in the Mongolian gerbil, *Meriones unguiculatus*. Lab Anim 6(3): 337–342.

Palm, D. K., and P. Holländer. 2007. A procedure for intravenous injection using external jugular vein in Mongolian gerbil (*Meriones unguiculatus*). Lab Anim 41(3): 403–405.

Payne, A. P. 1994. The harderian gland: A tercentennial review. J Anat 185(Pt 1): 1–49.

Percy, D. H., and S. W. Barthold. 2007. *Pathology of Laboratory Rodents and Rabbits*, 3rd ed. Ames, IA: Wiley-Blackwell.

Thiessen, D. D., A. Clency, and M. Goodwin. 1976. Harderian gland pheromone in the Mongolian gerbil *Meriones unguiculatus*. J Chem Ecol 2(2): 231–238.

Thiessen, D. D., M. Graham, J. Perkins, and S. Marcks. 1977. Temperature regulation and social grooming in the Mongolian gerbil (*Meriones unguiculatus*). Behav Biol 19(3): 279–288.

Vincent, A. L., G. E. Rodrick, and W. A. Sodeman Jr. 1979. The pathology of the Mongolian gerbil (*Meriones unguiculatus*): A review. Lab Anim Sci (5): 645–651.

Wightman, S. R., P. C. Mann, and J. E. Wagner. 1980. Dihydrostreptomycin toxicity in the Mongolian gerbil, *Meriones unguiculatus*. Lab Anim Sci 30(1): 71–75.

Womack, J. E. 1972. Red cell survival in the gerbil (*Meriones unguiculatus*). Comp Biochem Physiol 43(4): 801–804.

CHAPTER 6 REVIEW

Short Answer

1. What anatomic feature do gerbils have that make them an ideal stroke model?
2. Which gland is used for marking territory? How is it different in males vs females?
3. Which organ is quite large relative to total body weight in comparison to mice and rats?
4. What is the gestation length of a nonlactating gerbil?
5. True/False: Gerbil neonates are born precocious.
6. Why do gerbil cages often need less frequent changing than other rodents?
7. What natural behavior does providing deep bedding allow for in a gerbil enclosure?
8. What can result if a gerbil is restrained by the tail improperly?
9. What are the options for collection of small volumes of blood?
10. Why is urine collection particularly challenging in this species?
11. True/False: Preanesthetic fasting is not required in this species due to their high metabolic rate.
12. True/False: Just like hamsters, guinea pigs, and rabbits, many antibiotics are unsafe to use in gerbils due to the sensitivity of the intestinal microflora.
13. What bacterial disease are gerbils highly susceptible to?
14. Which pinworm species are gerbils the primary host for?
15. What husbandry-related changes can be made to treat and care for gerbils with nasal dermatitis?
16. Why is it particularly important to control excess noise in gerbil housing areas?

7 Hamsters

Hamsters are rodents of the family Cricetidae. There are over 50 species, subspecies, and varieties of hamsters. Only two are found in any significant number in laboratories: the golden or Syrian hamster (*Mesocricetus auratus*) and the Chinese or striped hamster (*Cricetulus griseus*). The Syrian is by far the most frequently used, and the specific information provided in this chapter refers primarily to this variety. The adult Syrian weighs approximately 114–140 g and comes in a variety of colors, including reddish golden brown with gray ventrum (wild-type), cinnamon, cream, white, piebald (patches of two or more colors, often including white), and albino. A long-haired variety also exists called a teddy bear; however, this type is not usually seen in research. Their life span is approximately 18–24 months, although they can live up to 3 years. Nearly all Syrian hamsters supplied by US commercial vendors are derived from three or four littermates captured in Syria in 1930. The Chinese hamster is much smaller than the Syrian, weighs approximately 30 g, and is gray-brown with a dark stripe down the back as shown in Figure 7.1. The Siberian or Djungarian hamster (*Phodopus sungorus*), also known as the dwarf or hairy-footed hamster, is infrequently utilized in research. The Siberian hamster is mouse-sized, weighing 30–50 g. This hamster has a short furred tail, grayish dorsal surface with a black dorsal stripe, and white ventrum.

USES

Hamsters are important research animals, although their use has decreased from their peak in the 1970s. Their small size, ease of handling, low care requirements, and relative freedom from spontaneous diseases are positive attributes. Syrian hamsters

Clinical Laboratory Animal Medicine: An Introduction, Fifth Edition.
Lesley A. Colby, Megan H. Nowland, and Lucy H. Kennedy.

Companion website: www.wiley.com/go/colby/clinical

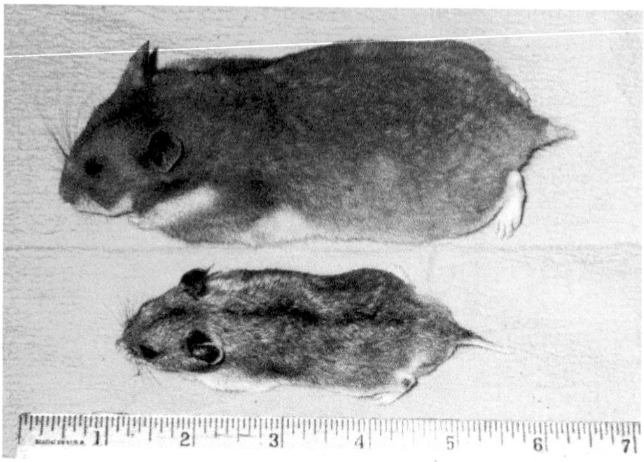

Fig 7.1. Size comparison of Syrian and Chinese hamsters. (*Source:* Photo courtesy of ACLAM.)

have proven valuable in a number of areas of biomedical research, particularly in studies of infectious diseases, cancer, immunology, hypothermia, dental caries, reproductive physiology, cardiomyopathy, thrombosis, prion disease, and circadian rhythm. Chinese hamsters are used as a model of type 1 juvenile-onset diabetes and in cytogenetic studies (the study of chromosomes and their role in heredity), which take advantage of their low diploid chromosome number of 22. Both Syrian and Chinese hamsters have been used in radiobiology research as they are radioresistant (resistant to the effects of radiation).

Multiple inbred strains of hamsters have been developed as animal models of human and animal disease conditions and other research uses. These include the following: BIO 1.50 (muscular dystrophy, carcinogenicity, and dental caries), BIO 2.4 (cystic prostatic hypertrophy), BIO 4.24 (obesity and adrenal cortical tumors), BIO 12.14 (paralysis and muscular dystrophy), BIO 14.6 (cardiomyopathy and muscular dystrophy), BIO 15.16 (carcinogenicity studies), BIO 87.20 (cystic prostatic hypertrophy and carcinogenicity studies), BIO F1D (carcinogenicity studies), and CHF148 (cardiomyopathy).

BEHAVIOR

Hamsters tend to be solitary rather than social animals. Studies have shown that group housing is stressful and can lead to aggression and obesity. Hamsters are generally aggressive and territorial toward unfamiliar hamsters of either sex, but are less apt to fight if housed together at the time of weaning or before they are sexually mature. Females, in particular, are prone to fight or kill other hamsters, especially when pregnant or lactating. Hamsters frequently exhibit agonistic postures but are not naturally aggressive to their handlers. However, they will often bite if suddenly disturbed or if handled roughly. They are easily tamed if handled gently and repeatedly.

In their natural desert environment, hamsters live in deep tunnels that provide cooler temperatures and higher humidity. Like most rodents, they are nocturnal although they do exhibit periods of activity during the day. They are sound sleepers and, upon casual observation, may appear dead. Healthy hamsters are active and spend time storing and transporting food in their distensible cheek pouches. When exercise wheels are provided, they readily run on them and are reported to run up to 8 km (5 mi) per day. They make very little noise except to chatter or screech when hurt, frightened, or fighting.

The hamster is considered a permissive hibernator; it may or may not hibernate, depending upon environmental conditions (Box 7.1). Low light intensity, short day lengths, quietness, and cooler temperatures of approximately 8°C (46°F) induce hibernation. During this period, the hamster has a decreased body temperature with extremely slow respirations and heart rate, yet it remains sensitive to touch. Hibernation is not continuous but consists of 2–3 days of inactivity alternating with short periods of arousal to normal alertness.

ANATOMIC AND PHYSIOLOGIC FEATURES

General biologic and reproductive data for the Syrian hamsters are listed in Table 7.1. The hamster has a stout body with short legs; large, bright black eyes; prominent dark ears; and a stubby tail. It has a large quantity of very loose skin that is covered with dense, soft, short fur. Hamsters have well-developed cheek (buccal) pouches that are located along the lateral neck and head and extend back to the shoulder region. Animals may fill the pouches with food. Females may place newborn pups in their pouches if stressed. When full, the check pouches can be mistaken as abnormal masses of the thorax. The cheek pouches are easily everted in an anesthetized animal, are devoid of glands, and are immunologically privileged sites as they largely lack lymphatic drainage. Transplantation of foreign tissue to the cheek pouch does not cause immunological rejection. Hamsters have a Harderian gland located posterior to each globe in the ocular orbit. These exocrine glands secrete lipid- and porphyrin-rich material that lubricates the eyes and conjunctiva.

Typical of rodents, hamsters have a dental formula of 2(I 1/1, C 0/0, P 0/0, and M 3/3) with fixed roots. The teeth turn yellow-orange with age due to the composition of the dental enamel and, secondary to their shape, tend to retain bits of food near the crowns, predisposing hamsters to dental caries. The mandibular symphysis may not fuse even in adulthood. The stomach is distinctly compartmentalized into a forestomach and a glandular stomach. The nonglandular forestomach acts like a rumen and has a higher pH than the glandular stomach. The digestive tract suggests an adaptation for

Box 7.1

The hamster is considered a permissive hibernator; it may or may not hibernate, depending upon environmental conditions.

Table 7.1. Biologic and reproductive data for Syrian hamsters

Adult body weight: Male	85–130g
Adult body weight: Female	95–150g
Life span	18–24mo
Body temperature	37°–38°C (98.6°–100.4°F)
Heart rate	250–500 beats per minute
Respiratory rate	35–135 breaths per minute
Tidal volume	0.6–1.4mL
Food consumption	8–12g/100g per day
Water consumption: Male	4.5–5mL/100g per day
Water consumption: Female	13.6–14mL/100g per day
Breeding onset: Male	10–14wk
Breeding onset: Female	6–10wk
Estrous cycle length	4d
Gestation period	15–16d
Postpartum estrus	Infertile
Litter size	5–9
Weaning age	20–25d
Breeding duration	10–12mo
Chromosome number (diploid)	44

Source: Adapted from Harkness et al. (2010) and Mulder (2012).

water conservation, having a long duodenum and jejunum, short ileum, large cecum, and long colon. The lungs consist of a large, single left lobe and five smaller lobes on the right side. The hamster kidney has an extremely long papilla that extends out into the ureter, which allows *in vivo* collection of urine samples from single collecting tubules.

Adult hamsters have prominent deposits of brown adipose tissue, the majority of which are located caudal to and between the scapulae. This tissue plays a thermogenic role, particularly in hibernating hamsters and in newborns. Two flank glands, also called hip or costovertebral glands, are present in both sexes but are much more developed in the male. These sebaceous glands are present in each flank region in areas of darkly pigmented and roughened skin that is covered with coarse hairs. The overlying fur may appear wet due to gland excretions. The glands are used to mark territory and are involved in mating behavior. In males, they also play a role in converting testosterone to dihydrotestosterone. They are frequently mistaken as an abnormal feature (e.g., tumor) by those unfamiliar with hamster anatomy.

Differentiation between adult males and females is rather simple and can be determined without handling the animal. When viewed from above, the male's hindquarters appear more pointed. The tail is elevated due to the presence of the underlying large scrotal sac. The female's hindquarters are broader and more rounded. Adult males have prominent testicles that can retract through the open inguinal canals. Applying gentle pressure to the male's caudal abdomen will cause the testicles to descend into the scrotal sac. Male hamsters have an os penis as well as large seminal vesicles that are located on each side of the bladder and resemble a ram's horns. Adult females are larger than males and have on average seven pairs (range = 6–11 pairs) of mammary glands with mammae visible on their ventral surface; males lack mammae. Two cervical canals lead to a duplex uterus. The female has three orifices in the anogenital area—the urethral, vaginal, and anal—and displays a shorter anogenital distance than the male. Newborns can be sexed by comparing the anogenital distance. The anogenital distance is greater in the male, and the genital papilla of the male is more prominent than that of the female.

There are several distinctive characteristics of the hematologic and urinary profiles of hamsters. Leukocyte counts are 5,000–10,000/μL, with the lymphocyte being the most dominant leukocyte. Polychromasia is relatively common in hamster erythrocytes. Hamsters excrete approximately 7 mL of urine daily. Their urine has a basic pH and appears turbid and milky due to the presence of calcium carbonate crystals. Select hematologic and biochemical values are listed in Appendix 1, "Normal Values."

BREEDING AND REPRODUCTION

Males and females reach sexual maturity at approximately 12 weeks of age and 90 g (males) or 90–100 g (females) of body weight. The female hamster is continuously polyestrous, cycling every 4 days. There is a normal seasonal breeding quiescence, however, in the winter months. Ovulation is spontaneous. A white, stringy, opaque, and odiferous postovulatory discharge is present on the second day of the cycle. This normal discharge indicates that the hamster reached peak estrus the day before and its presence can be used to predict optimal breeding time. The female can be successfully mated in the evening of the third day after the observance of the postovulatory discharge.

Females will generally attack newly introduced males except during estrus. Because of this behavior, it is best to observe the pair closely for compatibility and to leave them together for only 30 minutes, although a pair may be left together overnight if mating activity is observed within the first approximately 10 minutes of pairing. When a receptive female is placed with a male, after a short familiarization period, she will assume the lordosis position, an arching of the lower back with a wide rear leg stance that facilitates copulation. Mating is characterized by repeated intromissions and ejaculations. Signs of pregnancy include a distended abdomen and rapid weight gain at 10 days postmating. Pregnancy can be confirmed by the absence of a postovulatory discharge on days 5 and 9 after mating. The postpartum estrus is usually anovulatory. Pseudopregnancies do occur.

The gestation period is the shortest of any of the common laboratory animals at an average of 16 days. The female is frequently restless before parturition. A bloody vaginal discharge may be seen prior to delivery of the first fetus. Litter size is usually five to nine pups. At birth, pups are hairless, have closed eyes and ears, but have fully erupted incisors. Ears open at 4–5 days of age, hair growth is noticeable at 9 days, and eyes open at 14–16 days. Young hamsters start eating food and drinking water when they are 7–10 days of age. Care should be taken to ensure that they can reach the water supply and are provided with food on the floor of the cage. They are weaned at 3 weeks of age. A fertile estrus follows weaning by 2–18 days.

Cannibalism of the young and litter abandonment are common during the first pregnancy, the first week postpartum, and anytime a dam is stressed. To reduce this risk, the female should be placed in a clean cage with clean bedding, food, and nesting material at 14 days after mating to minimize the need to change the cage immediately before or soon after parturition. Housing in opaque or tinted cages and in a quiet area is also helpful. To minimize maternal stress, the dam and pups should be disturbed as little as possible during the most critical 7–10-day postdelivery period. If the cage must be disturbed during this period, it may be helpful to first provide the female with preferred food items. The food may be ingested to fill the cheek pouches, thereby deterring her from cannibalizing the young. The reproductive efficiency of both sexes decreases by 14 months of age.

HUSBANDRY

Housing and Environment

A variety of cages used for other laboratory rodents are satisfactory. Hamsters prefer solid-bottom cages with contact bedding. An adult hamster over 100 g requires a floor area of at least 123 cm^2 (19 in.^{2}) and a cage height of at least 15 cm (6 in.). Caging materials should be carefully selected to preclude destruction and escape as hamsters are noted escape artists. They frequently will dislodge cage lids and/or gnaw on caging materials, escape, and evade capture. They do not return to their cages as rats and gerbils do. Rigid plastic and stainless steel are acceptable caging materials. Ground corn cobs, paper products, and hardwood chips can be used as bedding materials. The use of cedar or untreated softwood bedding is not recommended as they emit aromatic hydrocarbons that can adversely affect liver metabolism. Additional items may be added to the cage to increase cage complexity (e.g., huts or tubes) or for the animal to gnaw or manipulate.

Environmental parameters for hamsters, recommended in the *Guide for the Care and Use of Laboratory Animals* (ILAR, 2011), include a temperature between 20° and 26°C (68° and 79°F), relative humidity between 30% and 70%, and 10–15 air changes per hour. Typically, 12–14 hours of light per day is provided (14 hours for breeders), most frequently controlled by automatic timers.

Sanitation

Hamsters are fastidious in that they will use different locations of the cage in which to store food, urinate, and defecate. Weekly cleaning of the cage usually suffices because hamsters produce little waste or odor. Cages, bottles, and feed hoppers should be disinfected with chemicals, hot water 61.6°–82.2°C (143°–180°F), or a combination of both. Detergents and chemical disinfectants enhance the effectiveness of hot water, but they must be thoroughly rinsed from all caging surfaces with fresh water. Soaking or rinsing the cages with an acid solution may help to remove urine scale (mineral) buildup. Refer to Chapter 4 for a more detailed description of disinfection methods.

Environmental Enrichment and Social Housing

An animal's social needs should be carefully considered when housing animals in the laboratory environment. Enrichment should increase the normal behavior for the species and decrease abnormal or stereotypic behaviors. Paper or plastic huts as well as tunnels (e.g., PVC piping) can provide hiding places and may, if appropriately designed, help to decrease cagemate aggression (Figure 7.2). Animals enjoy burrowing in deep bedding. Running wheels can provide a source of exercise; hamsters enjoy running on exercise wheels and have been reported to run up to 5 miles a day, mostly during dark hours. Items that can be directly manipulated by the animal may also be beneficial. Both males and females build nests, with nest-building activity increasing in females during pregnancy and lactation. Commercially prepared nesting material, such as compressed cotton fiber nestlets, may be provided. Clear communication among the principal investigator, the IACUC, and the facility veterinarian regarding the introduction or standard use of any enrichment item is vital to minimize introducing research variability.

Feeding and Watering

Fresh, properly stored commercial pelleted rodent diets that contain 15%–25% protein, 35%–40% carbohydrate, 4%–5% fat, and 5% crude fiber are adequate for hamsters. Mixed seed diets are not appropriate as hamsters are often selective when fed mixed seed diets, eating favorite items and not receiving a balanced diet. Examples of potential consequences include a nutritional myopathy caused by a vitamin deficiency and alopecia precipitated by a low-protein diet. These conditions are uncommon in modern research facilities in which animals are fed appropriate diets,

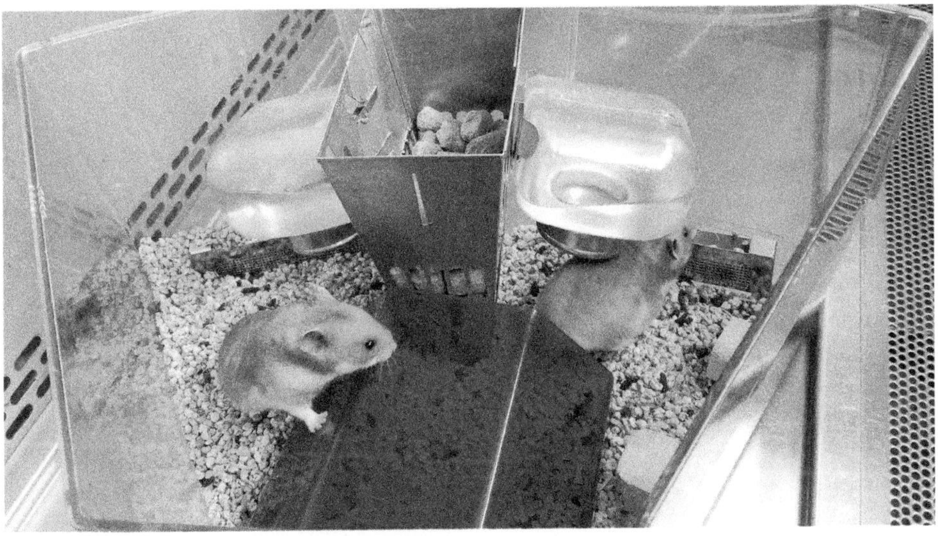

Fig 7.2. Pair-housed hamsters can benefit from plastic huts or tunnels as part of their enrichment. (*Source*: Photo courtesy of Crystal Johnson, Icahn School of Medicine Mount Sinai.)

but they are seen in pet hamsters. Hamsters eat an average of 8–12 g/100 g of body weight per day. Young hamsters start consuming solid food at 7–10 days of age. It is permissible by the Animal Welfare Act to place pelleted feed on the floor of a primary enclosure for this species. Alternatively, diet can be provided in a slotted, sheet metal hopper or a wire bar feeder. Slot widths of less than 11 mm in food hoppers, as may be used with mice or rats, should be avoided as hamsters have difficulty reaching food because of their broad noses. Hamsters hoard food and will frequently remove pellets from the feeder and store them on the cage floor or in a corner of the cage. Although hamsters enjoy fruits and vegetables, they are neither necessary nor suggested to supplement their diets. Fresh, potable water should be available *ad libitum*. Water can be provided by bottles, water pouches (e.g., Hydropac®, Sipper Sack®), or an automated watering system. On average, hamsters drink approximately 8–10 mL of water per 100 g of body weight per day although the range does differ between sexes (males, 4.5–5 mL/100 g per day; females, 13.6–14 mL/100 g per day). Hamsters are coprophagic and may consume their own feces as they are excreted from their rectum. Coprophagy serves to recycle B vitamins and other nutrients.

TECHNIQUES

Handling and Restraint

To avoid an aggressive startle response, it is important to ensure a hamster is awake and expects to be handled. A hamster can be transferred from one cage to another by cupping the hands under the animal (Figure 7.3), using a small cup or tube, or grasping a pinch of skin at the nape of the neck. Restraint may be accomplished by grasping all of the loose skin at the nape of the neck and back. It is important to immobilize the hamster fully to prevent handler injury. This restraint method is commonly referred to as scruffing, shown in Figure 7.4. Use of protective gloves and forceps is not recommended because they may cause aggressive behavior.

Identification

Cage cards are most often used as a form of general identification in a research setting. Ear punching, ear tagging, or subcutaneous microchip implantation may be used to permanently identify individual animals. Dyes, permanent markers, or fur clipping can be used as temporary identification methods.

Blood Collection

Assuming the animal is mature, healthy, and on an adequate plane of nutrition, the total blood volume of most species averages 7% of the body weight in grams. Table 7.2 lists approximate adult hamster blood volumes. A typical rule of thumb for blood withdrawal suggests that up to 10% of the circulating blood volume can be withdrawn from normal, healthy animals every 2–3 weeks with minimal adverse effect. Small amounts of blood can be obtained by capillary tube collection from limb veins (e.g., lateral metatarsal vein) of conscious animals or by retro-orbital bleeding of the orbital venous sinus or from the jugular of anesthetized animals. The retro-orbital

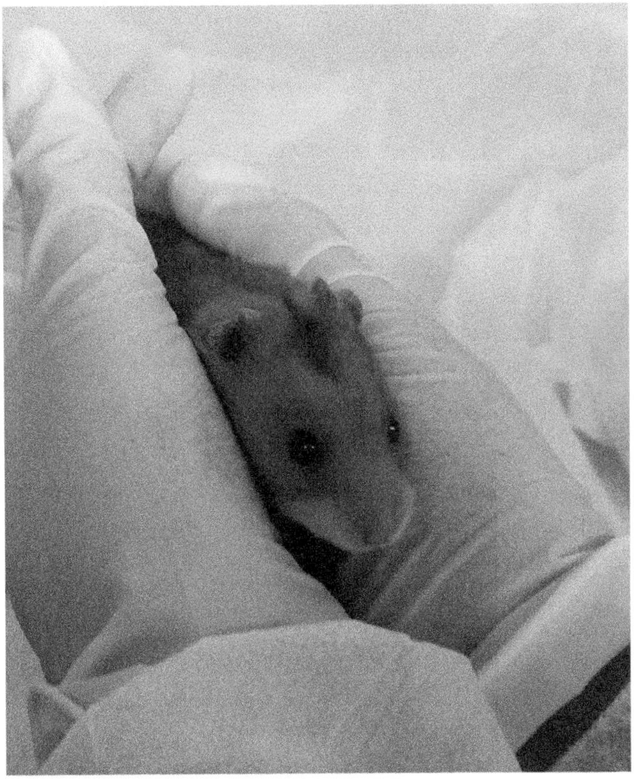

Fig 7.3. Gentle cupping of hands around a hamster for movement. (*Source*: Photo courtesy of Crystal Johnson, Icahn School of Medicine Mount Sinai.)

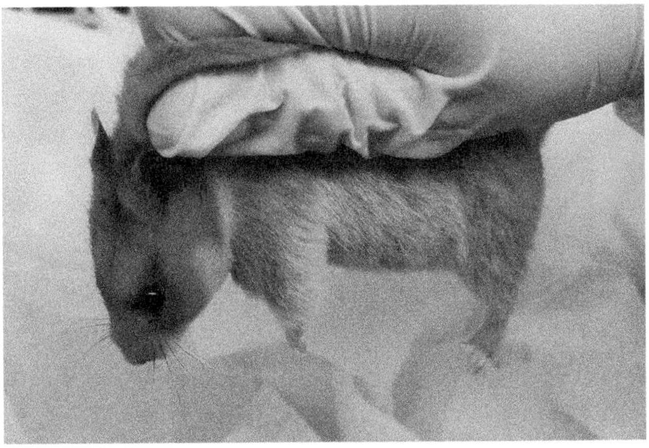

Fig 7.4. Restraint of the hamster using whole-hand grip. (*Source*: Photo courtesy of Crystal Johnson, Icahn School of Medicine Mount Sinai.)

bleeding technique is similar to the technique described in Chapter 4; as with the mouse, the retro-orbital sinus may be accessed from both the lateral and the medial canthus of the eye. When using the lateral canthus technique, the capillary tube should be directed medially. Use of a topical ophthalmic anesthetic is highly recommended to

Table 7.2. Adult hamster blood volumes and suggested sample size

	Volume (mL)
Total blood	6.8–12
Single sample	0.5–1.2
Exsanguination	3–5

Source: Adapted from Harkness et al. (2010).
Note: Values are approximate.

help alleviate postprocedural discomfort. Larger blood samples can be obtained via cranial (anterior) vena cava or cardiac puncture in an anesthetized animal. Cardiac sampling is associated with significant mortality and should be used only as a terminal blood collection method. Hamster blood quickly coagulates; therefore, care must be taken to use appropriate anticoagulants.

Urine Collection

Urine may be collected using a metabolic cage that separates the urine and fecal pellets. Other methods to collect 1–2 drops of urine include briefly restraining the hamster, placing it on a cold metal surface, or placing it in a plastic bag, each of which may stimulate urination.

Drug Administration

Most drug administration techniques used in small animal practice can be used with hamsters when modified to fit their smaller size. To avoid overdosing or underdosing medications, small scales are useful for obtaining accurate body weights for drug dose calculations. To increase dosing accuracy of small drug volumes, substances may be diluted to larger, more easily measured volumes and syringes designed for small volume administration (e.g., tuberculin syringe) may be used.

In some situations, medications can be administered orally by mixing them in the water or feed. Many factors may affect a hamster's willingness to drink or eat medicated water or food. Therefore, administration of all substances, especially analgesics, in feed or drinking water is discouraged unless it can be shown that all animals will consume required amounts. A tuberculin syringe can be used to administer a liquid into the oral cavity. For greater accuracy or for administering unpalatable liquids, a specialized gavage needle can be used to deliver a substance directly into the stomach. Both rigid metal and flexible plastic gavage needles are available. Use of a ball-tipped gavage needle helps ensure that the needle does not pass into the trachea. A maximum oral volume of 2 mL is suggested.

Small-gauge hypodermic needles, such as 23 or 25 gauge, should be used for injections. Medications can also be administered by subcutaneous (SC) injection, with a maximum volume of 3–4 mL, using the loose skin over the shoulders. Intramuscular injections are not frequently used because hamsters have such small muscle mass. Another drawback to the intramuscular route is that certain drugs such as ketamine can cause muscle necrosis and nerve irritation leading to self-mutilation of the affected area. If the intramuscular route must be used, a maximum volume of 0.1 mL is recommended.

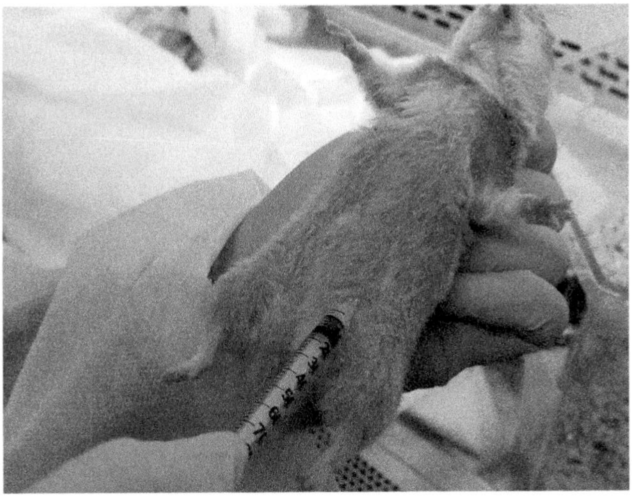

Fig 7.5. Intraperitoneal injection in a hamster. (*Source*: Photo courtesy of Crystal Johnson, Icahn School of Medicine Mount Sinai.)

In the hamster, as with other small rodents, medications and injectable anesthetics are most commonly administered by the intraperitoneal (IP) route. A maximum volume of 3–4 mL is suggested. When receiving an IP injection, some recommend that the animal's head be tilted downward in an effort to avoid puncture of the intestines. The injection is made immediately to the right or left of the midline in the lower half of the abdomen (Figure 7.5). Intravenous injections are most frequently made into the cephalic vein, the jugular vein, or the lateral metatarsal vein. A maximum volume of 0.3 mL is recommended for the intravenous route. Suggested maximum dosing volumes are listed in Table 7.3.

Anesthesia, Surgery, and Postoperative Care

A variety of agents that can be used to tranquilize and anesthetize hamsters are listed in Table 7.4. Preanesthetic fasting is not recommended as the hamster has a high metabolic rate and, as such, is prone to hypoglycemia and hypothermia. Single-injection anesthesia techniques are generally used to minimize handling stress. Fairly consistent anesthesia can be induced by the IP administration of a ketamine–xylazine mixture. Ketamine can also be combined with an inhalant anesthetic such as isoflurane.

Hamsters can be anesthetized through the use of an induction chamber or masked down with an inhalation anesthetic delivered from a precision vaporizer. Isoflurane and sevoflurane should be administered via a precision vaporizer with a mask or nosecone apparatus in conjunction with a nonrebreathing system. Alternatively, very brief (~1–2 minutes) anesthesia can be produced through the use of a simple anesthetic chamber. See Chapter 4 for additional information.

While anesthetized, hamsters should have bland, sterile ophthalmic ointment placed in their eyes to prevent exposure keratitis. The depth of anesthesia in hamsters can be estimated by observation of the righting reflex, muscle tone, pedal withdrawal reflex, abdominal skin pinch reflex, respiratory rate and depth, and color of mucous membranes and skin.

Table 7.3. Maximum adult hamster dosing volumes

Route	Amount (mL)
IP	3–4
SC	3–4
IM	0.1
IV	0.3
PO	2.0

Source: Adapted from Harkness and Wagner (1995) and Lukas (1999).

Table 7.4. Anesthetic agents and tranquilizers used in hamsters

Drug	Dosage	Route	Reference
Inhalants			
Isoflurane	1%–4% to effect	Inhalation	Wixson (1994)
Sevoflurane	To effect	Inhalation	Morrisey and Carpenter (2004)
Injectables			
Acepromazine	2.5 mg/kg	IP	Flecknell (2016)
Alphadolone/alphaxalone	150 mg/kg	IP	Flecknell (2016)
Dexmedetomidine	0.015–0.05 mg/kg	IP	Flecknell (2016)
Diazepam	5 mg/kg	IP	Flecknell (2016)
Fentanyl-fluanisone	0.3–0.6 mL/kg	IP	Flecknell (2016)
Fentanyl-fluanisone	1 mL/kg	IP	Flecknell (2016)
+ diazepam	5 mg/kg	IP	
Ketamine	50–100 mg/kg	IP	Flecknell (2016)
Ketamine	150 mg/kg	IP	Flecknell (2016)
+ acepromazine	5 mg/kg	IP	
Ketamine	100 mg/kg	IP	Harkness et al. (2010)
+ diazepam	5 mg/kg	IP	
Ketamine	100 mg/kg	IP	Flecknell (2016)
+ dexmedetomidine	0.125 mg/kg	IP	
Ketamine	200 mg/kg	IP	Flecknell (2016)
+ xylazine	10 mg/kg	IP	
Midazolam	5 mg/kg	IP	Flecknell (2016)
Pentobarbital	50–90 mg/kg	IP	Flecknell (2016)
Tiletamine-zolazepam	30 mg/kg	IP	Forsythe et al. (1992)
+ xylazine	10 mg/kg	IP	
Xylazine	1–5 mg/kg	IP	Flecknell (2016)

IP = intraperitoneal.

Surgery should be done in an aseptic manner. Prevention of blood loss is an important consideration. Surgical procedures are most frequently performed for experimental rather than for therapeutic purposes. Nephrectomy, adrenalectomy, thymectomy, and ovariectomy are a few of the surgeries most commonly performed in research. The hamster oocyte is the only rodent ovum that will accept sperm from other species. As a consequence, female hamsters may be ovariectomized and their oocytes utilized in human male fertility testing and research. When castrating a hamster, it is important to close the open inguinal canals.

The anesthetized hamster should be placed on a clean, dry paper or cloth towel and recovered in an escape-proof incubator. Use of a circulating-water heating blanket or self-regulating heating pad promotes euthermia and is recommended. Generic, electric heating pads should never be placed in direct contact with the animal as they may cause thermal burns. Small-particle bedding materials are contraindicated in recovery cages because they can stick to the eyes, nose, and mouth of the recovering animal and may be aspirated. Postoperative care should include hydration of the anesthetized animal (e.g., subcutaneous or intraperitoneal injection of a warmed solution such as saline, saline–dextrose, lactated Ringer's), and support of normal body temperature. Hypostatic pulmonary congestion should be prevented by turning the animal at least every 30 minutes. It is important to maintain hydration and nutrition levels in the postoperative period to support normal metabolic processes and gut physiology. Select commercially available supportive and critical care products for laboratory animals are provided in Appendix 3.

When in pain, hamsters are often reluctant to move, have a hunched body appearance, and are more aggressive. Carprofen is recommended for mild postoperative discomfort. Buprenorphine works well to control acute or chronic visceral pain but causes more sedation. Hamsters are markedly resistant to morphine's hypnotic and sedative effects, and require higher doses than usually required in other species. The nonsteroidal anti-inflammatory drug carprofen is a useful analgesic that requires only once-daily dosing and is effective against mild-to-moderate incisional, inflammatory, and visceral pain. Analgesic agents that can be used in hamsters are listed in Table 7.5.

Imaging Techniques

Great advances have been made in rodent and small animal imaging over the last decade. For a detailed description of current imaging modalities, see Chapter 3.

Euthanasia

Methods of euthanasia must be consistent with the most current American Veterinary Medical Association (AVMA) *Guidelines for the Euthanasia of Animals* (AVMA, 2013) and performed by trained personnel. Per AVMA Guidelines, "Carbon dioxide is acceptable with conditions for euthanasia in those species where aversion or distress can be minimized. Carbon dioxide exposure using a gradual fill method is less likely to cause pain due to nociceptor activation by carbonic acid prior to onset of unconsciousness; a displacement rate from 10% to 30% of the chamber volume/min is recommended.... CO_2 flow should be maintained for at least 1 minute after respiratory arrest." Conscious animals should never be placed in an area prefilled with 100% CO_2 as this can cause pain of the mucous membranes. Furthermore, only a pure form of

Table 7.5. Analgesic agents used in hamsters

Drug	Dosage	Route	Reference
Acetylsalicylic acid	240 mg/kg q24h	PO	Harkness et al. (2010)
Buprenorphine	0.1–0.5 mg/kg q8h	SC	Harkness et al. (2010)
Butorphanol	1–5 mg/kg q4h	SC	Harkness et al. (2010)
Carprofen	5 mg/kg q24h	SC	Pollack (2002)
Flunixin meglumine	2.5 mg/kg q12–24 h	SC	Heard (1993)
Ketoprofen	5 mg/kg	SC	Pollack (2002)
Meperidine	20 mg/kg q2–3h	SC	Heard (1993)
Morphine	2–5 mg/kg q2–4h	SC	Heard (1993)
Nalbuphine	4–8 mg/kg	SC	Mason (1997)
Oxymorphone	0.2–0.5 mg/kg q6–12h	SC	Heard (1993)
Pentazocine	10 mg/kg q2–4h	SC	Heard (1993)
Piroxicam	3 mg/kg q24h	PO	Harkness et al. (2010)
Tramadol	5–10 mg/kg q12–24 h	PO	Morrisey and Carpenter (2011)

PO = per os; and SC = subcutaneous.

CO_2 must be used, such as from a commercially supplied cylinder. Neonates are resistant to hypoxia and require greater duration of exposure. For this reason, other methods may be preferred for this age group. Studies have shown that the method of CO_2 euthanasia can result in significant differences in immunologic and hematologic variables; thus consistency of method may be important in accurate interpretation of research data. Other acceptable methods of euthanasia include overdose of an inhalant anesthetic and IP administration of a barbiturate anesthetic at three to four times the anesthetic dose.

THERAPEUTIC AGENTS

Suggested hamster antimicrobial and antifungal drug dosages are listed in Table 7.6. Antiparasitic agents are listed in Table 7.7 and miscellaneous drugs are listed in Table 7.8.

INTRODUCTION TO DISEASES OF HAMSTERS

Most laboratory rodent colonies today are relatively free of the viruses, bacteria, parasites, and fungi that cause clinical disease. However, sporadic outbreaks may still occur, and it is important for individuals to have a basic knowledge of the most common infectious agents and how to respond to them. Presented here is a general overview of common bacterial, viral, fungal, and parasitic agents of hamsters as well as standard diagnostic and treatment modalities.

Table 7.6. Antimicrobial and antifungal agents used in hamsters

Drug	Dosage	Route	Reference
Amikacin	2–5 mg/kg q8–12h	SC	Harkness et al. (2010)
Cephaloridine	10–25 mg/kg q24h	SC	Harkness et al. (2010)
Chloramphenicol	30–50 mg/kg q12h	SC, PO	Burgmann and Percy (1993)
Chlortetracycline	20 mg/kg q12h	PO, SC	Allen et al. (1993)
Ciprofloxacin	7–20 mg/kg q12h	PO	Harkness et al. (2010)
Doxycycline	2.5 mg/kg q12h	PO	Allen et al. (1993)
Enrofloxacin	5–10 mg/kg q12h	PO, SC	Harkness et al. (2010)
Gentamicin	5 mg/kg q24h	SC	Anderson (1994)
Griseofulvin	25–50 mg/kg q12h for 14–60 d	PO	Harkness et al. (2010)
	1.5% in DMSO for 5–7 d	Topical	Harkness et al. (2010)
Ketoconazole	10–40 mg/kg q24h for 14 d	PO	Rollin and Kesel (1995)
Metronidazole	7.5 mg/70–90 g animal q8h	PO	Collins (1995)
Neomycin	100 mg/kg q24h	PO	Burgmann and Percy (1993)
	16 mg/kg q24h	SC	Collins (1995)
Sulfadimethoxine	10–15 mg/kg q12h	PO	Harkness et al. (2010)
Tetracycline	10–20 mg/kg q8–12h	PO	Burgmann and Percy (1993)
Trimethoprim-sulfa	15–30 mg/kg q12–24h	PO, SC	Harkness et al. (2010)
Tylosin	2–8 mg/kg q12h	SC, PO	Burgmann and Percy (1993)
Vancomycin	20 mg/kg for 3+ months	PO	Boss et al. (1994)

DMSO = dimethyl sulfoxide; PO = per os; and SC = subcutaneous.

Table 7.7. Antiparasitic agents used in hamsters

Drug	Dosage	Route	Reference
Amitraz	1.4 mL/L water using cotton-ball application q14d for 3–6 treatments	Topical	Harkness et al. (2010)
Carbamate (5%)	Twice weekly	Topical	Harkness et al. (2010)
Fenbendazole	20 mg/kg q24h for 5 d	PO	Allen et al. (1993)
Fipronil	7.5 mg/kg q30–60 d	Topical	Richardson (1997)
Ivermectin	0.2–0.4 mg/kg q7–10 d	PO, SC	Harkness et al. (2010)
Lime sulfur	Dilute 1:40 with water, dip q7d for 6 wk		Anderson (1994)
Pyrantel pamoate	50 mg/kg	PO	Rollin and Kesel (1995)
Praziquantel	6–10 mg/kg	PO	Harkness et al. (2010)
Pyrethrin powder	Three times a week for 3 wk	Topical	Anderson (1994)
Thiabendazole	100–200 mg/kg	PO	Harkness et al. (2010)

PO = per os; and SC = subcutaneous.

General signs of illness include loss of coat and body condition, hunched posture, ocular discharge, weight loss, and extended periods of daytime inactivity. Hypothermia, dehydration, and anorexia are common and need to be treated aggressively with supportive care.

Table 7.8. Miscellaneous agents used in hamsters

Drug	Dosage	Route	Reference
Atipamezole	0.1–1 mg/kg	SC, IP, IV	Flecknell (2016)
Atropine	0.04 mg/kg	SC	Flecknell (2016)
	10 mg/kg q20 min for organophosphate overdose	SC	Harkness and Wagner (1995)
Cimetidine	5–10 mg/kg q6–12h	PO	Allen et al. (1993)
Dexamethasone	0.5–2.0 mg/kg then decreasing dose q12h for 3–14d	PO, SC	Harkness and Wagner (1995)
	0.6 mg/kg	IM	Anderson (1994)
Digoxin	0.05–0.1 mg/kg q12–24h	PO	Morrisey and Carpenter (2004)
Diphenhydramine	1–2 mg/kg q12h	PO, SC	Morrisey and Carpenter (2004)
Doxapram	5–10 mg/kg	IP, IV	Flecknell (2016)
Furosemide	1–4 mg/kg q4–6h	SC	Harrenstien (1994)
Glycopyrrolate	0.01–0.02 mg/kg	SC	Huerkamp (1995)
Lactobacilli	Administer during antibiotic treatment period, then 5–7d beyond cessation	PO	Collins (1995)
Lactulose syrup	0.5 mL/kg q12h	PO	Morrisey and Carpenter (2011)
Loperamide hydrochloride (Imodium A-D)	0.1 mg/kg q8h for 3d then q24h for 2d, given in 1 mL of water	PO	Harkness and Wagner (1995)
Naloxone	0.01–0.10 mg/kg	SC, IP	Huerkamp (1995)
Oxytocin	0.2–3 IU/kg	SC	Anderson (1994)
Prednisone	0.5–2.2 mg/kg	SC, PO	Anderson (1994)
Sulfacrate	25–50 mg/kg	PO	Morrisey and Carpenter (2004)
Vitamin B complex	0.02–0.2 mL/kg	SC	Anderson (1994)
Vitamin D	200–400 IU/kg	SC	Anderson (1994)
Vitamin E-selenium (Bo-Se)	0.1 mL/100–250 g	SC	Anderson (1994)
Vitamin K	1–10 mg/kg q24h for 4–6d	IM	Harkness and Wagner (1995)
Yohimbine	0.5–1 mg/kg	IV	Harkness and Wagner (1995)

IM = intramuscular; IP = intraperitoneal; PO = per os; SC = subcutaneous; and IV = intravenous.

chapter 7

Bacterial Diseases

Antibiotic-Associated Enterocolitis

The potential value of treating a hamster with an antimicrobial agent must be carefully weighed against the risk of inducing antibiotic-associated enterocolitis (Box 7.2). Care must be used in selecting the antibiotic and length of therapy. Discrepancies exist among reports of antimicrobial use in hamsters. Many antimicrobial agents are highly toxic for hamsters, even when the agent is given in a single, low dose. Lincomycin, clindamycin, ampicillin, vancomycin, erythromycin, cephalosporins, gentamicin, and penicillin have all been associated with enterocolitis.

Box 7.2

The potential value of treating a hamster with an antimicrobial agent must be carefully weighed against the risk of inducing antibiotic-associated enterocolitis.

Hamster intestinal microbial flora is predominantly of the bacterial genera *Lactobacillus* and *Bacteroides*, with few coliforms. Without external disruption, the normal flora controls the proliferation of other organisms and any toxins they may produce. Antibiotic-associated enterocolitis may develop when antibiotics (such as those listed in the preceding paragraph) are administered that disrupt the normal intestinal microbial flora, facilitating the proliferation of *Clostridium difficile* organisms and the toxins A and B that they produce. Clinical signs are similar regardless of the antimicrobial agent involved and include anorexia, ruffled fur, dehydration, and profuse diarrhea. Most affected hamsters die within 4–10 days of antibiotic administration. Some animals do not develop clinical signs but are found dead. The characteristic gross lesion on necropsy is a hemorrhagic ileocolitis. Treatment may consist of discontinuing antibiotic administration, providing a *Lactobacillus* supplement to help reestablish normal intestinal flora diversity, and providing supportive care. Gram-negative antibiotics should be continued if overgrowth of a specific Gram-negative organism (e.g., *C. difficile*) is confirmed through culture. It has been reported that hamsters could be protected against fatal *C. difficile* enteritis by long-term, daily oral administration of vancomycin or metronidazole although disease relapse may occur following antibiotic withdrawal due to the persistence of *C. difficile* spores, continuing environmental contamination, and lack of appropriate immunity. It is important to note that *C. difficile* toxin production with subsequent morbidity and mortality can occur, even when no antibiotics have been administered. In these situations, it is suspected that another stressful event has resulted in disruption of the intestinal flora. *C. difficile* can also induce a fatal disease in humans.

Proliferative Ileitis—Transmissible Ileal Hyperplasia, Hamster Enteritis, or Wet Tail

Proliferative ileitis is the most common spontaneous disease of hamsters (Box 7.3). The causative agent is the Gram-negative bacteria, *Lawsonia intracellularis*, the same agent that induces proliferative enteritis in swine, ferrets, and rabbits. The organism is predominantly transmitted by the fecal–oral route and disease is usually confined to young animals, 3–8 weeks of age. Mortality is often high (50%–90%); death usually occurs within 24–48 hours of symptom development although death may occur in the absence of clinical signs. Stress plays an important role in susceptibility to clinical disease, with weaning, improper diet, transportation, crowding, and poor sanitation serving as significant predisposing factors. Clinical signs include unkempt hair coat; anorexia; a moistened perineal area; foul-smelling, watery diarrhea; and dehydration. On abdominal palpation, the animal frequently seems uncomfortable, and distended bowel loops are noted. Intussusceptions and rectal prolapses can occur. Typical gross necropsy lesions include gas and yellow diarrhea in the distal intestinal tract as well as a segmentally thickened and edematous ileum.

Box 7.3

Proliferative ileitis is the most common spontaneous disease of hamsters.

Prognosis is grave. To be effective, antibiotics must be administered early in the course of disease. Tetracycline, metronidazole, enrofloxacin, and trimethoprim–sulfa combinations are recommended. Chloramphenicol has also been used with some success. Administering warmed fluids intraperitoneally or subcutaneously and increasing the room temperature may be helpful. Quarantine of affected hamsters and good sanitation practices are useful in controlling proliferative ileitis. The importance of correcting any management problems and eliminating stress factors should not be overlooked.

Tyzzer's Disease

Hamsters do not appear to be as susceptible as gerbils to *Clostridium piliforme*, the causative agent of Tyzzer's disease. Disease is most often seen in weanlings, with resultant high morbidity and mortality. Clinical signs may include a profuse watery diarrhea as well as nonspecific signs of illness including ruffled hair coat, lethargy, anorexia, and dehydration. Transmission is by the oral route. Characteristically, predominant lesions involve the liver, but enterocolitis without liver disease or heart lesions is sometimes seen. Hepatomegaly with numerous white or yellow pinpoint foci measuring 1–2 mm in diameter is typically observed at necropsy. Edema and hemorrhage of the intestines, particularly in the ileocecal area, may also be present. Oxytetracycline or tetracycline can be used to suppress infection. Supplemental fluid therapy can be provided if indicated, but in disease outbreaks it is recommended that infected animals be culled. Infectious spores can remain in the environment for prolonged periods of time. To eliminate spores, the environment should be cleaned and all cages and feeding and watering equipment should be sterilized.

Salmonellosis

Salmonellosis is rarely seen in laboratory hamsters although human outbreaks have been traced to infected pet and laboratory hamsters. *Salmonella* is transmitted by the fecal–oral route primarily through contaminated food and bedding material. Clinical signs are those of general illness as enteritis or diarrhea is frequently not observed in infected rodents. Pathologic findings may include multifocal necrosis of the liver, hepatosplenomegaly, and septic pulmonary thrombophlebitis. Small white foci may be seen on the liver and spleen at necropsy. Treatment is not recommended as it does not reliably eliminate the organism from infected animals but can result in an asymptomatic carrier state. Infected colonies are most frequently culled and contaminated equipment and environments sanitized.

Campylobacteriosis

There is a relatively high prevalence (nearly 100%) of *Campylobacter jejuni* colonization of hamsters. The organism is believed to be a normal commensal of the hamster intestinal tract, becoming an opportunistic pathogen presumably during periods of stress or intestinal flora disruption. Transmission is fecal–oral. Most infected hamsters are asymptomatic although a small proportion may develop diarrhea. Diagnosis is by culture or polymerase chain reaction (PCR). Hamsters should be considered a potential source for human infections.

Helicobacter

Many strains of helicobacter normally inhabit the hamster intestine and rarely cause disease in the hamster. *Helicobacter* strains of most note are *H. cinaedi*, a significant pathogen of immunocompromised humans, and *H. aurati*, a strain previously shown to induce chronic weight loss and poor body condition in 18- to 24-month-old hamsters. *H. cholecystus* has been shown to cause gallbladder and pancreatic disease in weanling hamsters.

Abscesses and Skin Ulceration

Abscesses and skin ulceration are most frequently caused by *Staphylococcus aureus*. Other less common organisms include *Streptococcus* spp. and *Pasteurella pneumotropica*. Systemic enrofloxacin, tetracycline, or ciprofloxacin can be used with local treatment of the area.

Pneumonia

Streptococcus spp. and *P. pneumotropica* infections may cause pneumonia. The illness is usually acute, with affected animals exhibiting sneezing, dyspnea, ocular discharge, and depression. Enrofloxacin, tetracycline, and chloramphenicol are useful antibiotics to treat pneumonia.

Viral Diseases

Few viral pathogens are recognized in the hamster. Two viruses, hamster polyomavirus and hamster parvovirus, may induce a clinical disease state. One virus, lymphocytic choriomeningitis virus, rarely induces clinical signs in naturally infected hamsters but does present a significant public health concern. In addition, hamsters are susceptible to infection by a number of murine viruses such as Sendai virus and pneumonia virus of mice. Clinical disease is rarely recognized in adult animals. However, infections may significantly affect research results and hamsters can serve as a reservoir of infection for other rodent species housed in the same facility.

Hamster Polyomavirus

Animals infected with hamster polyomavirus (HaPyV) typically develop one of two disease conditions. Animals that naturally contract the virus through exposure to contaminated environments or fomites may develop trichoepitheliomas on the face, feet, neck, back, flanks, or abdomen. These lesions are pathognomonic for the disease. Multiple masses may develop but then regress over time. Hamsters injected with the virus may develop lymphoma and clinical signs that pertain to the affected organ(s). The intestines, mesentery, and liver are most frequently affected. Infection can be diagnosed by PCR, histology, and immunohistochemistry. Treatment is not recommended. Colony depopulation, environmental decontamination, and repopulation with animals free of the disease are most commonly performed.

Hamster Parvovirus

Hamster parvovirus (HaPV) was first reported in 1982 in a hamster colony with high mortality in suckling and weaning animals. It has been hypothesized that the hamster is not the natural viral host and that the virus may have originated in a species in which it does not cause clinical disease. In fact, HaPV is nearly genetically identical to mouse parvovirus-3. Virus transmission is believed to be through ingestion or inhalation. Neonates and weanlings are clinically affected with runting, incisor abnormalities, domed craniums, small testicles, and a potbellied appearance. Diarrhea, ataxia, and hemorrhagic disease may also develop. Infected adults rarely develop clinical signs. Infections may persist for multiple weeks. Diagnosis is by PCR or serology. Colony depopulation followed by environmental decontamination is recommended.

Lymphocytic Choriomeningitis Virus

The natural host and reservoir of this virus is the wild house mouse (*Mus musculus*). Infection, however, can be transmitted readily to other species—including the hamster, which is especially susceptible to infection. Lymphocytic choriomeningitis (LCMV) is an important public health concern because the virus may be transmitted from infected animals to humans through contact with urine, feces, saliva, or infected tissues and cell lines. Aerosol transmission has been noted. Both pet and laboratory-reared hamsters have been the source of several hundred human cases in the United States. Currently, most research institutions actively test for and exclude this virus from their rodent colonies. However, animal infections are occasionally identified, most frequently in association with the exchange of infected animals or biologics from foreign institutions or pet suppliers that do not actively exclude the virus. Once infected, animals may transmit the virus both horizontally and vertically. Adult hamsters that contract the disease rarely develop clinical signs. Animals infected prenatally may remain subclinical for multiple months, but then develop a progressive wasting disease. Infected humans may display no clinical signs or a mild febrile illness or, less commonly, may develop aseptic meningitis, encephalitis, or meningoencephalitis. Human infection can be fatal. The virus may not be readily transmitted through dirty bedding exposure. Therefore, a dirty bedding sentinel system may not detect infected colonies. Contact sentinels or other diagnostics are recommended. Serologic testing results have been unreliable, but PCR can be diagnostic. Due to the public health concern, treatment of infected animals is not recommended; rather colony depopulation is routine. It is important that the virus be excluded from colonies, such as by the quarantine and testing of new animals and testing of all biologics. Animal facilities must preclude the unintended entry of wild rodents as they may also serve as a source of infection.

Parasitic Diseases

Demodex

Two species of mites, *Demodex criceti* and *D. aurati*, occur in hamsters. Demodex mites are very common in both research and commercial vendor colonies. The presence of demodex mites is not thought to constitute a disease state as a low number of mites are normally present on immunocompetent hamsters with no apparent ill effects. Disease is most frequently seen in older animals, particularly males, and in immunocompromised individuals. Affected hamsters may have a rough hair coat; proliferative or ulcerative dermatitis; and areas of alopecia over the back, neck, and rump. Demodex mites can be difficult to detect; a deep skin scraping is suggested to visualize the mite. Affected animals may be culled from the colony. If treatment is preferred, it is best to bathe the hamster in a mild soap and towel-dry prior to treating it with a dilute solution of amitraz applied with a cotton ball or other applicator and allowed to dry. Dipping the animal in an amitraz solution is not suggested. Oral ivermectin treatment may be efficacious.

Notoedres

The hamster ear mite, *Notoedres spp.*, can cause exudative crusting lesions not only on the ears, but also on the snout, extremities, anus, and genitalia. Infestations are treated with ivermectin although infections are extremely unusual in the modern laboratory animal facility.

Pinworms

Hamsters can be infected by *Syphacia* spp., *Aspiculuris* spp., and *Dentostomella* spp. *Syphacia mesocriceti* is specific to the hamster, but many of the other pinworms that infect hamsters infect other species as well. *Syphacia obvelata* can be transmitted between mice and hamsters and *Syphacia muris* between rats and hamsters through contact with the parasite's eggs. Immunocompetent hamsters rarely display clinical signs of infection; however, they may affect certain research projects. Diagnostic methods vary based upon the infecting species but may include perianal cellophane tape tests, fecal flotation, direct examination of intestinal contents, and PCR. Avermectins and benzimidazoles are reported to be effective treatments.

Tapeworms

Several species of cestodes readily infect hamsters. In small numbers, tapeworms are relatively nonpathogenic although heavy burdens may result in emaciation or mechanical obstruction of the intestines. Heavy infestations can cause diarrhea. The cestode *Rodentolepis nana*, the dwarf tapeworm, has been frequently identified in hamster colonies. Infections with *R. nana* are a concern because of its direct life cycle, transmission to other rodents, and zoonotic potential. Recommended treatments include praziquantel or thiabendazole.

Protozoa

Numerous protozoa, including *Spironucleus* spp., *Trichomonas* spp., and *Giardia* spp., are found in the intestines but are of no known clinical significance. Eradication of these parasites from a colony is difficult. Treatments known to be effective in mice are frequently ineffective in hamsters.

Neoplasia

The incidence of spontaneous tumors in hamsters is relatively low although they occur more frequently in females. The most common primary tumors are lymphomas as well as endocrine tumors (especially adrenal gland tumors) and intestinal tumors. The incidence and severity of tumors vary among colonies.

Miscellaneous Conditions

Malocclusion

Malocclusion and overgrowth of incisors occasionally occur in hamsters secondary to trauma or due to a genetic predisposition. If severe and undetected, overgrown incisors can lead to emaciation and death due to an inability to eat. Incisors can be trimmed with suture removal scissors or toenail clippers, but this practice may lead to fractures of the teeth. Use of a dental bur is less likely to cause tooth fractures.

Bedding-Associated Dermatitis

A dermatitis that primarily affects the footpads and digits has been reported in hamsters housed on wood shavings. Lesions may spread to the legs and shoulders. Disease etiology is thought to relate to a contact dermatitis and/or a physical irritation as fine wood pieces have been observed lodged in the dermis or subcutis of affected animals. A granulomatous inflammation with digit degeneration and atrophy may develop.

Nutritional Myopathy

A nutritional myopathy caused by a vitamin deficiency can occur in hamsters fed a nutritionally incomplete diet such as an all-seed diet. In mild cases, the hamster is able to move the hind legs but cannot support its weight. In more advanced cases, the hamster may have posterior paresis. Nutritional improvement, supplementation with vitamin E, and an opportunity to exercise are usually curative.

Trauma

Hamsters are prone to aggression and may inflict serious injuries upon each other. Cannibalism is common in stressed and young animals. Paralysis is most frequently the result of traumatic injuries such as a fall onto a hard surface. Serious trauma, including fractures, may occur with inappropriate handling and restraint. External splinting is often not satisfactory for fracture repair. Stainless steel hypodermic needles used as intramedullary pins may be preferable for repair of fractured long bones. Fine stainless steel wire or staples may be preferable for laceration repairs as they may resist an animal's attempt at removal.

Osteoarthritis

Osteoarthritis is frequently observed in hamsters older than 2 years and most commonly involves the femoral–tibial joint. As the characteristics of the disease are similar to those in humans, the hamster is a recognized animal model of the human condition.

Glomerulonephropathy

Progressive and degenerative renal disease is a common problem in aged hamsters and is an important cause of mortality. Females are more commonly affected. Uremia, proteinuria, and polyuria are seen in affected animals. Amyloid deposition frequently occurs concurrently.

Amyloidosis

Amyloidosis is a metabolic condition characterized by excessive, extracellular deposition of inert protein fibrils in a variety of organs. The incidence of the condition varies between animal colonies, and is most common in aged animals, especially females. The most frequently affected organs are the liver, kidney, stomach, adrenal gland, thyroid, and spleen. Animals may be asymptomatic; clinical signs that develop frequently result from the loss of function of the affected organ. No treatment exists.

Atrial Thrombosis

Both male and female geriatric hamsters frequently suffer from atrial thrombosis although the incidence varies across animal colonies. Most thromboses occur in the left atrium and are secondary to degenerative cardiomyopathy and amyloidosis. Clinical signs are suggestive of heart failure and may include hyperpnea, severe dyspnea, tachycardia, and cyanosis. Significant subcutaneous edema can also be seen with this disease. Temporary clinical improvement has been reported in some hamsters treated with digitalis and furosemide.

Polycystic Disease

Aged hamsters frequently develop cysts, most frequently in the liver. Less frequently, cysts are found in the pancreas, epididymis, and seminal vesicles. Usually, no clinical signs are associated with the cysts and their cause is unknown, although there appears to be a genetic component.

BIBLIOGRAPHY

Allen, D. G., J. K. Pringle, and D. A. Smith. 1993. *Handbook of Veterinary Drugs.* Philadelphia, PA: JB Lippincott.

American Veterinary Medical Association (AVMA). 2013. *AVMA Guidelines for the Euthanasia of Animals.* Available at http://www.avma.org/KB/Policies/Documents/euthanasia.pdf [accessed July 13, 2018].

Anderson, N. L. 1994. Basic husbandry and medicine of pocket pets. In *Saunders Manual of Small Animal Practice*, J. S. Birchard and R. G. Sherding (eds.), pp. 1363–1389. Philadelphia, PA: WB Saunders.

Boss, S. M., C. L. Gries, B. K. Kirchner, G. D. Smith, and P. C. Francis. 1994. Use of vancomycin hydrochloride for treatment of *Clostridium difficile* enteritis in Syrian hamsters. *Lab Anim Sci* 44(1): 31–37.

Burgmann, P., and D. H. Percy. 1993. Antimicrobial drug use in rodents and rabbits. In *Antimicrobial Therapy in Veterinary Medicine*, 2nd ed., J. F. Prescott and J. D. Baggot (eds.), pp. 524–541. Ames, IA: Iowa State University Press.

Burke, T. J. 1995. "Wet tail" in hamsters and other diarrheas of small rodents. In *Kirk's Current Veterinary Therapy XII: Small Animal Practice*, J. D. Bonagura (ed.), pp. 1336–1339. Philadelphia, PA: WB Saunders.

Collins, B. R. 1995. Antimicrobial drug use in rabbits, rodents, and other small mammals. In *Antimicrobial Therapy in Caged Birds and Exotic Pets*, pp. 3–10. Trenton, NJ: Veterinary Learning Systems.

Flecknell, P. A. 1997. Medetomidine and atipamezole: Potential uses in laboratory animals. *Lab Anim (NY)* 26(2): 21–25.

Flecknell, P. A. 2009. *Laboratory Animal Anaesthesia*, 3d ed. London: Academic Press.

Flecknell, P. A. 2016. *Laboratory Animal Anaesthesia*, 4th ed. Oxford: Academic Press.

Forsythe, D. B., A. J. Payton, D. Dixson, P. H. Myers, J. A. Clark, and J. R. Snipe. 1992. Evaluation of Telazol–xylazine as an anesthetic combination for use in Syrian hamsters. *Lab Anim Sci* 42(5): 497–502.

Harkness, J. E. 1993. *A Practitioner's Guide to Domestic Rodents*. Lakewood, CO: American Animal Hospital Association.

Harkness, J. E., P. V. Turner, S. VandeWoude, and C. L. Wheler. 2010. *Harkness and Wagner's Biology and Medicine of Rabbits and Rodents*, 5th ed. Ames, IA: Wiley-Blackwell.

Harkness, J. E., and J. E. Wagner. 1995. *Biology and Medicine of Rabbits and Rodents*, 4th ed. York, PA: Williams & Wilkins.

Harrenstien, L. 1994. Critical care of ferrets, rabbits, and rodents. *Semin Avian Exotic Pet Med* 3: 217–228.

Heard, D. J. 1993. Principles and techniques of anesthesia and analgesia for exotic practice. *Vet Clin North Am Small Anim Pract* 23: 1301–1327.

Huerkamp, M. J. 1995. Anesthesia and postoperative management of rabbits and pocket pets. In *Kirk's Current Veterinary Therapy XII: Small Animal Practice*, J. D. Bonagura (ed.), pp. 1322–1327. Philadelphia, PA: WB Saunders.

Institute of Laboratory Animal Resources (ILAR). 2011. *Guide for the Care and Use of Laboratory Animals*, 8th ed. ILAR, National Research Council. Washington, DC: National Academies Press.

Lukas, V. 1999. Volume guidelines for compound administration. In *The Care and Feeding of an IACUC*, M. L. Podolsky and V. S. Lukas (eds.), p. 187. Boca Raton, FL: CRC Press.

Mason, D. E. 1997. Anesthesia, analgesia, and sedation for small mammals. In *Ferrets, Rabbits, and Rodents: Clinical Medicine and Surgery*, E.V. Hillyer and K. E. Quesenberry (eds.), pp. 378–397. Philadelphia, PA: WB Saunders.

Miedel, E.L., and F. C. Hankenson. 2015. Biology and diseases of hamsters. In *Laboratory Animal Medicine*, 3rd ed., J.G. Fox, L.C. Anderson, G. Otto, K.R. Pritchett-Corning, and M.T. Whary (eds.), pp. 209–245. Amsterdam: Academic Press.

Morrisey, J. K., and J. W. Carpenter. 2004. Formulary. In *Ferrets, Rabbits, and Rodents: Clinical Medicine and Surgery*, K. E. Quesenberry and J. W. Carpenter (eds.), pp. 436–444. St. Louis, MO: WB Saunders.

Morrisey, J. K., and J. W. Carpenter. 2011. Drug formulary. In *Ferrets, Rabbits, and Rodents: Clinical Medicine and Surgery*, K. E. Quesenberry and J. W. Carpenter (eds.), pp. 566–575. St. Louis, MO: WB Saunders.

Mulder, G. B. 2012. Management, husbandry, and colony health. In *The Laboratory Rabbit, Guinea Pig, Hamster, and Other Rodents*, M. A. Suckow, K. A. Stevens, and R. P. Wilson (eds.), pp. 765–777. San Diego, CA: Academic Press.

Pollack, C. 2002. Postoperative management of the exotic animal patient. *Vet Clin North Am: Exotic Anim Pract* 5: 183–212.

Reid, W. D., C. Davies, P. D. Pare, and R. L. Pardy. 1989. An effective combination of anaesthetics for 6-hour experimentation in the golden Syrian hamster. *Lab Anim* 23: 156–162.

Richardson, V. C. G. 1997. *Diseases of Small Domestic Rodents*. Oxford: Blackwell.
Rollin, B. E., and M. L. Kesel. 1995. *The Experimental Animal in Biomedical Research. Vol II: Care, Husbandry, and Wellbeing: An Overview by Species*. Boca Raton, FL: CRC Press.
Thayer, C. B., S. Lowe, and W. C. Rubright. 1972. Clinical evaluation of a combination of droperidol and fentanyl as an anesthetic for the rat and hamster. *JAVMA* 161: 665–668.
Wixson, S. K. 1994. Rabbits and rodents: Anesthesia and analgesia. In *Research Animal Anesthesia, Analgesia and Surgery*, A. C. Smith and M. M. Swindle (eds.), pp. 59–92. Greenbelt, MD: Scientists Center for Animal Welfare.

FURTHER READING

American Association of Laboratory Animal Science (AALAS). Introduction to hamsters. Available at www.aalaslearninglibrary.org [accessed September 25, 2018].
Anton, P. M., M. O'Brien, E. Kokkotou, et al. 2004. Rifalazil treats and prevents relapse of *Clostridium difficile*–associated diarrhea in hamsters. *Antimicrob Agents Chemother* 48(10): 3975–3979.
Barthold, S. W., S. M. Griffey, and D.H. Percy. 2016. *Pathology of Laboratory Rodents and Rabbits*, 4th ed. Ames, IA: Wiley-Blackwell.
Bauck, L. 1989. Ophthalmic conditions in pet rabbits and rodents. *Compend Contin Educ Pract Vet* 11(3): 258–269.
Burr, H. N., L. Paluch, G. S. Roble, and N. S. Lipman. 2012. Parasitic diseases. In *The Laboratory Rabbit, Guinea Pig, Hamster, and Other Rodents*, M. A. Suckow, K. A. Stevens, and R. P. Wilson (eds.), pp. 839–866. San Diego, CA: Academic Press.
Cassano, A., S. Rasmussen, and F. R. Wolf. 2012. Viral diseases. In *The Laboratory Rabbit, Guinea Pig, Hamster, and Other Rodents*, M. A. Suckow, K. A. Stevens, and R. P. Wilson (eds.), pp. 821–837. San Diego, CA: Academic Press.
Frisk, C. S. 2012. Bacterial and fungal diseases. In *The Laboratory Rabbit, Guinea Pig, Hamster, and Other Rodents*, M. A. Suckow, K. A. Stevens, and R. P. Wilson (eds.), pp. 797–820. San Diego, CA: Academic Press.
Gaertner, D. J., K. R. Boschert, and T. R. Schoeb. 1987. Muscle necrosis in Syrian hamsters resulting from intramuscular injections of ketamine and xylazine. *Lab Anim Sci* 37(1): 80–83.
Hubrecht, R., and J. Kirkwood. 2010. *The UFAW Handbook on the Care and Management of Laboratory and Other Research Animals*, 8th ed. Ames, IA: Wiley-Blackwell.
Johnson-Delaney, C. 1999. Postoperative management of small mammals. *Exotic DVM* 1(5): 19–21.
Karolewski, B., T. W. Mayer, and G. Ruble. 2012. Non-infectious diseases. In *The Laboratory Rabbit, Guinea Pig, Hamster, and Other Rodents*, M. A. Suckow, K. A. Stevens, and R. P. Wilson (eds.), pp. 867–873. San Diego, CA: Academic Press.
LaRegina, M., W. H. Fales, and J. E. Wagner. 1980. Effects of antibiotic treatment on the occurrence of experimentally induced proliferative ileitis of hamsters. *Lab Anim Sci* 30(1): 38–41.

Lavin, L. M. 2007. Avian and exotic radiography. In *Radiography in Veterinary Technology*, 4th ed., pp. 294–301. St. Louis, MO: WB Saunders.

Meshorer, A. 1976. Leg lesions in hamsters caused by wood shavings. *Lab Anim Sci* 26: 827–829.

Murray, K. A. 2012. Anatomy, physiology, and behavior. In *The Laboratory Rabbit, Guinea Pig, Hamster, and Other Rodents*, M. A. Suckow, K. A. Stevens, and R. P. Wilson (eds.), pp. 753–763. San Diego, CA: Academic Press.

Peace, T. A., K. V. Brock, and H. F. Stills Jr. 1994. Comparative analysis of the 16S rRNA gene sequence of the putative agent of proliferative ileitis of hamsters. *Int J Syst Bacteriol* 44(4): 832–835.

Percy, D. H., and S. W. Barthold. 2007. *Pathology of Laboratory Rodents and Rabbits*, 3rd ed. Ames, IA: Wiley-Blackwell.

Silverman, J. 2012. Biomedical research techniques. In *The Laboratory Rabbit, Guinea Pig, Hamster, and Other Rodents*, M. A. Suckow, K. A. Stevens, and R. P. Wilson (eds.), pp. 779–795. San Diego, CA: Academic Press.

Silverman, J., M. Huhndorf, M. Balk, and G. Slater. 1983. Evaluation of a combination of tiletamine and zolazepam as an anesthetic for laboratory rodents. *Lab Anim Sci* 33(5): 457–460.

Smith, G. D. 2012. Taxonomy and history. In *The Laboratory Rabbit, Guinea Pig, Hamster, and Other Rodents*, M. A. Suckow, K. A. Stevens, and R. P. Wilson (eds.), pp. 747–752. San Diego, CA: Academic Press.

Streilein, J. W., W. R. Duncan, and F. Homburger. 1980. Immunogenetic relationships among genetically defined, inbred domestic Syrian hamster strains. *Transplantation* 30(5): 358–361.

Valentine, H., E. K. Daugherity, B. Singh, and K. J. Maurer. 2012. The experimental use of Syrian hamsters. In *The Laboratory Rabbit, Guinea Pig, Hamster, and Other Rodents*, M. A. Suckow, K. A. Stevens, and R. P. Wilson (eds.), pp. 875–906. San Diego, CA: Academic Press.

Van Hoosier, G. L. Jr., and C. W. McPherson (eds.). 1987. *Laboratory Hamsters*. Orlando, FL: Academic Press.

CHAPTER 7 REVIEW

Short Answer

1. What is the gestation period in the hamster and why is it unique?
2. What is the most commonly used hamster in biomedical research?
3. Name two inbred hamster strains that could be used for muscular dystrophy research.
4. True/False: Hamsters are social species and should be group housed.
5. What conditions are needed for a hamster to hibernate?
6. Why are the cheek pouches an ideal location for tumor implantation?

7. What normal structure can be found on each flank on the hamster, and what is its physiologic role?
8. What is the most ideal time to pair hamsters for successful breeding?
9. True/False: Per the Animal Welfare Act, it is acceptable to feed hamsters on the floor of the cage.
10. What are some enrichment items that are appropriate for hamsters and what natural behaviors do they promote?

Fill in the blank

11. Litter abandonment and ________________ of young are common during the first pregnancy.
12. Antibiotic-associated ________________ may develop when antibiotics that disrupt the normal intestinal microbial flora are given.
13. Proliferative ileitis is commonly called ________________.
14. ______________ is a condition characterized by excessive, extracellular deposition of inert protein fibrils in organs such as the liver, kidney, and spleen.
15. Hamsters have a high metabolic rate, and therefore ________________ is not recommended prior to anesthesia.
16. Hamsters are less susceptible than gerbils to ________________, but it can still cause high morbidity and mortality in weanlings.
17. ____________ can cause one of two presentations in the hamster; ________________ on the face, feet, neck, etc. or ______________ in the internal organs.
18. ___________ mites are found on healthy, immunocompetent hamsters, and thought only to cause a problem in older and immunocompromised animals.
19. Diets made up primarily of ___________ can lead to nutritional deficiencies.
20. Clinical signs of heart failure are often seen in older hamsters with ___________, which typically occurs secondary to amyloidosis or degenerative cardiomyopathy.

Critical Thinking

21. You are recently assigned responsibility for a hamster breeding colony in a biomedical research facility. The number of viable births has decreased over the past 4 months. In addition, there is a high percentage of litter abandonment and cannibalism by the dams. You visit the animal room and observe the following: all hamsters are housed in clear microisolation shoebox-style cages with ½ in. of corn cob bedding; 70°F room temperature; 45% humidity; 12 air changes per hour; and light timers that are set to deliver 12 hours of light per day. You check a number of the cage cards and discover many of the breeders are 16–18 months of age. Make suggestions to assist the researcher with her hamster breeding colony.

8

Guinea Pigs

Guinea pigs are caviomorph (New World hystricognath) rodents native to South America. Although they belong to the order Rodentia, guinea pigs are more closely related to porcupines and chinchillas than to mice and rats. The guinea pig is colloquially known as a "cavy," derived from its scientific name, *Cavia porcellus*. Guinea pigs historically have been, and continue to be, used as a common human food source in some South American countries. Three primary breeds of guinea pigs are recognized: English, Abyssinian, and Peruvian, and each can be distinguished by the length, texture, and direction of hair growth. English guinea pigs have uniformly short, straight hair, and are the breed seen most frequently in the research setting. Multiple genetic classifications used in research have been derived from the English breed, including outbred stocks (e.g. Dunkin-Hartley and Hartley), inbred strains (e.g. Strain 2 and Strain 13), and mutant strains (e.g. the IAF hairless strain developed following a spontaneously occurring genetic mutation of an outbred Hartley colony). Abyssinian guinea pigs have short, coarse hair arranged in whorls or rosettes, which gives them an untidy appearance. Peruvian guinea pigs have long, fine, silky hair. Guinea pigs may be monocolored, bicolored, or tricolored.

USES

The guinea pig has a long history as a research model. The number of guinea pigs used in the laboratory peaked in the 1960s, largely due to their central role in tuberculosis research. Although their use has significantly decreased, they are still a very valuable and unique resource in many areas of research.

Clinical Laboratory Animal Medicine: An Introduction, Fifth Edition.
Lesley A. Colby, Megan H. Nowland, and Lucy H. Kennedy.

Companion website: www.wiley.com/go/colby/clinical

Guinea pigs are an appealing animal model due to a body size conducive to surgical manipulation, wide commercial availability, a tractable disposition, and broad historical use. They share several features with humans, such as the need for dietary vitamin C and susceptibility to tuberculosis. They are a well-established model of anaphylaxis. Sensitized animals have a high incidence of anaphylaxis when injected with a small amount of antigen and subsequently develop lethal bronchiolar constriction in response to histamine release. Guinea pigs are also frequently used as a source of complement, which is used in complement fixation tests to diagnose infectious diseases, and are used in studies of immunology, otology, infectious disease, asthma, delayed hypersensitivity, nutrition, and toxicology.

BEHAVIOR

Guinea pigs are communal animals that live together amicably. When group housed, they tend to huddle together as a single unit. Like other rodents, they are thigmotactic, preferring to maintain contact with the cage periphery while avoiding the "open field" of the cage center. Providing a "shade" over the cage can result in increased utilization of the cage space (Byrd et al. 2016). Guinea pigs establish male-dominated social hierarchies. Once the hierarchy is formed, the group is usually stable. Introduction of a new male into a group, however, can provoke fighting. Dominant animals will frequently chew and barber the hair near the hip or rump of subordinate cagemates. Barbering is also associated with boredom and overcrowding. Adults, especially males, will chew the ears of the young.

Unlike the mouse and rat, guinea pigs are active during daylight hours and eat frequently during both light and dark hours. They are generally calm but can be easily excited by sudden noise or changes in their environment, tending to freeze at unfamiliar sounds and scatter when exposed to sudden movements. The immobility reaction can last from several seconds to 20 minutes. The scatter reaction can involve stampeding, jumping, or rapid circling of their cage, which can result in the trampling and serious injury or death of young within the cage. Guinea pigs exhibit the Preyer or pinna reflex, in which they cock their ears in response to a sound. Vocalization appears to be an important component of their behavioral repertoire; at least 11 different vocalizations have been recorded, some of which are inaudible to humans. The whistle is used in anticipation of feeding, a purr during social interactions, and a squeal or scream is elicited when injured or fearful. Guinea pigs develop rigid habits and have an aversion to change in diet and environment. Developing strong food preferences early in life, animals may refuse to consume novel food items or even previously accepted food or drink if it has been modified in any way (e.g. medication-supplemented food items) to the point of starvation. Indeed, feeding habits can be so strongly entrenched that they may refuse to eat or drink from novel food or water receptacles.

ANATOMIC AND PHYSIOLOGIC FEATURES

Guinea pig biologic and reproductive data are listed in Table 8.1. Guinea pigs have a compact body with short legs and a vestigial tail. Unlike other common laboratory rodents, these animals possess four digits on the forefeet and three on the hind feet. Guinea pigs have large tympanic bullae, which facilitates access to the internal structures of the ear. Hearing, olfaction, and color discrimination are well developed. Their dental formula, 2(I 1/1, C 0/0, P 1/1, and M 3/3), is unique among rodents, as most lack premolars. The opening of the oral cavity is small and a diastema, or gap, is present between the incisor and premolar teeth. All of the teeth are open rooted, growing continuously. The chisel-like incisors are white, unlike those of other rodents, and the upper pair of incisors is shorter than the lower pair. The anatomic structure of their pharynx is unique. The soft palate is continuous with the base of the tongue and possesses an opening called the palatal ostium: This arrangement forms the sole passage from the oropharynx to the distal pharynx (Timm et al. 1987). Due to this anatomical structure, and because their oral cavity is quite long and narrow, intubation is difficult. The thymus of the guinea pig lies in the ventral cervical region surrounding the trachea. This location facilitates its surgical removal in support of select immunological studies requiring thymectomy; however, accessory thymic tissue may be present in surrounding tissues. This differs from most other rodents in which the thymus is located in the thoracic cavity overlying the heart. The adrenal glands are bilobed and large. The guinea pig is monogastric and, unlike many other rodents, has an undivided stomach lined entirely with glandular epithe-

Table 8.1. Biologic and reproductive data for guinea pigs

Adult body weight: Male	900–1200 g
Adult body weight: Female	700–900 g
Life span	5–7 y
Body temperature	37.2–39.5°C (99–103.1°F)
Heart rate	230–380 beats per minute
Respiratory rate	40–130 breaths per minute
Tidal volume	2.3–5.3 mL/kg
Food consumption	6 g/100 g per day
Water consumption	10 mL/100 g per day
Breeding onset: Male	3–4 mo (600–700 g)
Breeding onset: Female	2–3 mo (350–450 g)
Estrous cycle length	15–17 d
Gestation period	59–72 d
Postpartum estrus	Fertile
Litter size	1–6
Weaning age	14–21 d
Breeding duration	18–48 mo
Chromosome number (diploid)	64

Source: Adapted from Harkness et al. (2010).

lium. The cecum is large and holds up to 65% of the gastrointestinal capacity, occupying most of the left midabdominal cavity. Guinea pigs are vigorously coprophagic, regularly consuming feces directly from the anus or from the cage floor. They have sebaceous marking glands located circumanally and on the rump and will often walk or sit while pressing the glands against a surface.

The guinea pig is the only common laboratory animal, other than nonhuman primates, that resembles the human in its dietary requirement of vitamin C. Vitamin C plays a significant role as an antioxidant, in collagen synthesis, and in support of the cardiovascular and immune systems. It must be provided in the diet as guinea pigs lack the enzyme L-gulonolactone oxidase required for endogenous synthesis (Box 8.1). Cavies (as well as ferrets and nonhuman primates) are steroid resistant: steroid administration does not induce as significant a reduction in lymphocyte numbers and function as occurs in steroid-sensitive species.

Sexing is done by manipulation and visualization. Male guinea pigs are larger than females and possess large testes and an os penis. The penis has two prongs at the tip and, with slight manual pressure, is easily extruded from the preputial sheath. The inguinal canals remain open in the male. Males have several accessory sex glands, including large, transparent, smooth seminiferous vesicles that extend 10 cm into the abdomen from the pubis and are commonly mistaken as uterine horns by those unfamiliar with guinea pig anatomy. Females have a bicornuate uterus with a single cervical os. Both sexes possess one pair of mammary glands in the inguinal region; however, the male's nipples are smaller. The female has a vaginal closure membrane that is open only during estrus and parturition. Females have a Y-shaped genital–anal opening with the rectal opening positioned at the base of the Y, the urethra positioned within the top branches of the Y, and the vaginal opening in the center. This is in contrast to the male's slit-shaped rectal opening as depicted in Figure 8.1.

Compared with other rodents, the packed cell volume, erythrocytes, and hemoglobin levels of the guinea pig are relatively low. Typical of rodents, the lymphocyte is the dominant leukocyte. Heterophils (like those of the rabbit) replace neutrophils and have distinct eosinophilic cytoplasmic granules. The guinea pig has a unique leukocyte, the Foa Kurloff or Kurloff cell, a mononuclear lymphocyte with a large intracytoplasmic inclusion (Figure 8.2). Kurloff cells proliferate with estrogenic stimulation and exhibit some natural killer cell activity. Although they can be found in the peripheral circulation of both males and nonpregnant females, elevated numbers are found in the circulation of pregnant females, with highest numbers in the placenta. Urine is normally alkaline (pH 8–9), opaque, and creamy yellow due to high concentrations of calcium crystals. Selected hematologic and biochemical values are listed in Appendix 1, "Normal Values."

Box 8.1

Vitamin C must be provided in the diet as guinea pigs lack the enzyme L-gulonolactone oxidase required for endogenous synthesis.

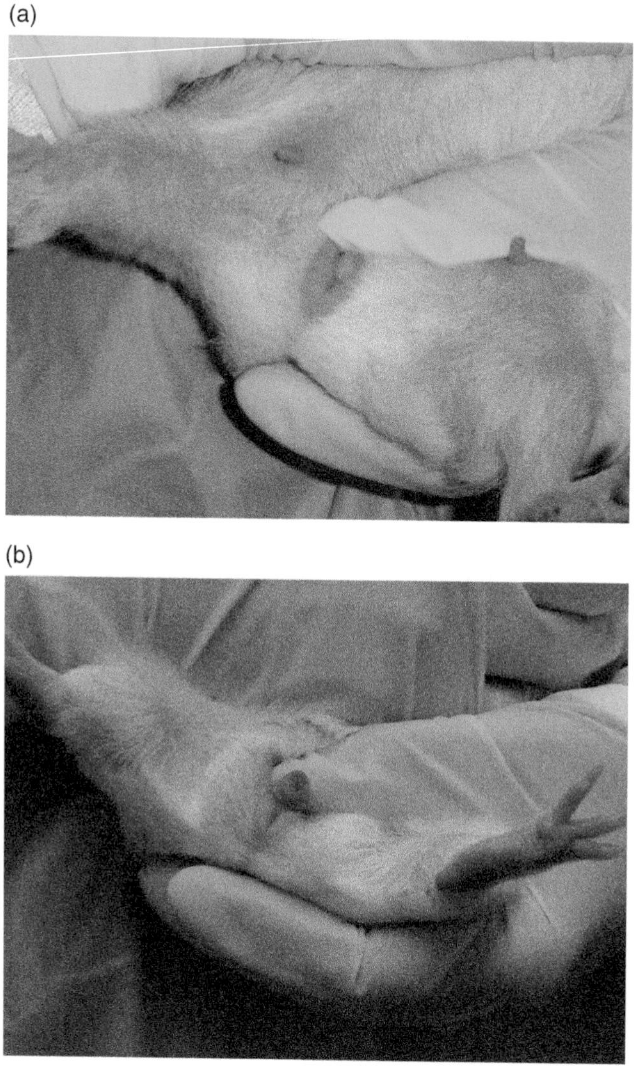

Fig 8.1. (a) Genitalia of female (Y-shaped) and (b) male (slit-shaped) with penis everted. (*Source:* Photo courtesy of ULAM, University of Michigan.)

BREEDING AND REPRODUCTION

The sow, or female, is usually bred at 2–3 months of age, which corresponds to a weight of 350–450 g. It is important that breeding occur prior to 7 months of age to prevent permanent fusion of the pelvic symphysis, which often results in dystocia (Box 8.2). The boar, or male, is bred at 3–4 months of age or 600–700 g body weight. The sow is a nonseasonal, continuously polyestrous breeder with a 15- to 17-day estrous cycle. Detection of estrus is not necessary unless timed matings are desired as guinea pigs are normally pair housed for mating. When in estrus, the sow displays a swollen, congested vulva and exhibits lordosis, characterized by extension of all four legs, straightening and arching of the back, and elevation of the pubic area.

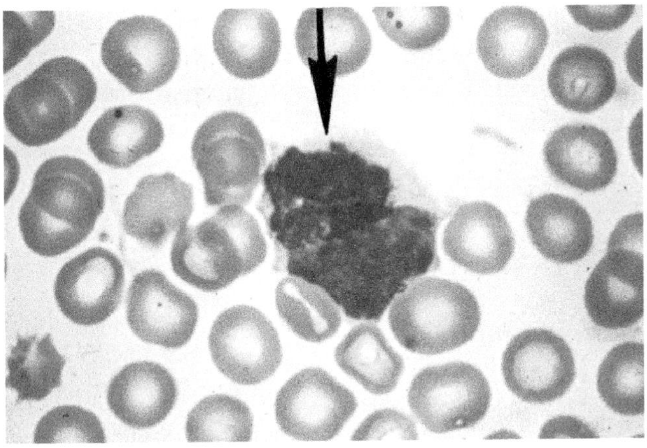

Fig 8.2. Kurloff cell, mononuclear lymphocyte with a large intracytoplasmic inclusion. (*Source:* Photo courtesy of ACLAM.)

Box 8.2

It is important that breeding occur prior to 7 months of age to prevent permanent fusion of the pelvic symphysis, which often results in dystocia.

The male will purr, circle the sow, and sniff and lick her anogenital area prior to mounting. Mating can be confirmed by the presence of a vaginal plug, a solid mass formed from ejaculate fluids that may be retained in the vagina for several hours after copulation. Pregnancy can be confirmed by palpating the fetal mass at 14–21 days of gestation. The fetal skeletons can be visualized radiographically at 6 weeks. A fertile postpartum estrus does occur from 2 to 10 hours after parturition.

It is important for the sow to remain active during pregnancy to maintain body condition and prevent obesity. Due to the normally large total fetal mass, a sow's body weight may nearly double during pregnancy. Guinea pigs have a labyrinthine hemomonochorionic placentation, as do humans. The gestation period ranges from 59 to 72 days, with an average of 68 days. The gestation length varies inversely with the size of the litter: longer for small litters and shorter for large litters. During the last week of gestation, the pelvic symphysis relaxes and separates due to the effects of the hormone relaxin. Unlike some other species, guinea pigs do not build nests. The sow farrows in a squatting position. Parturition normally takes approximately 30 minutes, with 5–10 minutes between pups. If a sow strains unsuccessfully for 20 minutes, strains intermittently over the course of 2 hours, or if a pup is not delivered within 10–15 minutes of an oxytocin injection, a cesarean section is indicated. Both the sow and the boar may consume the placenta. Unlike most other rodents, young are precocious: they are born fully haired, with teeth, and with their eyes and ears open. The pup receives all maternal antibodies from the placenta, none from the colostrum. The young do not nurse for the first 12–24 hours following birth.

They can begin eating solid food and drinking water during the first week of life and are nearly self-sufficient by 4–5 days of age. However, an approximate 50% mortality rate is observed in young that do not nurse within the first 3–5 days of life. Guinea pigs can be weaned at 14–21 days or when they weigh approximately 180 g.

HUSBANDRY

Housing and Environment

Guinea pigs may be housed individually or in groups. To reduce limb injuries, solid-bottom cages with bedding are preferred. Wire flooring should be avoided as the feet of smaller animals often fall through the mesh, lacerating or fracturing their limbs. Because guinea pigs are not inclined to climb or jump, most can be kept in open-top cages, provided the sides are at least 25 cm (10 in.) high. Rectangular cages are preferred over square as they tend to diminish the stampede response. Adult animals (greater than 350 g) should be provided with at least 652 cm^2 (101 $in.^2$) of floor space per animal with a cage height of at least 7 inches. The bedding material should be as dust free as possible. Ground corncobs, processed cellulose products, or other material of plant origin can be used. Wood shavings can adhere to the moist perineal region, causing irritation or obstructions and thus are not recommended. Housing temperatures range between 20°C and 26°C (68°F and 79°F), with 21°C (70°F) recommended. Having a compact body, low temperatures are better tolerated than high temperatures, especially if the humidity is high. The environmental humidity should be maintained between 30% and 70%, with at least 10–15 air changes per hour. Provide 12 hours of light per day, controlled through automatic timers. Guinea pigs are susceptible to *Bordetella bronchiseptica* and thus should be cared for prior to and ideally physically distanced from species such as rabbits, cats, and dogs that may be subclinically infected.

Sanitation

Cages should be cleaned at least two to three times weekly as these animals produce a significant volume of waste. Cages, water bottles, and feed hoppers should be disinfected with chemicals, hot water 61.6–82.2°C (143–180°F), or a combination of both. An acid rinse prior to cage washing facilitates removal of scale that develops from an accumulation of urine minerals. Detergents and chemical disinfectants enhance the effectiveness of hot water, but they must be thoroughly rinsed from all caging surfaces with fresh water. Refer to Chapter 3 and Chapter 4, for a more detailed description of disinfection methods.

Environmental Enrichment and Social Housing

Guinea pigs are social animals and do best when housed in small, compatible groups. The provision of enrichment items may benefit this species; objects should be nontoxic, nondigestible, sanitizable, and safe. The types of enrichment items most frequently provided to guinea pigs are those items that the animal can manually manipulate or gnaw on, items that provide increased cage complexity (e.g. partially enclosed structures or huts), or food treats commercially prepared for laboratory animal use. Given the guinea pig's rigid habits and tendency toward neophobia, introducing novel items may be stressful for these animals. Therefore, the use of all enrichment items must be critically evaluated before being routinely provided to a colony.

Feeding and Watering

Commercial pelleted diets manufactured specifically for laboratory guinea pigs can be fed ad libitum. It is important that the food be properly stored and used prior to the manufacturer's determined expiration date (usually within 6 months of milling), to help ensure adequate vitamin C content. Diets with questionable or inadequate levels of vitamin C should never be provided, regardless of any attempts to provide the vitamin via supplemental food items or vitamin C tablets. Rabbit chow is not appropriate for guinea pigs as it lacks vitamin C and has excess levels of vitamin D. Guinea pigs eat an average of 6 g/100 g of body weight per day. Feed is best provided in self-feeders, such as a J-feeder, mounted on the cage wall, as animals tend to sit, sleep, and defecate in bowls placed on the cage floor. Good-quality hay can be provided as a supplement to reduce boredom and decrease barbering. Kale, parsley, beet greens, kiwi fruit, broccoli, oranges, and cabbage are good sources of vitamin C and can be fed in small amounts not to exceed 10–15% by weight of the pelleted diet. Any fresh fruit or vegetable treats provided should be of a quality fit for human consumption and thoroughly cleaned prior to feeding to reduce potential of contamination with pathogenic organisms. Potential bacterial, viral, and parasitic contaminants of hay must be considered. To decrease this risk, some institutions provide autoclaved or sterilized hay. Uneaten items should be removed from cages daily. Fresh potable water should be available ad libitum by bottle or automated watering system. Adult guinea pigs drink an average of 10 mL/100 g of body weight per day. As with food receptacles, water bowls or crocks placed on the cage floor should not be used as they readily become contaminated with feces and bedding. Guinea pigs are untidy water drinkers; rather than lick, they often chew on and play with sipper tubes and valves and will waste a significant amount of water. Animals may inadvertently flood their own cages through the manipulation of water lixits with ends positioned within their cage. Guinea pigs will also push food particles up the sipper tube of water bottles and foul the water supply. The use of automated water systems with valves located outside the cage is therefore advantageous.

TECHNIQUES

Handling and Restraint

Guinea pigs should be handled gently but firmly. They should be lifted using two hands, grasping under the trunk with one hand while supporting the rear quarters with the other hand (Figure 8.3). Support is particularly important with adults and pregnant animals. Grasping a guinea pig too firmly around the thorax or abdomen can impede breathing and cause injury to the lungs, diaphragm, or liver.

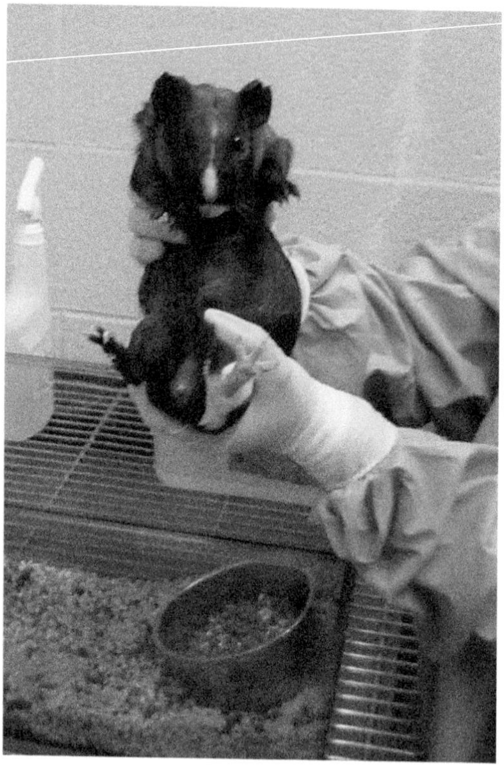

Fig 8.3. Appropriate guinea pig restraint: one hand around the trunk and one hand supporting the rear quarters. (*Source:* Photo courtesy of ULAM, University of Michigan.)

Identification

Cage cards or color pattern records can be used to identify guinea pigs. Permanent individual animal identification can be accomplished by ear notching, ear tagging, tattooing, or microchip placement. Dyes, shaving of the fur, and nontoxic markers can be used for temporary identification.

Blood Collection

Assuming the animal is mature, healthy, and on an adequate plane of nutrition, the blood volume (in milliliters) of most species averages 7% of the body weight in grams. Table 8.2 lists approximate adult guinea pig blood volumes. A typical rule of thumb

Table 8.2. Adult guinea pig blood volumes and suggested sample size

	Volume (mL)
Total blood	40–80
Single sample	4–8
Exsanguination	15–30

Source: Adapted from Harkness et al. (2010).
Note: Values are approximate.

for blood withdrawal suggests that up to 10% of the circulating blood volume can be withdrawn every 2–3 weeks from normal, healthy animals with minimal adverse effect.

Guinea pigs lack readily accessible peripheral veins. Small amounts of blood (<1 mL) can be obtained from the saphenous vein, cephalic vein, or a toenail bed. Larger quantities of blood can be obtained from the cranial vena cava or jugular vein, femoral artery or vein, or directly from the heart. The guinea pig must be sedated to obtain blood from the cranial vena cava or femoral vessels and must be anesthetized for cardiac puncture. Venipuncture of the cranial vena cava can cause bleeding into the thoracic cavity. Cardiac puncture involves a significant element of risk and is not recommended except as a terminal procedure. Alternatively, a catheter can be surgically implanted into the jugular vein to collect larger quantities or repeated blood samples.

Urine Collection

Urine may be collected by using a metabolic cage, gentle manual pressure on the bladder, cystocentesis, or placing the animal on a cold, clean surface.

Drug Administration

Palatable drugs can be incorporated into the food or water, but guinea pigs often refuse food or water with an unfamiliar taste. Liquids can be administered orally using a small syringe. Orogastric gavage with a metal dosing needle, which is easily accomplished in mice and rats, is not an option with guinea pigs due to the unique anatomy of the palate. Passing a 5- or 6-French infant feeding tube through the palatal ostium of an unanesthetized guinea pig is an option for administering drugs directly into the stomach; it requires the use of a plastic bite block to protect the tube. Subcutaneous (SC) injections require some force because guinea pig skin is tough, especially over the neck and back. A maximum volume of 20 mL/kg is recommended. Intramuscular (IM) injections with a maximum volume of 0.3 mL may be given in the lumbar musculature or quadriceps muscle to avoid the sciatic nerve. Intraperitoneal (IP) injections are made lateral to the midline in the lower right quadrant of the abdomen. Some recommend tilting the guinea pig's head toward the floor with the objective of shifting the abdominal organs forward, helping to prevent inadvertent injection into the intestine. A maximum volume of 20 mL/kg can be given IP. Intravenous (IV) injections can be made using the saphenous or the cephalic vein. Suggested maximum dosing volumes are summarized in Table 8.3.

Table 8.3. Maximum guinea pig dosing volumes

Route	Volume (mL/kg)
IP	20
SC	20
IM	0.3/site with maximum of two injections
IV	5 (bolus)/20 (infusion)
ID	0.05/site
PO	20

Sources: Huerkamp et al. (1996) and Lukas (1999).

Anesthesia, Surgery, and Postoperative Care

Guinea pigs should be fasted for 3–6 hours prior to anesthetic induction to decrease the amount of ingesta in the cecum and stomach that could otherwise restrict movement of the diaphragm and interfere with respiration. These animals frequently retain a considerable amount of feed in their buccal cavities, which can contribute to airway obstruction when they are anesthetized. Gently rinse the mouth with 10–20 mL of tap water to remove this material before induction. A variety of agents used to tranquilize and anesthetize guinea pigs are listed in Table 8.4. Anesthesia in the guinea pig

Table 8.4. Anesthetic agents and tranquilizers used in guinea pigs

Drug	Dosage	Route	Reference
Inhalants			
Isoflurane	2%–5% to effect	Inhalation	Harkness and Wagner (1995)
Sevoflurane	To effect	Inhalation	Morrisey and Carpenter (2004)
Injectables			
Acepromazine	0.5–1 mg/kg	IM	Harkness and Wagner (1995)
Diazepam	2.5 mg/kg	IM, IP	Flecknell (2009)
Fentanyl-droperidol	0.44–0.8 mL/kg	IM	Flecknell (2009)
Fentanyl-fluanisone	1 mL/kg	IM, IP	Flecknell (2009)
Fentanyl-fluanisone	1 mL/kg	IM, IP	Flecknell (2009)
+ diazepam	2.5 mg/kg	IP	
Ketamine	100 mg/kg	IM, IP	Flecknell (2009)
Ketamine	100 mg/kg	IM	Flecknell (2009)
+ acepromazine	5 mg/kg	IM	
Ketamine	40 mg/kg	IM	Clemens and Seeman (2011)
+ dexmedetomidine	0.15 mg/kg	IM	
Ketamine	60–100 mg/kg	IM	Gilroy and Varga (1980)
+ diazepam	5–8 mg/kg	IM	
Ketamine	40 mg/kg	IP	Flecknell (1997)
+ medetomidine	0.5 mg/kg	IP	
Ketamine	40–60 mg/kg	IP	Harkness et al. (2010)
+ xylazine	2–5 mg/kg	IP	
Ketamine	22–64 mg/kg	IM	Anderson (1994)
+ xylazine	2–5 mg/kg	IM	
+ acepromazine	0.75 mg/kg	IM	
Midazolam	5 mg/kg	IM, IP	Flecknell (2009)
Pentobarbital	25–35 mg/kg	IP	Harkness et al. (2010)
Tiletamine-zolazepam	40 mg/kg	IM	Buchanan et al. (1998)
+ medetomidine	0.5 mg/kg	IM	
Tiletamine-zolazepam	40 mg/kg	IM	Buchanan et al. (1998)
+ xylazine	5 mg/kg	IM	
Tiletamine-zolazepam	60 mg/kg	IP	Jacobson (2001)
+ xylazine	5 mg/kg	IP	
+ butorphanol	0.1 mg/kg	IM	

IM = intramuscular; IP = intraperitoneal.

chapter 8

is difficult for a number of reasons. This species has a variable response to drugs; thus there is a wide range of dosages for various agents reported in the literature. Care must be used when determining an appropriate dose of injectable agents, as the true or metabolically active body weight can be overestimated due to the proportionally high quantity and weight of cecal and intestinal contents and fecal mass. Under some anesthetics, such as pentobarbital and volatile agents, guinea pigs exhibit a peculiar squirming muscle movement that does not signify return to consciousness. When using agents such as ketamine–xylazine combination, use the lowest dose possible and dilute and/or reduce the amount injected per site. As such agents injected IM have been noted to cause muscle necrosis and/or self-mutilation of the injected limb, IP dosing is suggested.

Face masks are often used to administer inhalation agents as intubation is difficult due to the small size of the oral opening and trachea as well as the anatomy of the pharynx. Care must be taken during intubation attempts to not traumatize the soft tissue at the base of the tongue. As with orogastric gavage, intubation requires passage through the palatal ostium. A 14- to 16-gauge IV catheter can be used as an endotracheal tube. Isoflurane and sevoflurane should not be used with an open-drop method, because lethal concentrations of gases can be rapidly reached at room temperature. Inhalant anesthetics should always be used with appropriate waste gas scavenging systems.

The ear pinch, respiratory rate, and heart rate can be used to monitor the depth of anesthesia. Palpebral reflexes, eyeball position, and pedal reflexes are not reliable indicators of depth of anesthesia in guinea pigs. Unmedicated ophthalmic ointment should be instilled in the eyes of anesthetized animals to prevent exposure keratitis. Profuse salivary secretions are common and can be controlled by administering atropine or glycopyrrolate. Use of a circulating water heating pad or other precisely controlled heat source is recommended to maintain body temperature.

Surgery should be performed in an aseptic manner as guinea pigs, as well as other rodents, are susceptible to infection. Postoperative care should include hydration of the anesthetized animal (e.g. SC or IP injection of a warmed solution such as saline, saline–dextrose, lactated Ringer's), and support of normal body temperature. Hypostatic pulmonary congestion should be prevented by turning the animal at least every 30 minutes during recovery. It is important to maintain hydration and nutrition levels in the postoperative period to support normal metabolic processes and gut physiology (Box 8.3). Analgesics must be provided as a standard of care for alleviating pain associated with surgical or other painful procedures. If a procedure is known to cause pain in humans, it must be assumed to also cause pain in other animals unless proven otherwise. Scientific justification must be provided and approved by the IACUC if there is a need to withhold the use of analgesics.

Box 8.3

It is important to maintain hydration and nutrition levels in the postoperative period to support normal metabolic processes and gut physiology.

Table 8.5. Analgesic agents used in guinea pigs

Drug	Dosage	Route	Reference
Buprenorphine	0.05 mg/kg q8-12h	SC	Flecknell (2009)
Butorphanol	2 mg/kg q4h	SC	Flecknell (2009)
Carprofen	1–2 mg/kg q12-24h	PO	Morrisey and Carpenter (2004)
	4 mg/kg ~q24h	SC	Flecknell (2009)
Dexmedetomidine	0.15 mg/kg	IM	Clemens and Seeman (2011)
Flunixin meglumine	2.5–5 mg/kg q12-24h	SC	Heard (1993)
Ibuprofen	10 mg/kg q4h	PO	Harkness et al. (2010)
Ketoprofen	1 mg/kg q12-24h	SC, IM	Harkness et al. (2010)
Medetomidine	0.3 mg/kg	IM	Clemens and Seeman (2011)
Meloxicam	0.1–0.3 mg/kg q24h	PO, SC	Harkness et al. (2010)
Meperidine	10–20 mg/kg q2-3h	SC, IM	Flecknell (2009)
Syrup	0.2 mg/mL drinking water		Huerkamp (1995)
Morphine	2–5 mg/kg q4h	SC, IM	Flecknell (2009)
Nalbuphine	1–2 mg/kg q3h	IM	Heard (1993)
Oxymorphone	0.2–0.5 mg/kg q6-12h	SC	Harkness et al. (2010)
Piroxicam	6 mg/kg q24h	PO	Dobromylskyj et al. (2000)
Tramadol	5–10 mg/kg q12-24h	PO	Morrisey and Carpenter (2012)

IM = intramuscular; PO = per os; SC = subcutaneous.

Research rodents present some unique challenges for pain control, including the need to dose many rodents at a time, the difficulty of assessing postoperative pain, and the concern about effects on research. Recently, an ethogram to recognize pain in guinea pigs has been validated via video, but has not yet moved to a real-time cage-side evaluation. Animal care and research staff have an ethical responsibility to continue to look for better ways to reduce pain and distress in their research subjects. Providing analgesia prior to a painful event (preemptive analgesia) affords superior pain control over attempts to control pain once it develops. Guinea pigs that are in pain may have an abnormal posture, appear hunched, may salivate excessively, or may be reluctant to move. Table 8.5 lists analgesics commonly used in this species. Butorphanol is recommended for mild postoperative discomfort. Buprenorphine works well to control acute or chronic visceral pain. Administration of nonsteroidal analgesics such as carprofen, ketoprofen, and flunixin, are alternatives to the use of opioids. To produce a more balanced analgesia, nonsteroidal agents can be used in combination with opioids.

Imaging Techniques

Many imaging modalities once used only in humans [e.g., digital x-ray imaging, magnetic resonance imaging (MRI), computed tomography (CT), positron emission tomography (PET), dual-energy x-ray absorptiometry (DEXA) scan, and ultrasound] have been adapted for use with laboratory animal species. For more detailed information regarding imaging in laboratory animals, please see Chapter 3.

Euthanasia

Suitable methods for euthanasia include inhalant anesthetic overdose, IV or IP administration of pentobarbital (use three to four times the anesthetic dose or a commercial euthanasia solution), and exposure to a controlled release of carbon dioxide. Refer to Chapter 4 for more information on appropriate euthanasia methods.

THERAPEUTIC AGENTS

Guinea pigs are extremely sensitive to antibiotics with a Gram-positive spectrum. Disturbance of their predominantly anaerobic flora leads to overgrowth of clostridial organisms and other bacteria. Antibiotics should be used only when indicated and with extreme care. Suggested antimicrobial and antifungal drug dosages for the guinea pig are listed in Table 8.6. Antiparasitic agents are listed in Table 8.7, and miscellaneous agents are listed in Table 8.8.

Table 8.6. Antimicrobial and antifungal agents used in guinea pigs

Drug	Dosage	Route	Reference
Amikacin	2–5 mg/kg q8-12h	SC, IM	Harkness et al. (2010)
Amoxicillin	Not recommended—toxic		Flecknell (1987)
Ceftiofur sodium	1 mg/kg q24h	IM	Harkness (1993)
Cephalexin	50 mg/kg q24h	IM	Richardson (1992)
Cephaloridine	10–25 mg/kg q8-24h	IM	Anderson (1994)
Chloramphenicol	50 mg/kg q12h	PO, SC, IM	Harkness et al. (2010)
Ciprofloxacin	7–20 mg/kg q12h	PO	Harkness et al. (2010)
Doxycycline	2.5 mg/kg q12h	PO	Allen et al. (1993)
Enrofloxacin	0.05–0.2 mg/mL drinking water for 14 d		Harkness and Wagner (1995)
	5–10 mg/kg q12h	PO, SC, IM	Harkness et al. (2010)
Gentamicin	2–4 mg/kg q8-24h	SC, IM	Harkness et al. (2010)
Griseofulvin	25–50 mg/kg q12h for 14–60 d	PO	Harkness et al. (2010)
	1.5% in DMSO for 5–7 d	Topical	Harkness et al. (2010)
Itraconazole	2.5–10 mg/kg q24h	PO	Morrisey and Carpenter (2012)
Ketoconazole	10–40 mg/kg q24h for 14 days	PO	Adamcak and Otten (2000)
Lime sulfur dip	Dilute 1 : 40 with water; dip q7d for 4–6 wk	Topical	Harkness et al. (2010)
Metronidazole	20 mg/kg q12h	PO	Morrisey and Carpenter (2004)
Neomycin	12–16 mg/kg q12h	PO	Anderson (1994)
Sulfadimethoxine	10–15 mg/kg q12h	PO	Harkness et al. (2010)
Sulfamerazine	1 mg/mL drinking water		Anderson (1994)
Sulfamethazine	1 mg/mL drinking water		Anderson (1994)
Sulfaquinoxaline	1 mg/mL drinking water		Collins (1995)
Tetracycline	10–20 mg/kg q8-12h; use with caution, toxicities reported	PO	Allen et al. (1993)
Trimethoprim-sulfa	15–30 mg/kg q12h	PO, SC	Harkness et al. (2010)
Tylosin	10 mg/kg q24h; use with caution	PO, SC	Harkness et al. (2010)

DMSO = dimethyl sulfoxide; IM = intramuscular, PO = per os; SC = subcutaneous.

Table 8.7. Antiparasitic agents used in guinea pigs

Drug	Dosage	Route	Reference
Amitraz	0.3% solution q7d	Topical	Morrisey and Carpenter (2004)
Fenbendazole	20 mg/kg q24h for 5 d	PO	Allen et al. (1993)
Ivermectin	0.2–0.5 mg/kg q7d for 3 wk	PO, SC	Harkness et al. (2010)
Metronidazole	25 mg/kg q24h	PO	Morrisey and Carpenter (2004)
Piperazine citrate	2–5 mg/mL drinking water for 7 d, off 7 d, repeat		Anderson (1994)
Praziquantel	6–10 mg/kg	PO	Harkness et al. (2010)
Pyrethrin powder or shampoo	Dust/shampoo q7d for 3 wk	Topical	Harkness et al. (2010)
Selamectin	15 mg/kg	Topical	Eshar and Bdolah-Abram (2012)
Sulfadimethoxine	10–15 mg/kg q12h	PO	Harkness et al. (2010)
Sulfamerazine	1 mg/mL drinking water		Anderson (1994)
Sulfamethazine	1 mg/mL drinking water		Anderson (1994)
Sulfaquinoxaline	1 mg/mL drinking water		Collins (1995)
Thiabendazole	100 mg/kg q24h for 5 d	PO	Allen et al. (1993)

PO = per os and SC = subcutaneous.

INTRODUCTION TO DISEASES OF GUINEA PIGS

Most laboratory guinea pig colonies today are relatively free of the variety of agents that cause clinical disease. However, sporadic outbreaks may still occur, and it is important for those involved in their care to have a basic knowledge of the most common infections, their potential impact on research, and their management or eradication. Presented here is a general overview of common bacterial, viral, fungal, and parasitic agents of guinea pigs and some standard diagnostic and treatment modalities.

Disease conditions in guinea pigs are often difficult to reverse. Ill guinea pigs do not tolerate clinical procedures well and have a tendency to progressively decline rather than recover. As such, the early identification of health abnormalities is of great importance. Nonspecific signs of illness in the guinea pig include a hunched posture; a scruffy, unkempt coat; reduced appetite; and weight loss. Lethargy, disinterest in surroundings, discharge from the nose or eyes, and/or diarrhea may be present. Anorexia is a common, nonspecific sign of illness that necessitates aggressive support because it is a life-threatening condition. Nutritional support may be provided through the administration of food items (e.g. moistened food pellets and critical care formulas). Animals may be encouraged to eat by the provision of especially appealing food items or soft or gel-based diets; however, guinea pigs may refuse these items if they are unfamiliar. Sterile fluids may be administered to support hydration and to provide energy (e.g. dextrose solutions). Fluids can be administered SC, IP, IV, or intraosseously (IO) via the femur. A dehydrated animal should be given 10 mL of maintenance fluids per 100 g of body weight daily via a parenteral or oral route until it is drinking normally. Oral rehydration solutions are available commercially. The parenteral administration of vitamin C is recommended if sufficient dietary consumption cannot be assured.

Table 8.8. Miscellaneous agents used in guinea pigs

Drug	Dosage	Route	Reference
Aminophylline	50 mg/kg	PO, SC	Morrisey and Carpenter (2012)
Atipamezole	1 mg/kg	SC, IP, IV	Flecknell (1997)
Atropine	0.05–0.1 mg/kg	SC	Harkness and Wagner (1995)
	10 mg/kg q20 min (for organophosphate toxicity)	SC	Harkness and Wagner (1995)
Betamethasone	0.1–0.2 mL	IM, SC	Richardson (1992)
Calcium EDTA	30 mg/kg q12h	SC	Morrisey and Carpenter (2004)
Calcium gluconate	100 mg/kg	IM	Hoefer (1999)
Chlorpheniramine	5 mg/kg	SC	Borchard et al. (1990)
Cimetidine	5–10 mg/kg q6-12h	PO	Allen et al. (1993)
Cisapride	0.5 mg/kg q8-12h	PO	Morrisey and Carpenter (2004)
Dexamethasone	0.5–2 mg/kg, then decreasing dose q12h for 3–14 d	PO, SC	Harkness and Wagner (1995)
Doxapram	2–5 mg/kg	IP, IV	Harkness (1993)
Furosemide	1–4 mg/kg q4-6h	IM, SC	Harrenstien (1994)
Glycopyrrolate	0.01–0.02 mg/kg	SC	Huerkamp (1995)
Human chorionic gonadotropin	1000 IU per animal, repeat in 7–10 d	IM	Morrisey and Carpenter (2012)
Kaopectate liquid	0.2 mL q6-8h per adult	PO	Johnson-Delaney (1996)
Lactulose syrup	0.5 mL/kg q12h	PO	Morrisey and Carpenter (2012)
Loperamide hydrochloride (Imodium A-D)	0.1 mg/kg q8h for 3 d, then q24h for 2 d	PO	Harkness and Wagner (1995)
Metoclopramide	0.5 mg/kg q8h	SC	Johnson-Delaney (1996)
Naloxone	0.01–0.1 mg/kg	SC, IP	Huerkamp (1995)
Oxytocin	0.2–3 IU/kg	SC, IM, IV	Anderson (1994)
Potassium citrate	10–30 mg/kg q12h	PO	Morrisey and Carpenter (2004)
Prednisone	0.5–2.2 mg/kg	SC, IM	Anderson (1994)
Sucralfate	25–50 mg/kg q12h	PO	Morrisey and Carpenter (2004)
Vitamin B complex	0.02–0.2 mL/kg	SC, IM	Anderson (1994)
Vitamin C	50–100 mg q24h for deficiency	PO, SC	Morrisey and Carpenter (2012)
	10–30 mg/kg	SC, IM, PO	Morrisey and Carpenter (2012)
Vitamin E-selenium (Bo-Se)	0.1 mL/100–250 g	SC	Anderson (1994)
Vitamin K	1–10 mg/kg q24h for 4–6 d	IM	Harkness and Wagner (1995)
Yohimbine	0.5–1 mg/kg	IV	Harkness and Wagner (1995)

IM = intramuscular; IP = intraperitoneal; IV = intravenous; PO = per os; SC = subcutaneous.

Bacterial Diseases

Antibiotic Toxicity

Guinea pigs are highly sensitive to antibiotics, particularly those specific for Gram-positive organisms (Box 8.4). The normal intestinal microbiome of guinea pigs is predominantly composed of Gram-positive organisms such as streptococci and lactobacilli. Administration of antibiotics effective against Gram-positive bacteria destroys the normal flora and permits an overgrowth of Gram-negative and clostridial organisms. Penicillins, including ampicillin and amoxicillin, lincomycin, clindamycin, erythromycin, bacitracin, streptomycin, and the cephalosporins, can induce toxicity and should be avoided. The offending antibiotics can cause toxicity when administered orally, parenterally, and even topically. *Clostridium difficile* appears to play the primary role in the enterotoxemia that follows antibiotic treatment. *Escherichia coli* has also been observed to produce a bacteremia in treated animals. Treatment is generally unrewarding; the disease is almost always fatal. At necropsy, the cecal mucosa is edematous and frequently hemorrhagic. Fluoroquinolones, trimethoprim–sulfonamide combinations, tetracycline, and chloramphenicol are among the less hazardous antimicrobials. All antibiotics should be administered with caution, using the lowest effective dosage. Transfaunation with a slurry of fecal pellets freshly collected from healthy animals can be gavaged in an attempt to reestablish or maintain normal intestinal flora.

Ulcerative Pododermatitis

Ulcerative pododermatitis, or "bumblefoot," is frequently associated with *Staphylococcus* spp. infection. Predisposing factors include traumatic lesions of the feet such as may occur with rough, poorly sanitized flooring. Obese animals as well as animals housed on wire flooring are especially prone to the disease. Affected animals have swollen, painful granulomatous lesions on the ventral surface of their forefeet. Amyloid deposits may develop in multiple organs (e.g. liver, spleen, and adrenal glands) as a sequela of the disease. Affected animals should be moved to cages with solid floors and provided with soft, deep bedding. In mild cases, the feet can be treated with warm-water chlorhexidine soaks and the application of dimethyl sulfoxide (DMSO) containing a topical antibiotic and/or povidone iodine. Systemic antibiotics such as trimethoprim–sulfa, enrofloxacin, gentamicin, or chloramphenicol as well as dexamethasone should be given in severe cases. The feet should be treated with topical antibacterial ointment and bandaged. Analgesics should be provided to control pain from the foot lesions. In severe cases, bumblefoot can lead to osteomyelitis. Once it has progressed to this stage, prognosis is poor.

Box 8.4

Guinea pigs are highly sensitive to antibiotics, particularly those specific for Gram-positive organisms.

Pneumonia and Respiratory Diseases

Bordetella bronchiseptica and *Streptococcus pneumoniae* are the primary bacteria that cause respiratory disease in guinea pigs. *Klebsiella pneumoniae*, *Pasteurella multocida*, *Streptococcus zooepidemicus*, *Citrobacter freundii*, and *Pseudomonas aeruginosa* have also been implicated. *Bordetella* and *Streptococcus* are common commensal organisms that may proliferate and induce respiratory infections when an animal is compromised or stressed. Younger animals and pregnant sows are particularly at risk for disease. Affected animals may have no clinical signs or may exhibit dyspnea, nasal discharge, sneezing, and other nonspecific signs such as anorexia, ruffled fur, and weight loss. Alternatively, sudden death may be observed. Pregnant sows may abort or produce stillborn offspring.

Bordetella bronchiseptica is moderately prevalent in modern facilities and transmitted primarily by aerosol. Clinical symptoms are rare, however, even in cases in which the organism has been isolated. It is thought that prior outbreaks attributed to *B. bronchiseptica* may have in fact been combined infections with other agents. The organism may be transmitted to the guinea pig from other infected species such as rabbits. *B. bronchiseptica* typically produces gross lesions of rhinitis, tracheitis, and pulmonary consolidation. Purulent bronchitis and bronchopneumonia with large accumulations of neutrophils and intraluminal debris are typically seen on histopathology. Otitis media, accompanied by head tilt, may also occur with *Bordetella* infections. Diagnosis can be achieved through bacterial culture, enzyme-linked immunosorbent assay (ELISA), or polymerase chain reaction (PCR). Fluoroquinolones, trimethoprim–sulfa, and chloramphenicol can be used for treatment; however, it is often unrewarding.

Streptococcus pneumoniae is the causative agent of diplococcal pneumonia. This is primarily a historical disease in guinea pigs and it is thought that prior outbreaks may have resulted from combined infections with other agents. Clinical signs can be nonspecific, such as depression, anorexia, ruffled hair coat, and sudden death, or they may include nasal and ocular discharge, dyspnea, torticollis, and abortion or stillbirth. Fibrinous pleuritis, pericarditis, peritonitis, and marked consolidation of affected lung lobes are typical gross lesions. Otitis media, metritis, and other suppurative processes may also occur. Acute bronchopneumonia with fibrinous exudation and polymorphonuclear cell infiltration are typical microscopic changes. Diagnosis is by culture or PCR. Treatment may be approached as with *Bordetella* infections; however, a carrier state may be induced. Infected humans may serve as a source of infection. Face masks and other standard personal protective equipment should be employed, and workers with possible streptococcal infections should avoid any contact until a course of antibiotics has been completed. Zoonotic infection is possible.

Cervical Lymphadenitis

Commonly called “lumps,” cervical lymphadenitis, characterized by abscessation of the cervical lymph nodes, was once commonly seen in guinea pigs. It is now rare in a research setting. *Streptococcus equi* subspecies *zooepidemicus* of Lancefield's group C is the most common etiologic agent. *Streptobacillus moniliformis* (transmitted from wild rodents) and other *Streptococcus* spp., however, are sometimes implicated. Initially, the swollen lymph nodes (commonly the cervical lymph nodes) are firm in consistency. As the disease progresses, the lymphatic tissue is replaced by thick, creamy, purulent exudate, resulting in prominent soft swellings in the ventral cervical region. The infection is spread by various routes, including aerosols, bite wounds, contaminated cage equipment (e.g. food hoppers that require animals to repeatedly stretch over their edge), and abrasion of the oral mucosa by rough food. The animals generally do not appear to be clinically affected by the abscessed lymph nodes. In some instances, only an inapparent upper respiratory tract infection exists. Alternatively, an acute, fatal, septicemic disease or pneumonia may occur. Occasionally, otitis interna, torticollis, nasal or ocular discharges, or abortions or stillbirths are noted. Treatment may include surgical incision; drainage and lavage of lesions with chlorhexidine or povidone iodine; and systemic antibiotic therapy with enrofloxacin, trimethoprim–sulfa, gentamicin, or chloramphenicol. Control is best accomplished by culling affected animals prior to rupture of lesions and appropriate environmental sanitization.

Salmonellosis

Salmonellosis is a highly lethal disease in guinea pigs although it is very rarely detected in modern research colonies. *Salmonella typhimurium* and *S. enteritidis* are the most common isolates. The most likely source of infection in a colony is the ingestion of contaminated water or food, especially fresh vegetables and fruit that have been inadequately washed before feeding.

Salmonellosis usually occurs as an acute to subacute fatal septicemia. Clinical signs may include anorexia, weight loss, light-colored soft feces, conjunctivitis, dyspnea, and abortion. Diarrhea is uncommon. Inapparent carriers may exist within a colony. Gross lesions may be absent at necropsy in peracute and acute cases. Massive splenomegaly frequently occurs along with multiple yellow–white nodules in the spleen, liver, and other organs. Multifocal granulomatous hepatitis, splenitis, and lymphadenitis, with infiltration by histiocytic cells and polymorphs, are frequently seen. A definitive diagnosis depends on the presence of typical lesions on histopathology and on recovery of organisms from the spleen, blood, or feces.

Treatment is usually not recommended in an outbreak due to the danger of intra- and interspecies spread as well as its zoonotic potential. The most prudent approach is to euthanize all affected and contact animals and disinfect the environment thoroughly.

Tyzzer's Disease

Spontaneous cases of Tyzzer's disease, caused by *Clostridium piliforme*, have been reported in guinea pigs, though clinical disease is rare in modern laboratory facilities. Immunocompromised, stressed, and young animals are at highest risk. Affected animals may have a rough hair coat, appear lethargic or emaciated, develop diarrhea, and die suddenly. Typical gross necropsy findings include necrosis and inflammation of the ileum, cecum, and colon and multiple necrotic foci in the liver. Treatment with drugs in the tetracycline family or chloramphenicol may be attempted but is usually unrewarding and is not recommended.

Mastitis

Bacterial mastitis is common in lactating sows. *Pasteurella* spp., *Klebsiella* spp., *Staphylococcus* spp., *Streptococcus* spp., and others have been implicated. The mammary glands become warm, enlarged, and hyperemic and may produce blood-tinged milk.

The young should be weaned immediately and appropriate antibiotic therapy instituted in the sow. Hot packs applied to the mammary glands are also helpful. As this is generally a painful condition, analgesics should be provided.

Conjunctivitis

Chlamydophila caviae is the causative agent of guinea pig inclusion conjunctivitis. Cyclic outbreaks of severe disease are common in enzootically infected colonies. Adult animals are frequently asymptomatic. Overt signs of disease are primarily seen in 1- to 3-week-old guinea pigs. Transmission occurs via direct contact or aerosol. Clinical signs include a reddened conjunctiva, serous to purulent exudate, and photophobia. Definitive diagnosis is made from microscopic exam of conjunctival scrapings and identification of intracytoplasmic inclusion bodies in epithelial cells. The disease tends to be self-limiting, with lesions healing in 3–4 weeks. Sulfonamide ophthalmic ointments may be used to make the animal more comfortable. *C. caviae* should be considered a potential human pathogen.

Other agents have been implicated in conjunctivitis in the guinea pig, including *Streptococcus zooepidemicus*, coliforms, *Staphylococcus aureus*, and *Pasteurella multocida*. Concurrent infection with *C. caviae* is a possibility.

Cystitis and Urolithiasis

Urinary tract infections are most common in older sows, but uncommon in boars. Disease is often subclinical until urinary blockage or severe infection occurs. Blood may be noted on the vulva or in the cage. Trimethoprim–sulfa or enrofloxacin can be used for initial empirical treatment, but final antibiotic selection should be based on culture and sensitivity testing. Urinary calculi are common. Limit or avoid foods high in calcium (e.g. alfalfa, clover, select fresh fruits, and vegetables) because their ingestion may induce hypercalciuria with resultant urolithiasis. Occasionally, cystotomy is indicated for removal of a large urolith. Aged boars are prone to urethral blockage by proteinaceous plugs.

Mycotic Diseases

Encephalitozoon cuniculi

Classified until recently as a protozoan, *E. cuniculi* has since been re-categorized as a fungus. An incidental finding in guinea pigs, typically without clinical signs, more information about this organism can be found in Chapter 11.

Dermatophytosis

Trichophyton mentagrophytes is the most common etiologic agent of ringworm in the guinea pig. Clinical infections are uncommon; however, guinea pigs frequently harbor the organism asymptomatically. Stressed animals are susceptible. Irregular areas of alopecia usually arise on the face and spread to the trunk and limbs. The lesions may appear crusty or scaly. Microscopic examination of a skin scraping can be used in diagnosis. *T. mentagrophytes* does not fluoresce under ultraviolet light. Topical antifungal creams, griseofulvin in dimethyl sulfoxide applied topically, or griseofulvin administered orally can be used for treatment. *T. mentagrophytes* is infective to humans and other animals.

Viral Diseases

Several viral agents such as Sendai, pneumonia virus of mice, and reovirus 3 have the ability to replicate briefly in the guinea pig. These agents do not cause apparent disease but the guinea pig can serve as a reservoir of virus for other rodents. Guinea pigs may become infected with other (non-Sendai) paramyxoviruses (e.g. human influenza, simian virus 5). Infected animals can be detected through serologic testing, although they exhibit no clinical signs or apparent ill effects. Viral transmission is believed to be through human contact or exposure to contaminated biologic materials.

Cytomegalovirus

Cytomegalovirus (CMV) is a common pathogen of guinea pigs. It is a herpes virus and is species specific. Infections rarely cause detectable clinical disease unless the animal is immunosuppressed or stressed. Infected animals may exhibit swelling and tenderness of the salivary gland area. Large, intranuclear and intracytoplasmic inclusion bodies, characteristic of cytomegaloviruses, may be detected in the salivary glands. Transmission occurs through shedding of the virus in the saliva or urine or transplacentally. The virus may persist in the host for years as an inapparent or latent infection.

Adenovirus

Guinea pig adenovirus most frequently causes no clinical signs of illness but has been associated with outbreaks of fatal pneumonia. Young as well as stressed animals are most susceptible to disease; transmission occurs through direct contact. Pathologic lesions include lung consolidation with nonsuppurative necrotizing bronchitis and bronchiolitis. Prior exposure may be detected through immunofluoresence assay (IFA) or ELISA serology; active infections are diagnosed through PCR of lung tissue or feces. The virus can be eradicated from infected colonies through embryo rederivation and possibly through strategically testing and culling affected animals.

Lymphocytic Choriomeningitis Virus

Guinea pigs can become naturally infected with lymphocytic choriomeningitis virus (LCMV), an RNA arenavirus, through contact with saliva, nasal secretions, and urine. LCMV is also a frequent contaminant of transplantable tumor lines. Unlike in the mouse and hamster, the virus is not thought to propagate within the guinea pig. Naturally infected guinea pigs most frequently exhibit no clinical signs although experimentally infected animals may develop meningitis and paralysis. Lymphocytic choriomeningitis virus is zoonotic and can cause severe illness in humans, particularly those who are immunosuppressed.

Parasitic Diseases

Acariasis

Two species of mites, *Trixacarus caviae* and *Chirodiscoides caviae*, are the most common cause of acariasis in guinea pigs. These mites are commonly found on pet guinea pigs, but rarely in research facilities. *T. caviae* is a burrowing, sarcoptic mange mite that can produce alopecia, crusting, and severe pruritus that may lead to self-mutilation and debilitation. Severe infections can be fatal. Lesions are usually distributed on the neck, shoulders, lower abdomen, and inner thighs. The mite is not readily detected by skin scrapings. *C. caviae*, a fur mite that does not burrow into the skin but attaches to the hair shaft, causes few clinical signs. Alopecia and pruritus, when present, are concentrated in the lumbar region and lateral aspect of the hindquarters. In heavy infestations, mites can be seen moving on the hair shafts. Mites are spread by direct contact with the host, animal bedding, or hair and debris. Treatments include permethrin or carbamate compounds (*Chirodiscoides*) or ivermectin or selamectin (*Trixacarus*).

Pediculosis

Gliricola porcelli and *Gyropus ovalis* are biting lice that cause occasional alopecia, rough hair coat, and mild pruritus. Lice are spread by direct contact with the host or by contaminated bedding. Treatments include pyrethroid flea powder dusts, lime sulfur dips, and ivermectin.

Protozoans

Eimeria caviae, the intestinal coccidia of guinea pigs, is usually nonpathogenic but occasionally causes colitis, diarrhea, and death. Recently weaned animals are primarily affected. The sporulation time is 3–10 days; thus good sanitation will disrupt the life cycle of the parasite. Sulfonamides can be used to treat infected guinea pigs.

Cryptosporidium wrairi is infrequently found in research facilities; however, up to 50% morbidity and mortality has been seen in infected colonies. Juvenile animals are most frequently affected. Clinical signs include lethargy, rough hair coat, diarrhea, weight loss, a potbellied appearance, and emaciation. Affected animals often have a greasy-appearing hair coat. Transmission occurs through ingestion of oocysts in feces or indirectly through contact with contaminated water, food, or fomites. At necropsy, the small and large intestines usually contain watery ingesta. Hyperemia of the small intestine and serosal edema of the cecum may be seen. Smears of fresh feces or mucosal scrapings examined with phase contrast microscopy are generally the best method of diagnosis. There is no effective treatment; however, addition of sulfamethazine to the water supply has been reported to suppress outbreaks. The environment can be cleaned with 5% ammonia to destroy the oocysts. Although some *Cryptosporidium* spp. (e.g. *C. parvum*, *C. felis*) are believed to be zoonotic, *C. wrairi* has been shown to only infect guinea pigs and is not currently considered a zoonotic threat.

The cysts of *Balantidium caviae* are commonly found in the feces of guinea pigs, but the organism is relatively nonpathogenic. *Klossiella cobaye* is considered a nonpathogenic renal coccidian.

Nematode Infection

Paraspidodera uncinata are small worms that reside in the cecal and colonic mucosa of guinea pigs. Infections are usually considered insignificant; however, heavy infections can cause diarrhea and unthriftiness. Transmission is by ingestion of infective eggs. Sanitation is important in controlling infection. Ivermectin, piperazine, or thiabendazole are effective treatments.

Neoplasia

The prevalence of tumors in guinea pigs is low, even in aged animals, with respiratory and integumentary tumors predominating. Genetic factors appear to play an important role in the incidence of neoplasia. Bronchogenic neoplasms are the most frequently reported primary pulmonary neoplasia, with up to a 35% incidence in animals over 3 years of age. The most common bronchiogenic neoplasm is the benign papillary adenomas that may initially induce clinical signs suggestive of an infectious pneumonia. Trichofolliculomas are the predominant neoplasms of the integumentary system. Trichofolliculomas are benign basal cell epitheliomas that present as solid masses most commonly over the lumbosacral area. The skin growth can be easily removed surgically. Other commonly reported integumentary tumors include fibrosarcomas, lipomas, sebaceous gland adenomas, and hemangiomas. Mammary gland tumors, predominantly benign fibroadenomas, have been reported. Tumors of the reproductive system are not uncommon. Leiomyomas and leiomyosarcomas are the most frequently reported tumors of the uterus; teratomas are the most commonly reported ovarian neoplasia. Inbred guinea pig strains exhibit a significantly increased incidence of cavian leukemia compared with outbred strains. The disease develops most frequently in animals under 3 years of age, with resultant high mortality. Animals show enlarged peripheral lymph nodes, rough hair coat, lethargy, icterus, and dull eyes. A retroviral component may be involved in some of these cases, though the exact relationship is undetermined. Tumors of the cardiovascular, urinary, and alimentary systems are rare. It has been proposed that the low incidence of spontaneous tumors in guinea pigs may be partially due to tumor protective effects of both Kurloff cells and the serum enzyme asparaginase that has been credited for antitumor activity when administered to select other species.

Miscellaneous Conditions

Malocclusion

Tooth overgrowth in guinea pigs usually involves premolars and anterior molars (Box 8.5). Maxillary premolars and molars overgrow laterally, abrading the cheek, whereas the mandibular premolars and molars overgrow medially, causing abrasion of and/or entrapping the tongue. The condition is easily overlooked because the cheek teeth are difficult to see on clinical exam. Affected animals exhibit excessive salivation, halitosis, chronic weight loss, and tongue trauma. Malocclusion tends to be a lifelong problem, requiring continual observation and repeated treatment. The offending teeth can be trimmed with pediatric rongeurs or a dental bur in a sedated or lightly anesthetized animal. Affected animals should not be bred because there is a genetic predisposition to malocclusion.

> **Box 8.5**
>
> *Tooth overgrowth in guinea pigs usually involves premolars and anterior molars (cheek teeth). The condition is easily overlooked because the cheek teeth are difficult to see on clinical exam.*

Alopecia

Hair pulling and barbering are common behaviors in guinea pigs. Animals may chew their own hair or that of a cagemate. The location of hair loss can usually provide a clue about whether it is self-inflicted or a result of barbering by a dominant cagemate. Self-barbering occurs just caudal to the shoulders. Dominancy or agonistic barbering occurs on the rump, back, ears, and around the eyes. There is no specific treatment for barbering other than removing the offending animal from the group. Providing good quality hay or enrichment items may be of some benefit. Measures to reduce stress levels should also be considered.

Intensively bred sows frequently exhibit a bilateral alopecia over the back and rump during advanced pregnancy and lactation. Nutrition, genetic, and endocrine factors may be involved. Around the time of weaning, a thinning of hair occurs during the transition from juvenile fur to more mature hair.

Trauma

Animals, especially young, can suffer a leg fracture if their foot becomes trapped in wire flooring. Other fractures, diaphragmatic hernias, and liver contusions with hemorrhage into the peritoneal cavity may occur in animals that are improperly handled or dropped. Depending on the fracture location, a simple, lightweight splint may be used to support the fracture during bone healing.

Heat Stress

Guinea pigs are highly susceptible to heat stress. Heat stress may occur even in moderate temperatures in areas of high humidity and/or poor ventilation. Clinical signs include excessive salivation, rapid shallow breathing, hyperemia of extremities, and elevated body temperature. Rapid cooling with cool water or ice water, steroids, and supportive care may be attempted; however, treatment is often unrewarding.

Water Deprivation

Animals can die of water deprivation even when ample water appears available to them. This may occur when water is provided by a device unfamiliar to the animal; when water devices are placed too high or are otherwise inaccessible, particularly to weanlings; and when water is unpalatable. Other causes of dehydration include malfunctioning automated watering devices or sipper tubes (e.g. tubes that are plugged with foreign objects or air locks) as well as the actions of dominant individuals that prevent subordinate animals from drinking.

Scurvy

The guinea pig requires an exogenous source of vitamin C (6 mg daily for maintenance), due to a genetic deficiency of the enzyme L-gulonolactone oxidase, which is involved in the conversion of L-gulonolactone to L-ascorbic acid. Hypovitaminosis C (also known as scurvy) frequently occurs when guinea pigs are fed rabbit chow or outdated and/or improperly stored guinea pig chow. To ensure that appropriate nutrients, including vitamin C, are provided, guinea pig chow should be purchased only from reputable commercial vendors; stored in a cool, dry place; and used within the manufacturer's recommended time following milling. Vitamin C degrades rapidly in chow or in supplemented water. Most chows now contain microencapsulated vitamin

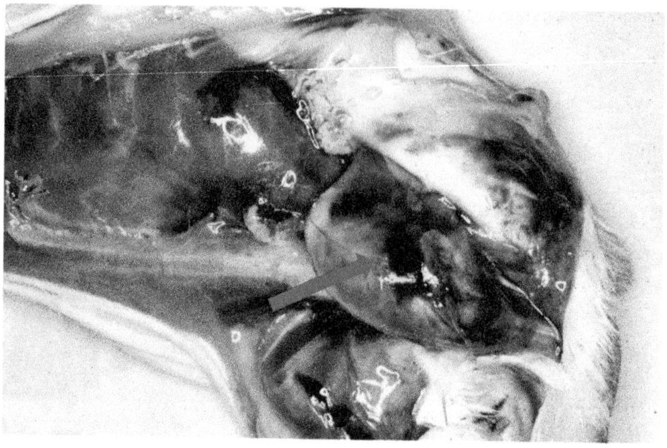

Fig 8.4. Typical scurvy lesion with hemorrhage in stifle area. (*Source:* Photo courtesy of ACLAM.)

C (L-ascorbyl-2-polyphosphate) and have a shelf life of approximately 6 months. Signs of scurvy usually appear within 2 weeks after guinea pigs have been deprived of vitamin C. Clinical signs include reluctance to move, unkempt appearance, swelling around the joints, and infrequently diarrhea. The most prominent gross lesions seen at necropsy are hemorrhages in the muscle and periosteum, particularly around the stifle joint (Figure 8.4) and rib cage, as well as epiphyseal enlargement at the costochondral junction. Affected guinea pigs should receive 30 mg/kg per day of parenteral (preferable) or oral ascorbic acid until recovery is evident. If vitamin C is supplemented in the drinking water, bottles should be changed daily to ensure adequate vitamin C is consumed. Animals may experience ill-effects with only marginal hypovitaminosis C such as may occur during periods of partial or full anorexia or feeding of improperly stored diets. These animals are more prone to upper respiratory disease, bacterial infections, and conjunctivitis.

Dystocia

The most common cause of dystocia is incomplete relaxation of the pubic symphysis due to fusion and ossification of the pubic symphysis. Normally, 2–24 hours before parturition, the pubic symphysis of a pregnant sow becomes separated, allowing the birth canal to increase in diameter. If sows are not initially bred prior to 7 months of age, the pubic symphysis will often fuse and ossify. Dystocia can also result from an excessively large or malformed fetus, large litter, obesity, pregnancy toxemia, and uterine inertia. A sow in dystocia often presents with a bloody or greenish-brown discharge. Uterine inertia may respond to oxytocin; however, if parturition has not begun within 15 minutes after administration, a cesarean section should be performed.

Pregnancy Toxemia (Ketosis)

Two different patterns of disease are associated with pregnancy toxemia in the guinea pig: the fasting or metabolic form and the circulatory or toxic form. The clinical signs are similar, and both forms usually occur in late pregnancy. Animals exhibit depression, acidosis, ketosis, proteinuria, and ketonuria. They produce clear urine with pH lowered from around pH 9 to pH 5–6.

The fasting or metabolic form, called ketosis, occurs in obese sows during the last 2–3 weeks of pregnancy. Sows during their first or second pregnancy are more frequently affected. Stress factors such as changes in feeding routines or environment may precipitate the disease. Affected animals usually become comatose and die within 5–6 days after onset of symptoms. A similar condition may be observed in obese, aged males. A reduced carbohydrate intake with subsequent mobilization of fat as a source of energy apparently is involved. Lesions seen at necropsy include fatty liver, fatty kidneys, ample fat stores, and an empty stomach. Common treatments include lactated Ringer's solution, calcium gluconate, 5% glucose, and corticosteroids; however, prognosis is poor. The incidence can be reduced in breeding sows by controlling food intake to prevent obesity and by breeding at a body weight of 450–500 g. Breeding sows should not be disturbed by changing diets, moving to new quarters, or other factors that might induce fasting.

In the circulatory or toxic form, a large gravid uterus compresses the aorta caudal to the renal vessels, which causes uteroplacental ischemia. Blood pressure is reduced in the uterine vessels, causing placental necrosis and hemorrhage, thrombocytopenia, ketosis, and death. The guinea pig has been identified as a possible animal model for preeclampsia in pregnant women.

Circumanal Sebaceous Accumulations

Excessive accumulations of sebaceous secretions occur in the folds of the circumanal and genital region in adult male guinea pigs. The sebaceous secretions can also form a plug that accumulates in the folds between the two halves of the scrotum.

Preputial Infection and Vaginitis

Male guinea pigs occasionally develop preputial infections caused by lodging of foreign material in the preputial folds. Breeding males housed on bedding may be affected when pieces of bedding adhere to the moist prepuce following copulation and are drawn into the preputial fornix. Treatment involves removing the bedding particles and cleansing the area.

Vaginitis in female guinea pigs is usually caused by entrapment of bedding material in the vagina, causing a foreign body reaction. Treatment includes washing the area carefully to remove the foreign material. It may be desirable to place the animal on a different type of bedding until the area has healed.

Gastric Dilation, Cecal Torsion, and Typhlitis

Gastric dilation, cecal torsion, and acute typhlitis occur sporadically in guinea pigs of all ages. Animals are usually found dead with no previous indication of disease.

Diabetes Mellitus

A spontaneous diabetes mellitus that occurs in animals 3–6 months of age has been reported. Affected animals are not clinically ill but have hyperglycemia, glycosuria, and rarely ketonuria. Exogenous insulin is not required for survival, though it can decrease glycosuria.

Soft Tissue Calcification

Soft tissue or metastatic calcification occurs most often in guinea pigs over 1 year of age. Affected animals may be unthrifty and exhibit muscle stiffness or lameness.

Mineral deposition may be confined to the soft tissue around the elbows and ribs or may be more widespread to the lung, trachea, heart, aorta, liver, kidney, stomach, uterus, and sclera. This syndrome is thought to be attributable to a dietary imbalance of two or more minerals—for example, low magnesium and high phosphorus—and is one reason why guinea pigs should not be fed diets formulated for other species. Multiple linear chalky deposits on affected organs can be seen grossly at necropsy.

Nutritional Muscular Dystrophy

A myopathy has been associated with vitamin E/selenium deficiency. Clinical signs may include depression, hindlimb weakness, conjunctivitis, and reduced reproductive performance in sows. Affected animals usually have elevated serum creatine phosphokinase (CPK) levels. Treatment with vitamin E/selenium injections may be of benefit.

Osteoarthritis

Spontaneous osteoarthritis of the stifle and other joints has been described. Obesity, hypovitaminosis C, and joint injury may contribute to joint degeneration.

Aging

Aged guinea pigs are prone to develop fecal impactions composed of soft, cecal feces within the anus. Loss of muscle tone and/or an inability to eat feces directly from the anus may play a role. Multiple ovarian cysts, fatty infiltration of the pancreas, and segmental nephrosclerosis are frequently observed at necropsy of aged animals.

BIBLIOGRAPHY

Adamcak, A. and B. Otten. 2000. Rodent therapeutics. *Vet Clin North Am: Exotic Anim Pract* 3: 221–237.

Allen, D. G., J. K Pringle, D. A. Smith, P. D. Conlon, and P M. Burgmann. 1993. Rodents and Rabbits. In *Handbook of Veterinary Drugs*, pp. 499–532. Philadelphia: JB Lippincott.

Anderson, N. L. 1994. Basic husbandry and medicine of pocket pets. In *Saunders Manual of Small Animal Pratice*, S. J. Birchard and R. G. Sherding (eds.), pp. 1363–1389. Philadelphia; WB Saunders.

Borchard, R. E., C. D. Barnes, and L. G. Eltherington. 1990. *Drug Dosage in Laboratory Animals: A Handbook*, 3rd ed. Caldwell, NJ: Telford Press.

Buchanan, K. C., R. R. Burge, and G. R. Ruble. 1998. Evaluation of injectable anesthetics for major surgical procedures in Guinea pigs. *Contemp Top Lab Anim Sci* 37(4): 58–63.

Byrd C. P., C. Winnicker, and B. N. Gaskill. 2016. Instituting dark-colored cover to improve central space use within Guinea pig enclosure. *J Appl Anim Welf Sci* 19(4): 408–413.

Clemens, D. and J. Seeman. 2011. *The Laboratory Guinea Pig*, 2nd ed. Boca Raton, FL: CRC Press.

Collins, B. R. 1995. Antimicrobial drug use in rabbits, rodents, and other small mammals. In *Antimicrobial Therapy in Caged Birds and Exotic Pets*, pp. 3–10. Trenton, NJ: Veterinary Learning Systems.

Dobromylskyj, P., P. A. Flecknell, B. D. Lascelles, et al. 2000. Management of postoperative and other acute pain. In *Pain Management in Animals*, P. Flecknell and A. Waterman-Pearson (eds.), pp. 81–145. London: WB Saunders.

Eshar, D. and T. Bdolah-Abram. 2012. Comparison of efficacy, safety, and convenience of selamectin versus ivermectin for treatment of *Trixacarus caviae* mange in pet Guinea pigs. *J Am Vet Med Assoc* 241(8): 1056–1058.

Flecknell, P. A. 1987. *Laboratory Animal Anaesthesia: An Introduction for Research Workers and Technicians*. London: Academic Press.

Flecknell, P. A. 1997. Medetomidine and atipamezole: potential uses in laboratory animals. *Lab Anim (NY)* 26(2): 21–25.

Flecknell, P. A. 2009. *Laboratory Animal Anaesthesia*, 3rd ed. pp. 282–285. Boston: Academic Press.

Gilroy, B. A. and J. S. Varga. 1980. Ketamine–diazepam and ketamine–xylazine combinations in guinea pigs. *Vet Med Small Anim Clin* 75(3): 508–509.

Harkness, J. E. 1993. *A Practitioner's Guide to Domestic Rodents*. Lakewood, CO: American Animal Hospital Association.

Harkness, J. E. and J. E. Wagner. 1995. *Biology and Medicine of Rabbits and Rodents*, 4th ed. York, PA: Williams & Wilkins.

Harkness, J. E., P. V. Turner, S. VandeWoude, and C. L. Wheler. 2010. *Harkness and Wagner's Biology and Medicine of Rabbits and Rodents*, 5th ed. Ames, IA: Wiley-Blackwell.

Heard, D. J. 1993. Principles and techniques of anesthesia and analgesia for exotic practice. *Vet Clin North Am Small Anim Pract* 23: 1301–1327.

Hoefer, H. 1999. Common problems in guinea pigs. In *Proceedings of the North American Veterinary Conference*, pp. 831–832.

Huerkamp, M. J. 1995. Anesthesia and postoperative management of rabbits and pocket pets. In *Kirk's Current Therapy XII: Small Animal Practice*, J. D. Bonagura (ed.), pp. 1322–1327. Philadelphia: WB Saunders.

Huerkamp, M. J., K. A. Murray, and S. E. Orosz. 1996. Guinea pigs. In *Handbook of Rodent and Rabbit Medicine*, K. Laber-Laird, M. M. Swindle, and P. Flecknell (ed.), pp. 103–104. Oxford: Elsevier.

Jacobson, C. A. 2001. A novel anesthetic regimen for surgical procedures in Guinea pigs. *Lab Anim* 35(3): 271–276.

Johnson-Delaney, C. A. 1996. *Exotic Companion Medicine Handbook for Veterinarians*. Lake Worth, FL: Wingers.

Lavin, L. M. 2007. Avian and exotic radiography. In *Radiography in Veterinary Technology*, 4th ed., pp. 294–301. St. Louis, MO: WB Saunders.

Lukas, V. 1999. Volume guidelines for compound administration. In *The Care and Feeding of an IACUC*, M. L. Podolsky and V. S. Lukas (eds.), p. 187. Boca Raton, FL: CRC Press.

Morrisey, J. K. and J. W. Carpenter. 2004. Formulary. In *Ferrets, Rabbits, and Rodents Clinical Medicine and Surgery*, 2nd ed. K. E. Quesenberry and J. W. Carpenter (eds.), pp. 436–444. St. Louis, MO: WB Saunders.

Morrisey, J. K. and J. W. Carpenter. 2012. Drug formulary. In *Ferrets, Rabbits, and Rodents: Clinical Medicine and Surgery*, K. E. Quesenberry and J. W. Carpenter (eds.), pp. 566–575. St. Louis, MO: WB Saunders.

Timm, K. I., S. E. Jahn, and C. J. Sedgwick. 1987. The palatal ostium of the Guinea pig. *Lab Anim Sci* 37(6): 801–802.

FURTHER READING

Allen, D. G., P. M. Dowling, D. A. Smith, et al. 2004. *Handbook of Veterinary Drugs*, 3rd ed. Philadelphia, PA: JB Lippincott.

Anderson, N. L. 2006. Pet rodents. In *Saunders Manual of Small Animal Practice*, 3rd ed., S. J. Birchard and R. G. Sherding (eds.), pp. 1881–1909. Philadelphia, PA: WB Saunders.

Bauck, L. 1989. Ophthalmic conditions in pet rabbits and rodents. *Compend Contin Educ Pract Vet* 11(3): 258–268.

Brabb, T., D. Newsome, A. Burich, and M. Hanes. 2012. Infectious diseases. In *The Laboratory Rabbit, Guinea Pig, Hamster, and Other Rodents*, M. A. Suckow, K. A. Stevens, and R. P. Wilson (eds.), pp. 637–683. San Diego, CA: Academic Press.

Carpenter, J. W. 2017. *Exotic Animal Formulary*, 5th ed. St. Louis, MO: Elsevier.

Dunbar, M. L., E. M. David, M. R. Aline, and J. L. Lofgren. 2016. Validation of a behavioral ethogram for assessing postoperative pain in Guinea pigs (*Cavia porcellus*). *J Am Assoc Lab Anim Sci* 55(1): 29–34.

Flecknell, P. A. 2015. *Laboratory Animal Anaesthesia*, 5th ed. London: Academic Press.

Gresham, V. C. and V. L. Haines. 2012. Management, husbandry, and colony health. In *The Laboratory Rabbit, Guinea Pig, Hamster, and Other Rodents*, M. A. Suckow, K. A. Stevens, and R. P. Wilson (eds.), pp. 603–619. San Diego, CA: Academic Press.

Hargaden, M. and L. Singer. 2012. Anatomy, physiology, and behavior. In *The Laboratory Rabbit, Guinea Pig, Hamster, and Other Rodents*, M. A. Suckow, K. A. Stevens, and R. P. Wilson (eds.), pp. 575–602. San Diego, CA: Academic Press.

Harrenstien, L. 1994. Critical care of ferrets, rabbits, and rodents. *Semin Avian Exotic Pet Med* 3: 217–228.

Hawkins, M. G. and C. R. Bishop. 2011. Disease problems of Guinea pigs. In *Ferrets, Rabbits, and Rodents: Clinical Medicine and Surgery*, 3rd ed., K. E. Quesenberry and J. W. Carpenter (eds.), pp. 295–310. St. Louis, MO: Saunders.

Hoefer, H. L. 2004. Skin diseases and treatment in small mammals. In *Proceedings of the North American Veterinary Conference*, pp. 1391–1392.

Huneke, R. 2012. Basic experimental methods. In *The Laboratory Rabbit, Guinea Pig, Hamster, and Other Rodents*, M. A. Suckow, K. A. Stevens, and R. P. Wilson (eds.), pp. 621–635. San Diego, CA: Academic Press.

Institute of Laboratory Animal Resources (ILAR). 2011. *Guide for the Care and Use of Laboratory Animals*, 8th ed. ILAR, National Research Council. Washington, DC: National Academies Press.

Kaiser, S., C. Kruger, and N. Sachser. 2010. The Guinea pig. In *The UFAW Handbook on the Care and Management of Laboratory and Other Research Animals*, 8th ed., R. Hubrecht and J. Kirkwood (eds.), pp. 380–398. Ames, IA: Wiley.

Lang, C. M. and B. L. Munger. 1976. Diabetes mellitus in the Guinea pig. *Diabetes* 25(5): 434–443.

McKellar, Q. A., D. M. Midgley, E. A. Galbraith, E. W. Scott, and A. Bradley. 1992. Clinical and pharmacological properties of ivermectin in rabbits and Guinea pigs. *Vet Rec* 130: 71–73.

Nakatani, T., Y. Suzuki, K. Yoshida, and H. Sinohara. 1995. Molecular cloning and sequence analysis of cDNA encoding plasma alpha-1 antiproteinase from Syrian hamster: Implications for the evolution of Rodentia. *Biochim Biophys Acta* 1263(3): 245–248.

Percy, D. H. and S. W. Barthold. 2007. *Pathology of Laboratory Rodents and Rabbits*, 3rd ed. Ames, IA: Wiley-Blackwell.

Pritt, S. 2012. Taxonomy and history. In *The Laboratory Rabbit, Guinea Pig, Hamster, and Other Rodents*, M. A. Suckow, K. A. Stevens, and R. P. Wilson (eds.), pp. 563–574. San Diego, CA: Academic Press.

Quesenberry, K. E., T. M. Donnelly, and C. Mans. 2011. Biology, husbandry, and clinical techniques of Guinea pigs. In *Ferrets, Rabbits, and Rodents: Clinical Medicine and Surgery*, 3rd ed., K. E. Quesenberry and J. W. Carpenter (eds.), pp. 13–26. St. Louis, MO: Saunders.

Richardson, V. C. G. 2011. *Diseases of Domestic Guinea Pigs*. 2nd ed. Oxford: Blackwell Scientific.

Ross, M. C., L. D. Zoeffel, J. D. McMonagle, and J. H. McDonough. 2000. Isoflurane anesthesia for Guinea pigs (*Cavia porcellus*) in a stereotaxic surgical apparatus. *Contemp Top Lab Anim Sci* 39(2): 43–46.

Shomer, N. H., H. Holcombe, and J. E. Harkness. 2015. Biology and diseases of Guinea pigs. In *Laboratory Animal Medicine*, 3rd ed., L. C. Anderson, G. Otto, K. R. Pritchett-Corning, M. T. Whary and J. G. Fox (eds.), pp. 247–283. San Diego, CA: Academic Press.

Smith, A. and D. J. Corrow. 2005. Modifications to husbandry and housing conditions of laboratory rodents for improved well-being. *ILAR J* 46(2): 140–147.

Smith, D. A. and P. M. Burgmann. 1997. Formulary. In *Ferrets, Rabbits, and Rodents: Clinical Medicine and Surgery*, E. V. Hillyer and K. E. Quesenberry (eds.), pp. 392–404. Philadelphia: WB Saunders.

Taylor, D. K. and V. K. Lee. 2012. Guinea pigs as experimental models. In *The Laboratory Rabbit, Guinea Pig, Hamster, and Other Rodents*, M. A. Suckow, K. A. Stevens, and R. P. Wilson (eds.), pp. 705–744. San Diego, CA: Academic Press.

Wheler, C. 2013. Antimicrobial drug use in rabbits, rodents and ferrets. In *Antimicrobial Therapy in Veterinary Medicine*, 5th ed., S. Giguere, J. F. Prescott and P. M. Dowling (eds.), pp. 601–622. Ames, IA: Wiley-Blackwell.

White, W. J. and K. J. Field. 1987. Anesthesia and surgery of laboratory animals. *Vet Clin North Am Small Anim Pract* 17(5): 989–1017.

Williams, B. 2012. Non-infectious diseases. In *The Laboratory Rabbit, Guinea Pig, Hamster, and Other Rodents*, M. A. Suckow, K. A. Stevens, and R. P. Wilson (eds.), pp. 685–704. San Diego, CA: Academic Press.

CHAPTER 8 REVIEW

1. Guinea pigs are thigmotactic. Define thigmotactic.
2. True/False: Guinea pigs are nocturnal animals.
3. Guinea pigs often vocalize in response to different situations. Describe three vocalizations and the reasons for each.
4. Guinea pigs develop strong preferences and routines. Why is this important to know in a laboratory setting?
5. What anatomical feature makes them a popular model for auditory research?
6. Intubation of a guinea pig is difficult. Give two anatomical reasons for this difficulty.
7. Guinea pigs lack the enzyme L-gulonolactone oxidase. What nutrient must be thus present in the diet and what disease can result if it is not?
8. What male guinea pig structure can be mistaken for uterine horns on necropsy?
9. On a blood smear from a guinea pig, what are two differences you may notice compared with other rodents such as mice and rats?
10. What complication can result from female guinea pigs bred after 7 months of age and why?
11. What are the indications of guinea pig dystocia and what are the possible treatments?
12. Young guinea pigs are precocious. What does this mean in comparison to animals such as mice or rats?
13. What locations can be used to give IM injections to guinea pigs?
14. Why should you rinse the oral cavity of guinea pigs at the beginning of an anesthetic procedure?
15. Why is it important to have early identification of health concerns in guinea pigs?
16. If an outbreak of Salmonellosis is identified in a guinea pig colony, why is treatment not typically recommended?
17. What diagnostic should be considered when a guinea pig presents with conjunctivitis?
18. What are the two common fur mites of guinea pigs?
19. Which teeth are often involved when malocclusion occurs in guinea pigs?
20. What is the main predisposing factor for pregnancy toxemia in guinea pigs?

Critical Thinking

21. A behavioral research wants to explore the preferences of guinea pigs for various housing set ups and enrichment including size and heights of caging; various toys, shelters, and huts; single vs. social housing; and a variety of chow presentations and food treats. What special considerations for guinea pigs should be made when setting up this study?

9 Chinchillas

The chinchilla is a caviomorph (New World hystricognath) rodent closely related to guinea pigs, degus, and porcupines. It belongs to the family Chinchillidae. The two most common species are *Chinchilla chinchilla* (formerly *C. brevicaudata*), the short-tailed chinchilla, and *C. laniger*, the long-tailed chinchilla. Specific information in this chapter refers to *C. laniger*, the species most commonly encountered in research. The word chinchilla is derived from the name Chincha, a native people of the Andes. Chinchillas are native to South America, once inhabiting the rocky slopes of the Andes Mountains in Peru, Bolivia, Chile, and Argentina. Extensive hunting for their pelts has rendered them nearly extinct in the wild; fortunately, these animals breed successfully in captivity. Average adult weights range from 400 to 600 g; females are slightly larger than males. They range from 25 to 35 cm (10–14 in.) in length. The standard color is a smoky blue–gray that ranges from very light to very dark. Selective breeding has produced a number of color mutations, including beige, white, black, brown, silver, and violet. They are virtually odorless and easy to maintain.

USES

The chinchilla is a common research model in otolaryngological investigations, specifically auditory studies, including otitis media, tinnitus, noise-induced hearing loss, and cochlear implants. Their cochlear size and affiliated neural connections closely approximate human anatomy and physiology, as do their auditory range and sensitivity. They have large tympanic bullae, capsules that contain an extension of the thin, bony cavities housing the middle ear, allowing easy surgical access to the middle ear, cochlea, and surrounding structures. Additionally, there is a lack of

Clinical Laboratory Animal Medicine: An Introduction, Fifth Edition.
Lesley A. Colby, Megan H. Nowland, and Lucy H. Kennedy.

Companion website: www.wiley.com/go/colby/clinical

susceptibility to naturally occurring middle ear infections. Chinchillas show a less pronounced presbycusis (age-related hearing loss) as they age; study of this phenomenon is facilitated by their relatively longer life span compared with other rodent species. This approximates the age-related hearing loss in the human male, thus providing a naturally occurring model for related otology studies. Chinchillas are also used in research investigations involving Chagas disease, listeriosis, and *Pseudomonas* infections.

BEHAVIOR

In their native environment, chinchillas live in groups of several hundred in rock crevices or burrows at elevations above 800 m (2600 ft). They are social, inquisitive animals, with family groups of two to five sharing the same burrow. They rarely fight, although females can be quite aggressive toward strange males during breeding. Chinchillas have several predator-avoidance mechanisms. One is referred to as fur slip, which allows them to escape perceived dangerous conditions. When fighting or handled roughly, they release a large patch of fur to "slip" away. Chinchillas will also spray urine at perceived intruders of their territory. Although normally nocturnal or crepuscular, chinchillas may engage in periods of activity including jumping and climbing during daylight hours. They are dexterous, using their front paws to grasp food in the manner of most other rodents. Chinchillas are not a particularly vocal species, but will elicit a number of communicative sounds. They produce a series of low-frequency chirps during exploratory behavior, a rapid series of grunts as a contact call, bark and growl when threatened, and squeal or shriek when injured. They do not hibernate. Chinchillas, like guinea pigs, are creatures of habit and do not adapt well to change.

Like most rodents, these animals possess an innate preference for contact with the vertical perimeter of a bounded space (i.e., wall following, corner burrowing, and group aggregation), avoiding the perceived threats of open areas. This orientation response is called thigmotaxis.

ANATOMIC AND PHYSIOLOGIC FEATURES

Chinchillas' biologic and reproductive data are listed in Table 9.1. Their compact bodies are covered with exceptionally dense velvet-like fur with up to 60 hairs from each follicle; their long, bushy tails aid in balance. Four toes are present on all feet, each with a small claw. The plantar surfaces are devoid of fur. Their coat grows in waves, starting at the head and progressing toward the tail. The position of a pale bar line present in each hair indicates the stage of growth of the coat. In the furrier industry, the pelt is most valuable when the bar line is at the end of the hair all over the body. Relative to the size of their bodies, they have large heads with long vibrissae, prominent eyes, and bat-like ears. The thymus gland is entirely intrathoracic. The dental formula is 2(I 1/1, C 0/0, P 1/1, M 3/3). The chinchilla's teeth are open rooted,

Table 9.1. Chinchilla biologic and reproductive data

Adult body weight: Male	400–500 g
Adult body weight: Female	400–600 g
Life span	9–18 y
Body temperature	37–38 °C (98.6–100.4 °F)
Heart rate	100–150 beats per minute
Respiratory rate	40–80 breaths per minute
Food consumption	30–40 g/d; 5.5 g/100 g per day
Water consumption	10–20 mL/d; 8–9 mL/100 g per day
Breeding onset: Male	7–9 mo
Breeding onset: Female	4–5 mo
Estrous cycle length	30–50 d
Gestation period	105–120 d
Postpartum estrus	Fertile
Litter size	1–6
Weaning age	6–8 wk
Breeding duration	3 y
Chromosome number (diploid)	64

Source: Adapted from Harkness et al. (2010) and Quesenberry et al. (2004).

growing throughout their life span, and incisors are yellowish in contrast to the molars, which are cream colored. The mandible and maxilla are differently sized, with the mandible being wider than the maxilla. The oral cavity is narrow, primarily filled by the tongue. As with the guinea pig, the soft palate of the chinchilla is continuous with the base of the tongue and possesses an opening called the palatal ostium. The gastrointestinal tract is remarkably long as they are hindgut fermenters. The jejunum nearly fills the entire abdomen, the cecum is large, and the proximal colon is highly sacculated, in contrast to the terminal colon, which is smooth. The cecum holds less intestinal contents than that of the rabbit or guinea pig. Typical of rodents, chinchillas cannot vomit and are coprophagic.

Sexing chinchillas can be difficult because the external genitalia of males and females are similar. The female's prominent, cone-shaped clitoris may be mistaken for a penis at a quick glance. Males have a greater anogenital distance and larger genital papilla. In the male, there is no true scrotum; rather, the testicles are located in the inguinal canals or subcutaneously in the anal region. The female chinchilla is unique in that the vagina has a separate external opening between the rectum and urethral openings that remains closed by the vaginal membrane except during estrus and parturition. The female has two uterine horns, two cervices, and three pairs of mammary glands; two lateral and one inguinal.

Hematologic values for chinchillas reported in the literature are extremely variable. There are, however, several distinctive characteristics of their hematologic and urinary profiles. A seasonal effect on hematologic values of laboratory-adapted chinchillas has been reported. The red blood cell count and hemoglobin levels are highest in the winter season, while the white blood cell count is highest in the winter and early spring when reproductive processes increase. The lymphocyte is the predominant

Box 9.1

The chinchilla is able to withstand long periods without water (8 days to 2 weeks) and thus can excrete highly concentrated urine.

white blood cell. Chinchillas have a higher oxygen–hemoglobin affinity than other rodents and rabbits, probably due to their natural mountainous habitat. Urine is normally alkaline, with a pH of 8.5, and contains varying amounts of calcium carbonate crystals. The chinchilla is able to withstand long periods without water (8 days to 2 weeks) and thus can excrete highly concentrated urine (Box 9.1). The specific gravity often exceeds 1.045. White and red blood cells are normally not present in the urine, and casts are rare. The presence of a few squamous epithelial cells is normal, especially in females. Selected hematologic and biochemical values are listed in Appendix 1.

BREEDING AND REPRODUCTION

Puberty occurs at 4–12 months of age, depending upon the sex and the time of year the chinchilla is born. Females reach puberty at 4–5 months of age and males at 7–9 months. If young are born in the spring, puberty occurs in the fall; if born in the fall, puberty occurs approximately 1 year later. The chinchilla is seasonally polyestrous, with the main breeding season occurring between November and May. A harem system is generally used whereby one male has access to as many as 12 females. Females (does) are quite selective in their choice of a male (buck) for breeding and can be very aggressive toward the male. For pair breeding, the female is dominant and should be taken to the male's cage. For harem systems, a collar can be placed around the female's neck and a small exit hole provided within the caging system for the male to escape the aggressive female if necessary. The estrous cycle is 30–50 days in duration with an average of 38 days. Breeding occurs at night and is characterized by multiple intromissions. Ovulation is usually spontaneous. Detection of the large vaginal plug either in the female or on the cage floor is a reliable indicator that mating occurred the previous day. Gestation is lengthy, with an average of 111 days. A postpartum estrus occurs 2–48 hours after parturition, with a postlactational estrus 35–84 days after parturition.

Near parturition, the chinchilla may become inactive and anorectic and the vagina begins to open and takes on a bluish color. The female chinchilla does not make a nest. Parturition normally occurs in the early morning with all kits born within several hours. Dystocia is uncommon, but if labor takes longer than 4 hours, a cesarean section is advisable. Chinchillas are prone to retained placentas or feti and should be evaluated by abdominal palpation after parturition. The normal litter size is two, but may be as high as six. A disproportionate number of males are born, with a ratio of 119 male births for every 110 female births. Newborns are precocious, fully furred, with teeth, with their eyes and ears open, and frequently vocal. Milk letdown is sometimes sluggish and may be treated with parenteral administration of oxytocin.

Lactating females can develop gastrointestinal stasis 2–3 weeks postpartum that results in gaseous distension of the stomach and intestines and is frequently accompanied by hindlimb paralysis. An intravenous or intraperitoneal dose of calcium gluconate has been reported to diminish symptoms. Young begin to eat solid food within 1 week of birth. The use of a dust bath is contraindicated in the presence of newborns to prevent dust from entering their eyes and oral cavities. Generally, chinchillas are weaned at 6–8 weeks of age, but can be weaned as early as 3 weeks.

HUSBANDRY

Housing and Environment

Chinchillas are active animals, a fact which should be considered during caging selection. Multilevel cages work well to accommodate their activity level. Solid-bottom cages with hardwood chips or recycled paper products are appropriate for chinchillas. If wire-mesh flooring is used, spaces should be small enough, for example, 0.5 in. × 0.5 in., to prevent limb injuries and a solid area for resting should also be provided. Floor space and cage height recommendations have not been published for laboratory chinchillas; breeders and fanciers have found 1–2 ft^2 per animal with a minimum height of 12 inches to be suitable. Rabbit caging can be used, but must be modified to prevent accidental escape of chinchillas through catch (drop) pan openings. When using rabbit caging, the spacing of metal floor bars or perforated flooring should be carefully evaluated. Optimal housing temperature and humidity parameters for chinchillas are 61–70°F and 30–60% humidity, which differ slightly from that of many other laboratory rodents, as they can be easily heat-stressed. Ten-to-fifteen room air changes per hour and 14 hours of light per day are recommended. It is important to avoid an environment with poor ventilation and high temperature and humidity as chinchillas are heat sensitive and prone to matted fur when housed in these conditions. Dust baths, which aid in the absorption of skin oils, are an important component of the chinchilla's normal grooming behavior and are necessary to maintain a healthy coat (Box 9.2). Enclosed or open pans with a dust depth of 2–3 centimeters should be offered several times weekly. Sanitized chinchilla dust is available commercially; alternatively, silver sand and fuller's earth at a 9:1 ratio can be used. Provision of playground sand and talc are not recommended. Figure 9.1 shows an example chinchilla housing set up.

Sanitation

The frequency of primary enclosure sanitation depends primarily on the type of housing used. Solid-bottom cages and feeding and watering receptacles should be cleaned weekly and disinfected with chemicals, hot water 143–180°F, or a combination of both. Detergents and chemical disinfectants enhance the effectiveness of hot water, but they must be thoroughly rinsed from all caging surfaces with fresh water. Suspended cages usually require less frequent sanitation. Catch pans from suspended cages should be changed three times a week. Refer to Chapter 4, for a more detailed description of disinfection methods.

Box 9.2

Dust baths, which aid in the absorption of skin oils, are an important component of the chinchilla's normal grooming behavior and are necessary to maintain a healthy coat.

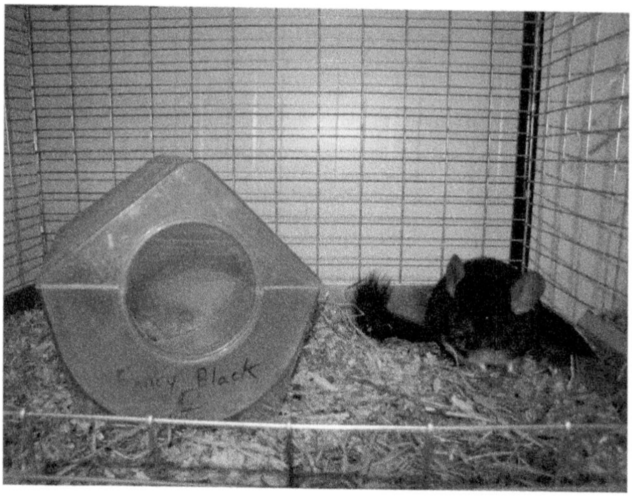

Fig 9.1. Chinchilla housing. (*Source:* Photo courtesy of Cathy Johnson-Delaney.)

Environmental Enrichment and Social Housing

An animal's social and psychological needs should be carefully considered when housing animals in the laboratory environment, with the aim to increase normal behavior and decrease abnormal or stereotypic behaviors. Chinchillas are frequently housed in pairs or small groups to address their social needs. Multilevel caging and feeding twice daily can be used to enrich the chinchilla's environment. A pumice gnawing stone to wear the teeth is available commercially and should be placed in the cage to promote normal gnawing behavior. Alternatively, fresh branches from willow, beech, hazelnut, or unsprayed fruit trees can also be used for gnawing enrichment. Items such as plastic dumbbells or balls placed in the cage or stainless steel chains (hung on the outside of the cage to minimize the chance for injury or choking) are well utilized by chinchillas. Huts with a flat top can be used to increase cage complexity and cage space utilization. PVC piping cut in small sections or aligned in an L-shaped design allow for seclusion. Formal approval should be secured from the researcher, the IACUC, and the facility veterinarian prior to the introduction of any enrichment items.

Feeding and Watering

Chinchillas should be fed a commercial pelleted laboratory chinchilla chow that contains 16–20% protein, 2–5% fat, and approximately 18% fiber. The pellets should contain a minimum of 2700 cal per kilogram of diet. Guinea pig or rabbit chow is adequate;

however, the smaller pellets in these diets are more difficult for the animal to grasp. Adults eat an average of 30–40 g of food per day, which should be offered from a J-feeder or other elevated self-feeder. Good quality grass hay, such as timothy or alfalfa, that is free of mold and insecticides, should be fed ad libitum from a hay rack. Cubed hay can be placed directly on the floor of the cage. The diet can be supplemented with small amounts of fresh fruits, vegetables, oatmeal, raisins, or sunflower seeds, but excessive supplementation can result in obesity and digestive tract upset and should be avoided. Dietary changes should be made slowly to avoid enteric problems. Chinchillas should be provided with fresh, potable water ad libitum by bottle or automated watering system.

TECHNIQUES

Handling and Restraint

Chinchillas are easy to handle and respond best to a light touch and gentle approach. They are not aggressive biters but will bite if agitated. To carry a chinchilla a short distance, lift it by the base of the tail and place the animal on the opposite forearm, up against the body with its head toward the elbow. To restrain a chinchilla, grasp the base of the tail with one hand and place the other hand over the shoulders and thorax as depicted in Figure 9.2. Figure 9.3 shows an alternative method of restraining a docile chinchilla. Care must be taken to avoid grasping the fur or rough handling as this can result in the loss of a patch of fur, called fur slip (Box 9.3). Additionally, never grasp a chinchilla by the end of the tail as this can result in a degloving injury.

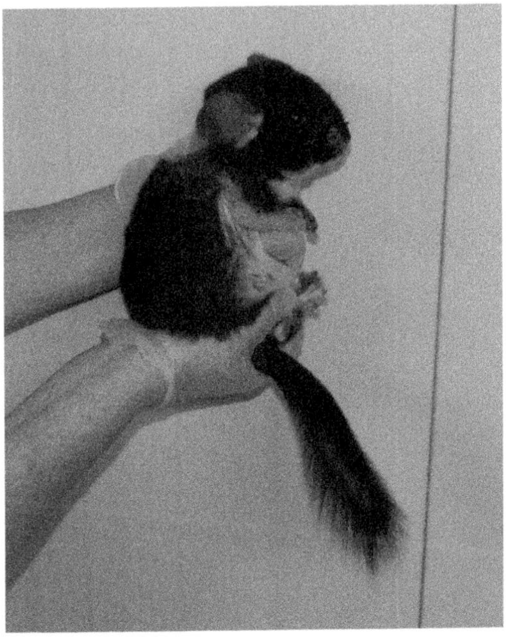

Fig 9.2. Restraint of the chinchilla. (*Source:* Photo courtesy of Cathy Johnson-Delaney.)

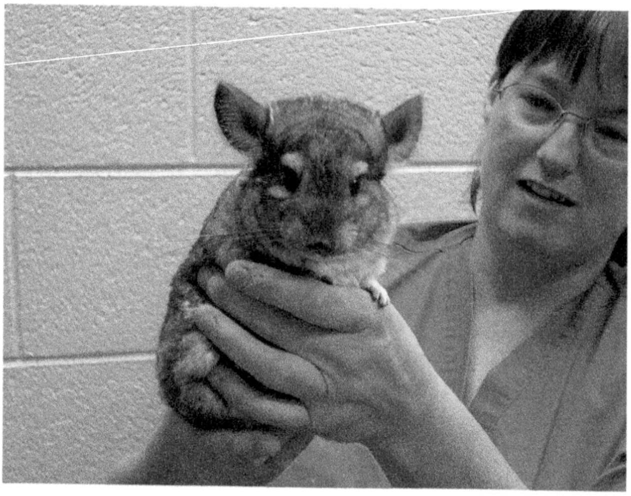

Fig 9.3. Restraint of a docile chinchilla.

> **Box 9.3**
>
> *Grasping the fur or roughly handling the chinchilla can result in fur slip and must be avoided.*

Identification

Cage cards are most often used as a form of general identification. There are several permanent methods of individual identification, including ear tagging or tattooing and subcutaneous (SC) placement of a microchip for electronic identification. In contrast, dyes, markers, or clipped fur can be used as temporary methods of individual identification.

Blood Collection

Assuming an animal is mature, healthy, and on an adequate plane of nutrition, the blood volume of most species averages 7% of the body weight. Table 9.2 lists approximate adult chinchilla blood volumes. A typical rule of thumb for blood withdrawal suggests that up to 10% of the circulating blood volume can be withdrawn from normal, healthy animals every 2–3 weeks with minimal adverse effect. In an adult chinchilla, small amounts of blood, 0.3–1 mL, can be collected from peripheral veins such as the lateral saphenous, cephalic, and femoral. The femoral vein is located at the medial aspect of the hind limb; blood can be collected using the technique employed to sample a cat's medial saphenous vein. The ventral tail artery is an alternate site. Larger quantities of blood can be collected from the jugular vein. For jugular venipuncture, anesthesia may be necessary; the chinchilla is positioned with the head and neck extended upward and the forelimbs extended downward over the edge of a table with a second person drawing the blood sample. Anesthesia is required for collection from the cranial vena cava transverse sinus (venous system encircling the auditory bullae) and heart.

Table 9.2. Adult chinchilla blood volumes and sample size

	Volume (mL)
Total blood	27–48
Single sample	3–5
Exsanguination	10–18

Source: Adapted from Harkness et al. (2010).
Note: Values are approximate.

Table 9.3. Maximum recommended injection volumes for adult chinchillas

Route	Volume (mL)
IP	10
SC	8–25
IM	0.3
IV	1
PO	5

Source: Adapted from Lukas (1999), Quesenberry et al. (2004), and Strake et al. (1996).

These sites involve greater risk due to the potential for vessel laceration and hemorrhage. Cardiac sampling is not recommended except as a terminal procedure.

Urine Collection

Urine can be collected using a metabolic cage, gentle digital pressure on the bladder, clean-catch method, or cystocentesis. Chinchillas that are annoyed will usually urinate, projecting their urine with accuracy for several feet.

Drug Administration

Palatable drugs can be incorporated into the food or water if it can be assured that therapeutic drug levels can be reached with this method. Liquids can be administered orally using a small syringe or directly into the stomach via a stomach tube. Subcutaneous injections with a maximum volume of 8 mL per site can be given between the shoulders or in the flank area. Intramuscular injections can be given in the epaxial muscles or in the quadriceps or semitendinosus muscle. Small-gauge needles, such as 23–25 gauge, should be used for intramuscular injections, and no more than 0.3 mL of a solution should be administered in one site. The intraperitoneal route can be used for volumes up to 10 mL. Intravenous injections are difficult but possible using the small peripheral vessels in the ears or legs. Suggested maximum dosing volumes are summarized in Table 9.3.

Anesthesia, Surgery, and Postoperative Care

A variety of agents that can be used to tranquilize and anesthetize chinchillas are listed in Table 9.4. Food should be withheld from chinchillas for 6 hours prior to anesthesia. Atropine can be administered 15 minutes before the induction of anesthesia to decrease

Table 9.4. Anesthetic agents and tranquilizers used in chinchillas

Drug	Dosage	Route	Reference
Inhalants			
Isoflurane	To effect	Inhalation	Hoefer (1994)
Sevoflurane	To effect	Inhalation	Morrisey and Carpenter (2004)
Injectables			
Acepromazine	0.5 mg/kg	IM	Johnson-Delaney (1996)
Diazepam	2.5 mg/kg	IP	Green (1982)
Fentanyl-droperidol	0.20 mL/kg	IM	Green (1982)
Ketamine	40 mg/kg	IM	Anderson (1994)
Ketamine	40 mg/kg	IM	Hoefer (1994)
+ acetylpromazine	0.5 mg/kg	IM	
Ketamine	4 mg/kg	IM	Parkinson and Mans (2017)
+ dexmeditomidine	0.015 mg/kg		
Ketamine	20 mg/kg	IP, IM	Flecknell (1987)
+ diazepam	5 mg/kg	IP, IM	
Ketamine	5–10 mg/kg	IM	Morrisey and Carpenter (2004)
+ midazolam	0.5–1 mg/kg	IM	
Ketamine	35–40 mg/kg	IM	Anderson (1994)
+ xylazine	4–8 mg/kg		
Tiletamine-zolazepam	20–40 mg/kg	IM	Hoefer (1994)

IM = intramuscular; IP = intraperitoneal.

salivary secretions. Ketamine administered alone is suitable for chemical restraint or noninvasive procedures or can be mixed with acepromazine or xylazine for longer and/or more painful procedures. Ophthalmic ointment should be used in the eyes of anesthetized or sedated chinchillas to prevent corneal drying.

Inhalation anesthetic agents (such as isoflurane or sevoflurane) can be administered via a chamber or face mask. A nose cone or face mask is generally used to maintain anesthesia as chinchillas are difficult to intubate. Care should be used during induction because some animals hold their breath and then take deep rapid breaths of the anesthetic agent, which can result in death if the concentration of anesthetic gases is high. Anesthetic depth can be monitored using toe pinch and palpebral reflexes. Care should be taken to scavenge waste anesthetic gases for the safety of personnel in the area.

Two of the most common clinical surgical interventions performed in chinchillas include a simple castration and opening and drainage of an abscess. Males have open inguinal canals that require closure during castration. A number of surgical procedures involving the auditory system are commonly performed for research.

Surgery should be done in an aseptic manner and blood loss should be minimized. Use of a circulating water blanket to support euthermia is highly recommended. Animals should be recovered on a clean, dry paper or cloth towel, separated from any direct bedding to prevent aspiration or ingestion of fine bedding particles. Anesthetized animals should never be placed in an enclosure with conscious cagemates. Postoperative care should include hydration maintenance and a method to prevent hypothermia; the

Table 9.5. Analgesia agents used in chinchillas

Drug	Dosage	Route	Reference
Buprenorphine	0.05 mg/kg q8-12h	SC	Morrisey and Carpenter (2004)
Butorphanol	0.2–2 mg/kg q4h	IM, SC	Morrisey and Carpenter (2004)
Carprofen	4 mg/kg q24h	SC	Richardson (1997)
	4 mg/kg q24h	PO	Harkness et al. (2010)
Flunixin meglumine	1–3 mg/kg q12h	SC	Hoefer (1999)
Ketoprofen	1 mg/kg q12-24h	SC	Harkness et al. (2010)
Meloxicam	0.1–0.3 mg/kg q24h	PO, SC	Harkness et al. (2010)
Morphine	2–5 mg/kg q2-4h	SC	Harkness et al. (2010)
Tramadol	5–10 mg/kg q12-24h	PO	Morrisey and Carpenter (2011)

IM = intramuscular; PO = per os; SC = subcutaneous.

administration of warmed lactated Ringer's or normal saline will help facilitate both thermoregulation and hydration during recovery. A nonambulatory animal should be turned every 30 minutes to prevent hypostatic pulmonary congestion. It is important to maintain hydration and nutrition levels in the postoperative period to support normal metabolic processes and gut physiology. In addition, it must be assumed that procedures which cause pain or distress in humans will cause pain or distress in other animals unless documented to the contrary. Therefore, unless approved by the IACUC, analgesics should be provided as a postprocedural standard of care. Analgesics that may be utilized in chinchillas are listed in Table 9.5.

Imaging Techniques

Many imaging modalities once used only in humans [e.g., digital x-ray imaging, magnetic resonance imaging (MRI), computed tomography (CT), positron emission tomography (PET, x-ray absorptiometry (DEXA) scan, and ultrasound] have been adapted for use with laboratory animal species. For more detailed information regarding imaging in laboratory animals, see Chapter 3.

Euthanasia

Chinchillas may be euthanized with inhalation anesthetic agent overdose, by injection of pentobarbital at three to four times the anesthetic dose, or with a commercial euthanasia solution given by the intravenous or intraperitoneal route. Although a controlled administration of carbon dioxide is an approved method of euthanasia, pre-sedation or the use of injectable agents provide a smoother and more esthetically acceptable euthanasia. Refer to Chapter 4 for a more detailed description of euthanasia methods.

THERAPEUTIC AGENTS

Suggested chinchilla antimicrobial and antifungal drug dosages are listed in Table 9.6. Antiparasitic agents are listed in Table 9.7, and miscellaneous agents are listed in Table 9.8.

Table 9.6. Antimicrobial and antifungal agents used in chinchillas

Drug	Dosage	Route	Reference
Amikacin	2–5 mg/kg divided q8h-12h	SC, IM, IV	Harkness et al. (2010)
Amoxicillin	Do not use		Morrisey and Carpenter (2004)
Ampicillin	Do not use		Morrisey and Carpenter (2004)
Cephalosporin	25–100 mg/kg q6h	PO	Johnson-Delaney (1996)
Chloramphenicol	50 mg/kg q12h	PO, SC, IM	Harkness et al. (2010)
Chlortetracycline	50 mg/kg q12h	PO	Allen et al. (1993)
Doxycycline	2.5 mg/kg q12h	PO	Johnson-Delaney (1996)
Enrofloxacin	10 mg/kg q12h	SC, IM, PO	Hoefer (1994)
Gentamicin	2 mg/kg q12h	SC, IM, IV	Harkness et al. (2010)
Griseofulvin	25 mg/kg q24h for 30–60 d	PO	Jenkins (1992)
Itraconazole	5 mg/kg q24h	PO	Mitchell and Tully (2009)
Metronidazole	10–20 mg/kg q12h; use with caution	PO	Harkness et al. (2010)
Neomycin	15 mg/kg q24h	PO	Burgmann and Percy (1993)
Oxytetracycline	50 mg/kg q12h	PO	Collins (1995)
Penicillin	Do not use		Morrisey and Carpenter (2004)
Sulfamerazine	1 mg/mL drinking water		Anderson (1994)
Sulfamethazine	1 mg/mL drinking water		Anderson (1994)
Tetracycline	0.3–2 mg/mL drinking water		Burgmann and Percy (1993)
	10–20 mg/kg q8-12h	PO	Harkness et al. (2010)
Trimethoprim-sulfa	30 mg/kg q12h	PO, SC, IM	Harkness et al. (2010)
Tylosin	10 mg/kg q24h	PO, SC, IM	Collins (1995)

IM = intramuscular; IV = intravenous; PO = per os; SC = subcutaneous.

Table 9.7. Antiparasitic agents used in chinchillas

Drug	Dosage	Route	Reference
Albendazole	25 mg/kg q12h for 2 d	PO	Donnelly (2004)
Fenbendazole	20 mg/kg q24h for 3–5 d	PO	Harkness et al. (2010)
Ivermectin	0.2 mg/kg q7d for 3 wk	PO, SC	Anderson (1994)
Metronidazole	25 mg/kg q12h for 5 d; use with caution	PO	Morrisey and Carpenter (2004)
Piperazine citrate	100 mg/kg q24h for 2 d	PO	Johnson-Delaney (1996)
Sulfadimethoxine	25–50 mg/kg q24h for 10 d	PO	Harkness et al. (2010)
Sulfamerazine	1 mg/mL drinking water		Anderson (1994)
Sulfamethazine	1 mg/mL drinking water		Anderson (1994)
Thiabendazole	50–100 mg/kg q24h for 5 d	PO	Allen et al. (1993)

PO = per os; SC = subcutaneous.

Table 9.8. Miscellaneous agents used in chinchillas

Drug	Dosage	Route	Reference
Atropine	0.05–0.1 mg/kg	SC	Harkness et al. (2010)
Calcium-EDTA	30 mg/kg q12h	SC	Hoefer (1994)
Calcium gluconate	100 mg/kg	IP	Richardson (1997)
Cisapride	0.5 mg/kg q8-12h	PO	Morrisey and Carpenter (2004)
Dexamethasone	0.6 mg/kg	IM	Anderson (1994)
Diphenhydramine	1–2 mg/kg q12h	SC, PO	Morrisey and Carpenter (2004)
Doxapram	5–10 mg/kg	IP, IV	Harkness (1993)
Fluoxetine	5–10 mg/kg q24h	PO	Donnelly (2004)
Furosemide	2–5 mg/kg q12h	PO, SC	Morrisey and Carpenter (2004)
Glycopyrrolate	0.01–0.02 mg/kg	SC	Huerkamp (1995)
Lactobacilli	Administer during antibiotic treatment period, then 5–7 days beyond cessation	PO	Collins (1995)
Lactulose syrup	0.5 mL/kg q12h	PO	Morrisey and Carpenter (2011)
Metoclopramide	0.5 mg/kg q8h	SC	Johnson-Delaney (1996)
Oxytocin	0.2–3 IU/kg	SC, IM, IV	Anderson (1994)
Prednisone	0.5–2.2 mg/kg	SC, IM	Anderson (1994)
Pseudoephedrine	1.2 mg/animal q12h	PO	Richardson (1997)
Sucralfate	25–50 mg/kg	PO	Morrisey and Carpenter (2004)
Vitamin B complex	0.02–0.2 mL/kg	SC, IM	Anderson (1994)
Vitamin K	1–10 mg/kg	IM	Johnson-Delaney (1996)
Yohimbine	0.5–1 mg/kg	IV	Harkness et al. (2010)

EDTA = ethylenediaminetetraacetic acid; IM = intramuscular; IP = intraperitoneal; IV = intravenous; SC = subcutaneous.

INTRODUCTION TO DISEASES OF CHINCHILLAS

The many improvements in environmental controls, preventative medicine, and husbandry for chinchillas have led to healthier laboratory chinchillas. Most are relatively free of the variety of agents that cause clinical disease; however, a decreased incidence does not mean that infections will not occur. Presented here is a general overview of common bacterial, viral, fungal, and parasitic agents of chinchillas and some standard diagnostic and treatment modalities.

The most common causes of disease in chinchillas relate to husbandry and feeding inadequacies. Poor housing conditions such as high humidity, poor ventilation, and overcrowding can contribute to respiratory disease, and a number of skin conditions are linked to poor diet. Like most rodents, chinchillas hide signs of disease as a survival mechanism. Healthy chinchillas are active and inquisitive and carry their tails high over their back, while ill animals tend to have a dull coat and be indifferent to their surroundings.

Bacterial Diseases

Respiratory Disease

Pasteurella spp., *Bordetella* spp., *Streptococcus* spp., and *Pseudomonas aeruginosa* alone or in combination can cause respiratory disease in chinchillas. Symptoms may include anorexia, depression, nasal discharge, and dyspnea. Young are particularly prone to disease of the lower respiratory tract or pneumonia. Predisposing factors include overcrowding, high humidity, drafty housing, poor ventilation, and stress. Tetracycline or drugs in the tetracycline family are antibiotics of choice except for *P. aeruginosa* infections, which are more sensitive to gentamicin. Prognosis is poor if chronic respiratory disease is present.

Bite Wounds and Abscess Formation

Bite wounds with secondary abscess formation can be seen in chinchillas housed in group arrangements. *Streptococcus* spp. and *Staphylococcus* spp. are most commonly involved. The wounds and/or abscesses should be drained and surgically debrided. Enrofloxacin or chloramphenicol is a good antibiotic to initiate therapy pending results of culture and sensitivity testing.

Enteritis

Enteritis is a common finding in chinchillas and can usually be traced to poor management. A number of conditions may be involved, including colic, intussusception, diarrhea, mucoid enteritis, fecal impaction, and rectal prolapse. *Pseudomonas* spp., *Pasteurella* spp., *Proteus* spp., *Salmonella* spp., and *E. coli* are frequently involved and can also cause a septicemia with or without enteritis. Affected animals can be listless, be dehydrated, produce soft or liquid feces, or have an absence of feces. Onset is often acute, with rapid disease progression making treatment unrewarding. Predisposing factors include a sudden diet change, inappropriate or prolonged antibiotic use, overcrowding, stress, and diets too low in fiber and too high in fat and protein. Antibiotic therapy and fluid replacement are recommended for treatment. Keeping a chinchilla clean and comfortable is an important part of nursing care. Gentamicin, sulfonamides, and neomycin are antibiotics of choice for enteritis.

Enterotoxemia

Clostridium perfringens type D has been reported to cause disease in chinchillas. The highest incidence occurs in young animals, 2–4 months of age. Animals may be found dead without signs of illness or may have diarrhea and exhibit signs of abdominal pain. Enterotoxemia has been prevented by immunization with toxoid. See the following section for additional information.

Antibiotic Toxicity

Care should be taken when selecting antibiotics for use in chinchillas because many agents can disrupt the normal intestinal microbiome. Avoid antimicrobials that have a selective Gram-positive spectrum, such as clindamycin, lincomycin, erythromycin, and ampicillin. Changes in enteric pH or normal intestinal microbiota can result in bacterial overgrowth and enterotoxemia such as that caused by *Clostridium* spp., resulting in severe diarrhea and sudden death. Broad-spectrum antibiotics used for only short periods of time are less likely to cause gastrointestinal concerns.

Supplementation with a lactobacillus product has been reported to help replenish favorable intestinal microbiota. Providing an oral electrolyte solution such as those used for human infants and/or fluids given subcutaneously or intravenously may also be beneficial.

Pseudomonas Infections

Chinchillas are very susceptible to *Pseudomonas aeruginosa* and are most often infected through contaminated drinking water. Clinical symptoms may include conjunctivitis, otitis, pneumonia, dermal pustules, enteritis, mesenteric lymphadenopathy, metritis, and septicemia with sudden death. Foci of necrosis are most commonly seen in the liver, kidney, and spleen at necropsy along with other general signs of septicemia. Gentamicin may be used to treat individual animals. Prevention includes chlorination, acidification, filtration, or autoclaving water provided to chinchillas. A polyvalent bacterin vaccine is available for chinchillas that provides effective protection from *P. aeruginosa* infection.

Listeriosis

Chinchillas are highly susceptible to infection with *Listeria monocytogenes*, which is no longer common in laboratory chinchillas. The disease can be sporadic in a colony or produce high mortality. All ages are affected, and encephalitic and enteric forms of the disease are seen. Clinical signs may include anorexia, diarrhea, depression, ataxia, circling, convulsions, and paralysis. Common disease syndromes include encephalitis, septicemia, and abortion. The disease is usually peracute in chinchillas, with death occurring within 48–72 hours after onset of signs. Treatment with chloramphenicol or tetracycline can be attempted; however, it is generally unrewarding due to rapid mortality. There has been some success with autogenous vaccines.

Pseudotuberculosis

Yersinia pseudotuberculosis can cause an acute or chronic contagious disease in chinchillas. The acute form is manifested as a septicemia. Anorexia, depression, progressive weight loss, intermittent diarrhea, or sudden death may be seen in the chronic form. Palpably enlarged mesenteric lymph nodes are a hallmark of this disease. Yellow–white foci of necrosis and caseous nodules are seen in the liver, spleen, mesenteric lymph nodes, and intestines. Tetracycline can be used, but treatment is usually ineffective.

Mastitis

Mastitis is fairly common and should be suspected if previously healthy neonates become restless, then lethargic from hunger as mammary glands become painful and edematous. Treat with antibiotics based on culture and sensitivity; sulfonamides may be effective. Local application of hot packs is usually beneficial. Neonates should be fostered to another female or hand-raised.

Metritis

Proteus vulgaris, *E. coli*, *Pseudomonas* spp., *Staphylococcus* spp., and *Streptococcus* spp. are the most common organisms that cause metritis, which is often precipitated by a retained placenta or fetus. Clinical signs include swelling and discoloration of the vulva, white to brown putrid exudate, and fever. The use of oxytocin to expel the placenta or fetus, flushing the vagina and uterus with saline, and parenteral antibiotic administration per culture and sensitivity are indicated. Offspring should be hand-reared to prevent cross-contamination.

Mycotic Diseases

Dermatophytosis

The most common cause of ringworm in the chinchilla is *Trichophyton mentagrophytes*. Lesions can occur anywhere on the body but typically appear as small, scaly areas of alopecia on the nose, ears, and feet. Ultraviolet light is not useful for diagnosis since *Trichophyton* does not fluoresce. Animals with lesions should be treated promptly or culled due to the zoonotic potential of this fungal agent. Treatment with oral itraconazole for a duration of 5–6 weeks is effective. Ensure each cage has its own dust bath to prevent this potential mode of fungal infection transmission.

Viral Diseases

There are few reports of viral agents causing disease. Lymphocytic choriomeningitis virus has been reported to affect chinchillas. Chinchillas infected with human influenza A virus are a model for childhood otitis media. Chinchillas are susceptible to human herpes virus 1.

Parasitic Diseases

Intestinal parasitism is generally uncommon. Infestation with coccidia, tapeworms, and nematodes are rare in well-managed facilities. Cystic subcutaneous masses caused by the intermediate stage of *Multiceps serialis* are occasionally seen; these masses may be surgically removed. The dog is the definitive host of this parasite, and the chinchilla functions as the intermediate host; transmission is by ingestion of contaminated feed. Chinchillas normally harbor high numbers of *Giardia* in their intestines. Stress and poor husbandry can cause numbers to increase and predispose animals to opportunistic infections. Affected animals usually have intermittent illness with sticky, black feces. Albendazole or fenbendazole are recommended treatments; metronidazole is contraindicated as it has been associated with liver failure in chinchillas.

Neoplasia

Neoplasia is uncommon in the chinchilla; there are few reports of its occurrence.

Miscellaneous Conditions

Malocclusion

Malocclusion ("slobbers") can be seen with the incisors or molars and results in overgrowth and abnormal wear of the teeth. Chinchillas may display selective appetite in the early stages of the condition that progresses to anorexia and excessive drooling. This causes the fur around the chin, chest, and forepaws to become wet. Malocclusion of the incisors is easy to visualize; however, sedation and careful examination may be necessary to examine the molars. Radiography is frequently required to evaluate the condition. Treatment involves trimming the overgrown teeth with a dental bur or rongeur, under sedation. Continued routine trimming of the teeth is usually necessary, and affected animals should not be bred because there may be a hereditary predisposition to the condition. Placement of a gnawing pumice stone in the cage is recommended.

Choke

Esophageal choke occurs when the entrance of the esophagus is occluded by a large piece of food or other foreign body. It is more common in animals that are fed raisins, fruits, and nuts or that consume bedding material. The chinchilla may cough, retch, and struggle in an effort to dislodge the offending material. The animal's condition will deteriorate rapidly if it is unable to free the obstruction.

Constipation

Constipation is a more frequent problem than diarrhea in chinchillas. It is evidenced by straining to defecate but producing only a few thin, short, hard pellets. Feeding a diet that is too low in fiber is the usual cause. Provision of a commercial, pelleted chinchilla diet or the provision of small amounts of fresh food such as apples, raisins, carrots, or lettuce and alfalfa cubes may resolve the problem.

Conjunctivitis

Conjunctivitis without clinical signs of respiratory infection is usually caused by irritation from the dust bath or dirty bedding. Treating with ophthalmic ointment, improving husbandry, and discontinuing dust baths for a few weeks are recommended.

Fur Chewing

Fur chewing is a serious problem in the chinchilla industry. The exact cause remains unknown; however, it appears to be a vice and seems to occur more in certain genetic lines. Loud noises, improper diet, hormonal imbalance, poor housing conditions, stress, and boredom have all been incriminated. Affected chinchillas are motley and have a lion's-mane appearance because they chew all of the fur within reach on their lower body to a short length. Hairballs are commonly found in the stomach at necropsy. These animals should not be bred.

Fur Slip

When chinchillas fight, are handled roughly, or become agitated during handling, the fur may be released in patches. The underlying skin appears clean and smooth. This release of fur occurs in response to the effect of adrenaline on the erector pili muscles. The fur may take up to 5 months to regrow.

Penile Hair Rings

Male chinchillas can accumulate a ring of twisted hair around the penis and under the prepuce. The condition can affect their breeding ability because the ring of hair can cause irritation, infection, and damage to the penis. Treat by applying a sterile lubricant to the penis and prepuce and gently rolling off the accumulated ring of hair.

Heat Stroke

Chinchillas are very prone to heatstroke, particularly if the humidity is high. Affected animals are usually found in a prostrate condition, panting, and have an elevated body temperature. Treatment involves cooling the animal's body with cold water until the temperature returns to normal. In addition, administering intravenous fluids can help to stabilize the cardiovascular system.

Fractures

Fractures of the tibia are commonly seen when a chinchilla is restrained by its hindlimb or catches its leg in the cage. This bone is very fragile as it is longer than the femur, and the fibula is nearly nonexistent, giving the tibia little support. Surgical repair can be a challenge because the bone cortices are thin and the lumen narrow; thus, wire or external fixation stabilized by bandages is more effective than an intramedullary pin. The chinchilla should be placed in a small cage to limit mobility until the fracture heals.

BIBLIOGRAPHY

Allen, D. G., J. K. Pringle, and D. A. Smith. 1993. *Handbook of Veterinary Drugs*. Philadelphia, PA: JB Lippincott.

Anderson, N. L. 1994. Basic husbandry and medicine of pocket pets. In *Saunders Manual of Small Animal Practice*, S. J. Birchard and R. G. Sherding (eds.), pp. 1363–1389. Philadelphia, PA: WB Saunders.

Boettcher, F. A., B. R. Bancroft, and R. J. Salvi. 1990. Blood collection from the transverse sinus in the chinchilla. *Lab Anim Sci* 40(2): 223–224.

Burgmann, P., and D. H. Percy. 1993. Antimicrobial drug use in rodents and rabbits. In *Antimicrobial Therapy in Veterinary Medicine*, 2nd ed., J. F. Prescott and J. D. Baggot (eds.), pp. 524–541. Ames, IA: Iowa State University Press.

Collins, B. R. 1995. Antimicrobial drug use in rabbits, rodents, and other small mammals. In *Antimicrobial Therapy in Caged Birds and Exotic Pets*, pp. 3–10. Trenton, NJ: Veterinary Learning Systems.

Donnelly, T. M. 2004. Disease problems in chinchillas and rodents. In *Ferrets, Rabbits, and Rodents: Clinical Medicine and Surgery*, K. E. Quesenberry and J. W. Carpenter (eds.), pp. 255–265. St. Louis, MO: WB Saunders.

Flecknell, P. A. 1987. *Laboratory Animal Anaesthesia*. London: Academic Press.

Green, C. J. 1982. *Laboratory Animal Handbooks 8: Animal Anesthesia*. London: Laboratory Animals, Ltd.

Hargett, C. E. Jr., J. W. Record, M. Carrier Jr., et al. 1989. Reversal of ketamine–xylazine anesthesia in the chinchilla by yohimbine. *Lab Anim (NY)* 18(7): 41–43.

Harkness, J. E. 1993. *A Practitioner's Guide to Domestic Rodents*. Lakewood, CO: American Animal Hospital Association.

Harkness, J. E., P. V. Turner, S. VandeWoude, and C. L. Wheler. 2010. *Harkness and Wagner's Biology and Medicine of Rabbits and Rodents*, 5th ed. Ames, IA: Wiley-Blackwell.

Hoefer, H. 1994. Chinchillas. *Vet Clin North Am Small Anim Pract* 24: 103–110.

Hoefer, H. 1999. Diagnosis and management of chinchilla diseases. *Proc North Am Vet Conf* 13: 833–835.

Huerkamp, M. J. 1995. Anesthesia and postoperative management of rabbits and pocket pets. In *Kirk's Current Veterinary Therapy XII: Small Animal Practice*, J. D. Bonagura (ed.), pp. 1322–1327. Philadelphia: WB Saunders.

Jankubow, K., J. Gromadzka-Ostrowska, and B. Zalewska. 1984. Seasonal changes in the haematological indices in peripheral blood of chinchilla (*Chinchilla laniger*). *Comp Biochem Physiol* 78A(4): 845–853.

Jenkins, J. R. 1992. Husbandry and common diseases of the chinchilla (*Chinchilla laniger*). *J Small Exotic Anim Med* 2: 15–17.

Johnson-Delaney, C. A. 1996. *Exotic Companion Medicine Handbook for Veterinarians*. Lake Worth, FL: Wingers.

Lukas, V. 1999. Volume guidelines for compound administration. In *The Care and Feeding of an IACUC*, M. L. Podolsky and V. S. Lukas (eds.), p. 187. Boca Raton, FL: CRC Press.

Merry, C. J. 1990. An introduction to chinchillas. *Vet Tech* 11(5): 315–322. Trenton, NJ: Veterinary Learning Systems.

Mitchell, M. A. and T. N. Tully. 2009. *Manual of Exotic Pet Practice*, pp. 474–492. Philadelphia, PA: Elsevier.

Morrisey, J. K. and J. W. Carpenter. 2004. Formulary. In *Ferrets, Rabbits, and Rodents Clinical Medicine and Surgery*, 2nd ed. K. E. Quesenberry and J. W. Carpenter (eds.) pp. 436–444. St. Louis, MO: WB Saunders.

Morrisey, J. K. and J. W. Carpenter. 2012. Formulary. In *Ferrets, Rabbits, and Rodents: Clinical Medicine and Surgery*, 3rd ed., K. E. Quesenberry and J. W. Carpenter (eds.), pp. 566–575. Philadelphia, PA: WB Saunders.

Parkinson, L. and C. Mans. 2017. Anesthetic and postanesthetic effects of alfaxalone–butorphanol compared with dexmedetomidine–ketamine in chinchillas (*Chinchilla lanigera*). *J Am Assoc Lab Anim Sci* 56(3): 290–295.

Quesenberry, K. E., T. M. Donnely, and E. V. Hillyer. 2004. Biology, husbandry, and clinical techniques of ghinea pigs and chinchillas. In *Ferrets, Rabbits, and Rodents: Clinical Medicine and Surgery*, 2nd ed. K. E. Quesenberry and J. W. Carpenter (eds.), pp. 392–403. Philadelphia: WB Saunders.

Quesenberry, K. E., T. M. Donnelly, and C. Mans. 2012. Biology, husbandry, and clinical techniques of Guinea pigs and chinchillas. In *Ferrets, Rabbits, and Rodents: Clinical Medicine and Surgery*, 3rd ed., K. E. Quesenberry and J. W. Carpenter (eds.), pp. 279–294. St. Louis, MO: WB Saunders.

Richardson, V. C. G. 1997. *Diseases of Small Domestic Rodents*. Oxford: Blackwell Scientific.

Strake, J. G., L. A. Davis, M. LaRegina, and K. R. Boschert. 1996. Chinchillas. In *Handbook of Rodent and Rabbit Medicine*, K. Laber-Laird, M. M. Swindle, and P. Flecknell (eds.), pp. 151–181. Oxford: Elsevier Science.

Timm, K. I., S. E. Jahn, and C. J. Sedgwick. 1987. The palatal ostium of the Guinea pig. *Lab Anim Sci* 37(6): 801–802.

Wohlsein, P., A. Thiele, M. Fehr, et al. 2002. Spontaneous human herpes virus type 1 infection in a chinchilla (*Chinchilla lanigera* f. dom.). *Acta Neuropathol* 104(6): 674–678.

FURTHER READING

Alworth, L.C., and S. B. Harvey. 2012. Anatomy, physiology, and behavior. In *The Laboratory Rabbit, Guinea Pig, Hamster, and Other Rodents*, M. A. Suckow, K. A. Stevens, and R. P. Wilson (eds.), pp. 955–966. San Diego, CA: Academic Press.

Carpenter, J. W. 2005. Rodents. In *Exotic Animal Formulary*, pp. 377–408. St. Louis, MO: Elsevier Saunders.

Hsu, C. C., J. A. Briscoe, and A. B. Keffer. 2012. Basic experimental methods. In *The Laboratory Rabbit, Guinea Pig, Hamster, and Other Rodents*, M. A. Suckow, K. A. Stevens, and R. P. Wilson (eds.), pp. 977–991. San Diego, CA: Academic Press.

Hsu, C. C, M. M.Chan, C. L. Wheler. 2015. Biology and diseases of Chinchillas. In *Laboratory Animal Medicine*, 3rd ed., J. G. Fox, L. C. Anderson, G. Otto, et al. (eds.), pp. 387–409. San Diego, CA: Academic Press.

Lavin, L. M. 2007. Avian and exotic radiography. In *Radiography in Veterinary Technology*, 4th ed., pp. 294–301. St. Louis, MO: WB Saunders.

Levin, S. I., D. M. Berger, and T. L. Gluckmann. 2012. Management, husbandry, and colony health. In *The Laboratory Rabbit, Guinea Pig, Hamster, and Other Rodents*, M. A. Suckow, K. A. Stevens, and R. P. Wilson (eds.), pp. 967–976. San Diego, CA: Academic Press.

Lopate, C. (ed.). 2012. *Management of Pregnant and Neonatal Dogs, Cats, and Exotic Pets*. Ames, IA: Wiley-Blackwell.

Martin, L. 2012. Chinchillas as experimental models. In *The Laboratory Rabbit, Guinea Pig, Hamster, and Other Rodents*, M. A. Suckow, K. A. Stevens, and R. P. Wilson (eds.), pp. 1009–1028. San Diego, CA: Academic Press.

Norton, J. N. and R. P. Reynolds. 2012. Diseases and veterinary care. In *The Laboratory Rabbit, Guinea Pig, Hamster, and Other Rodents*, M. A. Suckow, K. A. Stevens, and R. P. Wilson (eds.), pp. 993–1008. San Diego, CA: Academic Press.

Pollack, C. 2002. Postoperative management of the exotic animal patient. *Vet Clin North Am: Exotic Anim Pract* 5: 183–212.

Smith, A. and D. J. Corrow. 2005. Modifications to husbandry and housing conditions of laboratory rodents for improved well-being. *ILAR J* 46(2): 140–147.

CHAPTER 9 REVIEW

1. Why is the chinchilla a popular model for auditory studies? (Give three reasons)
2. What is presbycusis?
3. Why can sexing chinchillas be difficult?
4. What is the predominant leukocyte in the chinchilla?
5. How long is the gestation period of the chinchilla?
6. Why are the acceptable temperature and humidity ranges lower for chinchillas than for many other rodents?

7. How often should dust baths be offered to chinchillas and for what purpose?
8. What bacteria are most commonly isolated from abscesses or wounds originating from a chinchilla's bite?
9. What spectrum of antimicrobials should be avoided in chinchillas?
10. To what organism, spread through contaminated drinking water, are chinchillas very susceptible?
11. What are the clinical signs of malocclusion?

Critical Thinking

12. A researcher in your facility says that the chinchillas on study must be housed singly for research purposes. What might be good reasons to house animals singly? What other things might you provide to the animals to make up for the lack of social contact?

10 Zebrafish

Zebrafish have rapidly become a very popular model in the laboratory animal world. The zebrafish (*Danio rerio*) is a member of the minnow family, Cyprinidae. They are native to southeast Asia, and typically found in shallow slow moving waters in the areas of Nepal, India, and the Himalayan region. Their popularity began in the fish hobby world, and it's only been in the last few decades that technological advances have paved the way for them to become a powerful tool in the areas of developmental and genetic research. There are now numerous wildtype and transgenic lines available for researchers' use.

USES

The zebrafish began primarily as a model system of embryonic development. It is an ideal choice for studying embryonic development for several reasons: the large number of embryos a single female can produce in one spawning, the small size of the embryos, the rapid 3–4 day development from fertilized egg to larval stage, the transparent nature of the embryo during development, and the ease of both manipulating those embryos to create mutations and then observing the effects of those manipulations. Since zebrafish live in an aquatic environment, they also became an ideal model for screening chemicals and their effects on embryonic development.

Over time, researchers in many areas of biomedical research have realized how useful zebrafish could be for their studies, especially given the ability to alter the genome so readily. Zebrafish have been found to be useful in cancer studies, particularly in the area of carcinogenic compounds and their ability to induce cancer. Zebrafish also have unique tissue regeneration properties, and can regenerate cell

Clinical Laboratory Animal Medicine: An Introduction, Fifth Edition.
Lesley A. Colby, Megan H. Nowland, and Lucy H. Kennedy.

Companion website: www.wiley.com/go/colby/clinical

types that mammals cannot, including heart and spinal cord cells. Several diseases arising from single cell mutations have been seen to show similar phenotypes in zebrafish and humans. Muscular dystrophy is one such example and specific lines of fish have been developed to research this disease.

BEHAVIOR

In the wild, zebrafish are a social species, most commonly found in groups of 5–20 fish (Box 10.1). However, they can still exhibit aggressive behavior towards each other, especially during mating when biting, chasing, and circling behaviors are noted. Zebrafish may also exhibit aggression when housed in small groups (less than 5 fish per tank). They are diurnal, and sudden changes to the light cycle can have significant impacts on their behavior, especially related to breeding.

> **Box 10.1**
>
> *In the wild, zebrafish are a social species, most commonly found in groups of 5–20 fish.*

ANATOMIC AND PHYSIOLOGIC FEATURES

Zebrafish are bony fish with three unpaired fins (the dorsal, caudal, and anal) and two sets of paired fins (pelvic and pectoral). Their skin is covered by scales with a distinctive pigment pattern of horizontal stripes extending the length of their bodies. Zebrafish do not have a stomach; instead, the anterior portion of their intestine, or the intestinal bulb, is the main location for nutrient absorption and lipid and protein digestion. The zebrafish kidney has several differences from mammalian kidneys. Most notably, the kidney is divided into two portions (cranial and caudal). The cranial portion is the main hematopoietic organ of the zebrafish. The caudal portion (or trunk kidney) contains the majority of the nephrons and provides most of the renal filtering capacity. Zebrafish do not have a urinary bladder. Waste products from the gastrointestinal tract and the genitourinary tract exit at one location, called the urogenital pore.

During the larval stages of the zebrafish, gas exchange occurs across the skin; it is not until they fully develop to the juvenile stage that the gills take over this role. Gas and ion exchange occur in the gills of adult zebrafish. The gills are made up of several structures: the gill arches, the primary lamellae, and the secondary lamellae. Gas exchange occurs as water flows across the secondary lamellae. The gills are covered by a protective bony plate called the operculum. The zebrafish heart consists of only two chambers. Red blood cells and platelets are nucleated.

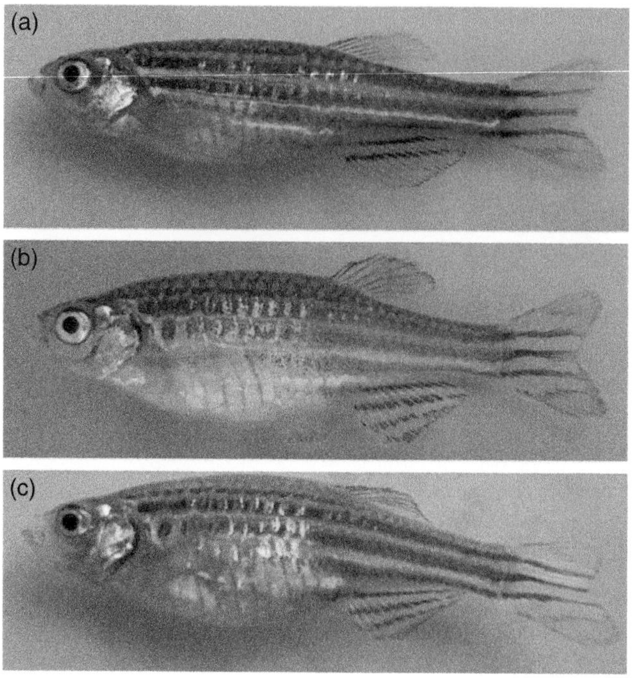

Fig 10.1. Photos of a male (a) and female (b and c) zebrafish. (*Source:* From Avdesh et al. (2012). Used with permission.)

Unlike mammals, a single genetic component for sex determination has not been found. Instead, it's thought that sex is determined by both endogenous (signals from other genes) and exogenous (environmental changes) factors. In general, adult female zebrafish are larger than males, have a rounded ventral surface, and are lighter colored. Male zebrafish tend to be more active and slender, and have more golden or yellow pigmentation on their fins (Figure 10.1).

Zebrafish have several specialized anatomic structures that are not present in mammals. The swim bladder is a gas-filled organ that fills a significant portion of the dorsal abdominal cavity. It is involved in buoyancy regulation and detection of vibrations. They also have a lateral line located in the skin along a horizontal line on either side of the body. The lateral line is a sensory structure made up of hair cells called mechanosensory neuromasts, which assists with detecting changes in water motion and can help with predator evasion and other normal behaviors in zebrafish.

REPRODUCTION AND LIFE STAGES

Zebrafish reproduction and development has been extensively characterized, as embryo manipulation is a primary research use for this species. Zebrafish are incredibly prolific, with the ability to produce thousands of embryos per female. Sexual maturity occurs around 3–6 months of age. Once sexually mature, female zebrafish have the ability to spawn continuously, and will do so if kept in mixed sex tanks. Zebrafish spawning is highly dependent on photoperiod, and occurs in the hour after dawn (Box 10.2). A light cycle of 14 hours of light to 10 hours of darkness (14:10) is ideal for most productive spawning. In the wild, zebrafish spawn mainly in shallow waters. Spawning tanks designed to provide a shallow area can promote breeding.

Box 10.2

Zebrafish spawning is highly dependent on photoperiod, and occurs in the hour after dawn.

Spawning can be set up either directly in their normal housing tank, typically connected to a larger system, or in separate static tanks. There are advantages and disadvantages to both. When spawning in the housing tank, a layer of marbles or a breeding box should be placed on the floor of the tank to allow fertilized embryos to fall safely to the bottom of the tank without risk of cannibalization by adult fish or removal by the water circulation. Male and female fish are paired and allowed to spawn for approximately an hour after the lights turn on, and then the fertilized eggs can be siphoned or lifted out of the tank. This method of spawning causes less distress to the fish overall, since they do not need to be moved. Removal of the eggs can be tedious, however, especially with a marble substrate. Static tanks used for spawning are very common in zebrafish facilities, and typically consist of an outer tank with an inset smaller tank that has a gridded floor to allow the eggs to fall through (Figure 10.2). The inner tank can easily be tilted to provide a shallow area for spawning. Challenges with this method are that the water is static and a small volume (typically), therefore water quality parameters can quickly change. In addition, fish need to be frequently moved, which is a stressful event for them.

Zebrafish embryos develop rapidly, with initial cell cleavage occurring in the first hour after fertilization and several subsequent cell cleavages over the next 2–3 hours. Since the egg is transparent, all phases of the embryonic period can be monitored through a microscope, allowing researchers to access and manipulate the embryo at specific stages. Embryos hatch around 3 days postfertilization (dpf) and are very limited in their movement until 5 dpf, at which point they gain functional swim bladders and also begin exogenous feeding (Figure 10.3). Larval zebrafish are housed in systems with low velocity of water flow so that they can easily feed. Their nutritional needs at this time are very high and they require a constant source of protein. Larval zebrafish continue progressing through a series of morphological changes until about 30–45 dpf, at which point they are considered juveniles. Juvenile zebrafish are morphologically similar to adult zebrafish; however, they are not considered to be adults until they reach sexual maturity at approximately 3 months of age. In captivity, zebrafish have an average lifespan of 3–4 years.

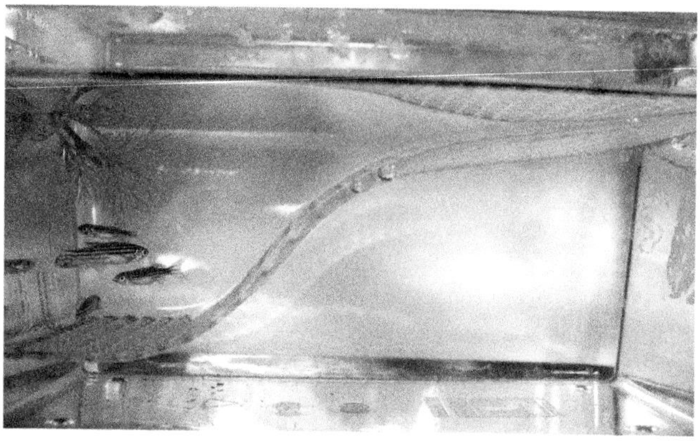

Fig 10.2. A zebrafish spawning tank. (*Source:* Photo courtesy of A. Skorupski.)

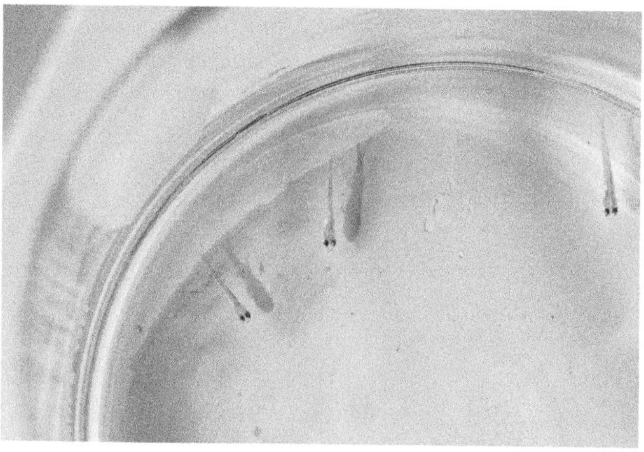

Fig 10.3. Larval zebrafish housed in a petri dish. (*Source:* Photo courtesy of A. Puffenberger.)

HUSBANDRY

Housing, Environment, and Sanitation

Although the Animal Welfare Act regulations do not apply to fish, the *Guide for the Care and Use of Laboratory Animals* (the *Guide*; ILAR, 2011) does contain sections and language dealing with housing of aquatic species. Any institution that is required to follow the PHS Policy is expected to follow the pertinent sections when setting up zebrafish housing in a biomedical research facility.

Zebrafish are typically housed in one of three aquaria configurations. These are recirculating, flow-through, or static/standalone systems. In recirculating systems, multiple tanks are connected to a single water source. Water flows into and out of the tanks at a rate controlled by the overall system. When the water exits the tanks, it enters a single large filtration system. Typically, water passes through four water treatment components before recirculating back into the animal housing tanks. In most systems, it first goes through a mechanical filter—a large sponge or similar material that catches large debris and removes it from the water. It then passes through

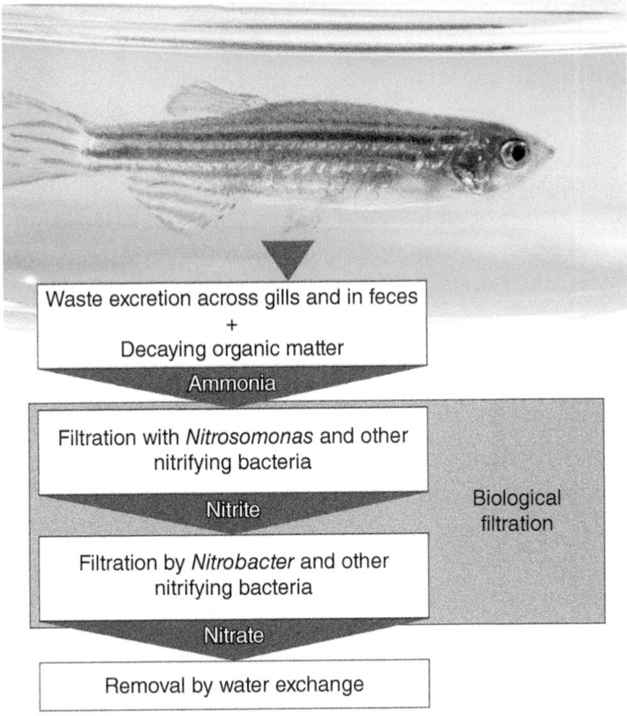

Fig 10.4. Components of the biological filter and nitrogen cycle. (*Source:* Courtesy of Austin Thomason, Michigan Photography—University of Michigan.)

biological and chemical filters. The biological filter is one of the most critical components for proper water filtration and maintaining health of the fish. In this section of the filtration system, *Nitrosomonas* spp. and *Nitrobacter* spp. convert toxic ammonia to nitrite and then again finally to the less toxic nitrate form (Figure 10.4). Without these bacterial assistants, a buildup of ammonia from fish and food waste can easily lead to the death of an entire colony. Often, the biological filters are filled with plastic balls, silicon beads, or sand in order to increase the amount of surface area available for bacterial growth. The chemical filter typically contains some form of carbon to inactivate organic compounds present in the water. Prior to re-entering the animal housing tanks, the water is then exposed to UV irradiation as UV light will damage or kill lingering bacteria, fungal, and viral pathogens.

Flow-through systems, like recirculating systems, may have multiple tanks on one rack; however, instead of passing through a filtration system and back into the animal housing tanks, water discharged from each tank is directed either into a drain or a collection basin. These flow-through systems are especially useful for administration of a drug or toxin in the water, animal quarantine, and studies that require the isolation of individual tanks. Standalone or static tanks are what one typically pictures when they think of aquariums—a single glass or acrylic tank housing a population of fish with a small filtration system affixed to the back of the tank or positioned underneath it. The filtration system typically still has all three filters: mechanical, biological, and chemical. The cost of labor to maintain static tanks can be high as the water needs to be changed manually on a regular basis. In contrast, with large recirculating or flow-through systems, water changes are typically automated and therefore labor costs may be lower.

The water source is an important factor in any fish facility, regardless of the housing system. Zebrafish systems can use municipal water, but due to variations in water contaminants and other factors, many facilities choose to use deionized or reverse osmosis water instead. If municipal water is used, at very minimum it must be treated to remove any chlorine or chloramine present in the water—both of which are common municipal water treatments and significantly toxic to zebrafish. If deionization or reverse osmosis is used to purify the water, then select salts and minerals that are removed through these processes need to be added back into the water prior to fish exposure in order to support normal biological functions.

Zebrafish can live in a fairly wide range of water temperatures, but their ideal range for growth and reproduction is 74–82 °F (23–28 °C). Commercial recirculating or flow-through systems used in biomedical research facilities are designed to maintain water temperature within an adjustable range. Individual aquarium heaters are typically placed in static tanks. Keeping the room air temperature within that range is also useful for helping prevent sudden fluctuations in water temperature, which can cause distress and illness in the fish colony. The light cycle should provide 12–16 hours of daylight; 14:10 is a common setting for zebrafish facilities. Other than temperature and light, the macroenvironment has few effects on the microenvironment for most zebrafish setups. One exception to that is the presence of aerosolized chemicals. The air that is used for zebrafish housing rooms should be free of all airborne contaminants, such as from chemicals used outside of the buildings. Additionally, chlorine-containing products should only be used in areas away from the main fish housing areas.

There is no suggested regular maintenance interval for cleaning the housing tanks. Algae may grow in tanks and is generally not harmful to the ecosystem. Zebrafish need to be clearly visible for daily health checks, so a good rule of thumb is to clean the tanks when approximately 50% of the surface is covered in algae. If chlorine-containing products, such as bleach, are used in any part of the cleaning process, the pieces must be rinsed with system water and left to air dry prior to coming in contact with any fish. Nets that are used to transfer fish from location to location are especially important to keep clean, as they can be a source for pathogen transmission. Two methods effective in sanitizing nylon nets are soaking them in sodium hypochlorite for 30 minutes or in potassium peroxymonosulfate + sodium chloride for 5 or 30 minutes. These methods also need to be followed with chlorine removal and air drying prior to coming in contact with any fish.

Water Quality

Water quality is one of the most important factors in maintaining zebrafish health, productivity, and welfare (Box 10.3). Although zebrafish can live in a range of conditions in the wild, they are sensitive to sudden shifts in quality or conditions. Regular testing of the system water should occur to ensure acceptable water parameters. Water testing should also be one of the first diagnostic steps for any health issue involving multiple fish. A brief overview of each parameter and its role in maintaining water quality will be discussed—more in depth information about this topic can be found in the references. Refer to Table 10.1 for recommended parameters and suggested testing frequencies.

Box 10.3

Water quality is one of the most important factors in maintaining zebrafish health, productivity, and welfare.

Table 10.1. Recommended water quality parameters and testing frequencies

Parameter	Ideal Range	Testing Frequency
Temperature	75–82 °F (24–28 °C)	Daily
pH	6.8–7.5	Daily
Conductivity	300–3800 μS (0.14–2.0 ppt)	Daily
Alkalinity	50–150 mg/L $CaCO_3$	Monthly
Hardness	50–100 mg/L $CaCO_3$	Monthly
Dissolved oxygen	>4 mg/L	Monthly
Carbon dioxide	<20 mg/L	Monthly
Ammonia	Zero	Daily to weekly
Nitrite	Zero	Daily to weekly
Nitrate	<50 mg/L	Weekly

Source: Adapted from Harper and Lawrence (2011) and Avdesh et al. (2012).

Fish waste products are composed primarily of ammonia, thus an increase in ammonia in the water can be due to normal fish metabolism, the presence of dead fish, and the presence of uneaten and decaying food. Ammonia is toxic to zebrafish at fairly low levels. As discussed earlier, recirculating water systems rely on a biofilter and bacterial species to remove ammonia and other nitrogenous wastes. It is important to note that the biofilter converts ammonia first to nitrite, which is also toxic to the fish. The nitrite must also be converted in the filter to the final product—nitrate, which fish can tolerate in higher levels. Nitrate is typically then removed by regular water changes. Healthy systems should have no measurable levels of ammonia or nitrite in the water.

pH, alkalinity, hardness, and salinity are important water parameters to monitor for zebrafish health. pH reflects the relative concentration of acids and bases in a solution. Neutral pH levels are generally ideal, although zebrafish can also do well in slightly alkaline water. Normal metabolic processes in the tanks (respiration, waste excretion) can cause the pH to drop over time, so supplemental buffer materials (typically sodium bicarbonate) are often added to maintain a neutral pH. Sudden large changes in pH should be avoided. Alkalinity represents the buffering capacity of the water. It is a measurement of the concentration of carbonate and bicarbonate ions in the water, which provide the ability to resist shifts in pH. Hardness refers to the presence of divalent ions in the water—mainly calcium and magnesium. These ions are important for various biological functions, and are provided to zebrafish through a combination of diet and concentration in the water. Salinity or conductivity is the measurement of all dissolved ions in the water and is important for maintaining normal osmoregulation. Zebrafish can tolerate a wide range of salinities, and adjusting salinity to a higher concentration can be beneficial for treatment of stress or disease states.

Dissolved gases are also present in water systems and are important to monitor. Most important is the availability of dissolved oxygen in the water for normal fish respiration. This parameter typically stays fairly stable in recirculating water systems, but may need more attention in static systems. Fish respiration converts oxygen to carbon dioxide, which can then be kept at lower concentrations by aeration of the water. Other dissolved gases (such as nitrogen) can be found in aquatic systems, and can cause disease if a buildup of the gas develops, such as during a system failure.

Environmental Enrichment and Social Housing

Zebrafish are a shoaling species, preferring to live in groups. As mentioned earlier, they can be territorial and aggressive at times. Aggression is more pronounced during breeding. Ideally, zebrafish should be housed in groups larger than five fish, but at an animal density of no more than five adult fish per liter of water.

The types of enrichment that zebrafish prefer are still unknown. Zebrafish enrichment is the focus of a number of current studies in zebrafish welfare. At this point, the best enrichment identified is group housing, which zebrafish have shown preference for over any single enrichment item. However, at times zebrafish may need to be housed singly for a research related purpose, and enrichment has been shown to potentially decrease the distress of single housing for these animals. Some options that have been used as enrichment in zebrafish tanks are plastic plants, marbles, mirrors, or gravel (Figure 10.5). As more studies are completed, there will be a better understanding of the ideal microenvironment for this species.

Feeding

Nutrition and feeding of zebrafish can be a complex subject. Precise nutritional requirements of zebrafish are still under investigation. Along with that, most zebrafish facilities are breeding and raising fish through their entire life cycle, and thus they need to take into account the nutritional requirements of larval, juvenile, and adult stage zebrafish. A combination of live and processed diets are fed in the majority of zebrafish facilities. Live diet options consist primarily of *Artemia* nauplii (the larval stage of brine shrimp) and smaller zooplankton such as *Paramecium* and rotifers of the *Brachionus* species. Processed feeds exist in flake and pellet formats, formulated specifically for zebrafish. Combinations of these diet options have led to successful growth and reproduction.

Appropriate food items are dependent on the life stage of the zebrafish. Zebrafish ingest their prey whole and cannot eat foods that are larger than their mouth (Box 10.4). Therefore, food items are limited in the earlier stages of life. Larval zebrafish begin to feed at around 5 dpf. Until they reach the juvenile stage (approximately 21–28 dpf), they require a constant source of nutrition to support the rapid growth and development during this phase of their life cycle. Live foods are often used at this stage for several reasons. Both rotifers and *Paramecium* are smaller than the maximum size larval zebrafish can eat (150–200 μM). Additionally, they swim through the water column where larval zebrafish are able to feed, and can live in tank water for a long time, reducing the need to constantly add more feed. They are high in protein and

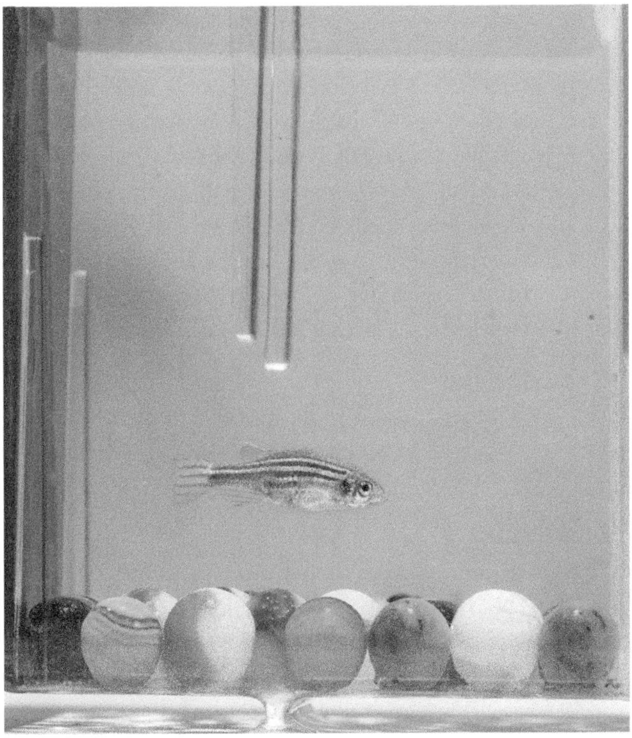

Fig 10.5. Marbles are one option for enrichment for singly housed zebrafish. (*Source:* Courtesy of Austin Thomason, Michigan Photography—University of Michigan.)

Box 10.4

Zebrafish ingest their prey whole and cannot eat foods that are larger than their mouth.

fulfill the nutritional needs of larval zebrafish. Processed feeds are available for the larval stage (with strategies to feed frequently, such as an automatic feeder), however, it has been shown that growth and performance are higher when larval zebrafish are fed live feed. That said, as processed feeds have improved in nutritional value, many facilities have chosen to move away from live food options, due to concerns of pathogen transmission and the challenges of producing large amounts of live food. Facilities need to assess the risks and benefits of both live and processed food options for the larval life stage, as it is currently possible to feed either, and a combination of both.

As zebrafish move into the juvenile life stage, they are able to consume foods of a much larger size—400–600 μM. They still need to be fed frequently (ideally 4–8 times a day), but can more readily obtain foods that have settled to the bottom of tanks. At this life stage, weaning from a live food to a pelleted food is easier to do. Live food, typically *Artemia* nauplii, is commonly fed. *Paramecium* are not considered nutritionally appropriate for juvenile zebrafish, although rotifers can still be fed.

Zebrafish are considered adults when they reach sexual maturity, starting at around 90 dpf. Adult zebrafish can be fed 1–3 times a day, and are easily and fully supported with processed formulated feeds. It is not uncommon to continue feeding adult zebrafish *Artemia* as well. Zebrafish should not be fed more than they can consume in 3–5 minutes, and excess food should be removed to minimize the amount of ammonia released into the water from decaying food. Adult zebrafish used for oocyte production may have higher nutritional needs, and can be fed up to 5 times a day. Adult zebrafish can easily eat foods larger than 600 μM in diameter, but it's generally considered safest to continue to feed items with a particle size of 400–600 μM.

TECHNIQUES

Handling and Restraint

As a fully aquatic animal, minimizing the amount of time that zebrafish are out of water is key to minimizing distress in handling. Additionally, the zebrafish body is covered by a mucus layer, which acts as a protective barrier against infection and should not be disrupted during handling. Nylon nets are typically used to gently catch and move zebrafish from one tank to another. If direct contact with the fish is necessary, personnel should wear powderless gloves to protect the fish's mucus layer and to protect personnel from exposure to *Mycobacterium* organisms that can cause zoonotic infection. Any procedure that removes the fish from water for longer than transfer to a second tank should be performed under general anesthesia and in such a way that the fish is kept wet and able to breathe.

Identification and Genotyping

Individual identification of zebrafish is not practical for most studies, so identification is typically limited to clear identification of groups of zebrafish housed in separate aquaria. As a large population of research zebrafish colonies are genetically modified, accurate genotyping and tank labeling is important for keeping colonies organized (Figure 10.6). Subcutaneous dyes have successfully been used to identify zebrafish, but are visible for only 30 days. The most common sampling technique for collecting tissues for genotyping is the fin clip or fin biopsy. This should be done under anesthesia and while wearing gloves. A small, sharp pair of scissors can be used to remove a small portion of the fin (most commonly the caudal fin). Zebrafish are able to regenerate the tissues of their fins and will regrow the tissue that was removed, so this method is not useful for identification purposes.

Blood Collection

Due to the size of the zebrafish circulatory system, survival collection of blood is impractical and difficult. Methods have been described for survival collection from the dorsal aorta, however, the amount that can safely be removed from the fish is too small for any real analysis other than a microscopic investigation of the cells present in the blood. Therefore, the majority of blood collection techniques in zebrafish are

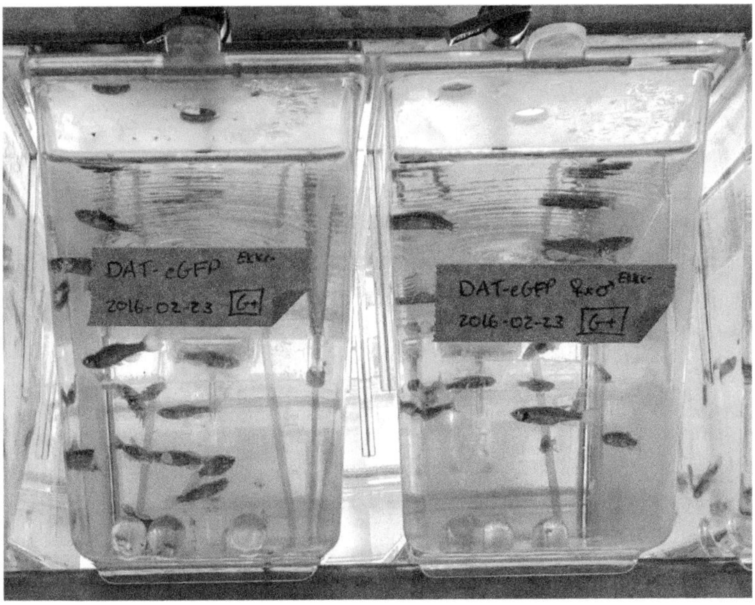

Fig 10.6. Identification of groups of fish by tank. (*Source:* Courtesy of Austin Thomason, Michigan Photography—University of Michigan.)

terminal techniques. Cardiac collection is straightforward, and involves exposing the heart immediately after euthanasia, followed by either removing the tip of the heart with scissors or inserting a 30-gauge needle into the ventricle. A heparinized capillary tube is used to draw up the blood either from the incised heart or from the needle hub. The dorsal aorta can also be used to collect blood at euthanasia, and can be accessed by making a transverse incision just caudal to the dorsal fin. Again, a heparinized capillary tube is then needed to draw up the blood.

Drug Administration

There are several methods available to administer drugs and other compounds to fish. Addition of compounds to the water can be a technically easy method of substance administration. Once placed in the water, zebrafish are exposed in two ways: through the gills (branchial diffusion) and through the gastrointestinal tract. All substances added to water within animal housing tanks must first be evaluated for their potential to negatively alter water quality parameters and influence fish health. Alternatively, oral administration alone can be accomplished by either dosing live feed (such as *Artemia*) with the substance, or by anesthetizing the zebrafish and orally gavaging up to 5 μL directly into the intestinal tract. Intraperitoneal (IP) and intramuscular (IM) injections are acceptable delivery techniques in zebrafish as well. IM injections can be performed in the dorsal epaxial muscles, and should be given slowly in order to minimize leakage back out through the skin. IP injections should be given after 24 hours of fasting to help avoid perforating the intestinal tract. IP injections are given on the midline in the area between the pectoral fin and the urogenital pore.

Anesthesia, Surgery, and Postoperative Care

Zebrafish are typically anesthetized by immersion in water treated with an appropriate anesthetic agent. Care should be taken to move the fish gently and quickly between water sources, and to protect the mucus layer during handling. A surgical plane of anesthesia is evidenced by a loss of all voluntary movement, a decrease in muscle tone, loss of tail-fin pinch reflex, and slow opercular movement. The most commonly used anesthetic agent in zebrafish is tricaine methanesulfonate, more typically known as MS-222. This drug is readily available, causes quick induction and recovery in zebrafish, and is currently approved by the FDA for fish anesthesia. MS-222 is acidic in solution, and does need to be buffered with sodium bicarbonate to a pH of 6–7 before the fish can be added to the anesthetic tank. MS-222 is highly dose dependent and can be used to induce mild sedation, a surgical plane of anesthesia, or euthanasia. Another alternative that has shown to be effective for surgical anesthesia is lidocaine hydrochloride, by itself and in combination with propofol. Metomidate hydrochloride has successfully been used for sedation and immobilization of zebrafish, but does not induce a surgical plane of anesthesia. Gradual cooling with ice to a temperature of 50–54 °F (10–12 °C) can be used for very brief and nonpainful procedures. The zebrafish cannot be in direct contact with the ice when this procedure is used. Typically, personnel will place ice water in a small container and then place a second container with holes inside the first, allowing the cold water to enter the inner container without any ice. Table 10.2 lists anesthetic drug doses that have been confirmed specifically in zebrafish.

Surgery in zebrafish comes with unique challenges. Many of the principles of mammalian surgery still apply. Aseptic technique, gentle tissue handling, hemostatic control, and proper selection of instruments and suture are the basis of proper surgical manipulation. Extra attention is needed to not damage the skin mucus layer and the scales, which need to remain moist throughout the procedure. Moistened sponges can help position the zebrafish for surgery while maintaining hydration of the skin and scales. Incisions should be closed with appropriate suture; for zebrafish, the suture material of choice is monofilament, such as nylon.

Recovery from anesthetic events should be done in tanks with a single fish at a time. To minimize postoperative infections or other complications, recovery tanks should be filled with clean water, and ideally not on a recirculating rack with the rest of the colony. Analgesic use in zebrafish is not common, due to the lack of understanding of the physiology of pain in fish species. Although the experience of pain in fish is still debated, it has been shown that analgesics can reduce behaviors in fish that are associated with a nociceptive response. Use of analgesics should be considered when performing painful procedures, and as more data is published showing their efficacy, it will likely become more common. Published information on the use of analgesics in zebrafish is scarce, however investigations into the use of various opioids and nonsteroidal anti-inflammatory drugs have been performed in other fish species. Specific to zebrafish, morphine and buprenorphine have been shown to ameliorate nociceptive response in larval or adult zebrafish. Aspirin has shown beneficial effects in adult zebrafish after fin clipping. Lidocaine hydrochloride may also have some efficacy as pre- and postoperative analgesia for fin clipping. Table 10.2 includes only analgesics that have shown beneficial effects in zebrafish specifically.

Table 10.2. Select anesthetic, analgesic, and euthanasia agents for use in zebrafish

Drug	Dosage	Route	Notes	Reference
Anesthesia				
Lidocaine hydrochloride	325 mg/L	Immersion	Surgical anesthesia	Collymore et al. (2014b)
Metomidate hydrochloride	6, 8, and 10 mg/L	Immersion	Sedation only	Collymore et al. (2014b)
Propofol + lidocaine hydrochloride	2.5 mg/L 50 mg/L	Immersion	Surgical anesthesia	Martins et al. (2016)
	1.25 μg/mL 100 μg/mL	Immersion	Surgical anesthesia	Martins et al. (2018a)
Tricaine methanesulfonate (MS-222)	150 mg/L	Immersion	Surgical anesthesia, must be buffered	Martins et al. (2016)
Analgesia				
Aspirin	1.0 and 2.5 mg/L	Immersion	Adult zebrafish	Chatigny et al. (2018)
Buprenorphine	0.1 μg/mL	Immersion	Larval zebrafish	Chatigny et al. (2018)
Lidocaine hydrochloride	2.0–5.0 mg/L	Immersion	Adult zebrafish	Martins et al. (2016)
Morphine	48 mg/L	Immersion	Larval zebrafish	Chatigny et al. (2018)
	3.0 and 6.0 mg/kg	IM	Adult zebrafish	Correia et al. (2011)
Euthanasia				
2-phenoxyethanol	0.3–0.4 mg/L	Immersion		AVMA (2013)
Benzocaine	>250 mg/L	Immersion	Must be buffered	AVMA (2013)
Clove oil (75–95% eugenol)	100 mg/L	Immersion		Davis et al. (2015)
Quinaldine sulfate	>100 mg/L	Immersion	Must be buffered	AVMA (2013)
Tricaine methanesulfonate	250–500 mg/L	Immersion	Must be buffered	AVMA (2013)

Euthanasia

Zebrafish are most commonly euthanized in biomedical research by an overdose of MS-222 in water. General principles for euthanasia are similar to anesthesia. Stress should be minimized by moving fish gently and rapidly between tanks, and water quality in the euthanasia tank should be the same level as the housing tank. The most ideal option is to use water directly from the housing system for euthanasia. Recall that MS-222 will need to be buffered to a neutral pH prior to use. Other immersion agents that are considered acceptable by the American Veterinary Medical Association's (AVMA) *Guidelines for the Euthanasia of Animals* (AVMA, 2013) include buffered benzocaine, quinaldine sulfate, and 2-phenoxyethanol. Rapid chilling in an ice water bath at 35–39 °F (2–4 °C) is an acceptable method of euthanasia for zebrafish and requires that fish not come in direct contact with the ice. For all immersion techniques, fish should be left in the euthanasia tank for at least 10 minutes after cessation of opercular movement. Decapitation or pithing may be used as secondary methods of euthanasia. Double pithing can be achieved through use of a small gauge needle to macerate brain and spinal cord tissue. Euthanasia of larval zebrafish is not reliable with either MS-222 or rapid chilling alone. The AVMA recommends a combination of rapid chilling followed by immersion in a dilute sodium hypochlorite solution as an acceptable and effective method of larval zebrafish euthanasia.

There are several additional methods of euthanasia that the AVMA labels acceptable with considerations. These include immersion in eugenol or clove oil, immersion in CO_2-saturated water, and decapitation followed by pithing. The following are unacceptable methods of euthanasia in any situation for finfish: flushing into the sewer system, slow cooling (e.g., placing a conscious fish into the freezer), and removal of the fish from water (anoxia). Lidocaine hydrochloride has recently been shown to be as effective and safe as MS-222 for zebrafish euthanasia, however, it is not yet discussed in the AVMA guidelines.

THERAPEUTIC AGENTS

Therapeutic agent use in the research of zebrafish is not common. The majority of diseases have underlying etiologies involving the water quality or housing system. Additionally, very few studies of antibiotic, antifungal, and antiparasitic use have been performed specifically in zebrafish. Since the majority of finfish being raised are used in the food industry for humans, use of drugs such as antibiotics are often not acceptable at all. Finally, many treatments consist of changing the temperature or adding sodium chloride to the water, as opposed to using a pharmaceutical drug. Treatments that have been found to assist in specific diseases will be discussed in the following section.

INTRODUCTION TO DISEASES OF ZEBRAFISH

Disease outbreaks in zebrafish facilities are often multifactorial and difficult to treat. Zebrafish used for biomedical research are acquired from a number of different sources, and many do not have a specific pathogen free program. Thus, the fish can arrive appearing healthy while still infected with a number of organisms. These can cause little or no disease until the fish are put under stress, typically due to a change in water quality. Because most institutions are using large recirculating water systems that share the water throughout up to hundreds of tanks, it is very easy for newly introduced organisms to be transferred throughout an entire colony. Use of quarantine racks and obtaining a clear pathogen history from shipping institutions can help minimize colony-wide exposure from new fish being added to an established facility. Bleaching embryos before entry to the colony is another common method of preventing pathogen exposure; however, this method does not protect against all *Pseudoloma* infections. In any disease outbreak, it is critical to do a full assessment of the housing system and the water quality, as well as perform necropsies of affected fish, in order to identify the underlying issue (Box 10.5). It is often not practical or

> **Box 10.5**
>
> *In any disease outbreak, it is critical to do a full assessment of the housing system and the water quality, as well as perform necropsies of affected fish, in order to identify the underlying issue.*

possible to treat large infectious disease outbreaks in zebrafish colonies outside of identifying and fixing any husbandry related problems.

Common signs of illness in zebrafish are often nonspecific and include lethargy, difficulty maintaining buoyancy, opercular flaring, clamped fins, change in color, flashing (rapid turning or rubbing themselves against the tank surfaces), scale loss, surface breathing, isolation from the school, mucus sloughing, abnormal body condition, and abnormal spinal curvature. Sudden death is also commonly seen in animals affected by a significant pathogen load or water quality issue.

Bacterial Diseases

Mycobacteriosis

Mycobacteriosis is commonly seen in zebrafish, caused by environmental species of *Mycobacterium* that are found in soil, water, or biofilms. Several species have been identified in zebrafish, including *M. marinum, M. chelonae, M. haemophilum, M. fortuitum, M. peregrinum,* and *M. abscessus*. These bacteria primarily cause opportunistic disease in zebrafish in the presence of several possible predisposing factors, such as poor water quality or overcrowding, immunosuppression, or genetic susceptibility. Disease presentation, morbidity, and mortality vary based on the infecting bacterial strain. Mycobacteriosis will often present with nonspecific signs such as lethargy, emaciation, skin ulceration, or coelemic distention. On gross necropsy, tan nodules can be seen in visceral organs—these are the granulomas that are characteristic of infection with *Mycobacterium* spp. Mycobacteriosis can be diagnosed by histologic identification of the acid-fast organism within granulomas. *Mycobacterium* species can also be cultured; however, some of the species will take up to 8 weeks to grow. Therefore, PCR has become an important tool in diagnosing mycobacteriosis in fish colonies. There is no treatment to completely eradicate mycobacteriosis, and affected or dead fish should be taken out of the systems as soon as possible, as they will shed the organism from their skin. Instead, facilities should focus on preventing outbreaks of mycobacteriosis by maintaining good water quality, removing sick fish promptly, keeping their systems sanitized and free of biofilms, and having a good quarantine program in place for bringing new fish into the facility. Recently, oral treatment of *M. chelonae* with tigecycline or clarithromycin has shown promise in reducing the severity of the infection, however, it does not eradicate it. Importantly, *Mycobacterium marinum* is a zoonotic agent that causes fish tank granuloma in humans. The disease typically presents as nodules or nonhealing ulcers on the skin and is contracted by handling infected fish, water, or tank materials with no gloves, especially with open wounds present on the hands and fingers. Proper PPE usage and hand washing should be followed at all times when handling zebrafish due to this pathogen.

Bacterial Gill Disease and Columnaris

Bacterial gill disease is caused by *Flavobacterium branchiophilum* and *Flavobacterium columnare*. These two opportunistic bacteria cause separate but similar disease presentations in zebrafish. *F. branchiophilum* targets only the gill epithelium, while *F. columnare* can effect both skin and gill epithelium. Affected fish may exhibit labored breathing or flared opercula. Abnormal skin presentation with *F. columnare* can range from loss of pigment to ulceration and necrosis. There may also be white lesions on the head, fins, and scales, which are often mistaken for a white fungus. These lesions are the reason that infection with *F. columnare* is also called "cotton wool disease." Like most bacterial infections in zebrafish, this is considered a husbandry or stress related disease, as it is associated with high stress situations such as poor water quality, handling or netting, shipping, or overcrowding. Rapid diagnosis can be performed by observing numerous long, rod-shaped, Gram-negative bacteria in wet mount preparations of gills or skin lesions. There is no treatment for either disease.

Aeromonad Infection

Outside of research zebrafish facilities, motile aeromonad infection is considered the most common bacterial disease of freshwater fish. In zebrafish, *Aeromonas hydrophila* and *Aeromonas sobria* are the causative agents of motile aeromonad septicemia (MAS). This disease is characterized by petechial hemorrhages of the skin, fins, oral cavity, and muscle. This is primarily a stress-induced disease, often associated with poor water quality. Specifically, high mortality events have been seen with water high in nitrite levels. MAS also may be associated with concurrent infections with common protozoal infections of zebrafish, such as with *Tetrahymena pyriformis*. Diagnosis is based on culture of the organism. Culture and sensitivity testing can provide guidance in potential treatment with appropriate antibiotics. Immunocompromised humans are at risk of zoonotic infection with these organisms.

Edwardsiellosis

Edwardsiella ictaluri is an emerging natural pathogen of zebrafish. It was previously believed to only cause disease in catfish, but recently has been identified as the causative agent of high morbidity and mortality events in zebrafish facilities. Affected fish present with signs consistent with acute septicemia, including lethargy, ascites, skin ulceration, and high mortality. *E. ictaluri* is susceptible to several antibiotics, however focus should be on preventing the entry of the organism into a colony by choosing appropriate vendors and utilizing a quarantine program for new fish.

Viral Diseases

No clinically significant and naturally occurring viral infections of zebrafish have yet been identified.

Mycotic Diseases

Saprolegniasis

Saprolegnia spp. are water molds that are ubiquitous inhabitants of water and soil and cause disease in zebrafish. They are not true fungi; instead they are currently classified in the Protista kingdom, and considered "pseudofungi." Infection in zebrafish requires an open wound; often rough handling or other diseases that cause skin ulceration can predispose zebrafish to infection with *Saprolegnia*. Affected zebrafish present with white, cottony tufts of growth on the damaged areas, which can also spread throughout the body. Visualization of the aseptate hyphae on a wet mount is a quick way to confirm the diagnosis. Although this organism has been successfully treated with prolonged immersion in saltwater baths, it is generally an unrewarding treatment. Facilities with disease outbreaks with this organism should instead focus on the husbandry conditions that likely led to the clinical presence of the disease.

Parasitic Diseases

Microsporidiosis

Microsporidial organisms were previously thought to be protozoal organisms, but have now been classified as a unicellular parasite in the Fungi kingdom. Microsporidiosis in zebrafish is primarily caused by *Pseudoloma neurophilia*, which is also considered the most common disease of research zebrafish. A second microsporidial organism, *Pleistophora hyphessobryconis,* is also capable of causing disease in zebrafish, however with much less significance than *P. neurophilia*. *P. neurophilia* primarily effects the central nervous system, where it forms cysts that are filled with spores. Along within the brain and spinal cord, these cysts can also be found in skeletal muscle, nerve ganglia, and ovaries. The potential to infect ovaries is particularly significant, as the organism has also been found to infect ova, thus promoting vertical transmission and complicating efforts to eradicate this pathogen from zebrafish colonies using traditional methods (such as bleaching embryos). Disease with *P. neurophilia* is also called “skinny disease” as the primary clinical sign seen is emaciation. Along with emaciation, changes to the spinal curvature are commonly seen. The disease tends to remain subclinical until times of high stress, such as during handling or shipping. PCR can be used to diagnose this disease, as well as looking for spore-filled cysts in wet mounts of the central nervous system. There are no treatments for this disease. As fish progress to severe scoliosis, ataxia, and emaciation, they should be removed and humanely euthanized.

Metazoan Infection

The primary metazoan parasite of interest in zebrafish is *Pseudocapillaria tomentosa*, a species of intestinal nematode. Intestinal capillariasis in zebrafish is characterized by the presence of adult worms in the lumen and wall of the intestinal tract. These worms are locally invasive, and can cause a range of pathology within the gastrointestinal wall, from mild inflammation to intestinal cell carcinomas or other neoplasms. Affected fish present with emaciation and reduced fecundity. Diagnosis is by histologic identification of worms within the gastrointestinal tract. *Pseudocapillaria tomentosa* infections have been successfully treated with *Artemia* that have been coated in a fenbendazole solution and an emamectin or ivermectin-impregnated pelleted diet. Zebrafish colonies may experience a drop in fecundity during treatment, which will then recover over time. Control and prevention of the disease revolves around good husbandry practices and regular maintenance of the system filters and UV lights (if applicable).

Neoplasia

Spontaneous neoplasia in zebrafish is a common clinical finding. Seminomas are the most common. Other frequently reported neoplasms include spindle cell carcinomas and various tumor types found in the intestine (often associated with *P. tomentosa* infection), ultimobranchial gland, and liver.

Miscellaneous Conditions

Diseases Associated with Poor Water Quality

Alterations to specific parameters in water quality can cause significant morbidity and mortality, regardless of concurrent infections. Water quality parameters most frequently associated with zebrafish morbidities include elevated ammonia, nitrite, and chlorine levels; and gas supersaturation. Identifying and fixing the water quality issue is the only treatment for affected fish.

Ammonia is the primary waste product of fish metabolism, and is also produced through the decay of uneaten food or other organic material. A low level of ammonia will always be present in a normal fish ecosystem; ammonia toxicity occurs when there is a buildup of the toxic form of ammonia (NH_3) in the water. As discussed previously, the bacteria living in the biological filter of a recirculating water housing system are responsible for converting ammonia to the more benign nitrate. Disruptions to the biological filter, or situations in which the amount of ammonia exceeds the capacity of the biological filter can lead to ammonia toxicity. Fish affected by ammonia toxicity show nonspecific signs, such as anorexia, lethargy, and decreased growth rate. If a high level of ammonia is seen in a system, at least 50% of the water within the system should be replaced immediately, and efforts should be made to reduce the biological load (decrease the density of the fish, remove any organic waste, and reduce feedings).

Nitrite toxicity is similarly caused by a disruption to the biological filter. Nitrite enters the zebrafish bloodstream and oxidizes hemoglobin into methemoglobin. The methemoglobin is unable to carry oxygen, and hypoxic damage occurs in the zebrafish. This disease is also called brown blood disease, and affected fish may have brown or tan gills. Affected fish will show signs of hypoxia, including increased respiratory rate and surface swimming. The addition of sodium chloride or calcium chloride to the water can reduce the amount of nitrite available for absorption by the gills, thus reducing the amount of methemoglobin produced. Water changes and establishing and maintaining a healthy biofilter are key to preventing this issue.

Chlorine and chloramine are commonly found in most city water sources and are both highly toxic to fish (Box 10.6). Chlorine can be removed from water through chemical filtration or through aeration for 24 hours before use in a zebrafish system; however, chloramine is not affected by aeration and must be removed by treatment with an activated carbon filter or a chemical neutralizer prior to entering any zebrafish housing system. Clinical signs of fish affected with chlorine toxicity include respiratory distress from gill necrosis and rapid death.

Supersaturation of zebrafish system water with either oxygen or nitrogen causes a characteristic gas bubble disease in fish, although especially high levels of supersaturation

Box 10.6

Chlorine and chloramine are commonly found in most city water sources and are both highly toxic to fish.

can cause death in minutes. Fish that are acutely affected will present with air bubbles in the gills, fins, eyes, skin, and oral cavity. They may also have exophthalmia. More chronically affected fish will have respiratory distress, and are often found at the bottom of the tank. The most common cause of gas supersaturation in a zebrafish system is mechanical in origin; specifically, leaks in the pipes connected to the water pump. If fish present with signs of gas bubble disease, the water circulation system should be thoroughly examined until the source of the leak is identified.

BIBLIOGRAPHY

American Veterinary Medical Association (AVMA). 2013. *AVMA Guidelines for the Euthanasia of Animals.* Available at http://www.avma.org/KB/Policies/Documents/euthanasia.pdf [Accessed November 5, 2018].

Avdesh, A., M. Chen, M. T. Martin-Iverson, et al. 2012. Regular care and maintenance of a zebrafish (*Danio rerio*) laboratory: An introduction. J Vis Exp (69):e4196.

Chang C. T., K. M. Doerr, and C. M. Whipps. 2017. Antibiotic treatment of zebrafish mycobacteriosis: tolerance and efficacy of treatments with tigecycline and clarithromycin. J Fish Dis 40(10): 1473–1485.

Chatigny, F., C. M. Creighton, and E. D. Stevens. 2018. Updated review of fish analgesia. J Am Assoc Lab Anim Sci 57(1): 5–12.

Cheung, E., D. Chatterjee, and R. Gerlai. 2014. Subcutaneous dye injection for marking and identification of individual adult zebrafish (*Danio rerio*) in behavioral studies. Behav Res Methods 46(3): 619–624.

Collymore, C., A. Tolwani, C. Lieggi, and S. Rasmussen. 2014b. Efficacy and safety of 5 anesthetics in adult zebrafish (*Danio rerio*). J Am Assoc Lab Anim Sci 53 (2): 198–203.

Collymore, C., R. J. Tolwani, and S. Rasmussen. 2015. The behavioral effects of single housing and environmental enrichment on adult zebrafish (*Danio rerio*). J Am Assoc Lab Anim Sci 54(3): 280–285.

Collymore, C., E. K. Banks, and P. V. Turner. 2016. Lidocaine hydrochloride compared with MS222 for the euthanasia of zebrafish (*Danio rerio*). J Am Assoc Lab Anim Sci 55(6): 816–820.

Correia, A. D., S. R. Cunha, M. Scholze, and E. D. Stevens. 2011. A novel behavioral fish model of nociception for testing analgesics. Pharmaceuticals 4(4): 665–680.

Davis, D. J., J. Klug, M. Hankins, et al. 2015. Effects of clove oil as a euthanasia agent on blood collection efficiency and serum cortisol levels in *Danio rerio*. J Am Assoc Lab Anim Sci 54(5): 564–567.

Esmail, M. Y., K. M. Astrofsky, C. Lawrence, and F. C. Serluca. 2015. The biology and management of the zebrafish. In *Laboratory Animal Medicine*, 3rd ed., J. G. Fox, L. Anderson, G. Otto, K. Pritchett-Corning, and M. Whary (eds), pp. 1015–1062. Amsterdam: Academic Press.

Gonzales, J. M., Jr. 2012. Preliminary evaluation on the effects of feeds on the growth and early reproductive performance of zebrafish (*Danio rerio*). J Am Assoc Lab Anim Sci 51(4): 412–417.

Grzelak, A. K., D. J. Davis, S. M. Caraker, et al. 2017. Stress leukogram induced by acute and chronic stress in zebrafish (*Danio rerio*). Comp Med 67(3): 263–269.

Harper, C. and C. Lawrence. 2011. *The Laboratory Zebrafish*. Boca Raton, FL: CRC Press.

Institute for Laboratory Animal Research (ILAR). 2011. *Guide for the Care and Use of Laboratory Animals*, 8th ed. Washington, DC: National Academies Press.

JoVE Science Education Database. 2019. Biology II: Mouse, Zebrafish, and Chick. Zebrafish Reproduction and Development. JoVE, Cambridge, MA.

Keck, V. A., D. S. Edgerton, S. Hajizadeh, et al. 2015. Effects of habitat complexity on pair-housed zebrafish. J Am Assoc Lab Anim Sci 54(4): 378–383.

Maley, D., A. S. Laird, S. Rinkwitz, and T. S. Becker. 2013. A simple and efficient protocol for the treatment of zebrafish colonies infected with parasitic nematodes. Zebrafish 10(3): 447–450.

Martins, T., E. Diniz, L. M. Felix, and L. Antunes. 2018a. Evaluation of anaesthetic protocols for laboratory adult zebrafish (*Danio rerio*). PLoS One 13 (5): e0197846.

Martins, T., A. Valentim, N. Pereira, and L. M. Antunes. 2018b. Anaesthetics and analgesics used in adult fish for research: A review. Lab Anim 4: 23677218815199 [Epub ahead of print]

Matthews, M. and Z. M. Varga. 2012. Anesthesia and euthanasia in zebrafish. ILAR J. 53(2): 192–204.

Meritet, D. M., D. M. Mulrooney, M. L. Kent, and C. V. Lohr. 2017. Development of quantitative real-time PCR assays for postmortem detection of *Mycobacterium* spp. common in zebrafish (*Danio rerio*) research colonies. J Am Assoc Lab Anim Sci 56(2): 131–141.

Singleman, C. and N. G. Holtzman. 2014. Growth and maturation in the zebrafish, *Danio rerio*: a staging tool for teaching and research. Zebrafish 11(4): 396–406.

Stoskopf, M. K. 2015. Biology and management of laboratory fishes. In *Laboratory Animal Medicine*, 3rd ed., J.G. Fox, L. Anderson, G. Otto, K. Pritchett-Corning, and M. Whary (eds), pp. 1063–1086. Amsterdam: Academic Press.

Strykowski, J. L. and J. M. Schech. 2015. Effectiveness of recommended euthanasia methods in larval zebrafish (*Danio rerio*). J Am Assoc Lab Anim Sci 54(1): 81–84.

Wafer, L. N., V. B. Jensen, J. C. Whitney, et al. 2016. Effects of environmental enrichment on the fertility and fecundity of zebrafish (*Danio rerio*). J Am Assoc Lab Anim Sci 55 (3): 291–294.

FURTHER READING

Collymore, C., G. Porelli, C. Lieggi, and N. S. Lipman. 2014a. Evaluation of 5 cleaning and disinfection methods for nets used to collect zebrafish (*Danio rerio*). J Am Assoc Lab Anim Sci 53(6): 657–660.

Collymore, C., V. Watral, J. R. White, et al. 2014c. Tolerance and efficacy of emamectin benzoate and ivermectin for the treatment of *Pseudocapillario tomentosa* in laboratory zebrafish (*Danio rerio*). Zebrafish 11(5): 490–497.

Fox, J., L. Anderson, G. Otto, et al. (eds). 2015. *Laboratory Animal Medicine*, 3rd ed. Amsterdam: Academic Press.

Harper, C. and C. Lawrence. 2011. *The Laboratory Zebrafish*. Boca Raton, FL: CRC Press.
Kent, M. and Z. Varga (eds.) 2012. Zebrafish health and husbandry. ILAR J 53(2).
Martins, T., A. M. Valentim, N. Pereira, and L. M. Antunes. 2016. Anaesthesia and analgesia in laboratory adult zebrafish: a question of refinement. Lab Anim 50(6): 476–488.
Noga, E. J. 2010. *Fish Disease: Diagnosis and Treatment*. Oxford: Wiley-Blackwell.
Ostrander, G. C. 2000. *The Laboratory Fish*. Academic Press.
University of Oregon. (1994–2018). The Zebrafish Information Network. https://zfin.org.
Westerfield, M. 2007. *The Zebrafish Book*, 5th ed. Eugene, OR: University of Oregon Press

CHAPTER 10 REVIEW

1. ____ What are the reasons that zebrafish are an ideal model for studies in embryonic development?
2. ____ What is an ideal zebrafish group size that will increase social interaction and minimize aggression?
3. ____ True/False: The zebrafish stomach has two compartments; a glandular and nonglandular.
4. ____ What is the primary hematopoietic organ of the zebrafish?
5. ____ What type of environment promotes spawning in zebrafish?
6. ____ Which type of aquaria set-up recycles water through several filters before delivering it back to many tanks?
7. ____ Which type of aquaria set-up sends water from the fish tanks straight into the drain or a dump tank?
8. ____ What is the role of *Nitromonas* and *Nitrobacter* spp. in a zebrafish environment?
9. ____ What is the difference between hardness and conductivity?
10. ____What are three types of live feed?
11. ____What is the typical tissue sample to collect for genotyping?
12. ____What is an appropriate method of euthanizing larval zebrafish?
13. ____What steps can a facility take to minimize introduction of pathogens into their facility when ordering new fish or embryos?
14. ____What is the causative agent of fish tank granuloma in humans?
15. ____What emerging pathogen of zebrafish was previously thought to only cause disease in catfish?
16. ____Why is it particularly difficult to eradicate *Pseudoloma neurophilia* from a colony?
17. ____True/False: Chlorine can be removed from water through aeration; chloramine cannot.

11

Rabbits

Rabbits, cottontails, and hares are of the order Lagomorpha and are collectively referred to as lagomorphs. Although often confused as a rabbit, hares belong to the genus *Lepus* and are in many ways quite dissimilar to rabbits. Cottontails are descendants of the North and South American rabbit and are classified in the genus *Sylvilagus*. Rabbits native to Europe have given rise to only one species, *Oryctolagus cuniculus*, which translates to "hare dug out of the earth." The laboratory rabbit is derived from this European rabbit. The three genera *Lepus*, *Sylvilagus*, and *Oryctolagus* cannot interbreed to produce viable offspring. Rabbit breeds can vary markedly in size, with a range of 1–9 kg (2.2–19.8 lb). There are numerous coat color variations, including albino, black, silver, and belted.

BREEDS

Though more than 50 breeds of rabbits are recognized in the United States, only 3 are commonly used in research: the New Zealand White (NZW), the Dutch Belted, and occasionally the Flemish Giant. The NZW is a medium-sized albino rabbit weighing between 3 and 5 kg (6.6–11.0 lb). It is the most commonly used breed in biomedical research. The Dutch Belted is a small breed, possessing a black or chocolate coat with a white belt encircling the thorax and a white facial blaze and feet. It weighs between 0.9 and 1.8 kg (2.0–4.0 lb) and is second in importance as a laboratory breed (Figure 11.1). The Flemish Giant is most often fawn or gray coated, weighs between 6.5 and 9 kg (14.3–19.8 lb), and is occasionally used for research.

Both spontaneously derived mutant strains of rabbits (e.g., Watanabe heritable hyperlipidemic rabbit, St. Thomas Hospital strain rabbit) and purposefully produced

Clinical Laboratory Animal Medicine: An Introduction, Fifth Edition.
Lesley A. Colby, Megan H. Nowland, and Lucy H. Kennedy.

Companion website: www.wiley.com/go/colby/clinical

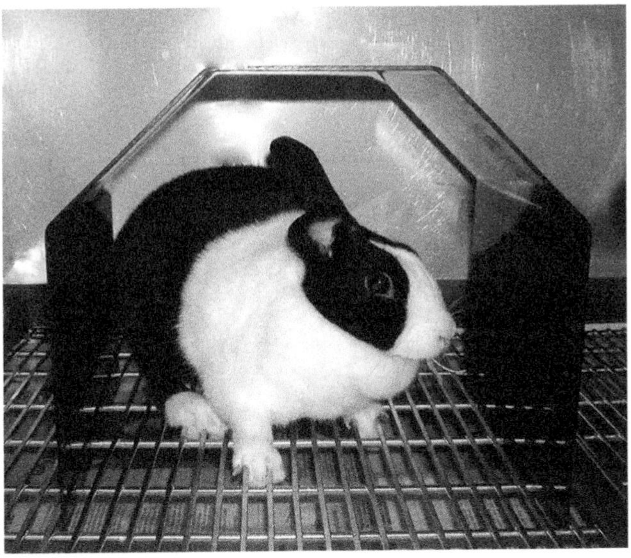

Fig 11.1. Dutch Belted rabbit in enrichment hut. (*Source:* Photo courtesy of Bio-Serv.)

transgenic rabbits are now commonly used and have expanded the use of rabbits as models of human disease and conditions.

USES

The rabbit has been, and continues to be, used extensively in biomedical research. Their popularity is partially due to their body size (between that of rodents and the larger mammals), their ease of handling, and their unique anatomical and physiological characteristics. In addition, rabbits are frequently selected due to their position on the evolutionary scale, closer to humans than rodents, but less evolved and with lower perceived sentience than nonhuman primates and other large mammals.

The rabbit has an extensive history of use and range of applications in biomedical research. Considerable research has been conducted to elucidate the mechanisms of lipid metabolism and hypercholesterolemia such as through study of the Watanabe heritable hyperlipidemic rabbit strain, which has a spontaneous genetic mutation of its low-density lipoprotein receptor, similar to human familial hypercholesterolemia. Rabbits have been used widely in the production of antibodies to characterize immune function as well as vaccine development. An interesting bit of history and an example of the use of one species (rabbit) to benefit another (dog) is the development of the rabies vaccine by Louis Pasteur in the late 1800s. Juvenile animals are susceptible to naturally occurring and induced mucoid enteropathy, a condition that facilitates investigation into human inflammatory bowel disease, cystic fibrosis, and cholera. Rabbits have also been used in the development of a wide range of surgical models (including the development of surgical laser use) and as models for acute respiratory distress syndrome, asthma, cerebral embolism, cardiovascular disease, endometriosis, and glaucoma. With the advent of CRISPR/Cas9 genetic modification technology, transgenic models are also becoming more available for studies in numerous areas of biomedical research.

BEHAVIOR

In general, rabbits are gentle and docile animals and are not normally aggressive toward human handlers. They tend to be curious but easily startled. When frightened or painful, they may emit a high-pitched scream or display in the form of foot stomping, growling, or snorting. As with other prey species, rabbits become still when frightened or stressed and may rarely show obvious signs of pain. Rabbits very rarely bite but may do so if painful. Other signs of pain include inactivity, dullness, a hunched stance, bruxism (tooth grinding), hiding, excessive or lack of grooming, aggression, and anorexia. Sexually mature rabbits are territorial and can fight if housed together without proper supervision. In contrast, if immature females are housed together at 3 months of age or younger, they often establish long-term stable groups. Trauma, pseudopregnancies, and infertility can, however, occur in group-housed rabbits. Rabbits can be effectively litter-box trained; they typically choose one area of their cage for defecation and urination.

Depending on environmental conditions, wild rabbits are either nocturnal or diurnal. They are crepuscular foragers, feeding predominantly at dusk and dawn, and hide in burrows or in thickets of brush during daylight hours. Rabbits housed indoors in controlled environments tend to have alternating periods of wakefulness and rest throughout the day and night. Nests for offspring are constructed from fur plucked from the abdomen and dewlap (ventral neck) area.

Rabbits prefer to occupy areas near the perimeter or walls of their enclosure, avoiding the perceived threats of open areas; this orientation response is called thigmotaxis. Knowledge of this behavioral preference can be employed to more quickly acclimate animals to handling by holding them securely with as much surface contact as possible.

ANATOMIC AND PHYSIOLOGIC FEATURES

Rabbit biologic and reproductive data are listed in Table 11.1. Rabbits have a compact body and heavily muscled back and rear legs. Their lightweight skeleton comprises only 7% of their total body weight. This muscle-to-skeletal bone ratio makes them particularly susceptible to fracture of their lumbar vertebrae (most often occurring at the L7–S1 junction). They have long ears with prominent vessels, have a short tail, and are covered with very fine, soft fur. Rabbits have five digits on the forelimbs, four digits on the hind limbs, and toenails capable of inflicting scratches to handlers. They have no footpads; fur covers the plantar and palmar surfaces of the tarsus and carpus. In addition to their use of feces and urine, rabbits have chin, anal, and inguinal glands that are used for territorial scent marking.

Each eye of the rabbits has an approximately 190° field of vision, but, due to the wide placement of eyes on their head, they possess only a very limited field of binocular vision. Harderian lacrimal glands are located behind the well-developed nictitating membranes and aid in lubrication. The blood flow through the large ears of the rabbits is a primary means of body temperature regulation.

Domestic rabbits resemble rodents in many respects. The principal anatomic feature differentiating them is an additional pair of incisors, known as peg teeth, which are smaller and positioned behind (posterior to) the upper incisors on the maxilla. The purpose of these short, cylindrical teeth is not clear. When the jaw is at rest, the mandibular incisors should be positioned between the two sets of maxillary incisors. The rabbit dental formula is 2(I 2/1, C 0/0, P 3/2, M 3/3); a diastema, or open space, is present between the incisors and the premolars. All of the teeth are open rooted, growing continuously throughout life. The incisors grow up to 10 cm (4 in.) in 1 year. The oral cavity is small and the tongue is relatively large, contributing to the difficulty of oral intubation. The esophagus of the rabbit is unique in that it has three striated muscle layers throughout the entire length, and mucous glands are absent. Rabbits cannot vomit due to anatomic positioning of their cardia and stomach. Unlike rodents, their stomachs are not divided and are thin walled, which may lead to postmortem stomach rupture secondary to significant gas accumulation following death or handling of abdominal contents at necropsy. The small intestine is relatively short, making up approximately 12% of the total length of the gastrointestinal tract. The large intestine consists of the cecum, the proximal colon, and the distal colon. Combined, the intestinal contents may account for up to 20% of the body weight,

Table 11.1. Biologic and reproductive data for rabbits

Adult body weight: Male	2–5 kg
Adult body weight: Female	2–6 kg
Life span	5–6 y or more
Body temperature	38.5°–40°C (101.3°–104°F)
Heart rate	130–325 beats per minute
Respiratory rate	30–60 breaths per minute
Tidal volume	4–6 mL/kg
Food consumption	5 g/100 g per day
Water consumption	5–12 mL/100 g per day
Breeding onset: Male	6–10 mo
Breeding onset: Female	4–9 mo
Estrous cycle length	Induced ovulator
Gestation period	29–35 d
Postpartum estrus	48 h
Litter size	4–10
Weaning age	4–6 wk
Breeding duration	1–3 y
Chromosome number (diploid)	44

Source: Adapted from Harkness et al. (2010).

Box 11.1

There are two types of feces produced by rabbits: firm, dry daytime fecal pellets and soft, moist nutrient-rich nighttime feces called cecotrophs that the rabbit normally ingests.

which is significant when calculating drug dosages based on body weight. For hindgut fermentation of their herbivorous diet, rabbits have a large, well-developed cecum that is approximately 10 times the size of the stomach and contains approximately 40% of the intestinal contents. There are two types of feces produced by rabbits: firm, dry, daytime fecal pellets and soft, moist, nutrient-rich, nighttime feces called cecotrophs (Box 11.1). The cecotrophs are covered with mucus to protect them from the acid pH of the stomach and are high in water, nitrogen, electrolytes, and B vitamins. These feces contain twice the protein and half the fiber of the firm, dry fecal pellets. Rabbits may ingest these from the cage floor or more frequently will ingest them directly from the anus. Healthy rabbits should never have empty stomachs due to their coprophagic behavior. Similar to guinea pigs, rabbits have bands of smooth muscle (taeniae) that course longitudinally along portions of the proximal colon resulting in the formation of sacculations (haustra) in this intestinal segment. The taeniae and haustra do not extend the entire length of the colon. The fusus coli separates the proximal and distal colon. It functions as a differential pacemaker for peristaltic waves of the proximal and distal colon and in the physical separation of colonic fiber contents. The distal colon, devoid of both taeniae and haustra, is smooth and loosely coiled in appearance.

Two lymphoid organs are associated with the gastrointestinal system of the rabbit: the sacculus rotundus at the ileocecal–colic junction, and the vermiform appendix at the tip of the cecum. The sacculus rotundus is considered to be analogous to the bursa of Fabricius in birds. These two lymphoid organs contain more than 50% of the total lymphoid tissue of the rabbit, accounting for the relatively small size of the spleen. The liver has four lobes with the gallbladder positioned between liver lobes to the right of the midline. Compared to other laboratory animals, rabbits produce relatively large quantities of bile that empty into the duodenum via the common bile duct.

Rabbits are obligate nose breathers. Their lungs have six lobes with each side having a cranial, a middle, and a caudal lobe. The right caudal lobe is further divided into a lateral and a medial lobe. The heart is small relative to their body size and their right atrioventricular valve is bicuspid instead of tricuspid, as occurs in other mammals. Their thymus persists into adulthood, not regressing as commonly occurs in many other adult mammals.

In contrast to most other mammals, the rabbit kidney is unipapillate rather than multipapillate, thus cannulating the rabbit kidney is more easily accomplished. Rabbits are the only known mammals in which the renal tubules can be dissected free from the kidney with an intact basement membrane, facilitating its use in renal physiology studies.

The genital tract of the female, like that of most domestic animals, is bicornate but differs in that the two horns of the uterus open into the vagina through separate cervices. The uterine horns are curled and lie in the caudal abdomen dorsal to the urinary bladder. The placenta is hemochorial, similar to the human. The female has four to five pairs of mammary glands and nipples. The males have only rudimentary nipples visible under their fur. In the mature male, the scrotal pouches are located anterior and lateral to the penis—unlike in most other mammals, where the scrotal sacs are caudal to the penis. Inguinal canals remain open for life. The testes generally descend around 12 weeks of age. Lateral to the external genitalia of both sexes are the paired, hairless inguinal pouches, which usually contain white-to-brown odiferous secretions from the inguinal glands. One unfamiliar with rabbit anatomy could conceivably mistake an inguinal pouch for the anus.

Mature female rabbits often have a prominent dewlap beneath their chin. Mature male rabbits normally have larger heads than females. Differentiating males from females can be accomplished readily in adults by gently pressing the skin back from the genital opening. The female has a short slit-shaped opening; pressing the skin back exposes the mucosal surface of the vulva. In the male, this procedure will cause the penis to evert and be readily visible. In the male, testicles may or may not be palpable due to the open inguinal canals. In the newborn, when pressure is applied against the genital orifice, the penis will evert, appearing as a cone-shaped protuberance, whereas the mucosa of the vulva protrudes only laterally and anteriorly, still maintaining the appearance of a slit-shaped opening. The posterior end of the vulva does not evert due to its close attachment near the anus.

There are several distinct characteristics of the hematologic, clinical chemistry, and urinary profiles of rabbits. Rabbit neutrophils, called pseudoeosinophils or heterophils, have intracytoplasmic eosinophilic granules that cause them to resemble eosinophils. Pelger–Huet anomaly may be observed, which is a hyposegmentation of the heterophil nuclei due to incomplete differentiation. True eosinophils have larger, darker granules than heterophils. Lymphocytes are the predominant leukocyte. Basophils are more common than in other mammals, making up 2%–7% of the leukocyte population. Serum calcium is not maintained within a tightly defined range, but rather fluctuates and reflects dietary intake and may be as high as 15 mg/dL. Aortic and kidney calcification may develop with prolonged, high dietary calcium carbonate levels. Rabbits produce approximately 50–75 mL/kg of urine daily that has an alkaline pH of approximately 8.2 and a specific gravity ranging between 1.003 and 1.036. It may appear cloudy due to the high quantities of calcium carbonate and ammonium magnesium phosphate crystals, which can be mistaken for a purulent discharge. Dietary porphyrins will occasionally cause the urine color to vary from dark red to orange. Porphyrin-stained urine can be differentiated from hematuria through microscopic identification of red blood cells in urine sediment or through observation of porphyrin fluorescence. Rabbits differ from most other mammals in that calcium and magnesium ions are excreted primarily in the urine rather than in the bile. Hematologic and biochemical parameters for the rabbit are listed in Appendix 1.

BREEDING AND REPRODUCTION

Adult females are known as does; adult males are bucks. Young rabbits are kits or kittens. The onset of puberty varies with breed. Smaller breeds generally mature earlier, and larger breeds mature later. Does tend to reach sexual maturity prior to bucks. NZW does are initially bred between 4 and 6 months at a weight of 3–4 kg. NZW bucks are first bred at approximately 6–7 months. Rabbits do not have a definite estrous cycle. Does have 7–10 days of receptivity followed by a short period, 1–2 days, during which they are not receptive to the male. They are induced ovulators like the cat and the ferret. The average reproductive life of a doe is approximately 3 years but may extend to 5–6 years. The average reproductive life of a buck is 5–6 years.

During breeding, agonistic behavior prevails, with chasing, squealing, tail flagging, enurination or urine spraying, and combat. In the wild, courtship chasing between adults is an early form of sexual activity. When rabbits are bred, the female should be taken to the male's cage as she may attack him in her own cage, and he may become distracted by scents in the female's environment. If the female is receptive, she will display lordosis (a flattening of the back and raising of the pelvis to position the perineum toward the male) and copulation will take place soon after introduction of the female. The buck elevates his hindquarters, walks stiff-legged, and lays his tail flat across his back. This maneuver supplies a visual stimulus to the doe. Additionally, inguinal gland secretions serve as an olfactory stimulus. The buck may turn his hindquarters and eject a small amount of urine toward a doe or at another male, followed by some form of circling about the cage. On occasion, a doe will refuse to mate with one buck but will readily accept another. She also may accept a buck once but refuse him a second time. Females may attempt to castrate males, so rabbits should be paired for only short periods and observed closely. It is normal behavior for the male to emit a cry at the time of copulation. After ejaculation, the male falls off the female to either side or backward as both feet are off the ground simultaneously at the time of ejaculation.

Ovulation occurs about 10 hours after mating. Approximately 25% of matings are anovulatory. To facilitate artificial insemination, ovulation can also be induced by administration of human chorionic gonadotropins or other luteinizing hormones. Pseudopregnancies are a common occurrence in rabbits and are caused by sterile matings, mounting by other does, or stimulation by a nearby male. Pseudopregnancy may extend over 16–22 days. Nest building may be observed during this time.

The gestation period is heavily influenced by breed, but it is also influenced by parity, nutritional status, and environmental factors. The range is from 29 to 35 days, with an average of 31 days. Most pregnancies maintained over 34 days result in stillbirths. Pregnancy can be detected by ultrasonography at day 7 postmating, radiography at day 11, and palpation at day 14. A nest box with appropriate contact bedding should be provided during the last few days of gestation and through the first month. Females begin building a nest 3–4 days prior to parturition by plucking fur from their dewlap and sides (Box 11.2). Parturition, or kindling, most frequently

Box 11.2

Females begin building a nest 3–4 days prior to parturition by plucking fur from their dewlap and sides.

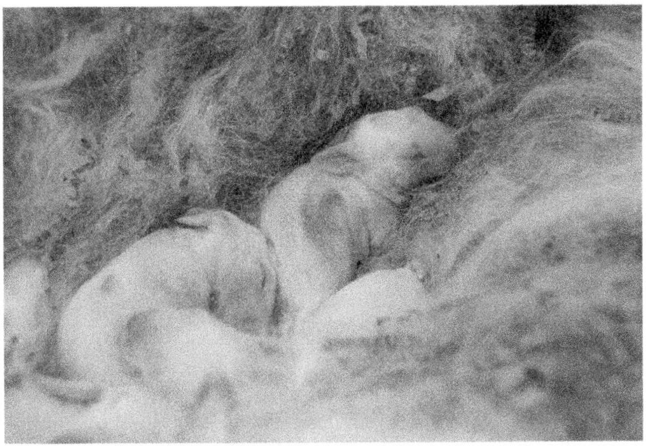

Fig 11.2. A litter of rabbit kits in a nest made of rabbit fur and nesting material. (*Source:* Courtesy of Austin Thomason, Michigan Photography—University of Michigan.)

occurs in the early morning and is usually rapid (approximately 10–15 minutes) but can last 1–2 days. Both anterior and breech presentations are normal. Dystocia, or difficult delivery, is uncommon. Does may breed immediately after parturition.

Litter size is influenced by breed and parity, with primiparous does producing smaller litters. NZW litters usually consist of seven to nine kits (Figure 11.2). Regardless of breed, kits nurse only once a day, either early in the morning or late in the evening, and usually for only 3–5 minutes. The young are altricial (blind, deaf, and hairless); their ears open at 8 days, eyes open at 10 days, and they begin to eat solid food at about 16–17 days of age. They are unable to self-regulate their body temperature until after 7 days of age. Does will not retrieve kits from outside of the nest box and will leave them to die. Kits may be weaned at 4–6 weeks of age. Orphaned rabbits should be fostered if at all possible. Colostrum is not a necessity as most passive immunity is acquired through the yolk sac prior to birth. Females may act savagely toward kits that are not their own. Therefore great care must be taken when introducing kits to unfamiliar females. Commercial milk replacer for lagomorphs is available; orphans may be fed via stomach tube or syringe.

HUSBANDRY

Housing and Environment

Rabbits are frequently housed in front-opening, stainless steel or plastic cages. Although metal grid or slatted flooring is still used, solid-bottom plastic flooring with perforated holes for excreta passage is more common. These cages are often designed as drawerlike units that can be slid out from the cage rack, facilitating animal examination. Excreta trays with or without paper liners are placed beneath the rabbit cages to facilitate cleaning. The provision of solid resting boards within a section of the cage may be beneficial for animal comfort and thermoregulation. Adult rabbits greater than 5.4 kg must be provided with at least 0.46 m^2 (5.0 ft^2) of floor space per rabbit and 40.5 cm (16 in.) of cage height to enable normal postural movements. See Table 11.2 for additional space requirement information. Additional cage space is required for does with litters. Newer caging designs allow for social housing by opening a panel between two adjacent cages. Group housing may be accomplished with select, compatible, same-sex animals. Females are more amenable to group housing if their social group is established prior to or soon after weaning (Figure 11.3). It is not advised to attempt to group house sexually intact adult males due to inter-animal aggression. Successful group housing of males, castrated prior to weaning, has been reported but should be approached with great caution. Group housing may be accomplished by using the animal housing room, or a component thereof, as the primary enclosure and providing the appropriate floor space per animal. Hardwood bedding, straw, paper products, or other suitable material may be placed on the floor to absorb urine and feces. Rabbits housed in groups will tend to use a consistent location for urination and defecation that should be at least spot-cleaned daily. Feed and watering devices should be elevated from the floor and sanitized weekly; the primary enclosure (room) should be sanitized at least every 2 weeks. Enrichment items such as open, small-animal carriers or plastic barrels can be added as "burrows," as can other enrichment devices

Table 11.2. Recommended cage space for rabbits

Weight (kg)	Floor area per animal (ft^2)	Height (in.)[a]
<2	1.5	16
Up to 4	3.0	16
Up to 5.4	4.0	16
>5.4	≥5.0	16

Source: Guide for the Care and Use of Laboratory Animals (ILAR, 2011).

[a] From cage floor to cage top.

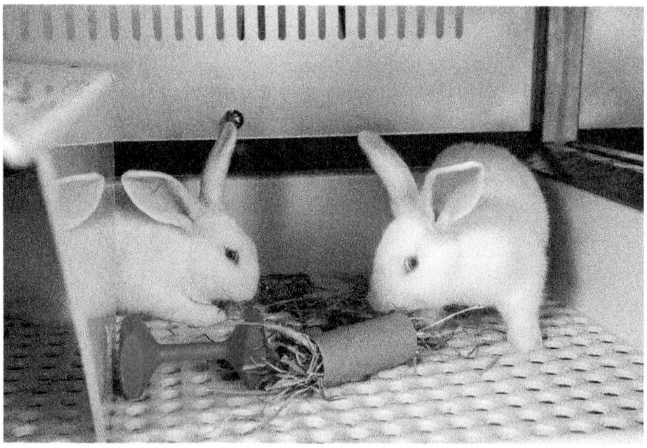

Fig 11.3. Pair housing of young rabbits. (*Source:* Courtesy of Austin Thomason, Michigan Photography—University of Michigan.)

chapter 11

specifically designed for laboratory animal use (see "Environmental Enrichment and Social Housing"). In all group housing arrangements, the provision of hiding places allows submissive animals to retreat if necessary.

As stated in the *Guide for the Care and Use of Laboratory Animals* (the *Guide*; ILAR, 2011), the room temperature should be maintained within a range of 16°–22°C (61°–72°F), a temperature lower than recommended for other species. Similar to other species, humidity levels between 30% and 70% are recommended. Rabbits are fairly resistant to cooler temperature, but they can quickly develop hyperthermia at increased temperatures. Ten to fifteen air changes per hour are suggested to maintain adequate ventilation. This, however, is only a guideline, and determination of optimal ventilation should include careful consideration of the amount of heat, humidity, and volatile compounds expected to be produced within the housing room. Room light timers should be programed to deliver a consistent duration of light each day (12–14 hours for maintenance; 14–16 hours for optimal breeding).

Sudden, loud noises may startle rabbits. Low-level background noise can be used to reduce their reaction to noises created by general husbandry practices. Elevated noise levels may produce physiologic changes, so rabbits should not be housed close to vocal species such as dogs, pigs, or nonhuman primates or near noisy equipment such as cage washers.

Environmental Enrichment and Social Housing

Rabbits tend to be social and should, if possible, be group- or pair-housed as described previously. Contact with personnel can be a form of enrichment for rabbits if they are gently and consistently handled when young. Novel objects or food items may also be used to enrich a rabbit's environment. Objects such as balls, plastic or metal chains, wooden blocks, Nylabones™, PVC tubing, huts, and other commercial items designed for use with laboratory animals may be provided (Figure 11.4). Even a simple metal bowl becomes an enrichment item as it is pushed around the cage. Studies have shown that interaction with items that the rabbit directly manipulates

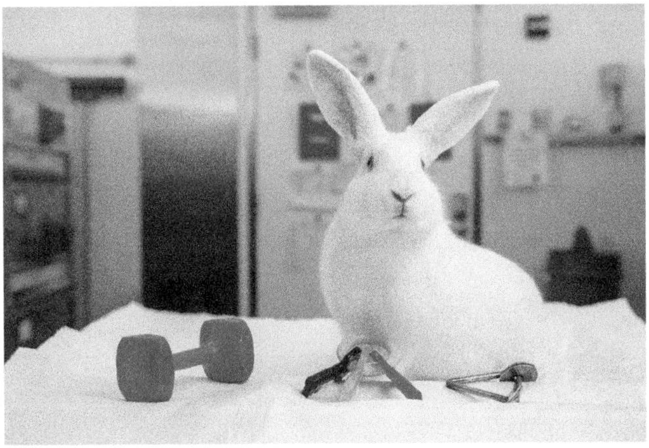

Fig 11.4. An assortment of enrichment devices appropriate for rabbits. (*Source:* Courtesy of Austin Thomason, Michigan Photography—University of Michigan.)

(manipulanda) decreases with time, and they should be frequently rotated to maintain novelty. These objects should be sturdy, sanitizable, and nontoxic. Rabbits tend to chew on enrichment items; these should be made of durable materials that are resistant to destruction and carefully observed for sharp edges or broken pieces. Food items such as carrots, lettuce, hay cubes, loose hay, or commercially produced consumables can be provided as treats and to eliminate boredom. They must be provided in limited quantities.

Feeding and Watering

Rabbits are strict herbivores and readily accept firm, dry pelleted commercial feed. Nutritional requirements vary with age, activity, and reproductive state. Maintenance diets for adult rabbits should contain at least 12% protein and 10% crude fiber. Higher-fiber diets that contain approximately 22.5% fiber are used to reduce obesity and prevent hairball, or trichobezoar, formation. All feed should be purchased from a reputable, commercial vendor, have a known mill date, and be appropriately stored to maintain nutritional content. Food consumption varies with age, ambient temperature, and water availability. Animals should be limit fed as *ad libitum* feeding will often lead to obesity, especially in NZW rabbits. Once-to-twice daily feeding of a total of approximately 5 g of commercial laboratory rabbit feed per 100 g of body weight per day will maintain an adult, medium-sized rabbit. During growth, gestation, or lactation, rabbits require an approximate 20% increase in caloric intake. Food pellets should be provided in elevated self-feeders (e.g., J-type hoppers attached to a cage side or door) rather than in an open bowl that becomes easily contaminated. Feeders should facilitate the addition of food without disturbing cage occupants. Offering a limited amount of high-fiber, low-calcium grass hay can help to maintain the health of the rabbit's gastrointestinal system. Alfalfa hay should be provided in only limited quantities due to its high calcium levels.

The average water consumption of a rabbit is 50–150 mL/kg of body weight per day, higher than many other species. Water consumption increases with ambient temperature, while food intake decreases. Rabbits readily accept water bottles as well as automated watering systems, which are much more efficient for production colonies and the research environment. Rabbits will not eat when water is unavailable.

Sanitation

Excreta trays should be cleaned as often as needed to control odor and ammonia levels. Daily cleaning is optimal. The carbonate and phosphate crystals from urine precipitate form a scale residue on cages and animal room floors. Soaking or rinsing with an acid solution (e.g., phosphoric acid, hydroxyacetic acid) is often required to remove urine scale. Primary enclosures, water bottles, automated watering systems, and feed hoppers should be disinfected with chemicals, hot water 61.6°–82.2°C (143°–180°F), or a combination of both. Detergents and chemical disinfectants enhance the effectiveness of hot water, but they must be thoroughly rinsed from all surfaces with fresh water. Refer to Chapter 4 for a more detailed description of disinfection methods.

TECHNIQUES

Handling and Restraint

Rabbits should be handled gently but firmly. They are prone to kick their hind limbs, which can cause deep scratches in their handlers. A rabbit should be lifted by obtaining a firm grip on the loose skin over the scruff of the neck with one hand; the other hand should be used to support the animal's hindquarters and limit back leg movement, as shown in Figure 11.5. If the hind limbs are not supported, the rabbit may kick out with such force as to fracture its lumbar spine, most commonly at the L7–S1 junction.

To carry a rabbit, a "football hold" provides a secure restraint technique and accommodates its need for physical contact. To accomplish this, one arm is used to cradle the rabbit and hold it firmly against the handler's body while concealing the rabbit's head in the bend of the elbow. The handler's other arm is placed over the rabbit's back and grasps the scruff of the neck to provide slight pressure so the rabbit is less likely to struggle (Figure 11.6). Rabbits may slip and slide on stainless steel examining tables and may try to jump. Using a towel for traction or as a wrap, coupled with a hand behind the rump and a firm grasp of the scruff ensures that the animal does not escape and sustain injury (Figure 11.7). Commercially available restraint devices—including metal or plastic restrainers as well as flexible, but snug-fitting, cloth bags (e.g., cat bags)—are available and primarily serve to control the body while the head or ears are manipulated. Caution must be exercised when using a restrainer as an improperly restrained rabbit may struggle and cause serious injury. A restrained animal should never be left unattended. Hypnosis may be used to examine the ventral

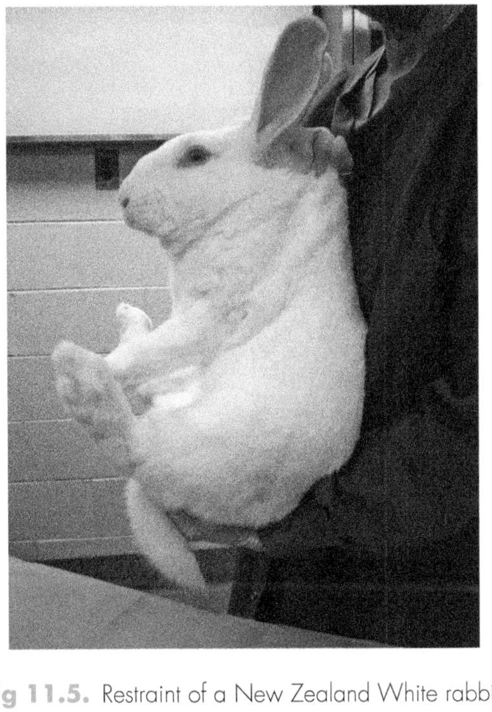

Fig 11.5. Restraint of a New Zealand White rabbit.

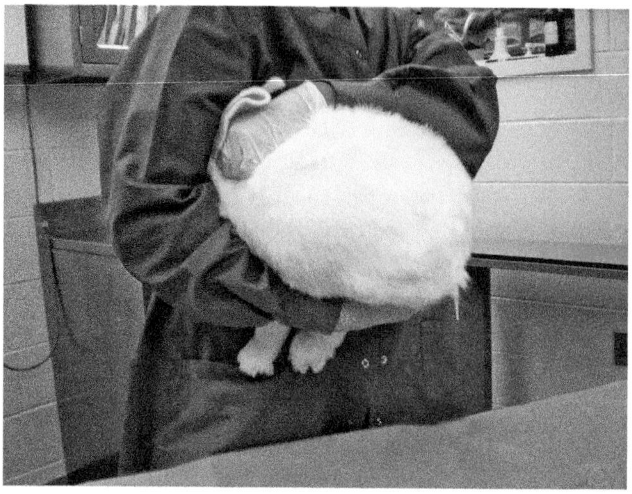

Fig 11.6. Football hold for carrying a rabbit.

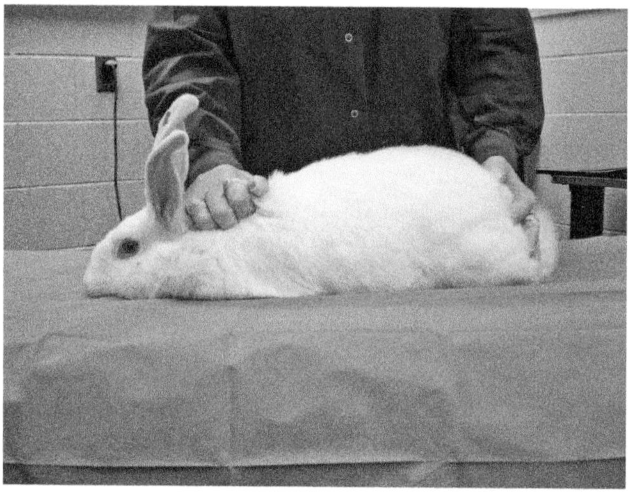

Fig 11.7. Restraint of rabbit for examination on a table.

aspect of the animal, to trim teeth or toenails, or to obtain a radiograph. Cover the rabbit's eyes and gently roll the animal onto its back; with the rabbit lying centered on its back, stroke the abdomen cranial to caudal. This will often have a calming or hypnotic effect, the degree of which will vary among individuals. Hypnosis should not be used for invasive or painful procedures.

Identification

Cage cards are commonly used as a form of general identification. Individual identification methods include ear tags, ear tattoos, or subcutaneous (SC) placement of a microchip. Fur dyes or clipped areas of fur as well as ear markings with a permanent pen can serve as temporary methods of identification.

Blood Collection

Approximate blood volumes for adult rabbits are listed in Table 11.3. Assuming the animal is mature, healthy, and on an adequate plane of nutrition, the blood volume of most species averages 7% of the body weight in grams. A typical rule of thumb for blood withdrawal suggests that up to 10% of the circulating blood volume (or 1% of the body weight) can be withdrawn every 2–3 weeks from normal, healthy animals with minimal adverse effect. A larger volume or more frequent blood collection may be possible if fluid replacement is provided and the hematocrit is monitored.

The marginal ear, cephalic, and lateral saphenous veins can be used to obtain small amounts of blood. These veins easily collapse with too much negative pressure. The auricular artery, also known as the central ear artery, is easily visible on the dorsal surface of the pinnae, where it extends from the ear base to the ear tip. It is one of the best sites for collection of larger blood samples. Individuals must be familiar with the anatomy of the auricular vessels (Figure 11.8). Warming the ear with a heat lamp or warm water and gently plucking the hair over the vessel stimulates blood flow. Topical application of an irritant such as 40% D-limonene or citrus oil can induce vasodilation but must be removed with 70% ethanol immediately postcollection to avoid undue skin irritation. Acepromazine, administered intramuscularly at a dosage of 1–5 mg/kg body weight, provides light sedation and also causes vasodilation. Infusing a small amount of local anesthetic such as 2% xylocaine, subcutaneously, or applying a topical

Table 11.3. Adult rabbit blood volumes and single sample size

	Volume (mL)
Total blood	160–480
Single sample	20–40
Exsanguination	60–160

Source: Adapted from Harkness et al. (2010).
Note: Values are approximate.

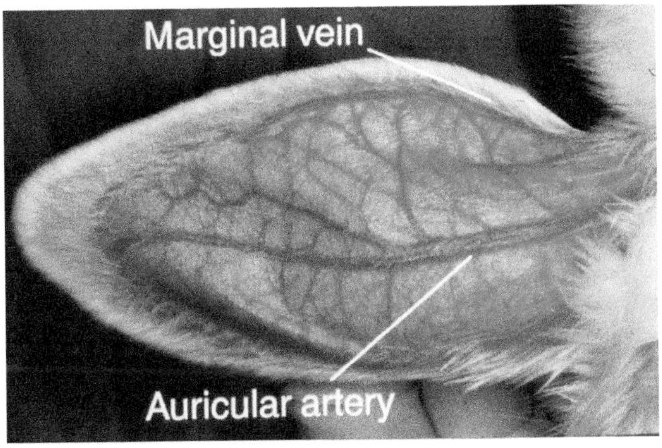

Fig 11.8. Blood vessels of the rabbit ear. (*Source:* Photo courtesy of ACLAM.)

chapter 11

anesthetic such as lidocaine–prilocaine cream (EMLA cream) 15 minutes to 1 hour prior to sampling can reduce discomfort at the collection site. Tubes that apply a slight vacuum allow a more rapid collection of up to 30–50 mL of blood. Hemostasis of the veins is easily achieved with slight pressure, but the artery must be held off for several minutes to prevent continued hemorrhage and hematoma formation. The application of a blood-clotting powder to the puncture site can speed hemostasis.

The jugular vein is another recommended site for blood collection that is often overlooked. The rabbit's head and front legs must be restrained securely to extend the neck, just as a cat would be restrained, to expose the jugular veins. Blood collection can also be performed with the rabbit in dorsal recumbency, but this method may be best facilitated with light sedation.

Cardiac puncture can be used to collect larger quantities of blood from an anesthetized rabbit. This technique should be performed only as a terminal procedure due to the high risk of lung laceration, pericardial bleeding, cardiac tamponade, and possible mortality. The rabbit is placed in dorsal recumbency and a 1.5-inch, 18-gauge needle can be inserted just to the left of the xiphoid process in a craniodorsal approach at a 30° angle from the surface of the thorax. Alternatively, the rabbit may be placed in right lateral recumbency and the chest palpated to locate the strongest heartbeat; the needle is introduced slowly between the ribs toward the opposite side of the chest.

Urine Collection

Urine can be collected as a clean catch sample or by gentle expression of the bladder. Cystocentesis provides another means of obtaining a clean urine sample. To perform this technique, the rabbit should be anesthetized or sedated. Using a V-trough or other restraint device, the rabbit is placed on its back and the lower abdomen is gently palpated to locate the bladder. Once the bladder is immobilized between the thumb and the forefinger, a small-gauge needle (22 or 23 gauge) attached to a syringe is slowly advanced from the midline into the bladder and urine is aspirated, and then the needle is withdrawn. Cystocentesis cannot be used if the bladder is not large enough to be manually isolated unless it is performed under ultrasound guidance. Care must be taken to ensure the needle is accurately placed; if blood or some other substance is aspirated, immediately withdraw the needle and recognize that a bowel or blood vessel may have been inadvertently entered.

Metabolic cages provide an efficient means of collecting both urine and feces as they are designed to separate the two forms of excreta. Finally, urethral catheterization may be used to collect urine from anesthetized rabbits. Catheters must always be handled aseptically to avoid the possible introduction of bacteria into the bladder, producing an infection.

Drug Administration

Maximum dosing volumes for the various routes are listed in Table 11.4. Palatable drugs may be administered to rabbits by incorporating them in the food or water. Medicated custom diets are available through commercial laboratory animal feed vendors. Liquid medications can be administered by placing the tip of a syringe in the corner of the mouth and slowly injecting small amounts repeatedly. Oral administration of unpalatable liquids may be accomplished using an orogastric tube. A bite block must be used to

Table 11.4. Approximate maximum dosing volumes in rabbits

Route	Amount
IP	20.0 mL/kg
SC	10.0–20.0 mL/kg
IM	0.5 mL per site
IV	2.0 mL/kg bolus
	10.0 mL/kg infusion
ID	0.05–0.1 mL per site
PO	15.0 mL/kg

Source: Diehl et al. (2001) and Suckow and Douglas (1997).

protect the orogastric tube. A simple bite block can be fashioned from a syringe casing modified with a hole for passage of the tube. Plastic blocks are available commercially and are smooth to ensure no injury to the tissues of the mouth. The placement of the tube into the stomach must always be verified prior to dosing to ensure drugs are not accidentally introduced into the trachea and lungs. Placement verification can usually be accomplished by using an empty syringe to gently aspirate; if the tube is in the trachea, the syringe will fill with air. A small volume of sterile water may also be introduced; a cough is usually elicited if the tube is in the trachea. An alternative method to check placement is to use a stethoscope pressed against the abdomen to listen for bubbles in the stomach as air is injected through the tube. Stainless steel feeding needles (13 gauge, 16 in.) can also be used to administer drugs orally. A nasogastric tube can be placed if continuous fluid administration into the stomach is required.

Subcutaneous injections should be administered under the loose skin between the shoulder blades or over the back, with a total maximum volume of 20 mL/kg delivered over multiple sites. Intramuscular injections with a maximum volume of 0.5–1.0 mL per site can be given in the large lumbar (epaxial) muscles along the spinal column and in the large muscles (quadriceps, thigh) of the hind limb. When injecting the thigh muscles, care must be taken to avoid the sciatic nerve that courses through the sciatic notch and along the posterior aspect of the hind limb (Figure 11.9). The lumbar muscle site is preferred for intramuscular injection.

Intravenous (IV) injections are most frequently given in the marginal ear vein. Application of a local anesthetic (e.g., lidocaine and prilocaine cream) at the puncture site can decrease animal discomfort. A maximum volume for bolus injection is approximately 2 mL/kg; up to 10 mL/kg may be given via a slow infusion. Continuous infusion of fluids or compounds can be performed using a venous catheter and a small automatic syringe pump that is contained in a jacket worn by the rabbit or by extending an IV line from a pump to the animal with use of a swivel-tether that permits normal movement. As an alternative to externalized catheters, a vascular access port (VAP) may be surgically implanted and used for both dosing and blood withdrawal. Aseptic technique and a defined operating procedure must be followed when accessing the VAP to minimize the chances for infection and to maintain catheter patency. Regardless of the route of administration, large volumes should be warmed to body temperature prior to administration.

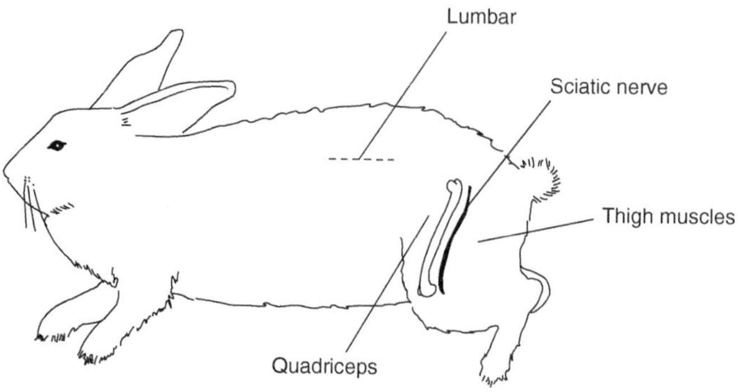

Fig 11.9. Intramuscular injection sites in the rabbit. (*Source:* Adapted from Timm and John (1980), © Regents University of California.)

Box 11.3

Intradermal (ID) injections are frequently used for the production of polyclonal antibodies.

Intradermal (ID) injections are frequently used for the production of polyclonal antibodies (Box 11.3). For ID skin injection, the skin should be clipped, cleaned with an antiseptic, held tautly, and the needle slowly advanced with the bevel facing up. The point of the needle (23 or 25 gauge) should enter just under the epidermal layer and into the dermis to produce a small, raised bleb. To stimulate a rabbit to produce a high titer of antibodies that can later be collected from its blood, purified antigens are suspended in a liquid medium and mixed with an antigenic stimulant (a component of the adjuvant) that induces a robust immune response. Historically, Freund's complete adjuvant (FCA) and Freund's incomplete adjuvant (FIA) were most frequently used. FCA is an oil-in-water suspension containing highly antigenic, killed *Mycobacterium* organisms. When used, FCA is mixed with the antigen of interest and injected in multiple ID locations along the animal's back and side, but avoiding the scruff region as this is where rabbits are frequently restrained. FCA is such a strong immunostimulant that it must only be administered one time per animal; injection site reactions often occur days to weeks later due to the body's reaction to the *Mycobacterium* component of the adjuvant. Skin lesions may include small nodules, diffuse swelling, and open abscesses or scabbing. Lesions are less likely to be significant if smaller injection volumes (0.05–0.1 mL) are used. If the animal's immune system must be further stimulated, FIA should be used in place of FCA. FIA is identical to FCA but lacks the *Mycobacterium* component. Given the complications associated with the use of Freund's adjuvants, alternative adjuvants including aluminum compounds, liposomes, and monophosphoryl lipid A have been developed and are now frequently used. Postimmunization monitoring for pain and distress is a necessary component of any antibody production protocol.

Anesthesia, Surgery, and Postoperative Care

Agents commonly used for anesthesia and tranquilization in rabbits are listed in Table 11.5. Although rabbits cannot vomit, withholding food for 2–6 hours before surgery allows for a more accurate body weight and can help decrease the pressure applied to the diaphragm by intestinal contents. Atropine esterase, which hydrolyzes atropine, is present in the serum of about one-third of the domestic rabbit population, significantly decreasing atropine efficacy. Glycopyrrolate, another anticholinergic, can be used instead of atropine to prevent bradycardia and decrease salivary and tracheobronchial secretions. Rabbits can be challenging to anesthetize because they may have variable responses to anesthetics, they are easily stressed and difficult to intubate, and many of their reflexes are unreliable indicators of the depth of anesthesia. With the correct technique and experience, most of these obstacles are easily overcome.

There are a number of injectable agents that can provide adequate anesthesia for short procedures. Ketamine, a dissociative anesthetic agent, can be mixed with a number of agents to prolong anesthesia and provide better analgesia. The ketamine/xylazine (K/X) combination remains a popular anesthetic choice. Dexmedetomidine combined with ketamine produces a slightly longer anesthetic period than is provided by K/X. Butorphanol or buprenorphine can be added to K/X or ketamine/dexmedetomidine (K/D) for better analgesia. The K/X combination has been implicated in several cases of myocardial fibrosis when used repeatedly in both Dutch and NZW rabbits. K/X has also been associated with sciatic nerve damage and self-mutilation, necessitating caution in hindlimb intramuscular injections. Xylazine and dexmedetomidine are alpha-2-adrenergic agonists that provide sedation and analgesia. Atipamezole can be given to reverse the effects of alpha-2 agonists and speed recovery. Ketamine/diazepam IV offers another option. A fentanyl/droperidol combination or acepromazine can be administered subcutaneously or intramuscularly for light sedation.

Propofol (5–15 mg/kg) IV has been used in rabbits and appears to be safe for very short-term (3–5 minutes) anesthetic maintenance. Long-term infusion of propofol has been reported to cause significant hypotension, hypoxemia, lipemia, and death in rabbits. Tiletamine hydrochloride has been associated with renal nephrotoxicity and should be avoided in rabbits. Caution should be exercised when using sodium pentobarbital or other barbiturates due to the narrow margin of safety between surgical anesthesia and death. In addition, barbiturates provide variable analgesia and cause respiratory and cardiovascular depression and hypothermia. Studies have shown that plasma levels of certain biochemical parameters may be significantly affected by anesthesia and should be interpreted with caution.

Inhalant agents, such as isoflurane and sevoflurane, are safe and commonly used in rabbits. Although rabbits can be induced via face mask, great care must be taken in restraining them to avoid injury. Administration of isoflurane to rabbits via a face mask or an anesthetic induction chamber is associated with apnea and a marked bradycardia. Premedication with acepromazine, diazepam, or another suitable sedative will allow for an easier and safer masking induction. A laryngeal mask airway (LMA) device can be used alternatively to deliver inhalant agents. The LMA is a device that is introduced through the oral cavity and pharynx and covers the laryngeal opening without entering the larynx or trachea. Additionally, a rabbit-specific supraglottic airway device called the V-Gel has been developed.

Table 11.5. Anesthetic agents and tranquilizers used in rabbits

Drug	Dosage	Route	Reference
Inhalants			
Isoflurane	1.5%–5% to effect	Inhalation	Gillett (1994)
Sevoflurane	To effect	Inhalation	Morrisey and Carpenter (2004)
Injectables			
Acepromazine	1 mg/kg	IM, SC	Flecknell (2016)
Acepromazine (for vasodilation with minimal sedation)	0.5–1 mg/kg	IM	Morrisey and Carpenter (2004)
Acepromazine	0.5 mg/kg	IM	Flecknell (2016)
+ butorphanol	0.5 mg/kg		
Bupivicaine	<1.5 mg/kg	Infiltrated SC	Harkness et al. (2010)
Dexmedetomidine	0.05–0.25 mg/kg	IM, SC	Flecknell (2016)
Diazepam	5–10 mg/kg	IM	Gillett (1994)
	1–5 mg/kg	IV	Gillett (1994)
Fentanyl–droperidol	0.22 mL/kg	IM	Flecknell (2016)
Fentanyl/fluanisone	0.2–0.5 mL/kg	IM	Flecknell (2016)
Fentanyl/fluanisone	0.3 mL/kg	IM	Flecknell (2016)
+ diazepam	1–2 mg/kg	IM, IV, IP	
Fentanyl/fluanisone	0.3 mL/kg	IM	Flecknell (2016)
+ midazolam	1–2 mg/kg	IV, IP	
Ketamine	50 mg/kg	IM	Flecknell (2016)
+ acepromazine	0.5–1 mg/kg		
Ketamine	25 mg/kg	IM	Flecknell (2016)
+ diazepam	5 mg/kg	IM	
Ketamine	10 mg/kg	IV	Gil et al. (2003)
+ diazepam	2 mg/kg	IV	
Ketamine	15 mg/kg	IM	Flecknell (2016)
+ dexmedetomidine	0.125 mg/kg	IM	
Ketamine	35 mg/kg	IM	Difilippo et al. (2004)
+ medetomidine	0.5 mg/kg	IM	
+ buprenorphine	0.03 mg/kg	IM	
Ketamine	25 mg/kg	IM	Stieve et al. (2008)
+ midazolam	5 mg/kg	IM	
Ketamine	30 mg/kg	IM	Vachon et al. (1999)
+ midazolam	0.2 mg/kg	IM	
+ xylazine	3 mg/kg	IM	
Ketamine	30–40 mg/kg	IM	Gillett (1994)
+ xylazine	3–5 mg/kg	IM	
Ketamine	10 mg/kg	IN	Robertson and Eberhart (1994)
+ xylazine	3 mg/kg	IN	
Ketamine	35 mg/kg	IM	Flecknell (2016)
+ xylazine	5 mg/kg	IM	
+ acepromazine	1 mg/kg	IM	

Table 11.5. *(Continued)*

Drug	Dosage	Route	Reference
Ketamine	35 mg/kg	IM	Marini et al. (1992)
+ xylazine	5 mg/kg	IM	
+ butorphanol	0.1 mg/kg	IM	
Lidocaine	<2 mg/kg	Infiltrated SC	Harkness et al. (2010)
Medetomidine	0.1–0.5 mg/kg	SC, IM	Flecknell (2009)
Medetomidine	0.25 mg/kg	IM	Ko et al. (1992)
+ midazolam	0.5 mg/kg	IM	
+ propofol	2 mg/kg	IV	
Medetomidine	0.25 mg/kg	IM	Ko et al. (1992)
+ propofol	4 mg/kg	IV	
Midazolam	0.5–2 mg/kg	IV, IM, IP	Flecknell (2016)
	2 mg/kg	IN	Robertson and Eberhart (1994)
Pentobarbital	20–45 mg/kg	IP, IV	Harkness and Wagner (1995)
Propofol	10 mg/kg	IV	Flecknell (2016)
Tiletamine–zolazepam	Generally not recommended (except IN) due to nephrotoxicity		Doerning et al. (1992)
Urethane	1000–2000 mg/kg	IP, IV	Flecknell (2016)
Xylazine	2–5 mg/kg	IM	Flecknell (2009)

IM = intramuscular; IN = intranasal; IP = intraperitoneal; IV = intravenous; and SC = subcutaneous.

Box 11.4

Rabbit intubation can be difficult due to the small size of the oral cavity and difficulty in visualizing the larynx.

Rabbit intubation can be difficult due to the small size of the oral cavity and difficulty in visualizing the larynx (Box 11.4). To intubate a rabbit, a long (40 mm), thin (size 0 or 1) laryngoscope blade or an otoscope can be used to allow visualization of the larynx. A flexible stylet inside the appropriately sized endotracheal tube (2–3 mm outside diameter in 1–3 kg rabbits; 3–6 mm outside diameter in larger rabbits) can be helpful in guiding the tube into the trachea. Rotating the tube as it passes over the epiglottis facilitates passage into the trachea. A topical spray of lidocaine can be used to anesthetize the epiglottis. Rabbits must be adequately anesthetized to avoid laryngospasm, which makes intubation even more difficult.

Alternatively, a blind intubation method can be used that, when properly performed, is both faster and less traumatic than the laryngoscope method. The rabbit's head is held with the palm of the hand on the back of the skull and the thumb and index finger placed along the length of each mandible. The most important step is to extend the neck adequately, with the nose pointing straight up or even slightly hyperextended so the path to the trachea is straight and minimally obstructed. The endotracheal tube is passed over the tongue until it is at the entrance to the larynx as evidenced by condensation in the tube when the rabbit exhales. During exhalation, the tube should be quickly and firmly passed forward while rotating it so that it enters the trachea. This method can be mastered with patience and practice.

The depth of anesthesia is best gauged by the rate and depth of respiration and the degree of jaw tension. Other indicators of the depth of anesthesia, in decreasing order of reliability, are the ear pinch, pedal reflex, and palpebral reflex. The ear pinch is more sensitive and persists longer than the others. If necessary, a drop of doxapram can be placed under the tongue to stimulate respiration. Rabbits are sometimes used in experimental studies that require surgical manipulations, including placement of indwelling vascular catheters, reproductive tract surgeries [ovariohysterectomies (OHEs) and castrations], orthopedic surgeries, and gastrointestinal surgeries.

For surgical prepping, clipping rabbit hair is difficult at best. Using a sharp 40 blade held flat against the skin, stretching the skin taut, and clipping slowly and carefully are important steps to avoid traumatizing the skin. The skin should be lightly scrubbed in preparation for surgery.

The incision for an OHE in a rabbit should be made lower on the abdomen, similar to an OHE approach in a cat. The bladder should be gently emptied prior to prepping the surgical site. The bladder is thin walled and may rupture if pressure is applied too vigorously. Rabbits have a very narrow linea alba and veins that tear easily. Additionally, care must be taken to ligate both cervices of the rabbit that enter into the vagina separately, especially in larger does. In the male, both inguinal canals remain open throughout life and must be sutured closed during a castration to avoid herniation of abdominal contents.

Rabbits are adept at removing sutures; it is best to use metal staples, clips, or a subcuticular pattern when closing the incision. After clipping, rabbit fur grows back in an uneven pattern. For optimal postoperative recoveries, surgeries should be performed with attention to aseptic technique, maintaining body temperature and blood pressure.

Analgesics must be administered for pain control in rabbits that undergo surgical procedures. Unless documented to the contrary and approved by the IACUC, it must be assumed that procedures that cause pain or distress in humans will cause pain and distress in other animals. Rabbits experiencing pain may show clinical signs, including depression, grinding of teeth, anorexia, and reluctance to move. They are notoriously stoic in response to pain; those unfamiliar with the species will often overlook subtle indications of a pain response. Analgesic agents for rabbits are listed in Table 11.6. Opiates such as butorphanol and buprenorphine are frequently used. Butorphanol is indicated for mild postoperative pain; buprenorphine is indicated for acute and chronic visceral pain. Buprenorphine can cause marked sedation if given too early in the anesthetic recovery period. Several drug options are available to stimulate the appetite of rabbits following surgery. Newer nonsteroidal anti-inflammatory agents, such as carprofen or meloxicam, provide good, long-lasting (up to 24 hours) analgesia for mild-to-moderate pain.

Postoperative care should include hydration support of the anesthetized animal (e.g., subcutaneous, intraperitoneal, or intravenous administration of a warmed solution such as saline, saline–dextrose, lactated Ringer's) and support of normal body

Table 11.6. Analgesic agents used in rabbits

Drug	Dosage	Route	Reference
Acetaminophen	200–500 mg/kg	PO	Gillett (1994)
Acetylsalicylic acid	100 mg/kg q4h	PO	Flecknell (2016)
Buprenorphine	0.01–0.05 mg/kg q8-12h	SC, IV	Flecknell (2016)
	0.5 mg/kg q12h	Per rectum	Huerkamp (1995)
Butorphanol	0.1–0.5 mg/kg q4h	SC, IV	Dobromylskyj et al. (2000)
Butorphanol	5 mg/kg	IM	Wixson (1994)
+ xylazine	4 mg/kg		
Carprofen	1.5 mg/kg q24h	PO	Flecknell (2016)
	4 mg/kg q24h	SC	Flecknell (2016)
Fentanyl	25 μg/h patch for up to 72 h		Foley et al. (2001)
Flunixin meglumine	1–2 mg/kg q12-24h	SC	Heard (1993)
Ibuprofen	2–7.5 mg/kg q12-24h	PO	Harkness et al. (2010)
	10 mg/kg ~q4h	IV	Flecknell (2016)
	2–7.5 mg/kg q4h	PO	Morrisey and Carpenter (2004)
	7.5 mg/kg q6-8h	PO	Smith and Burgmann (1997)
Ketoprofen	3 mg/kg q24h	SC, IM	Flecknell (2016); Heard (2009)
Meloxicam	0.6–1 mg/kg	SC, PO	Flecknell (2016)
	0.1–0.5 mg/kg q12-24h	PO, SC	Harkness et al. (2010)
Meperidine	5–10 mg/kg q2-3h	SC, IM	Harkness et al. (2010)
Morphine	2–5 mg/kg q2-4h	SC, IM	Flecknell (2009)
Nalbuphine	1–2 mg/kg q4-5h	IM, IV	Heard (1993)
Oxymorphone	0.05–0.2 mg/kg q6-12h	SC, IM	Harkness et al. (2010)
Pentazocine	5–10 mg/kg q4h	IM, IV	Flecknell (2016)
Piroxicam	0.2 mg/kg q8h	PO	Dobromylskyj et al. (2000)
Tramadol	10 mg/kg q24h	PO	Harkness et al. (2010)

IM = intramuscular; IV = intravenous; PO = per os; and SC = subcutaneous.

temperature through the use of a circulating water heating blanket. A nonambulatory animal should be turned at least every 30 minutes to prevent hypostatic congestion. It is important to maintain hydration and nutrition levels in the postoperative period to support normal metabolic processes and gut physiology.

Imaging Techniques

Great advances have been made in small-animal imaging over the last decade. For a detailed description of current imaging modalities, see Chapter 3.

Euthanasia

Rabbits are most frequently euthanized by an overdose of barbiturate or barbiturate-based euthanasia solution given intravenously. This method is painless, fast, easily accomplished, and relatively inexpensive. Inhalant anesthetic overdose can be used but is less favorable as the animal may experience an excitation phase during anesthetic induction. Rabbits that are used for polyclonal antibody production are usually exsanguinated under anesthesia for the terminal collection of blood and harvesting of the antibody-rich serum. Of note, many commercial supplies of sodium pentobarbital cause hemolysis because of high levels of alcohol, propylene glycol, or both. An alternate formulation should be obtained to avoid hemolysis.

THERAPEUTIC AGENTS

Table 11.7 lists a variety of antimicrobial and antifungal agents that can be used in rabbits. Refer to Table 11.8 for a list of antiparasitics for use in rabbits and to Table 11.9 for miscellaneous drugs used in rabbits.

Table 11.7. Antimicrobial and antifungal agents used in rabbits

Drug	Dosage	Route	Reference
Amikacin	2–5 mg/kg q8-12h	SC, IM	Harkness et al. (2010)
Amoxicillin	Do not use		Morrisey and Carpenter (2004)
Ampicillin	Do not use		Morrisey and Carpenter (2004)
Cephalexin	11–22 mg/kg q8-12h	PO, SC	Harkness et al. (2010)
Cephaloridine	11–15 mg/kg q12h	IM	Gillett (1994)
Cephalothin	12.5 mg/kg q6h for 6 d	IM	Russell et al. (1981)
Chloramphenicol	30 mg/kg q8-12h	PO, SC, IM, IV	Harkness et al. (2010)
Chlortetracycline	50 mg/kg q12h	PO	Morrisey and Carpenter (2004)
Ciprofloxacin	10–20 mg/kg q12-24h	PO	Morrisey and Carpenter (2004)
Clindamycin	Do not use		Morrisey and Carpenter (2004)
Doxycycline	2.5 mg/kg q12h	PO	Carpenter et al. (1995)
Enrofloxacin	5–15 mg/kg q12h; limit injections as they may cause muscle necrosis and sterile abscesses	PO, IM, SC	Morrisey and Carpenter (2004); Hernandez-Divers (2005)
Erythromycin	Do not use		Morrisey and Carpenter (2004)
Gentamicin	4 mg/kg q24h	SC, IM	Morrisey and Carpenter (2004)
Griseofulvin	12.5–25 mg/kg q24h for 30–45 d	PO	Hernandez-Divers (2005)
Ketoconazole	10–40 mg/kg q24h	PO	Morrisey and Carpenter (2004)

Table 11.7. *(Continued)*

Drug	Dosage	Route	Reference
Lime sulfur dip (2.5%)	Dip q7d for 4–6 wk		Morrisey and Carpenter (2004)
Metronidazole	20 mg/kg q12h	PO	Harkness et al. (2010)
Miconazole	q24h for 14–28 d	Topical	Harkness and Wagner (1995)
Minocycline	6 mg/kg q8h	IV	Nicolau et al. (1993)
Neomycin	30 mg/kg q12h	PO	Burgmann and Percy (1993)
Oxytetracycline	50 mg/kg q12h	PO	Burgmann and Percy (1993)
Penicillin G, benzathine	42,000–60,000 IU/kg q48h	SC, IM	Russell et al. (1981)
Penicillin G, procaine	40,000 IU/kg q24h	IM	Hernandez-Divers (2005)
Silver sulfadiazine 0.01% cream	q24h	Topical	Donnelly (2005)
Sulfadimethoxine	10–15 mg/kg q12h for 10 d	PO	Harkness and Wagner (1995)
Tetracycline	50 mg/kg q8-12h	PO	Burgmann and Percy (1993)
Trimethoprim-sulfa	30 mg/kg q12-24h	PO, IM, SC	Harkness et al. (2010)
Tylosin	10 mg/kg q12h	PO, SC, IM	Hernandez-Divers (2005); Harkness et al. (2010)
Vancomycin	50 mg/kg q8h	IV, IM	Harkness et al. (2010)

IM = intramuscular; IV = intravenous; PO = per os; and SC = subcutaneous.

INTRODUCTION TO DISEASES OF RABBITS

Improvements in environmental controls and husbandry have led to the identification and eradication of a majority of infectious agents in laboratory rabbits. Most laboratory rabbit colonies today are relatively free of the viruses, bacteria, parasites, and fungi that cause clinical disease. Basic knowledge of the variety of infectious agents that may infect a rabbit population is imperative to quickly and appropriately respond to a disease outbreak. Rabbits tend to be quite stoic, so detecting clinical signs can be a challenge. Some common signs include anorexia and refusal of treats, depression, hunched posture, and lethargy. Anorexic rabbits must be treated promptly to avoid the life-threatening condition of gastrointestinal stasis. Treatment includes fluid therapy (approximately 90–100 mL/kg per day) and nutritional support to maintain intestinal function and prevent dehydration. Oral rehydration solutions and critical care products are available commercially. Presented here is a general overview of common bacterial, viral, fungal, and parasitic agents of rabbits and some standard diagnostic and treatment modalities.

Table 11.8. Antiparasitic agents used in rabbits

Drug	Dosage	Route	Reference
Albendazole	7.5–20 mg/kg q24h (use with caution)	PO	Morrisey and Carpenter (2011)
Carbaryl powder (5%)	Twice weekly	Topical	Harkness and Wagner (1995)
Doramectin (1%)	0.2 mg/kg repeat in 10 d	SC	Voyvoda et al. (2005)
Fenbendazole	10 mg/kg, repeat in 2 wk prn	PO	Hillyer (1994)
	50 ppm in feed for 2–6 wk		Okerman (1994)
Fipronil	Do not use, toxic		Morrisey and Carpenter (2004)
Ivermectin	0.4 mg/kg q7-14d	PO, SC	Hillyer (1994)
Lasalocid	120 ppm in feed		Harkness and Wagner (1995)
Lime sulfur (2%–3%)	Dip q7d for 4–6 wk		Jenkins (1995)
Lufenuron	30 mg/kg q30d	PO	Morrisey and Carpenter (2004)
Mebendazole	50 mg/kg	PO	Harkness and Wagner (1995)
	1 g/kg of feed		Harkness and Wagner (1995)
Metronidazole	20 mg/kg q12h	PO	Harkness et al. (2010)
Monensin	0.002%–0.004% in feed		Harkness et al. (2010)
Piperazine	200 mg/kg, repeat in 2–3 wk	PO	Hillyer (1994)
Praziquantel	5–10 mg/kg, repeat in 10 d	PO, SC, IM	Allen et al. (1993)
Pyrantel pamoate	5–10 mg/kg, repeat in 2–3 wk	PO	Quesenberry (1994)
Pyrethrin	Shampoo/powder weekly for 4–6 wk		Harkness et al. (2010)
Selmectin	6 mg/kg	Topical	Morrisey and Carpenter (2004)
Sulfadimethoxine	50 mg/kg once, then 25 mg/kg q24h for 10–20 d	PO	Hillyer (1994)
Sulfamethazine	100 mg/kg q24h	PO	Gillett (1994)
	0.5%–1% in feed		Harkness et al. (2010)
Sulfaquinoxaline	125–250 ppm in feed		Harkness et al. (2010)
Thiabendazole	50–100 mg/kg q24h for 5 d	PO	Morrisey and Carpenter (2004)
	50 mg/kg q24h, repeat in 3 wk	PO	Hernandez-Divers (2005)
Tilmicosin	25 mg/kg once	SC	McKay et al. (1996)

IM = intramuscular; PO = per os; and SC = subcutaneous.

Bacterial Diseases

Bacterial Pneumonia and Respiratory Diseases

Pasteurellosis is the single most common and troublesome disease of domestic rabbits. It is caused by *Pasteurella multocida*, a Gram-negative coccobacillus. Rabbits may harbor the organism in the upper respiratory tract without showing clinical signs. From the respiratory tract, the organism may spread along the nasolacrimal ducts, eustachian tubes, down the trachea, hematogenously, and venereally. Following stress, a variety of syndromes may develop, including rhinitis, conjunctivitis, bronchopneumonia, otitis media and interna, genital infections, abscesses, and septicemia. *P. multocida* is readily spread from one rabbit to another by direct contact, fomites contaminated with nasal secretions, and even aerosolization within a room. A variety

Table 11.9. Miscellaneous agents used in rabbits

Drug	Dosage	Route	Reference
Atipamezole	1 mg/kg	SC, IP, IV	Flecknell (2016)
Atropine	0.1–3 mg/kg	SC	Harkness et al. (2010)
Barium	10–14 mL/kg	PO	Quesenberry (1994)
Bromelin enzyme	1–2 tablets q24h for 3–5 d	PO	Quesenberry (1994)
Calcium-EDTA	27 mg/kg q6h for 2–5 d (make at 10 mg/mL in 5% dextrose or saline)	SC	Johnson-Delaney (1996)
Calcium gluconate (10% solution)	5–10 mL	PO	Raphael (1981)
	3–5 mL	IV	
Cholestyramine	2 g per animal q24h for 18–21 d, gavage with 20 mL water	PO	Harkness and Wagner (1995)
Cimetidine	5–10 mg/kg q8–12h	PO, SC, IM, IV	Morrisey and Carpenter (2004)
Cisapride	0.5 mg/kg q8–24h	PO	Smith and Burgmann (1997)
Dexamethasone	0.2–0.6 mg/kg	SC, IM, IV	Gillett (1994)
Dexamethasone	0.5–2 mg/kg	IM, IV	Paul-Murphy and Ramer (1998)
Digoxin	0.005 mg/kg q12-24h	PO	Pariaut (2009)
Diltiazem	0.5 mg/kg q8-24h	PO	Pariaut (2009)
Diphenhydramine	2 mg/kg q8-12h	PO, SC	Morrisey and Carpenter (2004)
Doxapram	2–5 mg/kg q15min	IV	Huerkamp (1995)
Enalapril	0.5 mg/kg q12-24h	PO	Pariaut (2009)
Flumazenil	0.1–10 mg/kg	IV	Flecknell (2009)
Furosemide	2–5 mg/kg q12h	PO, SC, IM, IV	Paul-Murphy and Ramer (1998)
Glycopyrrolate	0.01 mg/kg	IV	Flecknell (2009)
	0.1 mg/kg	IM, SC	Flecknell (2009)
Human chorionic gonadotropin	20–25 IU per animal	IV	Harkness and Wagner (1995)
Iron dextran	4–6 mg/kg once	IM	Morrisey and Carpenter (2004)
Lactobacillus	1 notch daily of paste; or 1/4–1/2 tsp powder, or per package label; mix into food	PO	Johnson-Delaney (1996)
Loperamide hydrochloride (Imodium A-D)	0.1 mg/kg q8h for 3 d, then q24h for 2 d	PO	Harkness and Wagner (1995)
Meclizine hydrochloride (Antivert)	2–12 mg/kg q24h	PO	Harkness and Wagner (1995)
Metoclopramide	0.2–1 mg/kg q6-8h	PO, SC	Harkness and Wagner (1995)

(Continud)

Table 11.9. (*Continued*)

Drug	Dosage	Route	Reference
Naloxone	0.01–0.1 mg/kg	IV, IM	Gillett (1994)
Oxytocin	0.1–3 IU/kg	SC, IM	Harkness and Wagner (1995)
Pancreatic enzyme concentrate (Viokase-V)	Mix 1 tsp with 3 tbsp yogurt, let stand 15 min, then give 2–3 mL q12h	PO	Allen et al. (1993)
Polysulfated glycosaminoglycan	2.2 mg/kg q3d for 21–28 d, then q14d	IM, SC	Jenkins (1995)
Prednisolone	0.25–0.5 mg/kg q12h for 3 d, then q24h for 3 d, then q48h	PO	Quesenberry (1994)
	0.5–2 mg/kg q12h	PO	Morrisey and Carpenter (2004)
Prochlorperazine	0.2–0.5 mg/kg q8h	PO	Harcourt-Brown (2002)
Ranitidine	2–5 mg/kg q12h	PO	Harcourt-Brown (2002)
Simethicone	65–130 mg/animal q1h for 2–3 treatments	PO	Krempels et al. (2000)
Sodium bicarbonate	2 mEq/kg	IV, IP	Harrenstien (1994)
Stanozolol	1–2 mg	PO	Harkness and Wagner (1995)
Sucralfate	25 mg/kg q8–12h	PO	Harkness and Wagner (1995)
Verapamil (Calan)	0.2 mg/kg q8h for 9 treatments	SC	Harkness and Wagner (1995)
Vitamin A	500–1000 IU/kg once	IM	Johnson-Delaney (1996)
Vitamin B complex	0.02–0.4 mL/kg q24h	IM	Johnson-Delaney (1996)
Vitamin E-selenium (Bo-Se)	0.25 mL per rabbit	IM	Johnson-Delaney (1996)
Vitamin K	1–10 mg/kg prn	IM	Johnson-Delaney (1996)
Yohimbine	0.2–1 mg/kg	IM, IV	Gillett (1994)

EDTA = ethylenediaminetetraacetic acid; IM = intramuscular; IP = intraperitoneal; IV = intravenous; PO = per os; and SC = subcutaneous.

of *P. multocida* isolates appear to differ in virulence. Some forms are associated with a rapidly fatal septicemia, whereas other strains induce a slowly progressive rhinitis.

Sneezing and the presence of a serous to mucopurulent nasal discharge characterize the upper respiratory form of pasteurellosis, also known as snuffles. This is the most common clinical presentation of infection. Exudate is often seen on the inner aspect of the forelegs. Turbinate atrophy may be a sequela with some strains of *P. multocida*. A subacute to chronic suppurative conjunctivitis with epiphora may also be a clinical manifestation. The infection results in loss of fur around the medial canthus of the eye and is usually seen in conjunction with rhinitis. Animals may live for many months with these symptoms or the disease may progress to one of the other clinical forms.

The pulmonary form of pasteurellosis may be acute or chronic. The acute disease appears as a bronchopneumonia with variable consolidation of the lungs; cyanosis is often a prominent feature. Chronic pneumonia is often asymptomatic. At times, laboratory rabbits die of pneumonia without observable clinical signs because their limited exercise allows them to mask the severity of disease. Alternatively, rabbits with severe pneumonia may exhibit signs such as anorexia, depression, dyspnea, moist lung sounds (rales), and death.

Suppurative otitis media and otitis interna are common manifestations of this organism. Otitis interna causes vestibular derangements and torticollis, commonly called head tilt or wryneck. The head tilt may be so severe that the head is rotated nearly 180°.

Reproductive tract infections in rabbits include pyometra in the doe and orchitis in the buck. Venereal transmission has been described. Large, subcutaneous abscesses may be seen with *P. multocida* infections. The pyometra or abscess contents tend to be yellow–white and have a very thick, creamy consistency that is difficult to aspirate. Incising the abscess and removing the thick purulent material may be necessary to initiate successful treatment of the infection although means to minimize environmental contamination should be considered.

Definitive diagnosis is most often made by culture of the organism. Screening colonies through use of enzyme-linked immunosorbent assays (ELISA) or polymerase chain reaction (PCR) tests can also be a helpful, but not fully reliable means of identifying infected animals. To exclude the adverse effects of this organism on research results, only *Pasteurella*-free rabbits should be used; these animals are readily available. There is no commercially available vaccine. Eradication of the organism is extremely difficult with antibiotic treatment as the organism is harbored in the nasal passages, pharynx, and tympanic bullae. Antibiotics often used in treating pasteurellosis include penicillin G, enrofloxacin, and tilmicosin. No antibiotic treatment will reliably eliminate the carrier state. A degree of caution should be exercised in using antibiotics such as penicillin G for prolonged periods because rabbits are susceptible to developing a fatal diarrhea caused by clostridial enterotoxemia (Box 11.5).

Bordetella bronchiseptica has been recovered from the respiratory tracts of both normal and diseased rabbits. Thus, its status as a pathogen is not well established. It may facilitate *P. multocida* infections of the lower respiratory tract and should be regarded as a potential pathogen in young rabbits 4–12 weeks of age. Rabbits are frequently asymptomatic carriers of *Bordetella* spp. and should not be housed near guinea pigs because they may inadvertently infect them.

Cilia-associated respiratory (CAR) bacillus isolates from rabbits differ significantly from isolates obtained from infected rodents, suggesting that isolates may be host-specific. The organism appears to be an opportunistic invader of the respiratory tract and is found

Box 11.5

A degree of caution should be exercised in using antibiotics such as penicillin G for prolonged periods because rabbits are susceptible to developing a fatal diarrhea caused by clostridial enterotoxemia.

between the cilia of the respiratory epithelium. Naturally occurring infections are usually asymptomatic but may cause a slight nasal discharge. Histologically, there is slight hypertrophy and hyperplasia of the laryngeal, tracheal, and bronchial epithelium. Antimicrobial treatments for the CAR bacillus have not been evaluated for efficacy in rabbits.

Bacterial Enteritis and Miscellaneous Enteric Diseases

As a group, enteric diseases are second only to pasteurellosis as a health problem in domestic rabbits. Of the common diseases encountered, the enteric diseases are probably the least understood. In some cases, diarrhea is associated with a specific, well-defined agent, but in many cases, the cause of enteric disease is obscure. Specific enteric diseases include coccidiosis, enterotoxemia, Tyzzer's disease, and salmonellosis. Those of uncertain etiologies include colibacillosis and mucoid enteropathy.

Symptomatic treatment may be the best initial step in treating individual rabbits with acute diarrhea. Maintaining hydration and body temperature as well as changing the diet to one containing higher fiber and lower protein should be the focus of treatment. It is important to keep the rabbit's anus free from fecal impaction and the hindquarters clean and dry. Analgesics may be indicated in depressed, anorexic rabbits.

Colibacillosis

Colibacillosis might appropriately be classified as a specific enteric disease; however, the role of the *Escherichia coli* organism is not completely understood. The type of *E. coli* that most frequently causes disease in rabbits is known as enteropathogenic *E. coli* (EPEC). Enteropathogenic organisms do not produce enterotoxins, and they do not invade the intestinal mucosa. Rather, the EPECs adhere to receptors on the enterocytes and use a group of effector proteins to interfere with cell function. Enterohemorrhagic *E. coli* (EHEC) has also been reported as a natural infection in Dutch Belted rabbits, and is characterized by production of Shiga toxins. It is known that *E. coli* is either absent or present in low numbers in the gut of normal rabbits. In some cases of severe diarrhea, the organisms are isolated in large numbers. Due to this finding, it was once thought that *E. coli* was not a primary pathogen of rabbits, but this has since been disproven. Outbreaks of colibacillosis may be seen in sucklings (1–2 weeks old) or weanlings (4–6 weeks old) because of the prevalence of receptors which allow EPEC attachment.

Clinical signs are nonspecific and may be attributed to any of the enteric pathogens. Gross findings include an edematous and hemorrhagic cecum. Histologically, there may be villous atrophy, edema, congestion, hemorrhage, and characteristic attaching and effacing intestinal lesions with large numbers of Gram-negative coliform bacilli attached to the epithelium. Tentative diagnosis can be made through observation of the characteristic histologic lesions and by identification of nonhemolytic, facultatively anaerobic *E. coli* on fecal culture. A definitive diagnosis can be made with microscopy, serotyping, or biotyping.

Treatment is largely symptomatic. Systemic antibiotics (gentamicin, chloramphenicol, and neomycin), intestinal protectants such as bismuth subsalicylate, fluids and electrolytes, and other supportive measures may be beneficial. Alteration of the diet to reduce the amount of concentrates fed to no more than 2–3 oz per day and providing added roughage, such as hay, is often more effective than are antibiotics in reducing mortality.

Enterotoxemia

Clostridium spiroforme is the most common pathogen associated with enteritis in recently weaned (4- to 8-week-old) rabbits. Sporadic infections are most common, but epizootics do occur. In addition, *C. perfringens* and *C. difficile* have also been implicated in this disease complex but are lesser pathogens. It is now known that clostridial species are either absent or found in low numbers in the large intestine of rabbits. A disruption of the normal microflora of the gut appears to play an important role in the disease process of adult rabbits. Clostridial organisms may be isolated as the sole cause of enteric disease, but concurrent infections with *E. coli*, *C. piliforme*, or rotavirus are not uncommon. Changes in feed, weaning, antibiotic therapy, and concurrent infections may all be stressors that allow colonization of *C. spiroforme* and enterotoxin production. Weaning causes a change in gut flora, which most likely allows the pathogen to proliferate. A depression in antibacterial resistance favors the increased growth of toxin-producing bacteria. The enterotoxins cause damage to the enterocytes, with functional impairment and subsequent diarrhea, dehydration, and death.

A hemorrhagic and edematous cecum is typically seen in these cases. Gram stains of a smear of cecal contents can be helpful in identifying curved or coiled Gram-positive bacilli. Anaerobic cultures are also indicated for obtaining a presumptive diagnosis of clostridia-mediated diarrhea. A definitive diagnosis requires the demonstration of the enterotoxin (iota toxin) or causative organism. Cytotoxicity assays, ELISAs, and PCR tests are *in vitro* tests that can identify *Clostridia* spp.—associated toxins in the fecal material of rabbits. Treatment consists mainly of supportive therapy since there is little evidence that enterotoxemia can be effectively treated with antibiotics. Adding copper sulfate to the diet may reduce toxin production by *Clostridia* species. The administration of oral probiotics may have beneficial effects in weanlings as this may help reestablish a normal gut flora.

Several antibiotics have been associated with outbreaks of enterotoxemia, including erythromycin, clindamycin, lincomycin, and streptomycin. Penicillin and its derivatives are routinely used in rabbits but have also been associated with enterotoxemia and must be used with caution. Parenteral administration is preferred over oral administration. Antibiotics that are generally considered to be safe in rabbits include chloramphenicol, enrofloxacin, trimethoprim/sulfa, gentamicin, neomycin, vancomycin, and metronidazole. Preventive measures for animals receiving antibiotics include the oral administration of *Lactobacillus* spp. preparations to inhibit toxins or cholestyramine to absorb toxins.

Proliferative Enteropathy

Proliferative enteropathy (PE) is caused by infection with *Lawsonia intracellularis*, which is an obligate, intracellular, curved rod–shaped, argyrophilic bacterium located within the apical cytoplasm of infected crypt epithelial cells. PE has a worldwide distribution and affects a wide variety of species (e.g., hamsters, ferrets, and pigs). Since *L. intracellularis* isolates from different species have little genetic variation, intraspecies and interspecies transmission appears likely. Epizootics of the disease are usually confined to younger animals. Infection occurs primarily in weanlings, when passive maternal immunity declines. Transmission is fecal–oral, and then the organisms infect intestinal proliferating crypt epithelial cells and multiply. The intestine appears to be the only tissue infected. Most animals develop subclinical infection but shed the bacterium in feces, contributing to environmental contamination. Stressors, such as overcrowding, transport, change in diet, and experimental manipulations, may predispose rabbits to clinical infection.

Clinical signs include abdominal distention with sloshing sounds from the intestines, hunched posture, depression, polydipsia, anorexia, hypothermia 37°–38.5°C (99°–101°F), and constipation followed by profuse mucoid diarrhea. Affected animals may be emaciated and/or dehydrated. Grossly, rabbits have proliferative jejunitis and/or ileitis characterized by thickening and corrugation of the small intestinal mucosa and the presence of semifluid mucinous contents of the colon and cecum. Microscopically, intestinal crypts are elongated and often branched and lined by multilayered immature enterocytes. Special stains (Warthin-Starry silver stain, PAS stain) can be used to demonstrate the curved bacteria consistent with *L. intracellularis* in apical cytoplasm of enterocytes and within crypt lumens.

Diagnosis should be made based on the combination of clinical signs and results of necropsy, histopathology, bacteriology, and/or demonstration of intralesional organisms by histochemistry, electron microscopy, immunohistochemistry, ELISA, and/or PCR. Bacterial culture and isolation must be performed by use of cultured enterocytes because *L. intracellularis* does not proliferate in cell-free media.

Treatment is usually ineffective, although intense fluid therapy and broad-spectrum antibiotics may help rabbits in the early stages of this disease. Antibiotics must be administered with caution due to their potential impact on the intestinal flora. Provision of a heat source to prevent hypothermia is another important part of supportive therapy. Preventive measures include decreasing food intake when shipping and for 48 hours after arrival.

Tyzzer's Disease

Clostridium piliforme is a Gram-negative, spore-forming bacillus and is the etiologic agent of Tyzzer's disease. It is an obligate intracellular pathogen that can cause an acute hemorrhagic typhlocolitis, and is difficult to grow *in vitro*. Infections are most frequently observed in epizootic outbreaks of weanling rabbits between 6 and 12 weeks of age; morbidity and mortality can be very high. Though asymptomatic infections with fecal shedding are not uncommon, clinically affected animals present with acute and profuse diarrhea, anorexia, dehydration, lethargy, and fecal staining of the hindquarters. Death follows in 12–48 hours. Rabbits with chronic infections may show weight loss and muscle wasting. Stressors such as overcrowding, shipping, poor ventilation, and improper nutrition are precipitating factors that elicit an acute diarrheal disease. At necropsy, focal necrosis of the liver and intestinal mucosa is seen.

A diagnosis is based upon identifying Periodic Acid–Schiff stained or silver-positive intracytoplasmic filamentous bacilli in histologic sections of the liver, heart, or cecum. Alternatively, a Giemsa-stained impression smear of the hepatic lesions may reveal the typical bacilli. ELISA, immunofluoresence assay (IFA), and PCR assays can also be used to identify the presence of antibodies to the bacterium.

Oxytetracycline is suggested for treatment; however, the prognosis for animals showing clinical signs of Tyzzer's disease is grave. Institution of sound husbandry practices and elimination of environmental stress factors are crucial in controlling an outbreak in a rabbit colony. Spores can persist in the environment for extended periods; thus 1% peracetic acid, 0.3% sodium hypochlorite, or a vaporized sterilant should be used to clean laboratory surfaces.

Salmonellosis

Salmonella spp. infections are a relatively uncommon cause of enteric disease in laboratory rabbits, but are acutely fatal and characterized by septicemia. Diarrhea or abortions may be noted. Although various antibiotics may be effective in eliminating clinical signs of salmonellosis, treatment of affected animals is contraindicated due to the zoonotic potential of this organism and the possibility of inapparent carriers.

Miscellaneous Bacterial Infections

Staphylococcus aureus is considered a normal bacterial inhabitant of the rabbit nasopharynx, conjunctiva, and skin. It is one of the most common causes of conjunctivitis in rabbits. Pathogenic infections may occur and manifest in the forms of septicemia, dermatitis, and abscesses. Staphylococcal mastitis often causes septicemia in the doe and multiple abscesses in nursing kits maintained in unsanitary conditions. The organism can be identified through culture and its relative virulence assessed by PCR. Penicillin, enrofloxacin, cephalosporins, aminoglycosides, and chloramphenicol, in conjunction with topical treatment, are sometimes effective. Antibiotic treatment of staphylococcal infections, however, is frequently discouraging.

Mastitis occurs sporadically in lactating does and occasionally during pseudopregnancy. Blue breast is a common term for mastitis as the skin over the mammary gland changes from pink to red then to bluish purple. Several microorganisms, including *S. aureus*, *Pasteurella* spp., and *Streptococcus* spp., are causative agents. Causative organisms may be introduced by means of splinters from nest boxes, trauma from the teeth of nursing young, or unsanitary housing conditions. Treatment involves isolating the affected doe and treating her with appropriate antibiotics; lancing and flushing abscesses may be necessary. The young should be removed from the doe but not foster nursed on another doe because of the probability of spreading the disease to a healthy animal.

Necrobacillosis or Schmorl's disease, caused by *Fusobacterium necrophorum*, is characterized by ulceration of the skin and by subcutaneous swellings of the face, neck, and oral cavity. Septicemia with infection of the jugular vein can occur as a secondary infection. Although the organism is commonly present in the digestive tract of rabbits, the incidence of disease is low. Infection is thought to develop through fecal contamination of skin wounds. The recommended treatment for affected rabbits includes debridement, drainage of abscesses, provision of systemic antibiotics such as penicillin, tetracycline, or metronidazole, and improved sanitation. Lesions frequently reoccur. *Fusobacterium necrophorum* is transmissible to humans.

Pseudomonas aeruginosa is an uncommon pathogen in rabbits. Skin infections with blue-green discoloration may occur around the dewlap and in other areas in which the skin is in contact with moisture; infection may extend to other organs. Treatment involves removing the fur from the affected region, cleaning the lesion, and administering topical or systemic antibiotics. Affected animals' drinking water should be cultured and evaluated as the possible source of contamination.

Tularemia is caused by *Francisella tularensis*. It is a Gram-negative coccobacillus that infects vertebrates, especially rabbits and rodents, and usually causes sudden death of affected animals. Typical lesions at necropsy are small foci of necrosis in the spleen and liver. The organism can be transmitted by direct contact, via aerosols or ingestion, or by bloodsucking arthropods. The disease is seen in wild rabbits but is rare in domestic rabbits because of lack of exposure to the appropriate arthropod vectors. *Francisella tularensis* can cause a potentially fatal zoonotic disease in humans, seen primarily in hunters and wildlife personnel. It is classified as a select agent by the Federal Select Agent Program and is a reportable disease in the United States.

Spirochete Infections: Venereal Spirochetosis

Venereal spirochetosis, also known as rabbit syphilis, vent disease, and treponematosis, is caused by *Treponema paraluiscuniculi*, a Gram-negative, spiral-shaped rod that can be propagated only *in vivo*. Rabbit syphilis is uncommon in the research environment. The organism is serologically and morphologically similar to *T. pallidum*, which causes syphilis in humans. *T. paraluiscuniculi*, however, is nonpathogenic for humans. The disease is characterized by the presence of raised, crusted, occasionally hemorrhagic, ulcerative foci on the external genitalia, perineal region, and face. The disease may be confused with lesions caused by urine scald, ear mites, and sarcoptic mange. Asymptomatic infections are common in infected colonies.

The disease is transmitted by direct contact, usually venereally but occasionally by extragenital routes. Affected rabbits should be isolated during the acute disease. Treponematosis can be differentiated from other cutaneous diseases by dark-field examination of scrapings from the lesions. A *T. pallidum* ELISA can be used to diagnose *T. paraluiscuniculi* infections. Three doses of benzathine procaine penicillin intramuscularly administered at weekly intervals are reportedly effective in eliminating the infection. Penicillin derivatives should be used with great caution because of the possibility of inducing a fatal enterotoxemia.

Viral Diseases

Myxomatosis

Rabbit myxomatosis is caused by a poxvirus, the myxoma virus. Multiple viral strains exist with differing associated levels of pathogenicity. The myxoma virus is endemic on four continents: Australia, Europe, South America, and North America. The natural host in the United States is wild cottontails (*Sylvilagus* spp.), although it is also enzootic in wild *Oryctolagus* in the western United States. Transmission is usually by arthropod vectors (e.g., mosquitoes and fleas) but can be by direct contact. Aerosol transmission has been suspected in at least one outbreak. The initial clinical signs are growth of gelatinous, occasionally indistinct, subcutaneous masses. Several days later, a mucopurulent conjunctivitis with generalized subcutaneous edema develops, which causes the rabbit's eyes to swell shut and the ears to droop. Diagnosis of active infection is by virus isolation or PCR of infected tissues. Disease survivors can be detected through multiple serologic assays. A vaccine is available in Europe but is not approved for use in the United States.

Papillomatosis

Rabbit oral papillomavirus infection can stimulate papillomas (small white growths) on the underside of the tongue and elsewhere within the oral cavity. The domestic rabbit, *Oryctolagus*, is the natural host, with disease transmission through abraded oral mucosa such as from rough, contaminated feed. Lesions are usually seen in rabbits 2–18 months of age. Papillomas spontaneously regress within a few weeks.

Rotavirus

Rotavirus causes enteritis with mild to severe diarrhea in young rabbits. Weanlings are particularly susceptible. Fecal–oral transmission occurs although aerosol transmission is also suspected. Outbreaks occur in naive colonies, with high morbidity and mortality; infections tend to be acute and self-limiting in animals that survive. Maternal antibodies play a significant role in protecting suckling rabbits against the disease. Diagnosis is based on clinical signs, histologic findings, viral detection, and serological assays. The only treatment is supportive therapy.

Rabbit Hemorrhagic Disease (RHD)

The etiologic agent of rabbit hemorrhagic disease is a calicivirus. It is highly contagious and is spread by direct contact or aerosols. It has been reported in Asia, Europe, Africa, Australia, New Zealand, the United States, and Mexico. It is a reportable disease in the United States.

The disease is seen in rabbits older than 2 months; younger rabbits are not clinically affected. Transmission is by direct and fecal–oral contact, through fomites, and possibly through insects. Onset is acute; however, symptoms may include nervous system signs such as shaking, incoordination, and prostration. Morbidity and mortality range from 80% to 100%. Gross lesions include diffuse hemorrhage of the trachea, lungs, liver, spleen, kidneys, thymus, and peritoneum. The cause of death is most commonly disseminated intravascular coagulation (DIC) with deep venous thromboses. The disease can be presumptively diagnosed by clinical signs, pathological findings, and outbreak characteristics. Definitive diagnosis can be made through ELISA testing or PCR of infected tissues and rabbit inoculation. The virus cannot be reliably isolated *in vitro*. Infected colonies should be culled. Various types of vaccines are now available to protect valuable colonies.

Miscellaneous Viral Diseases

Rare reports of other viruses in rabbits include adenovirus, parvovirus, herpesvirus, and coronavirus. These viruses have been identified to cause disease only in very isolated cases and are not yet considered to be common pathogens of rabbits.

Mycotic Infections

Dermatophytosis

Ringworm is rarely encountered in laboratory rabbits. Infections with multiple dermatophytes have been documented; however, ringworm is most frequently caused by the zoonotic agent *Trichophyton mentagrophytes*. As *T. mentagrophytes* does not fluoresce under ultraviolet light, microscopic examination or culturing of hair or skin scrapings is usually required to establish a diagnosis. Lesions are pruritic, crusty, and hairless and in most cases first appear on the head, ears, or toes. Lesions may be treated with topical antifungal creams applied twice daily or by administration of griseofulvin orally.

Encephalitozoonosis

Encephalitozoonosis is usually a latent disease of rabbits caused by the fungal organism *Encephalitozoon cuniculi*. This agent was once considered a protozoal organism and is uncommon in rabbits produced for biomedical research. *Encephalitozoon* organisms are capable of infecting a wide range of mammals, including humans—where it is most frequently identified in immunocompromised individuals. In the rabbit, transmission most commonly occurs through ingestion of spores in the urine. Intrauterine and aerosol transmission have also been documented.

Infections are typically asymptomatic with mild lesions noted only on postmortem examination. While the organism can affect multiple organs and systems, the three most frequently affected are the kidneys, the central nervous system, and the eye. Infection of the kidneys may induce chronic renal failure but more frequently causes fibrosis and pitting of the renal cortex with no notable loss of kidney function. A pyogranulomatous encephalitis may develop with related clinical signs such as head tilt, seizures, depression, ataxia, swaying, and posterior paresis. Ocular lesions (e.g., uveitis and cataracts) may develop. Recognizing lesions induced by *E. cuniculi* is particularly important so that they are not mistakenly identified as experimental sequelae.

A tentative clinical diagnosis can be made with positive serology (e.g., multiplex fluorescent immunoassay, ELISA, IFA) or PCR of kidney tissue or urine. Definitive diagnosis is made with histologic observation of the organism in affected tissues. Acute infections of *E. cuniculi* have been successfully treated with fenbendazole-medicated pellets. Treatment of chronic infections is frequently unsuccessful.

Parasitic Diseases

Ear Mites

Psoroptes cuniculi, the rabbit ear mite, is a nonburrowing mite that chews on the epidermal skin of the inner ear and causes an intense inflammatory response. A dry, brown, crusty material accumulates on the inner surface of the ear. This condition is common in rabbits raised for the agricultural or pet industries but is exceedingly rare in research colonies.

Severe mite infestations induce inflammation and intense pruritus of the inner pinnae. Affected rabbits may shake their heads and intensely scratch their ears, possibly resulting in self-mutilation. Crusty lesions may be observed on the back of the neck from scratching. Rarely, a secondary bacterial infection occurs, leading to otitis media or interna. The mites can easily be seen with the aid of an otoscope or by placing the crusts in mineral oil on a slide and examining with a microscope. All life cycle stages of the mite are found on the rabbit; mites may survive in the environment for up to 3 weeks.

There are several options for treatments, including ivermectin, moxidectin, or selamectin. Cleaning of the pinnae and ear canal in severe cases is controversial. While removal of the crusty material will decrease the mite load, ear tissues and blood vessels may inadvertently be damaged. The use of analgesics should be considered in severely affected animals.

Fur Mites

Cheyletiella parasitovorax, the dandruff mite, causes thinning of the fur and scaly lesions, usually over the scapulae. The term "walking dandruff" has been used to describe the easily visualized mites that remain in contact with the keratin layer of the skin to feed on tissue fluid. Pruritus is not associated with infestation as the mite does not burrow. Transmission occurs through direct contact and fomites; adults may survive up to 10 days in the environment. Treatment is accomplished through multiple subcutaneous doses of ivermectin or by topical application of selamectin, permethrin, and carbaryl products. *C. parasitovorax* can infest multiple species, including dogs, cats, and humans.

Mange Mites

Although rabbits are susceptible to *Notoedres cati* and *Sarcoptes scabiei*, these mites do not commonly cause infestation. Clinical signs may include pruritus, alopecia, hyperemia, and epidermal crust formation. Pruritus may be so severe as to result in self-mutilation and trauma. Diagnosis is by observation of the mites on deep skin scrapings. Ivermectin, doramectin, and moxidectin can be used to treat mange mites.

Fleas

Rabbits can be infested with multiple species of fleas, including the rabbit flea (*Spilopsyllus cuniculi*) and the dog and cat fleas (*Ctenocephalides canis* and *C. felis*). Their presence must be strongly considered with wild-caught rabbits due to the possible transmission of multiple zoonotic agents (e.g., plague, Rocky Mountain spotted fever) as well as agents of special concern to rabbit colonies (e.g., myxoma virus, rabbit hemorrhagic disease). Effective treatments have included use of imidacloprid, selamectin, and lufenuron. The environment must also be treated to eliminate the parasite.

Cuterebra

Myiasis (from the Greek word for "fly," *myia*) is defined as the infestation of live vertebrate animals with fly larvae, which feed on the host's dead or living tissue or liquid body substances. Such infestation is rarely seen in laboratory rabbits but may be found in rabbits housed outdoors. *Cuterebra* spp., commonly called bot flies, parasitize rabbits and rodents to cause myiasis. The larvae live in the subcutaneous tissue and appear as large lumps with perforated breathing holes, usually on the neck or upper extremities. They grow up to 1 in. in length. Application of a heavy oil or occlusive ointment interrupts the larva's respiration, forcing it to migrate to the surface of the lesion, where it can be removed easily. Surgical treatment consists of incising the skin and removing the larvae. Care must be taken to avoid crushing the larvae, which can result in acute shock and death in the rabbit.

Pinworms

The rabbit pinworm, *Passalurus ambiguus*, is a whitish hairlike worm that can be seen in the rabbit's cecal contents and colon. Pinworms are generally nonpathogenic to rabbits, and infections are typically asymptomatic. There is no zoonotic potential for humans. Transmission is fecal–oral. Embryonated eggs pass in the feces and are immediately infective. Once ingested, the eggs hatch in the small intestine and larvae molt. Adult worms are found in the cecum. Definitive diagnosis requires identification of the typical egg in the feces. They can be treated with piperazine citrate or fenbendazole. Environmental decontamination is recommended to eliminate infectious adults and ova.

Tapeworms

Rabbits can be infested with tapeworms such as the rabbit tapeworm, *Cittotaenia ctenoides*. Rabbit tapeworms require the presence of an intermediate host (mite), therefore are virtually nonexistent in rabbit research colonies.

Coccidiosis

Coccidiosis is much less common in laboratory rabbits today but is still commonly found in pet rabbits. Two forms of coccidiosis have been identified in *Oryctolagus cuniculus*: intestinal and hepatic. The intestinal form is most prevalent and is caused by at least 11 species of *Eimeria*, including *E. magna*, *E. perforans*, *E. media*, and *E. irresidua*. The hepatic form is caused by *E. stiedae*.

Hepatic coccidiosis: Adult rabbits usually show no clinical signs from infection with *E. stiedae*, but heavy infections in young animals may cause weight loss, diarrhea, a potbellied appearance (due to marked hepatomegaly), liver failure, and death. Following fecal–oral transmission, the organism migrates either hematogenously or via the lymphatic system from the intestinal tract to the bile duct in which it reproduces. At necropsy, hepatomegaly with irregularly shaped, slightly raised yellow–white foci is noted. Microscopically, bile duct hyperplasia and inflammation are apparent.

Intestinal coccidiosis: Some species of intestinal coccidia are nonpathogenic while others can induce varying degrees of disease and target different regions of the intestine. Concurrent infections with multiple species are common. In mild cases of intestinal coccidiosis, few if any clinical signs are evident. In moderate to severe cases, weight gain may be poor and an odiferous, profuse, and soft to watery diarrhea with traces of blood may develop. Intussuception may be noted. Mortality is more common in young animals.

Eimeria has a direct life cycle. Fecal–oral transmission occurs most commonly through ingestion of sporulated oocysts in contaminated food or water, or via contact with contaminated fomites. Sporulation can occur in as little as 2 days if the ambient temperature and humidity are optimal. Reingestion of the soft nighttime fecal pellets does not allow time for sporulation; therefore, infection by this route is unlikely. With both intestinal and hepatic coccidiosis, oocysts appear in the feces except in animals that die very soon after onset of illness. Oocysts remain infectious in the environment for several months. The yeast *Saccharomycopsis guttulatus* is commonly found in rabbit feces and should not be incorrectly identified as a coccidial oocyte.

Prevention and control of coccidiosis is achieved by (1) strict cleaning and disinfection procedures; (2) use of cages with nonsolid flooring with a catch pan, J-type feeders, and water bottles or automated watering devices to reduce autoinfection; (3) medicated feed or water; and (4) in some cases, culling of infected animals. There is no effective treatment for elimination of *E. stiedae* from the liver. Drugs used for treating coccidiosis include sulfamethazine, sulfadimethoxine, sulfaquinoxaline, amprolium, monensin, robenidine, decoquinate, and lasalocid.

Neoplasia

The most common neoplasm of domestic rabbits is uterine adenocarcinoma, with a high incidence in does 5 years of age and older (Box 11.6). A doe's reproductive performance generally declines several months before the tumor can be detected clinically. Other clinical signs may include a bloody vaginal discharge or bloody urine. Masses may be found by gentle palpation of the abdomen. Metastasis to the lungs and other organs occurs frequently. Because of the frequency of uterine neoplasia in mature does, an ovariohysterectomy should be considered for laboratory rabbits that are held long-term and not used for breeding.

> **Box 11.6**
>
> *The most common neoplasm of domestic rabbits is uterine adenocarcinoma.*

Other neoplasias commonly identified in the rabbit, in decreasing order of frequency, are as follows: lymphoma/lymphoid leukemia; mammary papilloma and adenocarcinoma; and neoplasms of the skin, including trichoblastoma and collagenous hamartoma. Other neoplasias occasionally reported in the literature include uterine leiomyosarcoma, embryonal nephroma, and pituitary adenoma. Prolactin-secreting pituitary adenomas have been described in aged, nulliparous NZW rabbits. These tumors secrete prolactin and are associated with mammary gland abnormalities, including enlarged, nonpainful teats that are frequently engorged with fluid.

Miscellaneous Conditions

Buphthalmia

Buphthalmia, also known as congenital glaucoma, is one of the more common inherited diseases of domestic rabbits and is commonly seen in NZW laboratory rabbits. It is associated with an abnormal production and removal of aqueous fluid from the anterior chamber and may occur unilaterally or bilaterally. Clinical signs include an increase in the size of the anterior chamber, corneal opacity, and increased prominence of the eyeball. Vision will eventually be reduced and rabbits may show a slight head tilt to allow better visualization from a normal eye. The condition has a slow onset but, with continued progression, can result in a painful condition due to corneal ulceration and self-trauma. No treatment is necessary in the early stages, although enucleation is an option. Affected animals should not be bred.

Lumbar Spinal Fracture or Luxation

Fractures or luxations of the caudal lumbar spine are common, particularly at the L7–S1 junction (Box 11.7). The condition is strongly suggested by the sudden onset of posterior paralysis and is usually caused by a handler's failure to support an animal's hindquarters or when a rabbit falls or is dropped. The prognosis after back injury depends on the location and severity of the cord lesion but is usually unfavorable. Therapeutic criteria are similar to those for dogs and cats and may include steroids, frequent rotation of the animal to prevent pressure sores, and at least twice-daily manual expression of the bladder. Rarely, an animal will recover with cage rest, but in most cases posterior paralysis with urinary and fecal incontinence persists and euthanasia is recommended.

> **Box 11.7**
>
> *Fractures of the caudal lumbar spine are common, particularly at the L7–S1 junction.*

Hairballs (Gastric Trichobezoars)

Gastric hairballs should be suspected in rabbits that suddenly stop eating and drinking and pass no fecal material but otherwise appear alert and in good health. The presence of a hairball can usually be detected by palpation, but in some cases a radiograph may be necessary to confirm the diagnosis. Care must be taken in attributing clinical signs to the presence of hairballs as significant-sized hairballs are frequently present in the stomach of asymptomatic animals. Hairballs may be the result of excessive self-grooming secondary to boredom or low-fiber feeds, but dehydration, stress, pain, and *ad libitum* feeding have been suggested as contributing causes.

Restoring and maintaining hydration is of utmost importance. Mineral oil administered by a stomach tube and metoclopramide may be effective. Metoclopramide use must be approached with extreme caution due to the chance of gastric rupture. Administration of bromelin enzyme may be of some value as a treatment and preventive. Most treatments are ineffective, but medical treatment is usually preferred over surgical intervention, which is associated with a high mortality rate. Death following blockage of the stomach by a hairball is usually attributable to ketosis.

Feeding a high-fiber (up to 20%) pelleted diet in restricted amounts is one of the best ways to prevent hairballs. Providing roughage such as alfalfa or timothy hay may also be beneficial in prevention.

Heat Stroke

Rabbits are highly susceptible to overheating. Young rabbits in nest boxes, as well as older, obese, or pregnant rabbits, are particularly prone to heat prostration. Other predisposing factors include a high ambient temperature over 29.5°C (85°F), high humidity (70% or higher), poor ventilation, and crowding. Treatment is aimed at quickly reducing the body temperature and providing supportive care such as steroids and intravenous fluids. Prognosis is guarded to poor.

Ketosis (Pregnancy Toxemia)

Ketosis occasionally occurs in rabbits and in most cases is seen in obese does a few days prior to parturition. It is analogous to ketosis in guinea pigs and sheep in terms of etiology, treatment, and prevention. See the discussion on ketosis in Chapter 8, "Guinea Pigs."

Malocclusion

Tooth overgrowth results when open-rooted teeth are misaligned and therefore do not appropriately wear against other teeth or food items. Overgrowth is most commonly seen in the incisors. Mandibular prognathism, a common genetic condition in which the maxilla is abnormally short relative to the length of the mandible, causes the lower incisors to grow anterior instead of posterior to the large, primary upper incisors. Other causes of malocclusion include trauma and tooth root infection. Overgrowth of the cheek teeth may be underdiagnosed because of the difficulty in viewing these teeth. Use of an otoscope in a conscious rabbit or a dental bite block in a sedated rabbit allows improved visualization. A motorized dental bur or Dremel drill can be used to trim overgrown teeth. The use of nail clippers is best avoided because it can cause tooth fractures. Repeat trimming is indicated as needed, typically twice monthly to monthly. Culling of an affected animal and its offspring is the only successful means of eradication in a breeding group.

Moist Dermatitis

A moist dermatitis may occur in rabbits affecting either the area ventral to the dewlap or the anogenital region. Moisture from malocclusion-induced hypersalivation or the use of water bowls, and prolonged contact with urine or diarrhea in obese animals lend to colonization by a variety of opportunistic bacteria. Clipping and cleaning the affected areas and correction of environmental contributors will produce an uneventful resolution.

Splay Leg or Hip Dysplasia

Splay leg is an abnormality in which one or more limbs are abducted and cannot be maintained in a normal position. It may be caused by a recessive inherited trait although environmental conditions, including inappropriate flooring, can cause or contribute to the condition. The most common form is subluxation of the hip. Affected animals sit with their legs splayed out sideways. There is no effective treatment. Provision of flooring with good traction during the postnatal period is critical in preventing development of hip dysplasia in rabbits. Culling animals carrying this trait can help to reduce the incidence in a breeding colony.

Ulcerative Pododermatitis

Ulcerative pododermatitis is commonly called sore hock, but it actually involves the ventral metatarsal region rather than the hock. It usually occurs in heavy rabbits maintained on rounded wire-mesh floors rather than on flat-bar floors or in animals housed on solid floors that become urine soaked. The lesion consists of a circumscribed ulcerated area of the skin covered by a dry crusty scab. Abscesses, caused by organisms such as *S. aureus*, may form under the scab. Affected individuals may lose weight and sit in a hunched position or shift weight on their hind feet.

Treatment consists of providing soft, clean, dry bedding in a solid-bottom cage or providing a commercially available resting board. Animals should be limit-fed to prevent obesity, a contributing factor to the condition. Lesions may be treated by application of a topical ointment such as zinc oxide. A bandage affords protection against further trauma. If abscesses are present, broad-spectrum systemic antibiotics are indicated.

BIBLIOGRAPHY

Adam, H. K., J. B. Glen, and P. A. Hoyle. 1990. Pharmacokinetics in laboratory animals of ICI 35 868, a new I.V. anaesthetic agent. *Br J Anaesth* 52(8): 743–746.

Allen, D. G., J. K. Pringle, and D. A. Smith. 1993. *Handbook of Veterinary Drugs*. Philadelphia, PA: JB Lippincott.

Broome, R. L. and D. L. Brooks. 1991. Efficacy of enrofloxacin in the treatment of respiratory pasteurellosis in rabbits. *Lab Anim Sci* 41(6): 572–576.

Burgmann, P. and D. H. Percy. 1993. Antimicrobial drug use in rodents and rabbits. In *Antimicrobial Therapy in Veterinary Medicine*, J. F. Prescott and J. D. Baggot (eds.), pp. 524–541. Ames, IA: Iowa State University Press.

Carpenter, J. W., T. Y. Mashima, E. J. Gentz, and L. Harrenstien. 1995. Caring for rabbits: An overview and formulary. *Vet Med* (April): 340–364.

Diehl, K. H., R. Hull, D. Morton, et al. 2001. A good practice guide to the administration of substances and removal of blood, including routes and volumes. *J Appl Toxicol* 21: 15–23.

Difilippo, S. M., P. J. Norberg, U. D. Suson, et al. 2004. A comparison of xylazine and medetomidine in an anesthetic combination in New Zealand White rabbits. *Contemp Top Lab Anim Sci* 43(1): 32–34.

Dobromylskyj, P., P. A. Flecknell, B. D. Lascelles, et al. 2000. Management of postoperative and other acute pain. In *Pain Management in Animals*, P. Flecknell and A. Waterman-Pearson (eds.), pp. 81–145. London: WB Saunders.

Doerning, B. J., D. W. Brammer, C. E. Chrisp, and H. G. Rush. 1992. Nephrotoxicity of tiletamine in New Zealand White rabbits. *Lab Anim Sci* 42(3): 267–269.

Donnelly, T. M. 2005. Wet fur and dermatitis in a rabbit. *Lab Anim (NY)* 34: 23–25.

Flecknell, P. A. 1997. Medetomidine and atipamezole: Potential uses in laboratory animals. *Lab Anim (NY)* 26(2): 21–25.

Flecknell, P. A. 2009. *Laboratory Animal Anaesthesia*, 3d ed. London: Academic Press.

Flecknell, P. A. 2016. *Laboratory Animal Anaesthesia*, 4th ed. London: Academic Press.

Foley, P. L., A. L. Henderson, E. A. Bissonette, et al. 2001. Evaluation of fentanyl transdermal patches in rabbits: Blood concentrations and physiologic response. *Comp Med* 51(3): 239–246.

Gil, A. G., J. C. Illera, and G. Silvan. 2003. Effects of the anaesthetic/tranquillizer treatments on selected plasma biochemical parameters in NZW rabbits. *Lab Anim* 37(2): 155–161.

Gillett, C. S. 1994. Selected drug dosages and clinical reference data. In *The Biology of the Laboratory Rabbit*, 2nd ed., P. J. Manning, D. H. Ringler, and C. E. Newcomer (eds.), pp. 467–472. San Diego, CA: Academic Press.

Harcourt-Brown, F. M. 2002. *Textbook of Rabbit Medicine*. Oxford, UK: Butterworth-Heineman.

Harkness, J. E. and J. E. Wagner. 1995. *Biology and Medicine of Rabbits and Rodents*, 4th ed. Media, PA: Williams & Wilkins.

Harkness, J. E., P. V. Turner, S. VandeWoude, and C. L. Wheler. 2010. *Harkness and Wagner's Biology and Medicine of Rabbits and Rodents*, 5th ed. Ames, IA: Wiley-Blackwell.

Harrenstien, L. 1994. Critical care of ferrets, rabbits, and rodents. *Semin Avian Exotic Pet Med* 3: 217–228.

Heard, D. J. 1993. Principles and techniques of anesthesia and analgesia for exotic practice. *Vet Clin North Am Small Anim Pract* 23(6): 1301–1327.

Heard, D. J. 2009. Anesthesia, analgesia, and sedation of small mammals. In *Ferrets, Rabbits, and Rodents: Clinical Medicine and Surgery*, K. E. Quesenberry and J. W. Carpenter (eds.), pp. 356–365. St. Louis, MO: Saunders.

Hernandez-Divers, S. 2005. Rabbits. In *Exotic Animal Formulary*, J. W. Carpenter (ed.), pp. 409–444. St. Louis, MO: Elsevier Saunders.

Hillyer, E. V. 1994. Pet rabbits. *Vet Clin North Am Small Anim Pract* 24(1): 25–65.

Huerkamp, M. J. 1995. Anesthesia and postoperative management of rabbits and pocket pets. In *Kirk's Current Therapy XII: Small Animal Practice*, J. D. Bonagura (ed.), pp. 1322–1327. Philadelphia: WB Saunders.

Institute of Laboratory Animal Resources (ILAR). 2011. *Guide for the Care and Use of Laboratory Animals*, 8th ed. ILAR, National Research Council. Washington, DC: National Academies Press.

Jenkins, J. R. 1995. Rabbit drug dosages. In *Exotic Animal Formulary*, L. Bauck, T. H. Boyer, and S. A. Brown (eds.), pp. 13–17. Lakewood, CO: American Animal Hospital Association.

Johnson-Delaney, C. A. 1996. *Exotic Companion Medicine Handbook for Veterinarians*. Lake Worth, FL: Wingers.

Ko, J. C., J. C. Thurmon, W. J. Tranquilli, et al. 1992. A comparison of medetomidine–propofol and medetomidine–midazolam–propofol anesthesia in rabbits. *Lab Anim Sci* 42(5): 503–507.

Krempels, D., M. Cotter, and G. Stanzione. 2000. Ileus in domestic rabbits. *Exotic DVM* 2(4): 19–21.

Lipman, N. S., R. S. Marini, and S. E. Erdman. 1990. A comparison of ketamine/xylazine and ketamine/xylazine/acepromazine anesthesia in the rabbit. *Lab Anim Sci* 40(4): 395–398.

Marini, R. P., D. L. Avison, B. F. Corning, and N. S. Lipman. 1992. Ketamine/xylazine/butorphanol: A new anesthetic combination for rabbits. *Lab Anim Sci* 42(1): 57–62.

McKay, S. G., D. W. Mork, J. K. Merrill, et al. 1996. Use of tilmicosin for treatment of pasteurellosis in rabbits. *Am J Vet Res* 57: 1180.

Morrisey, J. K. and J. W. Carpenter. 2004. Formulary. In *Ferrets, Rabbits, and Rodents: Clinical Medicine and Surgery*, K. E. Quesenberry and J. W. Carpenter (eds.), pp. 436–444. St. Louis, MO: WB Saunders.

Morrisey, J. K. and J. W. Carpenter. 2011. Drug formulary. In *Ferrets, Rabbits, and Rodents: Clinical Medicine and Surgery*, K. E. Quesenberry and J. W. Carpenter (eds.), pp. 566–575. St. Louis, MO: WB Saunders.

Nicolau, D. P., C. D. Freeman, C. H. Nightingale, and R. Quintiliani. 1993. Pharmacokinetics of minocycline and vancomycin in rabbits. *Lab Anim Sci* 43(3): 222–225.

Nowland, M. H., D. W. Brammer, A. Garcia, and H. G. Rush. 2015. Biology and diseases of rabbits. In *Laboratory Animal Medicine*, 3rd ed. J. G. Fox, L. Anderson, G. Otto, K. Pritchett-Corning, and M. Whary (eds), pp. 411–461. Amsterdam: Academic Press

Okerman, L. 1994. *Diseases of Domestic Rabbits*, 2nd ed. Oxford: Blackwell Scientific.

Pariaut, R. 2009. Cardiovascular physiology and diseases of the rabbit. *Vet Clin North Am Exotic Anim Pract* 12: 135–144.

Paul-Murphy, J., and J. C. Ramer. 1998. Urgent care of the pet rabbit. *Vet Clin North Am Exotic Anim Pract* 1: 127–152.

Quesenberry, K. E. 1994. Rabbits. In *Saunders Manual of Small Animal Practice*, S. J. Birchard and R. G. Sherding (eds.), pp. 1345–1362. Philadelphia, PA: WB Saunders.

Raphael, B. L. 1981. Pet rabbit medicine. *Compend Contin Educ Pract Vet* 3: 60–64.

Robertson, S. A. and S. Eberhart. 1994. Efficacy of the intranasal route for administration of anesthetic agents to adult rabbits. *Lab Anim Sci* 44(2): 159–165.

Russell, R. J., D. K. Johnson, and J. A. Stunkard. 1981. *A Guide to Diagnosis, Treatment, and Husbandry of Pet Rabbits and Rodents*. Edwardsville, KS: Veterinary Medicine.

Smith, D. A. and P. M. Burgmann. 1997. Formulary. In *Ferrets, Rabbits, and Rodents: Clinical Medicine and Surgery*, E. V. Hillyer and K. E. Quesenberry (eds.), pp. 392–403. Philadelphia, PA: WB Saunders.

Stieve, M., H. Hedrich, H. Mojallal, P. Behrens, P. Müller, and T. Lenarz. 2008. Normative data of multifrequency tympanometry in rabbits. *Lab Anim* 42(3): 320–325.

Suckow, M. A., and F. Douglas. 1997. *The Laboratory Rabbit*. Boca Raton, FL: CRC Press.

Timm, K. I., and S. Jahn. 1980. Practical methodology of the rabbit. In *Practical Methodology* [slide series].

Vachon, P., J. Dupras, R. Prout, and D. Blais. 1999. EEG recordings in anesthetized rabbits: Comparison of ketamine–midazolam and Telazol with or without xylazine. *Contemp Top Lab Anim Sci* 38(3): 57–61.

Voyvoda, H., B. Ulutas, H. Eren, et al. 2005. Use of doramectin for treatment of sarcoptic mange in five Angora rabbits. *Vet Dermatol* 16(4): 285–288.

FURTHER READING

Aeschbacher, G., and A. I. Webb. 1993. Propofol in rabbits. 1. Determination of an induction dose. *Lab Anim Sci* 43(4): 324–327.

Baneux, P. J. and F. Pognan. 2003. In utero transmission of *Encephalitozoon cuniculi* strain type I in rabbits. *Lab Anim* 37(2): 132–138.

Brabb, T. and R. F. DiGiacomo. 2012. Viral diseases. In *The Laboratory Rabbit, Guinea Pig, Hamster, and Other Rodents*, M. A. Suckow, K. A. Stevens, and R. P. Wilson (eds.), pp. 365–400. San Diego, CA: Academic Press.

Britt, S., K. Cohen, and H. Sedlacek. 2012. Parasitic diseases. In *The Laboratory Rabbit, Guinea Pig, Hamster, and Other Rodents*, M. A. Suckow, K. A. Stevens, and R. P. Wilson (eds.), pp. 415–442. San Diego, CA: Academic Press.

Butt, M. T., R. E. Papendick, L. G. Carbone, and F. W. Quimby. 1994. A cytotoxicity assay for *Clostridium spiroforme* enterotoxin in cecal fluid of rabbits. *Lab Anim Sci* 44(1): 52–54.

Christensen, N. D. and X. L. W. Peng. 2012. Rabbit genetics and transgenic models. In *The Laboratory Rabbit, Guinea Pig, Hamster, and Other Rodents*, M. A. Suckow, K. A. Stevens, and R. P. Wilson (eds.), pp. 165–184. San Diego, CA: Academic Press.

Clifford, R. H., M. P. Ruth, and T. A. Liberati. 2003. 24-hour intravenous infusion via the marginal ear vein in the New Zealand White rabbit. *Contemp Top Lab Anim Sci* 42(5): 44–46.

Cranney, J. and Zajac, A. 1991. A method for jugular blood collection in rabbits. *Contemp Topics* 32 : 6.

Cundiff, D. D., C. L. Besch-Williford, R. R. Hook, et al. 1995. Characterization of cilia-associated respiratory bacillus in rabbits and analysis of the 16S rRNA gene sequence. *Lab Anim Sci* 45(1): 22–26.

Davis, H. and J. A. Gibson. 2000. Can rabbits tell humans apart?: Discrimination of individual humans and its implications for animal research. *Comp Med* 50(5): 483–485.

Delong, D. 2012. Bacterial diseases. In *The Laboratory Rabbit, Guinea Pig, Hamster, and Other Rodents*, M. A. Suckow, K. A. Stevens, and R. D. Wilson (eds.), pp. 303–347. San Diego, CA: Academic Press.

Flecknell, P. A. 1991. Postoperative analgesia in rabbits and rodents. *Lab Anim (NY)* 20: 34–37.

Flecknell, P. A., I. J. Cruz, J. H. Liles, and G. Whelan. 1996. Induction of anaesthesia with halothane and isoflurane in the rabbit: A comparison of the use of a face-mask or an anaesthetic chamber. *Lab Anim Sci* 30(1): 67–74.

Gil, A. G., G. Silván, M. Illera, and J. C. Illera. 2004. The effects of anesthesia on the clinical chemistry of New Zealand White rabbits. *Contemp Top Lab Anim Sci* 43(3): 25–29.

Guarniere III, V. J., D. G. Schabdach, D. A. Stock, and L. S. Keller. 1999. The effects of commercially available sodium pentobarbital formulations on plasma hemoglobin levels in New Zealand White rabbits. *Contemp Top Lab Anim Sci* 38(3): 54–56.

Halliday, L. C., J. E. Artwohl, C. Hanly, et al. 2000. Physiologic and behavioral assessment of rabbits immunized with Freund's complete adjuvant. *Contemp Top Lab Anim Sci* 39(5): 8–13.

Halliday, L. C., J. E. Artwohl, R. M. Bunte, et al. 2004. Effects of Freund's complete adjuvant on the physiology, histology, and activity of New Zealand White rabbits. *Contemp Top Lab Anim Sci* 43(1): 8–13.

Harris, L. D., L. B. Custer, E. T. Soranaka, et al. 2001. Evaluation of objects and food for environmental enrichment of NZW rabbits. *Contemp Top Lab Anim Sci* 1(40): 27–30.

Heavner, J. E. 2001. Anesthesia update: Agents, definitions, and strategies. *Comp Med* 51(6): 500–503.

Hedenqvist, P., H. E. Orr, J. V. Roughan, L. M. Antunes, and P. A. Flecknell. 2002. Anaesthesia with ketamine/medetomidine in the rabbit: Influence of route of administration and the effect of combination with butorphanol. *Vet Anaesth Anal* 29(1): 14.

Hubrecht, R. and J. Kirkwood. 2010. *The UFAW Handbook on the Care and Management of Laboratory and Other Research Animals*, 8th ed. Ames, IA: Wiley-Blackwell.

Johnson, C. A., W. A. Pallozzi, L. Geiger, et al. 2003. The effect of an environmental enrichment device on individually caged rabbits in a safety assessment facility. *Contemp Top Lab Anim Sci* 42(5): 27–30.

LaBreck, J. C., Y. H. An, and R. J. Friedman. 1998. Chronic use of propofol for multiple minor procedures in the rabbit. *Contemp Top Lab Anim Sci* 37(2): 84–85.

Lavin, L. M. 2007. Avian and exotic radiography. In *Radiography in Veterinary Technology*, 4th ed., pp. 294–301. St. Louis, MO: WB Saunders.

Lipman, N. S., Z-B. Zhao, K. A. Andrutis, et al. 1994. Prolactin-secreting pituitary adenomas with mammary dysplasia in New Zealand White rabbits. *Lab Anim Sci* 44(2): 114–120.

Lukas, V. 1999. Volume guidelines for compound administration. In *The Care and Feeding of an IACUC*, M. L. Podolsky and V. S. Lukas (eds.), p. 187. Boca Raton, FL: CRC Press.

Marini, R. P., X. Li, N. K. Harpster, and C. Dangler. 1999. Cardiovascular pathology possibly associated with ketamine/xylazine anesthesia in Dutch belted rabbits. *Comp Med* 49(2): 153–160.

Mctier, T. L., J. A. Hair, D. J. Walstrom, and L. Thompson. 2003. Efficacy and safety of topical administration of selamectin for treatment of ear mite infestation in rabbits. *J Am Vet Med Assoc* 223(3): 322–324.

Owiny, J. R., S. Vandewoude, J. T. Painter, et al. 2001. *Hip dysplasia in rabbits: Association with nest box flooring*. *Comp Med* 51(1): 85–88.

Peeters, J. E., R. Geeroms, H. Varewyck, et al. 1983. Immunity and effect of clopidol/methyl benzoquate and robenidine before and after weaning on rabbit coccidiosis in the field. *Res Vet Sci* 35(2): 211–216.

Percy, D. H. and S. W. Barthold. 2007. *Pathology of Laboratory Rodents and Rabbits*, 3rd ed. Ames, IA: Wiley-Blackwell.

Perkins, S. E., J. G. Fox, N. S. Taylor, et al. 1995. Detection of *Clostridium difficile* toxins from the small intestine and cecum of rabbits with naturally acquired enterotoxemia. *Lab Anim Sci* 45(4): 379–384.

Radi, Z. A. 2004. Outbreak of sarcoptic mange and malasseziasis in rabbits (*Oryctolagus cuniculus*). *Comp Med* 54(4): 434–437.

Shomer, N. H., S. Peikert, and G. Terwilliger. 2001. Enrichment-toy trauma in a New Zealand White rabbit. *Contemp Top Lab Anim Sci* 40(1): 31–32.

Smith, J. C., L. D. Robertson, A. Auhll, et al. 2004. Endotracheal tubes versus laryngeal mask airways in rabbit inhalation anesthesia: Ease of use and waste gas emissions. *Contemp Top Lab Anim Sci* 43(4): 22–25.

Steinleitner, A., H. Lambert, C. Kazensky, et al. 1990. Reduction of primary postoperative adhesion formation under calcium channel blockade in the rabbit. *J Surg Res* 48(1): 42–45.

Suckow, M. A., D. W. Brammer, H. G. Rush, and C. E. Chrisp. 2002. Biology and diseases of rabbits. In *Laboratory Animal Medicine*, 2nd ed., J. G. Fox, L. C. Anderson, and F. M. Lowe (eds.), pp. 329–364. San Diego, CA: Academic Press.

Suter, C., U. U. Muller-Doblies, J. M. Hatt, and P. Deplazes. 2001. Prevention and treatment of *Encephalitozoon cuniculi* infection in rabbits with fenbendazole. *Vet Rec* 148(15): 478–480.

Vachon, P. 1999. Self-mutilation in rabbits following intramuscular ketamine–xylazine–acepromazine injections. *Can Vet J* 40(8): 581–582.

Wagner, R. and U. Wendlberger. 2000. Field efficacy of moxidectin in dogs and rabbits naturally infested with *Sarcoptes* spp., *Demodex* spp. and *Psoroptes* spp. mites. *Vet Parasitol* 93(2): 149–158.

Weinstein, C. H., J. L. Fujimoto, R. E. Wishner, and P. O. Newton. 2000. Anesthesia of six-week-old New Zealand White rabbits for thoracotomy. *Contemp Top Lab Anim Sci* 39(3): 19–22.

CHAPTER 11 REVIEW

Short Answer

1. What are the three most common rabbit breeds used in research? Which ones are not albinos?
2. What is the Watanabe rabbit a model for and why?
3. In what way is rabbit dentition different from rodents?
4. What nutritional requirements do cecotrophs fulfill for rabbits?
5. How are heterophils different from the neutrophils seen in other species?
6. What are often present in the urine, causing it to appear cloudy?
7. True or False: Rabbits are induced ovulators, similar to cats and ferrets.
8. What behavior do female rabbits show approximately 3–4 days prior to giving birth?
9. True or False: Rabbit kits need to nurse every 2 hours for the first several weeks.
10. How do temperature requirements for rabbits differ from other species such as mice?
11. How can handlers prevent traumatic spinal fractures in rabbits?
12. What small blood vessel is easily accessible and useful for both blood withdrawal and intravenous injections?
13. What are the possible side effects of Freund's Complete Adjuvant?
14. Why are rabbits difficult to intubate?

(Continued)

Multiple Choice

15. Which of the following is a zoonotic agent?
    A. *Pasteurella multocida*
    B. *Treponema paraluiscuniculi*
    C. *Fransicella tularensis*
    D. *Clostridium spiroforme*
16. Which protozoa causes hepatic coccidiosis?
    A. *Eimeria magna*
    B. *Eimeria perforans*
    C. *Eimeria media*
    D. *Eimeria stediae*
17. What is the most common neoplasm of rabbits?
    A. Uterine adenocarcinoma
    B. Lymphosarcoma
    C. Bile duct adenoma
    D. Mammary adenocarcinoma
18. Which of the following is a reportable disease in the United States?
    A. Tyzzer's disease
    B. Rabbit hemorrhagic disease
    C. Rabbit papilloma virus
    D. Encephalitozoonosis
19. Which pathogen is associated with enteritis in 4–8-week-old kits?
    A. *Clostridium difficile*
    B. *Clostridium spiroforme*
    C. *Clostridium tetani*
    D. *Clostridium perfringens*
20. Which of the following is not due to a genetic mutation?
    A. Mandibular prognathism
    B. Splay leg
    C. Buphthalmia
    D. Sore hock

Critical Thinking

21. A new investigator is about to receive 6 New Zealand White rabbits in the 2.2–2.4 kg weight range. Rabbit cages with the following dimensions are available in the storage room: 21 in. in length, 18 in. in width, and 14 in. in height. Calculate the floor space available. Can these cages house the incoming rabbits?

12 Ferrets

The domestic ferret belongs to the order Carnivora and the family Mustelidae. Its scientific name is *Mustela putorius furo*, which appropriately translates into "stinky weasel thief." The domestic ferret is believed to be derived from the wild European polecat and is related to the skunk, weasel, otter, badger, and mink. The domestic ferret is a separate species from the native North American black-footed ferret, *Mustela nigripes*. There are two predominant varieties of domestic ferret based upon coat color and pattern: fitch (also known as sable or wild-type) and albino. The fitch, most commonly used in biomedical research, has a buff-colored coat with black mask, limbs, and tail. The albino, due to a recessive mutation, lacks all pigmentation and is therefore white with pink eyes. Male ferrets are referred to as hobs, females as jills, and the young as kits. A spayed female is a sprite and a neutered male is a gib, whereas a group of ferrets is called a business. Adult male ferrets weigh 1–2 kg; females are about half the size, weighing 0.5–1 kg.

USES

Although not used in large numbers for research, ferrets are valuable in a number of areas of study, including reproductive physiology, virus-induced neoplasms, bacterial infections, and viral diseases of humans and other animals. They have been particularly useful for studies of canine distemper, vesicular stomatitis, *Helicobacter pylori* gastritis, human influenza, and severe acute respiratory syndrome (SARS)–associated coronavirus. Ferrets have been used as an alternative carnivore for toxicology studies, replacing dogs and cats. Ferrets have a strong emesis (vomiting) response and thus are used to screen compounds for emetic potential. Because they have an oropharyngeal

Clinical Laboratory Animal Medicine: An Introduction, Fifth Edition.
Lesley A. Colby, Megan H. Nowland, and Lucy H. Kennedy.

Companion website: www.wiley.com/go/colby/clinical

anatomy similar to that of human infants, ferrets have also been used for neonatal intubation training.

BEHAVIOR

Ferrets are inquisitive, extroverted, and playful by nature. Most are docile and easily handled, particularly if acclimated to gentle handling when young, but may bite if excited, frightened, or hungry, or if handled only occasionally. Sexually intact males will fight with other males during the breeding season (periods of extended daylight hours), and females may defend their young. Ferrets are crepuscular and nocturnal, spending 15–20 hours per day sleeping; they are often slow to rouse when awakened. Similar to other mustelids, they engage in burrowing and digging behavior and prefer to use a nest box for seclusion and sleep. A corner or two of the cage is selected for urination and defecation; thus they may be trained to use a litter pan if this is preferred. Vocalizations include a chattering or screech, which occurs during playful activity; a hiss, which is used as a warning; and a whine, which may indicate discomfort. Ferrets will also emit a high-pitched scream in response to pain. During normal ambulation, the back is carried in an arched position, similar to other mustelids; a more horizontal carriage reflects clinical illness or pain, and it may result in mild ataxia. A shivering behavior may be noted, which is not clearly understood; however, it occurs most frequently when the ferret is awoken or excited and is regarded as normal behavior.

ANATOMIC AND PHYSIOLOGIC FEATURES

Ferret biologic and reproductive data are listed in Table 12.1. Ferrets have long, thin bodies with short legs, a medium-length tail, and thick, soft fur. Five clawed digits are present on all limbs; the nails are not retractable. Substantial seasonal fluctuations in weight are due to the accumulation of subcutaneous fat during the autumn months and its subsequent loss in the spring and summer. Significant sexual dimorphism, with males being larger than females, is evident (Figure 12.1). The albino coat color becomes tinged yellow as the ferret matures due to sebaceous secretions from the apocrine skin glands; these secretions are primarily responsible for the distinct musky odor. The ferret also has paired anal glands, one on either side of the anus, that are used for scent marking. If the animal becomes frightened, angry, or amorous, the glands may discharge their odiferous contents. It should be emphasized that descenting ferrets may reduce odor, especially in males, but will not eliminate it as the skin still produces the sebaceous secretions (Box 12.1).

Normal rectal temperature is in the range 38°–39°C (100°–102°F), but excitement may raise it to 40°C (104°F). Well-developed sweat glands are absent, and as a result these animals are prone to heat exhaustion at temperatures approaching 32°C (90°F). Heat is dissipated primarily through the respiratory system.

The dental formula, 2(I 3/3, C 1/1, P 3/3, M 1/2), is unique among carnivores, with three premolars per quadrant rather than the typical four. Supernumerary teeth are common in adults. They have a simple stomach similar to that of humans. The

Table 12.1. Biologic and reproductive data for ferrets

Adult body weight: Male	1–2 kg
Adult body weight: Female	0.5–1 kg
Life span	5–11 y
Body temperature	37.8°–40°C (100°-104°F)
Heart rate	200–400 beats per minute
Respiratory rate	33–36 breaths per minute
Food consumption	140–190 g/d (semimoist diet)
Water consumption	75–100 mL/d
Breeding onset: Male	8–12 mo
Breeding onset: Female	7–10 mo
Estrous cycle length	Continuous until intromission
Gestation period	42 + 2 d
Postpartum estrus	Occasional
Litter size	8, avg. (1–18 range)
Weaning age	6–8 wk
Breeding duration	2–5 y
Chromosome number (diploid)	40

Source: Adapted from Fox (1998).

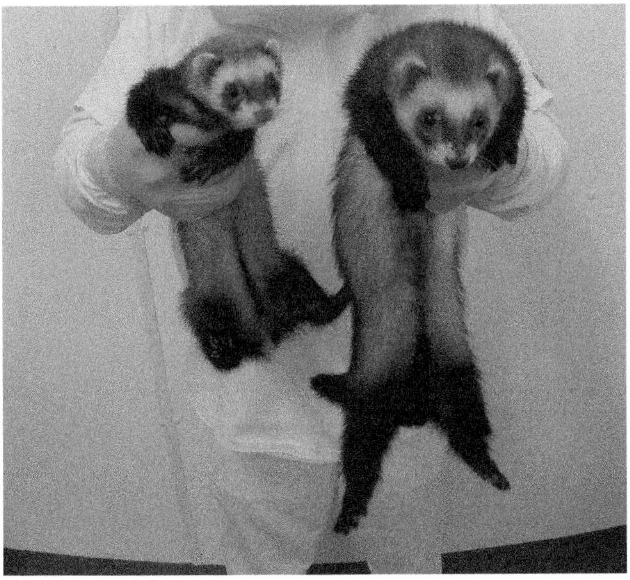

Fig 12.1. Male ferrets are significantly larger than female ferrets. (*Source:* Photo courtesy of Marshall BioResources.)

intestinal tract is short, having a transit time of 3–4 hours. There is no cecum, appendix, taeniae coli, or ileocolonic sphincter.

Ferrets have a very long trachea and large-diameter airways, which results in lower airway resistance. The lungs are relatively large compared with other small mammals, with approximately three times the lung capacity relative to their body size. Their

Box 12.1

Descenting ferrets may reduce odor, especially in males, but will not eliminate it as the skin still produces the sebaceous secretions.

lungs have two left lobes and four right lobes. Small, pale yellow, slightly elevated lesions may be seen on the surface of the lungs at necropsy; these are foci of alveolar histiocytosis and are of no known clinical significance. A single, brachiocephalic artery arising from the aortic arch is present in place of the bilateral common carotid arteries and may represent a functional adaptation to ensure cerebral blood flow when the head rotates 180°.

The reproductive systems of both males and females are similar to those of other carnivores, with a few exceptions. The female has a bicornate uterus with only one cervical os. Females have four pairs of mammary glands. Males retain open inguinal canals throughout their lives. During the nonbreeding season, August to November, spermatogenesis ceases, testicular size decreases, and the testes retract into the abdomen. Males lack seminal vesicles and a bulbourethral gland but do have a prostate gland and an os penis. Sexing of both adult and neonatal ferrets is accomplished without difficulty as the penis is situated on the ventral abdomen and the anogenital distance is greater in the male. The female vulva is readily visible just ventral to the anus.

There are several distinct characteristics of the physiologic and laboratory profiles of ferrets. Hematocrit values, hemoglobin levels, erythrocyte counts, and reticulocyte counts tend to be somewhat higher in ferrets than in other species of laboratory animals. The average values for males are slightly higher than for females in all except reticulocyte counts. Female ferrets in estrus tend to have lower platelet and leukocyte counts. Hematologic values may be altered by isoflurane anesthesia for both sexes, which should be a consideration in the interpretation of samples collected during or shortly after anesthesia. During the nonbreeding season, males have reduced plasma testosterone levels. The normal urine pH ranges between 6.5 and 7.5. Slight to moderate proteinuria is common. Males have naturally dark urine that may present difficulty in interpretation of urine chemistry tests using colorimetric methods. Hematologic and biochemical parameters for the ferret are listed in Appendix 1.

BREEDING AND REPRODUCTION

Ferrets normally reach sexual maturity in the spring after their birth or at approximately 9–12 months of age. The breeding season is light-dependent and in the Northern Hemisphere usually lasts from March to August for females and from December to July for males. Artificial illumination (16 hours light and 8 hours dark) can be used to produce an earlier onset of estrus for intensive breeding purposes.

Females are seasonally polyestrous and are induced ovulators. Marked swelling of the vulva, two to three times larger than the anestrous diameter, signals the start of estrus. Female ferrets that are not bred may remain in estrus for up to 6 months, which is characterized by weight loss, increased susceptibility to uterine infections, and aplastic anemia. Male sexual maturity precedes that of females to allow for sperm maturation. The enlargement and descent of the testicles into the scrotum marks the period of sexual activity in the male.

Mating should occur 2 weeks after the onset of vulvar swelling. The female should be taken to the male's cage and observed for fighting. Mating in ferrets is frequently noisy and energetic, with rolling, jumping, and the female submitting to being dragged around by the scruff of the neck. Leaving the pair together for 2 days is typical. Both neck restraint and intromission are required for ovulation, which occurs 30–40 hours after mating, with release of 5–13 ova. The female's enlarged vulva will regress to normal size quickly if she is pregnant, but slowly (5–6 days) if breeding was unsuccessful. Unlike other mustelids, delayed implantation does not occur in the ferret. The average gestation length is 42 days. Nonfertile matings result in a pseudopregnancy, which also lasts 42 days. Fetuses can be detected via ultrasound as early as 10 days, palpated by 14 days, or detected radiographically at 30 days. Females in estrus may be induced to ovulate via stimulation by other females, by vasectomized males, or by injections of human chorionic gonadotropin (hCG) or gonadotropin-releasing hormone (GnRH).

Jills should be single-housed and provided a nest box with bedding within 2 weeks of delivery. Appropriate bedding includes pieces of soft fabric or shredded paper. Litter size ranges from 1 to 18 kits with an average of 8. The young weigh approximately 8–10 g at birth and are altricial. Deciduous teeth erupt at 14 days; eyelids and external ear canals open at 28–35 days of age; and permanent canines erupt between 47 and 52 days. Kits begin eating solid food at about 3 weeks of age. They are weaned at 6–8 weeks and reach their adult weight at about 4 months. Weaned ferrets should be group-housed until sexually mature. Differences in size of males and females, due to sexual dimorphism, are apparent by week 7 and persist throughout life.

Depending on the time of year, the female will return to estrus about 2 weeks after the young are weaned or the following March. Jills can either be rebred or be administered hCG to terminate estrus. Ferrets can produce two to three litters per year if maintained on a stimulatory photoperiod and provided adequate nutrition.

HUSBANDRY

Housing and Environment

Ferrets can be housed in a variety of caging suitable to other small mammals, such as cats or rabbits. Care must be taken to modify caging to ensure secure containment of these smaller animals, known to be great escape artists. Solid-bottom cages are more suitable for their small feet than are those with slotted or wire mesh flooring. If wire mesh must be used, it should be 0.25 inch, and a sanitizable, commercially available resting board or platform can be placed in the cage to help protect the feet (Figure 12.2).

Adequate space must be provided to permit the animal to move around freely; a 24 in. × 24 in. × 18 in. cage is suitable to house a pair of adult ferrets. Hardwood chips or recycled paper products can be used in solid-bottom cages; a waste pan is employed under suspended cages with wire-grid floors. Ferrets seem to prefer a den or nest box

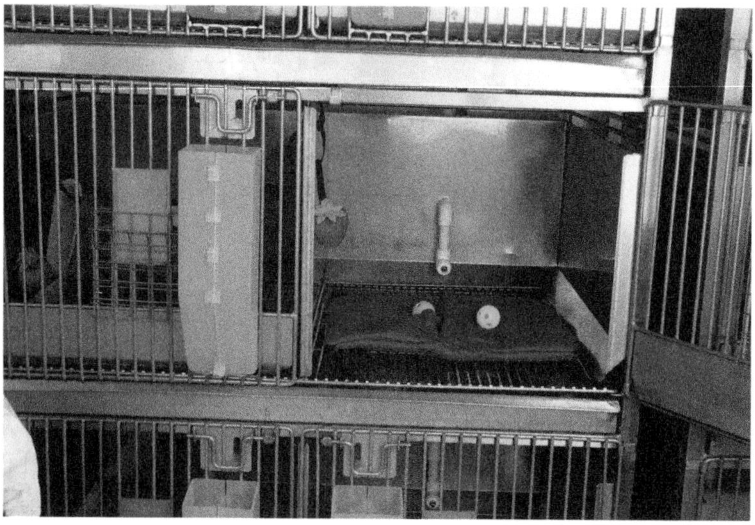

Fig 12.2. A typical ferret housing set up. (*Source:* Photo courtesy of Marshall BioResources.)

with a small entry hole and will use soft fleece materials commercially produced for the laboratory animal environment. Large-diameter PVC elbows and huts may also be used to provide an area of seclusion or as enrichment. Ferrets tolerate low temperatures without difficulty. A temperature range of 4°–18°C (39°–64°F) is generally optimal, but the young should not be kept at temperatures below 15°C (59°F). A humidity range between 40% and 65% and at least 10–15 air changes per hour are recommended. Photoperiods should be controlled through timed lighting and provide a 12:12 cycle of light and dark, with 14 hours of light for breeding animals.

Environmental Enrichment and Social Housing

Social housing is optimal for compatible animals of the same sex. Commercially available enrichment devices for ferrets include shaded polycarbonate huts, hammocks (Figure 12.3), PVC tunnels, certified items for gnawing or carrying, and balls that may be manipulated or filled with food treats designed for laboratory animal consumption. To stimulate their natural digging behavior, consider providing a box filled with an appropriate substrate such as rice, or crumpled paper. Due to their proclivity for gnawing and object ingestion, these items should be limited to those expressly designed for use with the ferret in a laboratory setting. Positive interaction with human handlers is also a viable form of enrichment. Release into a safe enclosure for periods of exercise is also a valuable addition to an enrichment program. Ferrets will readily use a shallow pool fashioned from common facility items (e.g., shoebox-style cages) for swimming activity; supervision should be provided.

Feeding and Watering

Ferrets are obligate carnivores and require a diet high in protein and fat and low in fiber. Commercially prepared, extruded diets intended for all life cycles are produced for use with laboratory ferrets and provide a guaranteed analysis of at least 38% protein (usually derived from chicken), 20.5% fat, and not more than approximately 4%

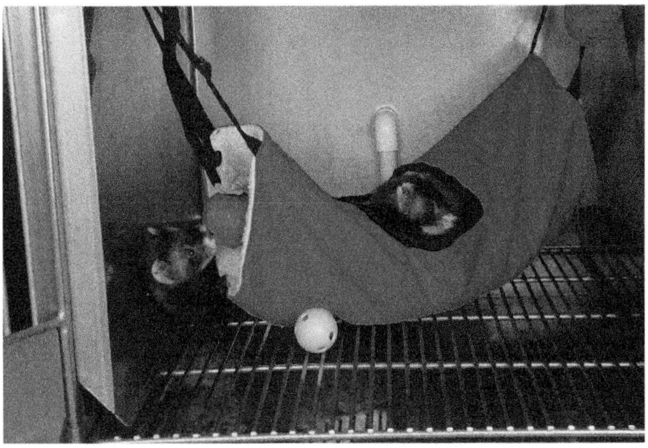

Fig 12.3. Fleece tube for enrichment and sleep. (*Source:* Photo courtesy of Marshall BioResources.)

fiber. These diets are available in a certified (screened for common environmental contaminants) or an irradiated form. Due to their high energy requirements, a documented range of 200–300 kcal per kg of body weight is required daily. Feeding is usually *ad libitum* and provided via a J-type feeder; these may require modification to prevent escape. Adult animals will consume approximately 6% of their body weight in feed daily. Due to their short gastrointestinal tract transit time, fasting over 3 hours is generally contraindicated and may result in hypoglycemia. Ferrets consume about 75–100 mL of water per day. They should have fresh, potable water available *ad libitum* via water bottles or an automated watering system.

Sanitation

Ferrets habitually use one or two corners of the cage for defecation and urination, and they can learn to use a litter pan, which should be cleaned daily and sanitized two to three times weekly. If used, direct bedding should be replaced as often as is necessary to keep the animals clean and dry; primary enclosures should be sanitized at least every 2 weeks. Water bottles are sanitized at least weekly and feeders every 1–2 weeks. Cages, water bottles, and feed hoppers should be disinfected with chemicals, hot water 61.6°–82.2°C (143°–180°F), or a combination of both. Detergents and chemical disinfectants enhance the effectiveness of hot water, but they must be thoroughly rinsed from all caging surfaces with fresh water. Refer to Chapter 3 for a more detailed description of disinfection methods.

TECHNIQUES

Handling and Restraint

Frequent, gentle handling of ferrets will promote tractability. They can be picked up from behind with one hand placed under the chest and the other supporting their hindquarters (Figure 12.4). Ferrets may be "tucked" into the crook of one's elbow for noninvasive procedures such as obtaining a rectal temperature.

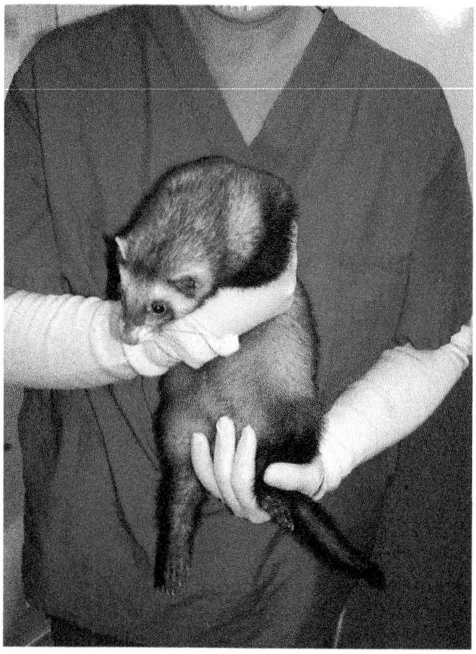

Fig 12.4. Restraint for carrying a ferret. (*Source:* Photo courtesy of C. Medina.)

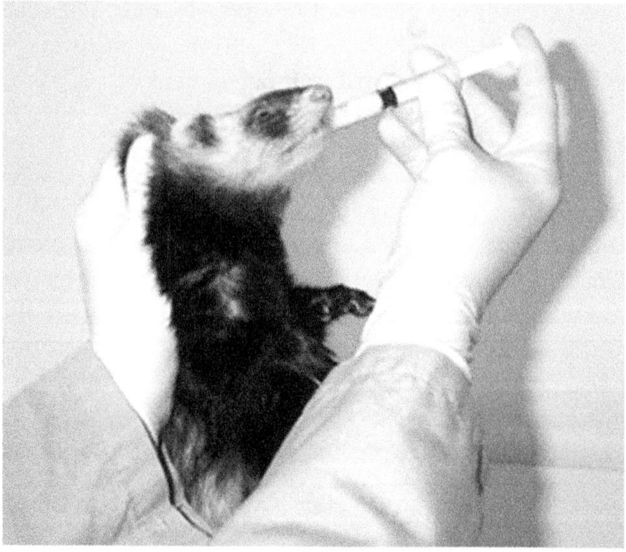

Fig 12.5. Oral dosing of a scruffed ferret. (*Source:* Photo courtesy of Marshall BioResources.)

Most ferrets can be manually restrained using exam gloves; gentle restraint is usually adequate for physical examinations. For more invasive procedures, one method is to scruff the loose skin at the nape of the neck with one hand (Figure 12.5), which appears to relax and immobilize ferrets. Scruffing will often induce a yawning behavior, which is considered a normal response. Most simple procedures, such as nail clipping, ear cleaning, chest auscultation, intramuscular and subcutaneous injections, and abdominal palpation can be performed using this technique. Another method is the placement of a hand across the shoulders with the thumb under the chin, the forefinger around the neck, and the other fingers around the chest caudal to the forelimbs. The other hand can be used to support the lower back. If a more secure hold is required, the other hand is placed around the pelvis cranial to the hind limbs. Ferrets should not be "stretched out" as doing so may cause them to vigorously resist. Ill animals or females with young may bite and should be handled with caution.

Identification

Cage cards may be used as a general means of identifying caged ferrets. Ear tags, ear punches, tattoos, or a subcutaneous microchip may be used for permanent identification of individual animals.

Blood Collection

Approximate blood volumes for ferrets are listed in Table 12.2. Assuming the animal is mature, healthy, and on an adequate plane of nutrition, the blood volume of most species averages 7% of the body weight in grams. A typical rule of thumb for blood withdrawal suggests that up to 10% of the circulating blood volume can be withdrawn every 2–3 weeks from normal, healthy animals with minimal adverse effect. Small amounts of blood, approximately 0.5 mL, can be obtained from the lateral saphenous or cephalic veins and can be accessed with a 25-gauge needle and tuberculin syringe. The superficial veins are not readily discernible and, for best success, the hair should be clipped and a small elastic tourniquet used.

The superficial caudal tail artery on the ventral side of the tail can be used to obtain blood from a restrained or sedated ferret. The hair should be clipped and the vessel dilated with warm water. Using a 22- to 25-gauge needle attached to a 3-mL syringe, the needle is inserted at a 30° angle to the skin about 2–3 mm caudal to the anus. The needle is advanced until it reaches the vertebra and then slowly withdrawn while aspirating until blood flows; 1–3 mL of blood may be collected from this site.

The jugular vein is the most accessible site for collection of larger blood volumes; up to 10 mL may be obtained via this route. For jugular access, the ferret can be restrained with the forelimbs held over the end of a table and the chin restrained upward, much like restraining a cat for the same procedure. Alternatively, the caudal approach can be used: with the animal in dorsal recumbency, grasp the scruff to extend the neck with one hand and use the other to restrain the forelimbs. Exceptionally

Table 12.2. Adult ferret blood volumes

	Volume (mL)
Total blood	60–120
Single sample	6–12
Exsanguination	24–60

Source: Adapted from Hillyer and Brown (1994).
Note: Values are approximate.

tractable animals may tolerate a gentle "towel and scruff" restraint while distracted with a nutritional supplement paste (e.g., Ferretone, Nutrical). For fractious ferrets, light sedation may be necessary. Clipping the fur and occluding the jugular at the thoracic inlet optimizes visualization of the vein. The cranial vena cava is an additional site that can be used to collect larger amounts of blood in a sedated or an anesthetized ferret, with an assistant to facilitate restraint. The animal is held in dorsal recumbency, with the head extended and the forelegs directed caudally. The needle is inserted between the first rib and the manubrium at a 45° angle to the body and directed toward the opposing rear limb, nearly to the hub. Aspirate as the needle is slowly withdrawn until blood enters and fills the syringe. This site carries a higher risk of hemorrhage and should be performed with caution.

Refinements in blood collection techniques include the use of a surgically placed vascular access port or an indwelling catheter. Although these have not been used extensively with ferrets, the technology is available and results in less repeated stress to ferrets and handlers. As with any intravascular device, aseptic technique and maintenance of patency with an appropriate anticoagulant flush are important.

Cardiac puncture can be used to collect a large terminal blood sample in anesthetized ferrets. The needle should be directed at the point of maximal heart beat intensity by palpation; it can be inserted either intercostally through the lateral chest wall or just lateral to the xiphoid process and directed craniodorsally at an approximately 30° angle into the heart.

Blood transfusions may be necessary for ferrets suffering from anemia of chronic disease, estrogen toxicity, or blood loss due to trauma or severe ulceration. Transfusions are usually indicated when the packed cell volume (PCV) falls below 15% for acute blood loss, below 12% with chronic disease, or below 25% for estrogen-induced anemia. There is a low risk of transfusion reaction, and there is no need to cross-match blood donors and recipients because ferrets have no detectable blood groups. Large male ferrets should be used as donors. To facilitate the blood collection process, administer atropine IM, then anesthetize the animal with isoflurane or sevoflurane via a face mask or an induction chamber. Approximately 10 mL of blood may be collected from an average male via the jugular vein or cranial vena cava. Blood should be collected into a syringe with an anticoagulant, at a ratio of 1 mL of CPDA-1 for 6 mL of blood. Fresh whole blood, 13–22 mL/kg, may be administered immediately at a rate of 0.25–0.5 mL/min.

Urine Collection

Urine may be collected using a metabolism cage, urinary catheter, cystocentesis, or by free catch. Urinary catheters can be placed in all hobs and most jills. A 3.5-French catheter is recommended, and sterile technique must be used. The urethral orifice of hobs is located on the ventral surface of the penis. Catheterization is easily accomplished but may require sedation or light anesthesia. To place a catheter in a jill, a vaginal speculum or otoscope is used to help visualize the urethral opening, which is about 1 cm cranial to the clitoral fossa.

The cystocentesis approach is similar to that used in cats, using ultrasound visualization, a 22-gauge needle, and a 3-mL syringe. The needle is introduced at a 90° angle just cranial to the pubic bone. Excited ferrets will often void on the table and samples can be used for simple dipstick urinalysis but cannot be used for culture.

Nail Trimming

Ferret nails are quite sharp, grow continuously, and should be kept trimmed to reduce the likelihood of scratches during restraint.

Drug Administration

Maximum dosing volumes are listed in Table 12.3. Oral dosing with palatable solutions is easy to accomplish by placing a syringe at the corner of the ferret's mouth and slowly depositing the liquid on the back of the tongue. As ferrets lack a cough reflex, caution is warranted in administration of compounds in a struggling animal. Unpalatable drugs can be given by an orogastric tube using a commercial bite block. The proper placement of the tube should always be verified by aspirating stomach contents or by placing the external end of the tube into a cup of water. If air is easily drawn into the syringe or bubbles are observed in the cup containing the submerged tube, it is likely in the trachea rather than the stomach. The maximum recommended volume for orogastric administration is 40 mL/kg.

Subcutaneous (SC) injections with a maximum volume of 20 mL/kg can be administered under the loose skin over the dorsum. Intramuscular (IM) injections with a maximum volume of 0.5 mL are given as in a dog or cat, in the semimembranosus or quadriceps thigh muscles. IM injections are easily administered when a ferret is scruffed or wrapped in a towel with a leg exposed. During the fall, allowance should be made for the thicker layer of subcutaneous fat, which may require a longer needle to deliver an injection. Placing a small amount of nutritional supplement paste (e.g., Nutrical or Ferretone) on their abdomen may provide a distraction for injections. Intraperitoneal (IP) injections with a maximum volume of 10 mL/kg can be administered just off of the midline in the lower abdominal quadrant. Care must be taken to aspirate before injecting the solution to ensure that the needle has not entered the bladder, bowel, or other organ. The cephalic or lateral saphenous veins can be used to deliver small volumes, 2 mL/kg, intravenously. Intravenous administration of larger volumes should be delivered at a maximum rate of 10 mL/kg either through a temporary indwelling catheter in the cephalic or saphenous veins or through a subcutaneous vascular access port supplying an indwelling catheter in the jugular vein.

Table 12.3. Maximum dosing volumes in ferrets

Route	Amount (mL/kg)
IP	10.0
SC	20.0
IM	0.5/site
IV	2.0 (bolus)/10.0 (infusion)[a]
PO	40.0

Source: Adapted from Harkness and Wagner (1995) and Lukas (1999).
[a] Infusion volumes are extrapolated from the R.M. Hull article (Hull, 1995) on guideline limit volumes, which states that generally the volume administration on a single occasion will be less than 10% of the circulating blood volume.

Immunization

Obtaining a vaccination history from the supplier for newly arrived ferrets is important to maintain immunity and not over-vaccinate. Only monovalent vaccines labeled for use in ferrets are recommended. Ferrets must be routinely protected against canine distemper by vaccination with a modified live vaccine. Kits should be vaccinated starting at 8 weeks of age, with two additional boosters given at 3-week intervals until 14 weeks, then annually. Hypersensitivity reactions ranging from skin erythema and pruritus to vomiting/diarrhea to anaphylaxis have been reported. As a precaution, it is prudent to observe the ferret for at least 15–20 minutes after vaccination. Diphenhydramine at 0.5–2.0 mg/kg IV or IM can be given prior to vaccination to prevent a repeat reaction or in response to clinical symptoms. Epinephrine (20 μg/kg IV, IM, or SC) and a short-acting corticosteroid such as dexamethasone sodium phosphate at 1–2 mg/kg IV or IM may also be used.

A killed rabies vaccine labeled for use in ferrets is available and should be administered at 3 months of age and annually thereafter. Vaccine reactions have also been observed but the incidence is markedly lower than with the canine distemper vaccine. Ferrets do not appear to be natural hosts for feline panleukopenia, canine parvovirus, canine parainfluenza virus, mink enteritis virus, transmissible mink encephalopathy, respiratory syncytial virus, or pseudorabies, although they have been experimentally infected with these agents.

Anesthesia, Surgery, and Postoperative Care

Agents commonly used for anesthesia and tranquilization in ferrets are listed in Table 12.4. Ferrets should not be fasted for longer than 3–6 hours due to rapid gastrointestinal tract transit time (3–4 hours) and physiology (Box 12.2). A number of injectable agents can provide adequate anesthesia for short procedures. Atropine at 0.05 mg/kg IM or SC or glycopyrrolate at 0.01 mg/kg IM or SC should be administered as a preanesthetic to reduce salivation and gastrointestinal secretions and to prevent bradycardia. The ketamine–acepromazine combination is safe and effective; however, it should be noted that the ketamine–xylazine combination has been associated with a significant number of premature ventricular contractions and death. It is advisable to use inhalant anesthetics rather than injectable agents in ill or debilitated animals. For optimal care a small induction chamber can be used to anesthetize a clinically ill animal, quickly intubate it, administer oxygen, and place an IV catheter to provide fluid support during an anesthetic procedure.

Inhalants, including isoflurane and sevoflurane, are safe and commonly used in ferrets; they are preferred for most surgical procedures as they provide rapid induction and recovery. Ferrets can be placed in a small induction chamber or masked for anesthetic induction. Premedication with acepromazine or other suitable sedative allows for an easier induction if a mask is used. Animals should be intubated with an uncuffed tube (2.0–3.5 mm internal diameter) for longer procedures. A degree of jaw tension is retained (and thus is not a good indicator of anesthetic depth); gauze may be used to retract the jaws to facilitate intubation. A topical anesthetic spray such as 2% lidocaine can be applied to help prevent laryngospasm. Due to their small body size, a nonrebreathing system should be used. Rate and depth of respiration, heart rate, and pedal and palpebral reflexes are useful in monitoring the depth of anesthesia.

Table 12.4. Anesthetic agents and tranquilizers used in ferrets

Drug	Dosage	Route	Reference
Inhalants			
Isoflurane	2%–5% to effect	Inhalation	Brown (1993)
Sevoflurane	To effect	Inhalation	Morrisey and Carpenter (2012)
Injectables			
Acepromazine	0.1–0.5 mg/kg	SC, IM	Morrisey and Carpenter (2012)
Diazepam	0.5–2 mg/kg	IM, IV	Morrisey and Carpenter (2012)
Fentanyl/droperidol	0.15 mL/kg	IM	Flecknell (1987)
Fentany/fluanisone	0.5 mL/kg	IM	Flecknell (2009)
Ketamine	30–60 mg/kg	IM	Fox (1998)
Ketamine	20–35 mg/kg	SC, IM	Hillyer and Brown (1994)
+ acetylpromazine	0.2–0.35 mg/kg	SC, IM	
Ketamine	25–35 mg/kg	IM	Brown (1993)
+ diazepam	2–3 mg/kg	IM	
Ketamine	4–8 mg/kg	IM	Flecknell (2009)
+ medetomidine	0.05–0.1 mg/kg	IM	
Ketamine	5 mg/kg	IM	Evans and Springsteen (1998)
+ medetomidine	0.08 mg/kg	IM	
+ butorphanol	1 mg/kg	IM	
Ketamine	5–10 mg/kg	IM, IV	Morrisey and Carpenter (2012)
+ midazolam	0.25–0.5 mg/kg	IM, IV	
Ketamine	10–25 mg/kg	IM	Hillyer and Brown (1994)
+ xylazine	1–2 mg/kg	IM	
Medetomidine	0.1–0.2 mg/kg	SC, IM	Morrisey and Carpenter (2012)
Medetomidine	0.08 mg/kg	IM	Ko and Heaton-Jones (1997)
+ butorphanol	0.1–0.2 mg/kg	IM	
Midazolam	0.25–0.5 mg/kg	SC, IM, IV	Morrisey and Carpenter (2012)
Propofol	3–6 mg/kg	IV	Morrisey and Carpenter (2012)
Tiletamine–zolazepam	12–22 mg/kg	IM	Payton and Pick (1989)
Tiletamine–zolazepam	3 mg/kg	IM	Ko et al. (1996)
+ ketamine	2.4 mg/kg	IM	
+ xylazine	0.6 mg/kg	IM	
Xylazine	1 mg/kg	SC, IM	Fox (1998)

IM = intramuscular; IV = intravenous; and SC = subcutaneous.

chapter 12

Box 12.2

Ferrets should not be fasted for longer than 3–6 hours due to rapid gastrointestinal tract transit time and physiology.

Table 12.5. Analgesic agents used in ferrets

Drug	Dosage	Route	Reference
Buprenorphine	0.01–0.03 mg/kg q8-12h	SC, IM, IV	Flecknell (2009)
Butorphanol	0.1–0.5 mg/kg q4-6h	IM, SC, IV	Cantwell (2001)
Carprofen	1 mg/kg q12-24h	PO	Morrisey and Carpenter (2012)
	4 mg/kg	SC	Flecknell (2009)
Flunixin meglumine	0.5–2 mg/kg q12-24h	SC	Flecknell (2009)
Ketoprofen	1–3 mg/kg q12-24h	PO, SC, IM	Morrisey and Carpenter (2012)
Meperidine	5–10 mg/kg q2-4h	SC, IM, IV	Heard (1993)
Meloxicam	0.1–0.2 mg/kg	SC, PO	Flecknell (2009)
Morphine	0.5–2 mg/kg q6h	SC, IM	Flecknell (2009)
Nalbuphine	0.5–1.5 mg/kg q2-3h	IM, IV	Heard (1993)
Oxymorphone	0.05–0.2 mg/kg q8-12h	IM, IV, SC	Heard (1993)
Pentazocine	5–10 mg/kg q4h	IM	Heard (1993)
Tramadol	5 mg/kg q12-24h	PO	Morrisey and Carpenter (2012)

IM = intramuscular; IV = intravenous; PO = per os; and SC = subcutaneous.

Commercial breeders typically neuter and descent ferrets at 3–4 weeks of age. Surgical approaches used in cats can be used in ferrets. Scrotal incisions with an open or closed technique can be used for castration. When performing an ovariohysterectomy (OHE), note that the ovarian pedicles normally contain large amounts of fat. Neutering reduces aggression in males and diminishes the musky scent released from the sebaceous skin glands by the action of estrogen and testosterone. An OHE prevents aplastic anemia caused by a prolonged state of estrus in the female. As in all animals, use of aseptic technique, prevention of hypothermia, and attention to hydration status increase the number of successful postoperative outcomes.

Analgesics should be administered for all surgical procedures unless there is scientific justification to withhold them, and as with humans and other mammals, preoperative administration of analgesics is preferred for optimal pain control. Acceptable analgesic agents for ferrets are listed in Table 12.5. Butorphanol is indicated to control mild postoperative discomfort. Buprenorphine works well to control acute or chronic visceral pain but causes more sedation. For musculoskeletal pain and inflammation, nonsteroidal anti-inflammatory drugs (NSAIDs) such as flunixin and carprofen work well in ferrets, but all NSAIDs may cause gastrointestinal upset and should be used with caution. It is particularly important that postprocedural care for ferrets ensure a rapid return to food and water intake due to rapid gastrointestinal tract transit time and to prevent a hypoglycemic state. Warmed lactated Ringer's and the use of a circulating water heating blanket will help ensure hydration and preservation of euthermia.

Imaging Techniques

Many imaging modalities once used only in humans [e.g., digital x-ray imaging, magnetic resonance imaging (MRI), computed tomography (CT), positron emission tomography (PET), x-ray absorptiometry (DEXA) scan, and ultrasound] have been adapted for use with laboratory animal species. For more detailed information regarding imaging in laboratory animals, please see Chapter 3.

Euthanasia

The most common and acceptable method of euthanasia for ferrets is the administration of an IV or IP overdose of a barbiturate or commercial euthanasia solution. Other acceptable methods include an overdose of inhalant anesthetic or IV administration of a supersaturated solution of potassium chloride (1–2 mmol/kg) bolus in conjunction with a surgical plane of anesthesia to induce cardiac arrest. All euthanasia methods must be in compliance with the current *AVMA Guidelines on Euthanasia* (AVMA, 2013).

THERAPEUTIC AGENTS

Antimicrobial and antifungal agents and their recommended dosages in ferrets are listed in Table 12.6. Antiparasitic agents for use in ferrets can be found in Table 12.7, and miscellaneous drugs and dosages for ferrets are listed in Table 12.8.

INTRODUCTION TO DISEASES OF FERRETS

Improvements in environmental quality as well as advanced understandings of both preventive medicine and husbandry programs for ferrets have resulted in healthier laboratory ferret colonies. Most ferrets today are relatively free of the variety of agents that cause clinical disease. However, a decreased incidence does not mean that infections will not occur, so it is imperative to be able to diagnose, treat, and control the spread of pathogenic agents if they are present. Presented here is a general overview of common bacterial, viral, fungal, and parasitic agents of ferrets and some standard diagnostic and treatment modalities.

Bacterial Diseases

Proliferative Bowel Disease

Lawsonia intracellularis is an intracellular campylobacter-like organism that causes proliferative bowel disease in numerous species, including ferrets, rabbits, hamsters, and pigs. Transmission is likely fecal–oral. The disease in ferrets, primarily seen in the young, is characterized by protracted intermittent diarrhea of greater than 6 weeks' duration, severe weight loss, rectal prolapse, and dehydration. Diarrhea is often green in color and may contain mucus or blood. In severe cases, ataxia and muscle tremors may occur.

Diagnosis is based upon clinical signs, a palpably thickened colon, and colonic biopsy with identification of the intracellular organisms via a silver stain. Mucosal thickening and glandular epithelial hyperplasia of the colon are characteristic histologic findings in ferrets, in contrast to hamsters and pigs, in which it is primarily in the ileum.

Several reports indicate that ferrets respond well to treatment with chloramphenicol at 50 mg/kg twice daily or metronidazole at 20 mg/kg twice daily for 2 weeks. Ferrets must also receive supportive care, including parenteral fluids and nutritional support for the best outcome. Severe cases may occasionally result in death despite supportive care.

Table 12.6. Antimicrobial and antifungal agents used in ferrets

Drug	Dosage	Route	Reference
Amikacin	10–15 mg/kg q12h	SC, IM	Brown (1993)
Amoxicillin	20 mg/kg q12h	PO, SC	Hillyer and Brown (1994)
Amoxicillin	10 mg/kg q12h	PO	Hoefer and Bell (2012)
+ metronidazole	20 mg/kg q12h	PO	
+ bismuth subsalicylate	1 mL/kg q12h for 14 d	PO	
Amoxicillin-clavulanate	13–25 mg/kg q8-12h	PO	Hillyer and Brown (1994)
Amphotericin B	0.4–0.8 mg/kg q7d (total dose 7–25 mg)	IV	Besch-Williford (1987)
Ampicillin	5–30 mg/kg q8-12h	SC, IM, IV	Morrisey and Carpenter (2012)
Cefadroxil	15–20 mg/kg q12h	PO	Brown (1995)
Cephalexin	15–30 mg/kg q8h	PO	Hillyer and Brown (1994)
Clarithromycin	12.5–25 mg/kg q12h	PO	Morrisey and Carpenter (2012)
Clarithromycin	12.5 mg/kg q8h	PO	Marini et al. (1999)
+ ranitidine	24 mg/kg q8h for 14 d	PO	
Chloramphenicol	50 mg/kg q12h	PO, SC, IM, IV	Hillyer and Brown (1994)
Ciprofloxacin	10 mg/kg q12h	PO	Brown (1995)
Clindamycin	5.5–10 mg/kg q12h	PO	Brown (1995)
Cloxacillin	10 mg/kg q6h	PO, IV, IM	Johnson-Delaney (1996)
Enrofloxacin	5–10 mg/kg q12h	PO, SC, IM	Brown (1995)
Erythromycin	10 mg/kg q6h	PO	Besch-Williford (1987)
Gentamicin	2–4 mg/kg q12h	SC, IM	Brown (1999)
Griseofulvin	25 mg/kg q24h	PO	Hillyer and Brown (1994)
Ketaconazole	10–30 mg/kg q8h	PO	Besch-Williford (1987)
Lincomycin	11 mg/kg q8h	PO	Besch-Williford (1987)
Metronidazole	50 mg/kg q24h	PO	Collins (1995)
Neomycin	10–20 mg/kg q6h	PO	Besch-Williford (1987)
Oxytetracycline	20 mg/kg q8h	PO	Besch-Williford (1987)
Penicillin, procaine	40,000–44,000 IU/kg q24h	SC	Morrisey and Carpenter (2012)
Sulfadimethoxine	30–50 mg/kg q12-24h	PO	Collins (1995)
Sulfamethazine	1 mg/mL drinking water		Collins (1995)
Tetracycline	25 mg/kg q12h	PO	Morrisey and Carpenter (2012)
Trimethoprim-sulfa	15–30 mg/kg q12h	PO, SC	Hillyer and Brown (1994)
Tylosin	10 mg/kg q8-12h	PO	Collins (1995)
	5–10 mg/kg q12h	IM, IV	Collins (1995)

IM = intramuscular; IV = intravenous; PO = per os; and SC = subcutaneous.

Table 12.7. Antiparasitic agents used in ferrets

Drug	Dosage	Route	Reference
Amitraz	0.3% solution q7–14d for 3–6 treatments	Topical	Morrisey and Carpenter (2012)
Amprolium	19 mg/kg q24h	PO	Brown (1999)
Carbaryl (5%)	Once weekly for 3–6 wk	Topical	Fox (1998)
Fenbendazole	20 mg/kg q24h for 5 d	PO	Morrisey and Carpenter (2012)
Fipronil	1 pump of spray or 1/5 of cat tube q60d	Topical	Morrisey and Carpenter (2012)
	0.2–0.4 mL q30d		Williams (2000)
Imidacloprid	1 cat dose q30d	Topical	Morrisey and Carpenter (2012)
Ivermectin	0.4 mg/kg, repeat in 2–4 wk	PO, SC	Hillyer and Brown (1994)
	0.05 mg/kg/mo	PO	Hillyer and Brown (1994)
	0.5 mg/kg, half dose in each ear, repeat in 2 wk	Topical	Hillyer and Brown (1994)
Lufenuron	30–45 mg/kg q30d	PO	Morrisey and Carpenter (2012)
Melarsomine dihydrochloride	2.5 mg/kg once, repeat in 30 d with 2 treatments 24 h apart	IM	Brown (1999)
Metronidazole	15–20 mg/kg q12h for 2 wk	PO	Brown (1993)
Milbemycin oxime	1.15–2.3 mg/kg/mo	PO	Johnson-Delaney (1996)
Piperazine citrate	50–100 mg/kg repeat in 14 d	PO	Morrisey and Carpenter (2012)
Praziquantel	5–10 mg/kg, repeat in 10–14 d	SC, PO	Morrisey and Carpenter (2012)
Pyrantel pamoate	4.4 mg/kg repeat in 2 wk	PO	Brown (1993)
Pyrethrin powder	Once weekly for 3 wk	Topical	Fox (1998)
Selmectin	6 mg/kg	Topical	Morrisey and Carpenter (2012)
Sulfadimethoxine	30–50 mg/kg q12–24h	PO	Collins (1995)

IM = intramuscular; PO = per os and SC = subcutaneous.

Helicobacter spp. Infection

Nearly 100% of ferrets are infected with *H. mustelae* shortly after weaning. Most animals remain asymptomatic. Fecal–oral transmission is likely. The organism can infect young ferrets as early as 5–6 weeks of age. Those ferrets that become clinically affected develop gastritis and gastroduodenal ulcers; observable signs include vomiting, weight loss, and melena. Gastroduodenal ulcers can hemorrhage, resulting in a large amount of blood loss; this should be treated as an emergency, providing supportive care and blood transfusions as necessary. Gastric adenocarcinoma may occur secondary to infection and also may present with vomiting, anorexia, and weight loss.

Diagnosis is challenging but can be accomplished by mucosal biopsy and endoscopy. *H. mustelae* can be cultured in a microaerobic atmosphere to allow identification of the organism by Gram-stain and morphology, as well as resistance or sensitivity to antibiotics. There are a few treatment regimens that require multidrug, multiday dosing including a 7–10-day regimen of triple therapy: oral amoxicillin (30 mg/kg) and metronidazole (20 mg/kg) combined with bismuth-subsalicylate (17.5 mg/kg) three times a day for 3–4 weeks. Cimetadine and sucralfate may also be administered to

Table 12.8. Miscellaneous agents used in ferrets

Drug	Dosage	Route	Reference
Activated charcoal	1–3 g/kg	PO	Richardson and Balabuszko (2001)
Aminophylline	4.4–6.6 mg/kg q12h	PO, IM	Hillyer and Brown (1994)
Anastrazole	0.1 mg/kg q24h	PO	Weiss et al. (1999)
Apomorphine	5 mg/kg	SC	Besch-Williford (1987)
Atenolol	6.25 mg per animal q24h	PO	Brown (1995)
Atipamezole	1 mg/kg	SC, IP, IV	Flecknell (1997)
Atropine	0.04 mg/kg	SC, IM, IV	Hillyer and Brown (1994)
	5–10 mg/kg (organophosphate toxicity)	SC, IM	Brown (1995)
Azathiprine	0.9 mg/kg q24-72h	PO	Burgess and Garner (2002)
Barium (20%)	15 mL/kg	PO	Hillyer and Brown (1994)
Bicalutamide	5 mg/kg q24h	PO	Weiss and Scott (1997)
Bismuth-subsalicylate (Pepto-Bismol)	0.25 mL/kg q4-6h	PO	Hillyer and Brown (1994)
Calcium EDTA	20–30 mg/kg q12h	SC	Morrisey and Carpenter (2012)
Captopril	1/8 of 12.5 mg tablet per animal q48h, increase to q12-24h	PO	Hillyer and Brown (1994)
Chlorpheniramine	1–2 mg/kg q8-12h	PO	Hillyer and Brown (1994)
Cimetidine	10 mg/kg q8h	PO, IV	Hillyer and Brown (1994)
Cisapride	0.5 mg/kg q8-12h, increase to 1 mg/kg if needed	PO	Morrisey and Carpenter (2012)
Dexamethasone	0.5–2 mg/kg	SC, IM, IV	Brown (1995)
Diazoxide	10 mg/kg/d or divided q8-12h	PO	Hillyer and Brown (1994)
Digoxin	0.005–0.01 mg/kg q12-24h	PO	Brown (1995)
Diltiazem	3.75–7.5 mg per animal q12h	PO	Brown (1995)
Diphenhydramine	0.5–2 mg/kg q8-12h	PO, IM, IV	Brown (1995)
Doxapram	5–10 mg/kg	IV, IM, IP	Flecknell (2009)
Enalapril	0.25–0.5 mg/kg q24-48h	PO	Brown (1995)
Epinephrine	0.02 mg/kg	SC, IM, IV, IT	Morrisey and Carpenter (2012)
Epoetin alfa	50–150 IU/kg	PO, IM	Brown (1995)
Famotidine (Pepcid)	0.25–0.5 mg/kg q24h	SC, PO, IV	Brown (1999)
Flutamide	10 mg/kg q12-24h	PO	Brown (1999)

Table 12.8. (*Continued*)

Drug	Dosage	Route	Reference
Furosemide	2 mg/kg q8-12h	PO, SC, IM, IV	Hillyer and Brown (1994)
Glycopyrrolate	0.01 mg/kg	IM	Heard (1993)
Gonadotropin-releasing hormone	20 μg/animal, repeat in 2 wk prn	SC, IM	Hillyer and Brown (1994)
Hairball laxative, feline	1–2 mL/animal q48h	PO	Brown (1993)
Heparin	200 IU/kg q12h for 5 d	SC, IM	Hillyer and Brown (1994)
Human chorionic gonadotropin	100 IU per animal, repeat in 1–2 wk prn	IM	Hillyer and Brown (1994)
Hydrocortisone sodium succinate	25–40 mg/kg	IV	Besch-Williford (1987)
Hydroxyzine	2 mg/kg q8h	PO	Morrisey and Carpenter (2012)
Insulin, NPH	0.5–6 IU/kg or to effect	SC	Besch-Williford (1987)
Iron dextran	10 mg/kg once	IM	Morrisey and Carpenter (2012)
Kaolin-pectin	1–2 mL/kg q2-6h prn	PO	Johnson-Delaney (1996)
Lactulose syrup	0.15–0.75 mg/kg q12h	PO	Brown (1999)
Leuprolide acetate	0.1 mg/animal <1 kg q4-6 wk	IM	Johnson-Delaney (1996)
	0.2 mg/animal >1 kg q4-6 wk	IM	Johnson-Delaney (1996)
Loperamide	0.2 mg/kg q12h	PO	Brown (1999)
Megestrol acetate	Do not use, predisposes ferret to pyometra		Johnson-Delaney (1996)
Melatonin	0.5–1 mg/animal q24h prn	PO	Paul-Murphy (2001)
Metaclopramide	0.2–1 mg/kg q6-8h	PO, SC, IM	Morrisey and Carpenter (2012)
Mitotane	50 mg per animal q24h for 7 d, then q72h	PO	Hillyer and Brown (1994)
Naloxone	0.04–1 mg/kg	IM, SC, IV	Dobromylskyj et al. (2000)
Nitroglycerin 2% ointment	1/16–1/8 inch per animal q12-24h		Brown (1993)
Omeprazole	0.7 mg/kg q24h	PO	Fox (1998)
Oxyglobin	6–15 mL/kg over 4h	IV	Orcutt (2001)
Oxytocin	0.2–3 IU/kg	SC, IM	Brown (1993)
Prednisone	0.6 mg/kg q24h, gradually taper dose	PO	Besch-Williford (1987)
Prednisolone sodium succinate	22 mg/kg	IV	Hillyer and Brown (1994)
Propanolol	0.2–1 mg/kg q8-12h	PO	Hillyer and Brown (1994)

(*Continued*)

Table 12.8. (Continued)

Drug	Dosage	Route	Reference
Prostaglandin	0.1–0.5 mg per animal	IM	Brown (1999)
Ranitidine bismuth	24 mg/kg q8h	PO	Burke (1988)
Ranitidine HCl	3.5 mg/kg q12h	PO	Burke (1988)
Stanozolol	0.5 mg/kg q12h	PO, SC	Brown (1993)
Sucralfate	1/8 of 1 g tablet per animal q6h	PO	Hillyer and Brown (1994)
Theophylline elixir	4.25 mg/kg q8-12h	PO	Johnson-Delaney (1996)
Thyroxin	0.2–0.4 mg/kg q12-24h	PO	Johnson-Delaney (1996)
Vitamin B complex	1–2 mg/kg prn	SC, IM	Morrisey and Carpenter (2012)
Yohimbine	0.2–1 mg/kg	IM, IV	Morrisey and Carpenter (2012)

IM = intramuscular; IV = intravenous; IP = intraperitoneal; PO = per os; and SC = subcutaneous.

increase stomach pH and coat ulcers, respectively. Sucralfate requires an acidic pH to function properly and therefore must be administered at least 2 hours prior to cimetidine administration. Alternatively, ranitidine bismuth (24 mg/kg) and clarithromycin (12.5 mg/kg) dosed orally three times per day for 2 weeks has resulted in eradication of the organism. Another reportedly efficacious regimen includes oral clarithromycin (50 mg/kg) once daily and oral amoxicillin (35 mg/kg) once daily for 2 weeks. In addition, both omeprazole (0.7 mg/kg, orally, once daily) and cimetidine (10 mg/kg, orally, three times per day) can be given to ferrets to reduce acid secretions. Ferrets proven free of *H. mustelae* infections are available commercially.

Campylobacteriosis

Campylobacter jejuni is a Gram-negative, spiral bacterium associated with enteritis and diarrhea in humans and many different animals, including dogs, cats, pigs, cows, goats, sheep, and ferrets. The organism, however, has also been isolated from asymptomatic ferrets. *C. jejuni* has been identified in zoonotic disease outbreaks in people recently in contact with young puppies or kittens that had diarrhea. Transmission is fecal–oral through direct contact or by ingestion of contaminated food and water. Experimental oral inoculation of the organism to young ferrets resulted in a self-limiting, mild to watery, mucinous diarrhea, with anorexia, dehydration, and/or tenesmus developing in some animals. Experimental inoculation of pregnant females has resulted in reproductive failure. Diagnosis depends on clinical signs and culture of affected animals. *C. jejuni* has special culture requirements, including thermophilic and microaerophilic conditions. Ferrets with known *C. jejuni* infection should be isolated to control spread, provided supportive care, and given antibiotics based on culture and sensitivity.

Salmonellosis

Salmonella spp. are Gram-negative rod-shaped bacteria associated with bloody diarrhea in humans and animals. Transmission is fecal–oral through direct contact or by ingestion of contaminated feed or water. Clinical cases have been rare, but several serotypes have been isolated from the feces of ferrets in a research colony. Typical clinical signs include melena anorexia, dehydration, and weight loss; abortion may be induced in pregnant females. Diagnosis is based on clinical signs and culture of the organism. Treatment includes antibiotic and fluid therapy, nutritional support, and reduction of stress. Due to the public health significance of this zoonotic organism, infected animals must be handled with caution and may be culled in lieu of treatment.

Tuberculosis

Ferrets are highly susceptible to certain avian, bovine, and human strains of the Gram-positive, acid-fast *Mycobacterium* spp. Most reports of this disease occurred in the early 1900s and were probably associated with the feeding of infected raw meat. Today, the risk of tuberculosis infections in US ferret research colonies is extremely low due to its relatively low incidence in humans and agricultural animals. However, as tuberculosis is recognized as a reemerging disease in humans, the incidence of infections in ferrets could increase. The organism can be transmitted by inhalation, ingestion, or wound infection. The body system affected (e.g., gastrointestinal, respiratory, lymphatic) is heavily influenced by the infecting *Mycobacterium* spp. Tuberculosis should be suspected in cases of lymphomegaly, especially in the mesentery. Definitive diagnosis requires isolation and identification of the organism. A subcutaneous tuberculin test regimen has not been defined for ferret use. Infected ferrets should be euthanized due to the zoonotic potential.

Mastitis

Staphylococcus aureus, *Streptococcus* spp., and hemolytic *Escherichia coli* are frequently associated with mastitis in nursing jills. Transmission is most likely associated with a contaminated environment, trauma from nursing kits, and stress of lactation. The acute form occurs within the first few weeks following parturition. Clinical signs include swollen, darkened, painful glands that may become gangrenous and proceed to septicemia and death. The chronic form develops as a sequela to the acute form or approximately 3 weeks after parturition and is characterized by firm mammary glands. Initial treatment includes the administration of analgesics as well as a broad-spectrum antibiotic (e.g., enrofloxacin, 2.5 mg/kg orally twice a day) that may then be refined based on culture and antibiotic sensitivity testing of the milk. Surgical debridement of the affected glands may be necessary for gangrenous lesions. Kits may need to be supplemented with milk replacer or cross-fostered because jills are often too painful to nurse. Antibiotic treatment of the kits is also warranted.

Pneumonia

Ferret pneumonia has been associated with a primary or secondary infection of multiple bacterial organisms, including *Streptococcus zooepidemicus*, *Streptococcus pneumoniae*, *Klebsiella pneumoniae*, and *Pseudomonas aeruginosa*. Noninfectious primary causes of pneumonia include megaesophagus or the accidental dosing of substances into the lungs during oral gavage. Clinical signs may include nasal discharge, dyspnea, increased lung sounds, anorexia, and pyrexia. Diagnosis is made by a combination of clinical signs, hematology, radiographs, and culture of tracheal wash. Treatment of this potentially fatal disease includes appropriate antibiotics, oxygen, fluids, and nutritional support.

Miscellaneous Bacterial Infections

Vaginitis is common in the female during estrus, especially when housed on hay or straw as the bedding may stick to the swollen vulva or enter the vagina and act as a nidus for a secondary bacterial infection. *Staphylococcus* spp. and *Streptococcus* spp. have been cultured from bite wound abscesses resulting from fighting or mating. Treatment of localized infections includes the administration of antibiotics (based on culture and sensitivity assays) and may require lancing.

Mycotic Diseases

Dermatophytosis (Ringworm)

Dermatophytosis caused by both *Microsporum canis* and *Trichophyton mentagrophytes* has been reported in ferrets, with cases involving *M. canis* predominating. Both zoonotic and interspecies disease transmission can occur. In ferrets, this fungal infection primarily affects young or older, immunosuppressed animals. Infection is influenced by geographic location and/or climate as cases are more frequently reported in the southern United States. Transmission is by direct contact or fomites, such as infected bedding. Ferrets housed in overcrowded or unsanitary conditions are predisposed to developing the disease. Clinically, ferrets may exhibit the typical ringlike lesions of alopecia and inflammation on any part of their body. Crusting and erythema may be evident, and pruritus may lead to scratching and secondary bacterial infections.

A tentative diagnosis may be based on typical clinical signs, but a fungal culture of the skin or hair or examination of a skin scraping partially digested with 10% KOH is needed to confirm the diagnosis. Use of a Wood's lamp is of limited diagnostic value as less than 50% of *M. canis* isolates and no *T. mentagrophytes* isolates fluoresce under UV light. Treatment consists of shaving the hair around the lesions, cleaning the affected animal with keratolytic baths and povidone iodine scrubs, and then applying topical antifungal ointments. Griseofulvin may also be administered per os at 25 mg/kg/day for 21–30 days, but this treatment is rarely needed. Environmental decontamination is important.

Viral Diseases

Canine Distemper

Distemper is a significant disease of ferrets due to their high susceptibility to canine distemper virus and an approximately 100% case mortality rate (Box 12.3). Transmission of the paramyxovirus is usually by aerosols or fomites, with an average incubation period of 7–9 days. Two disease phases may develop: a catarrhal phase and a neurological phase. In the catarrhal phase, infected ferrets initially develop anorexia,

> **Box 12.3**
>
> *Distemper is a significant disease of ferrets due to their high susceptibility to the disease and an approximately 100% case mortality rate.*

a serous-to-mucopurulent nasal and ocular discharge, and a rash beneath the chin and in the inguinal region. Edematous, hyperkeratotic footpads, and anal prolapse may later develop. Ferrets that survive the catarrhal phase may die in a neurotropic episode with hyperexcitability, hypersalivation, muscular tremors, convulsions, and coma. As treatment is usually unsuccessful, and death commonly occurs within 2–5 weeks of disease exposure, euthanasia is recommended over symptomatic supportive therapy. A suggestive diagnosis is based on clinical observations, known or suspected viral exposure, and a history of no prior vaccination. Confirmatory diagnosis is based on the observation of eosinophilic, intracytoplasmic, and intranuclear inclusions of tracheal, bronchial, epithelial, and bile duct tissues with Pollack's trichrome stain. Young ferrets should be routinely vaccinated for the disease at a frequency recommended by the vaccine manufacturer. Animal caretakers who have young puppies or work with dogs not vaccinated against canine distemper virus should not be assigned to care for ferrets.

Human Influenza

Ferrets are susceptible to several strains of human influenza virus, an orthomyxovirus. Influenza viruses are transmitted by aerosols, are highly infectious, and may cause initial signs similar to those of distemper. Within 48 hours of exposure, ferrets become listless and anorexic and develop a sharp rise in rectal temperature. Sneezing attacks occur and may be accompanied by a mucoserous nasal discharge. Ferrets may also develop conjunctivitis, photosensitivity, and otitis. Uncomplicated clinical disease usually largely resolves in approximately 4–5 days although disease complicated by a secondary bacterial pneumonia or in an immunocompromised animal may persist for multiple weeks. Recovery by day 4 differentiates uncomplicated influenza infection from the early stages of distemper. Congestion may be relieved by use of antihistamines. Cough suppressants may also be helpful for symptomatic relief. Influenza viruses may be freely transmitted between humans and ferrets. Animal caretakers with upper respiratory infections should wear respiratory protection and gloves when handling ferrets, and exercise extreme caution with neonatal kits, which are especially susceptible to the disease.

Aleutian Disease

Ferrets are susceptible to Aleutian disease virus (ADV), the parvovirus that causes Aleutian disease (AD) in mink. In contrast to the disease in mink, AD usually progresses slowly in ferrets. Infection may be subclinical for years; infected animals may serve as a source of infection for other ferrets during this time. ADV induces an immune-mediated disease in which a robust humoral immune response is stimulated, generating an overwhelming number of antigen–antibody complexes that then deposit in tissues, resulting in systemic vasculitis. Transmission is by direct contact, fomites, or via aerosol of saliva, urine, blood, or feces. Clinical signs may include a slow wasting of body condition, melena, splenomegaly, episodic fevers, posterior paresis, tremors, and eventually death. A presumptive diagnosis is made based on clinical signs and the finding of a characteristic hypergammaglobulinemia. Diagnosis is confirmed by polymerase chain reaction (PCR), immunofluoresence assay (IFA), and histologic findings, although an increase in gammaglobulins greater than 20% of total proteins is often considered diagnostic. Typical histopathologic lesions include lymphocytic and plasmacytic infiltrates of the kidney, liver, spleen, and meninges. There is no treatment or vaccine to prevent AD. Ferrets with clinical disease should be culled and their environment thoroughly disinfected.

Rabies

Ferrets are susceptible to infections with rabies virus, a rhabdovirus. There is an exceptionally low risk of rabies infection in laboratory ferrets unless they are allowed to roam freely outdoors in a rabies endemic area. There are a few reports of rabies in pet ferrets in the United States. Central nervous signs predominate with anxiety, lethargy, and posterior paresis. If vaccination is indicated based on the risk of rabies exposure and applicable regional and state regulations, ferrets should be administered a USDA-approved killed rabies vaccination at 3 and 12 months of age and then annually. There is no treatment for rabies. Regardless of vaccination status, ferrets that bite humans may be subject to euthanasia and a rabies screen depending on the state regulations.

Epizootic Catarrhal Enteritis

Epizootic catarrhal enteritis (ECE) is a coronaviral disease with up to 100% morbidity but low mortality. Transmission is likely fecal–oral. Ferrets become dehydrated secondary to fluid lost through vomiting and diarrhea. Most deaths occur in older animals with concurrent illnesses. Clinical signs include vomiting, diarrhea, dehydration, and depression. The stool changes through the course of the infection. Initially it may appear bright green and slimy because of abundant mucus, or it may skip that phase and appear as a yellow–gold, bubbly diarrhea. During the recovery phase, stools look like golden jelly filled with "bird seeds," an indication of intestinal malabsorption. In addition, teeth grinding, indicative of pain, may be observed.

Diagnosis is based on the typical clinical signs and histologic findings. Some ferrets may have elevated liver enzymes. Histologically, intestinal villar tip necrosis with moderate-to-marked crypt hyperplasia is observed. Immunohistochemistry can be performed for a definitive diagnosis. RT-PCR can also be performed on a fecal sample. Treatment is primarily supportive, including aggressive fluid therapy to combat the dehydration, administration of a gastrointestinal protectant, and feeding a soft, palatable food to sustain a positive energy balance.

Ferret Systemic Coronavirus

Reported in both research and pet ferrets, ferret systemic coronavirus (FRSCV) is a fatal disease of ferrets that closely resembles the dry form of feline infectious peritonitis and is closely related to the ferret epizootic catarrhal enteritis virus. Clinical signs are often nonspecific and include lethargy, weight loss, anorexia, diarrhea, vomiting, and neurologic signs (e.g., ataxia, tremors, head tilt, and seizures). However, palpable abdominal masses are frequently reported that may involve the mesentery, mesenteric lymph nodes, and abdominal viscera. Pyrexia is occasionally observed. Transmission is suspected to be fecal–oral with disease quickly spreading between grouped animals. As such, environmental decontamination is important in preventing disease spread. Diagnosis is by histology (characteristic granulomatous inflammation), immunohistochemistry (to identify the specific coronavirus antigen), and PCR. Prognosis is poor and currently no highly effective treatment has been identified. Current treatment efforts are centered on the provision of supportive care while multiple drugs are being evaluated for their effectiveness in suppressing or controlling the body's immune system response to the virus. FRSCV should be kept in mind as a differential for abdominal masses in young, ill ferrets.

Rotavirus

Rotaviruses may cause diarrhea in 1–4-day-old kits. Secondary bacterial infections may cause more severe diarrhea. Mortality is reduced if kits continue nursing and are given appropriate supportive care.

Parasitic Diseases

Sarcoptic Mange

Sarcoptes scabiei induces generalized or pedal mange. In the generalized condition, focal or widespread alopecia with intense pruritus develops; in pedal mange, the feet may become hyperemic, edematous, variably pruritic, and ulcerated from irritation and chewing. Although rare in the research setting, the organism can be transmitted by direct contact or contact with contaminated fomites. Diagnosis is by observation of the organism in skin scrapings or crusts partially digested in 10% KOH. Treatment consists of subcutaneous ivermectin (0.2–0.4 mg/kg) administered every 2 weeks until the mite is no longer detectable. Soaking or shampooing the feet in warm water may help relieve foot pruritus. Antibiotics may be indicated if a secondary bacterial infection develops. All animals showing clinical signs or in contact with an affected animal should be treated and the environment decontaminated. The mite may transiently infect humans.

Demodectic Mange

Demodex spp. mites have been reported rarely in ferrets, typically associated with some immunosuppressive event. Clinical signs include pruritus, alopecia, and discoloration of the skin. Diagnosis is by deep skin scraping. Treatment with amitraz dips, three times at weekly intervals, successfully eradicates the infestation.

Fleas

Ctenocephalides spp., especially the cat or dog flea, are common in pet ferrets but are rarely found in research colonies. If present, topical preparations used for elimination of fleas in cats (e.g., imidacloprid, fipronil, or selamectin) may be used for the effective and safe treatment of ferrets.

Ear Mites

Otodectes cyanotis infestation causes an accumulation of dark, waxy ear exudate, and inflammation of the ear canal. Mites can be acquired from, or transmitted to, dogs, cats, and other ferrets. The life cycle, from egg to mature mite, is about 3 weeks. Diagnosis is made by direct microscopic observation of the adult mites or their eggs in ear exudate. Mite eggs are resistant to treatment; thus one treatment kills only the mature mites and multiple weekly treatments are required to eliminate infection. Ears should be cleaned of exudate prior to treatment. Topical and subcutaneous treatments of ivermectin have been used successfully, but topical treatment appears to be more effective. For topical treatment, 1% ivermectin diluted 1:10 in propylene glycol at a dosage of 400 μg/kg, divided between both ears and repeated in 2 weeks, is most effective.

Heartworms

Ferrets are susceptible to natural and experimental infection with *Dirofilaria immitis*. Heartworm disease is unlikely to be found in a laboratory setting but is becoming more prevalent in pet ferrets, especially in the southern United States. Microfilaremia is characteristically of low concentration and transient in nature, similar to that seen in heartworm-infected cats. Ferrets seemingly have little ability to tolerate the presence of adult parasites in the heart without lethal consequences. Clinical signs of heartworm infection in ferrets may include lethargy, anorexia, dyspnea, pale mucous membranes, and ascites. A definitive diagnosis can be made with a combination of assays that detect heartworm antigen or antibodies, and echocardiography.

Coccidiosis

The most common parasite identified in ferrets is coccidia (*Eimeria* spp. or *Isospora* spp.). While most infections are subclinical, young or stressed animals as well as intensively managed colonies are prone to develop clinical disease to include diarrhea, lethargy, dehydration, rectal prolapse, and death. Disease is diagnosed through high-magnification fecal examination for detection of coccidial oocysts; however, fecal shedding is often intermittent and may be difficult to identify. Treatment with sulfadimethoxine at 50 mg/kg orally once and then 25 mg/kg daily for 9 days may be effective although altered doses and treatment duration may be required. Environmental cleaning and good husbandry practices should lower the oocyst burden and reduce the likelihood of spread through the ingestion of sporulated oocysts.

Cryptosporidiosis

Cryptosporidium spp. are protozoans that can infect a wide range of species, including ferrets, cattle, dogs, cats, and humans. To date, both immunocompetent and immunodeficient ferrets diagnosed with *Cryptosporidium* infection have failed to develop clinical signs. Transmission is by ingestion of sporulated oocysts in the feed, water, or environment. Autoinfection can also occur. Diagnosis is through observation of the small, spherical oocysts in a stained fecal preparation. There is no known treatment. *Cryptosporidium* spp. pose a zoonotic risk; thus children and immunosuppressed individuals should be restricted from access to infected ferrets. Good hygiene after handling any animal should also help to reduce the potential for human infection.

Miscellaneous Helminth Intestinal Parasites

Many types of intestinal parasites have been reported in ferrets, including *Toxascaris leonina*, *Toxocara cati*, *Ancylostoma* spp., *Dipylidium caninum*, *Mesocestoides* spp., and *Filaroides* spp. Identification of specific parasites is established by fecal examination. Treatments recommended for elimination of intestinal parasites are generally the same as for cats and dogs and include ivermectin and praziquantel.

Neoplasia

Pancreatic Beta Cell Tumors (Insulinomas)

Pancreatic beta cell tumors, also called insulinomas, are the most commonly reported neoplasm of ferrets. Four- to five-year-old ferrets are most commonly affected, although disease has been reported in ferrets as young as two. The cancerous cells produce high levels of insulin that drive glucose into the cells, resulting in a severe hypoglycemia, below the normal fasting blood glucose of 90–125 mg/dL. Clinical signs are secondary to hypoglycemia and include intermittent and progressive episodes of weakness, posterior paresis, ataxia, stupor or "star gazing" (short trancelike state), head bobbing, lethargy, weight loss, and vomiting. Ptalism (drooling) and pawing at the mouth may be observed as these are signs of nausea in the ferret. In severe cases, ferrets may develop seizures, become comatose, and die.

Diagnosis is based on clinical signs and blood glucose and blood insulin levels. Ferrets with 4-hour fasting blood glucose values between 60 and 85 mg/dL are suspect, whereas blood glucose less than 60 mg/dL may be diagnostic. Blood insulin levels greater than 350 pmol/L aids in the diagnosis. Small, well-defined tumor nodules are often palpable within the pancreas at necropsy or during surgical exploration. Tumor metastasis rarely occurs. Surgical debulking with partial pancreatectomy is the treatment of choice as it often produces a disease-free state and is associated with increased survival time. Unfortunately, about a 40% recurrence of the tumor over 10 months is reported. Medical treatment involves using drugs such as prednisone that inhibit glucose uptake and stimulate gluconeogenesis. Alternatively, diazoxide suppresses insulin secretion as well as inhibits glucose uptake and stimulates gluconeogenesis. Prognosis depends on whether metastasis has occurred and on how aggressively treatment is pursued. Most cases are chronic and usually fatal, but proper treatment can prolong the life of the ferret.

Adrenal Tumors

Adrenal cortical tumors are the second most common neoplasia of ferrets. Ferrets between 3 and 6 years of age are most commonly affected, with females more commonly affected than males. While adrenocortical adenomas and adenocarcinomas can both occur, adenomas are most common. Metastasis can occur. Adrenocortical hyperplasia is extremely common in ferrets greater than 4 years of age and induces the same clinical signs as are seen with neoplasia. It is notable that cortisol is rarely increased in ferrets although an excess production of adrenal steroids does occur.

Typical clinical signs include alopecia, swollen vulva in spayed females, prostatic enlargement in males, and increased sexual behavior in neutered ferrets. Pruritus is occasionally observed. In addition, hind-limb weakness may be apparent in chronic cases. Hair loss is the most common sign observed in ferrets with adrenal disease. Bilaterally symmetrical alopecia often begins at the tail and progresses forward over the hindquarters and abdomen until hair is present only on the neck, head, and extremities. Typical signs associated with hyperadrenocorticism in dogs, such as polyuria, polydypsia, polyphagia, pot-bellied appearance, and thin skin, are rarely seen in ferrets.

The clinical signs may be so characteristic that additional diagnostics may not be necessary. Ultrasound can be used to detect adrenal gland enlargement. Surgical removal of the abnormal adrenal gland is usually curative although a 10%–12%

mortality is associated with the surgical intervention. The left gland is affected 50% more often than the right. If both adrenals are enlarged, removal of the larger adrenal plus a subtotal adrenalectomy on the other gland is usually effective. A medical treatment regimen using mitotane has been described but is not specific for the tumor cells and thus causes unwanted side effects. A commercially manufactured subcutaneous implant of deslorelin acetate (Suprelorin F, Virbac Animal Health, Fort Worth, TX) is also available that provides approximately 12 months of nonsurgical management of the disease.

Lymphoma

There is a high incidence of lymphoma reported in ferrets, with two typical clinical presentations. The first form, juvenile lymphosarcoma, is seen in young ferrets less than 2 years of age that develop an acute lymphoblastic disease, frequently without lymph node enlargement. Large, immature lymphocytes quickly infiltrate the viscera, including the thymus, spleen, liver, and many other organs. One of the more common clinical signs is dyspnea due to a rapidly growing thymic mass that compresses the lungs. This condition has similar clinical signs to cardiomyopathy or pneumonia. Less commonly, extensive infiltration of the liver by neoplastic lymphocytes may result in marked increases in hepatic enzymes and icterus. Lymphoblastic lymphosarcoma should always be on the differential list for young ferrets presenting with serious illness. Clusters of lymphoma cases have been reported that suggest a potential infectious etiology (e.g., an unidentified retrovirus or Aleutian disease virus variant), but this possibility has not been confirmed.

The second form of lymphoma, "classic" lymphosarcoma, is seen in ferrets older than 3 years. These ferrets have a slowly progressive but chronic lymphocytic disease with lymphadenopathy. Classic lymphosarcoma is usually insidious, resulting in little clinical debility until extensive infiltration of visceral organs has occurred, which ultimately results in organ failure and death. Leukemia, increased numbers of circulating lymphocytes in the blood, can occur with either form but is uncommon. Clinical signs are nonspecific and include anorexia, weight loss, and lethargy.

Diagnosis should rely on microscopic evaluation of a lymph node aspirate or biopsy by an individual experienced with cell cytology. Biopsies or aspirates of visceral organs may also help in the diagnosis, with the spleen yielding the most consistent number of positive specimens. An elevated lymphocyte count on a complete blood count (CBC) is not definitive for lymphosarcoma and should not be used as the sole criterion for initiating treatment.

Prognosis is usually poor but depends on the stage at diagnosis and response to therapy. Treatments vary but include the administration of prednisone at 1 mg/kg orally once daily. This may initially lead to clinical improvement, but within 4–6 weeks, the majority of ferrets will develop disseminated disease that is refractory to further treatment. A more aggressive treatment protocol includes multiple-week (e.g., 14-week) IV administration of a combination of chemotherapeutic agents (e.g., vincristine, asparaginase, cyclophosphamide, and doxorubicin), often following treatment protocols developed for treatment of dogs and cats. Radiation therapy has also been used in the treatment of ferret lymphoma. This level of treatment is often not practical in a research setting.

Mast Cell Tumors

Ferrets frequently develop mast cell tumors. The masses intermittently appear and are associated with alopecia and variable pruritus. Tumors are described as firm, small (2–10 mm), tan or erythematous, slightly raised, and circumscribed. A black, crusty exudate is often present around the mass. Most tumors are benign, in contrast to the more malignant mast cell tumors described in other species. Complete surgical excision is usually curative.

Miscellaneous Neoplasia

Other types of spontaneous neoplasms are uncommon in ferrets. Ovarian leiomyomas, chordomas, squamous cell carcinomas, adenocarcinomas, and malignant megakaryocytic myelosis have been reported.

Miscellaneous Conditions

Estrus-Associated Aplastic Anemia

Female ferrets that are not bred and remain in persistent estrus will develop an aplastic anemia attributable to prolonged estrogenic exposure that suppresses both red and white blood cell production in the bone marrow. The common practice of spaying female ferrets at commercial vendors prior to their sale has greatly decreased the incidence of this condition over time. Clinical examination of affected animals typically reveals pale mucous membranes, vulvar enlargement, alopecia, petechial hemorrhages, anorexia, and marked depression. Hematologic findings include severe anemia, thrombocytopenia, granulocytopenia, and hypocellularity of the bone marrow. Death is usually due to thrombocytopenia with resultant uncontrolled hemorrhage or severe leukopenia with secondary bacterial infections.

An ovariohysterectomy is the treatment of choice for ferrets diagnosed early in the condition and with normal blood parameters. If a ferret is anemic or thrombocytopenic, then one or two injections of 100 IU of human chorionic gonadotropin or 20 μg of gonadotropin-releasing hormone (GnRH) can be given to induce ovulation and return the ferret to anestrus. B vitamins, iron, and blood transfusions may help to correct the anemia and stabilize the patient. Once blood parameters have returned to normal, the ferret should be spayed. Prognosis is usually based on the severity of anemia, with a PCV of less than 20% indicating a guarded prognosis and a PCV of less than 14% considered a poor prognosis. Supportive care that includes the use of steroids, force feeding, and vitamin supplementation may improve the chances of survival. Because of the high incidence of this disease in unmated female ferrets and the poor response to even the most vigorous therapy, ovariohysterectomy prior to the first estrus is advisable for females not intended for breeding.

Cardiomyopathy

There are two types of cardiomyopathy: dilatative and hypertrophic. The dilatative form is the most common in ferrets, usually affecting middle-aged or older ferrets. With dilatative cardiomyopathy, the heart muscles become flaccid, weak, and thin with the condition progressing until the heart can no longer effectively pump blood. Hypertrophic cardiomyopathy consists of progressively thickened heart muscles that also become ineffective in pumping blood. The cause of cardiomyopathy is unknown in ferrets. It has been shown that in cats and dogs, dilatative cardiomyopathy may be linked to insufficient amounts of select dietary amino acids, specifically taurine for cats and carnitine for dogs. It had been proposed, but not proven, that a dietary insufficiency may contribute to this disease in ferrets.

Both dilatative and hypertrophic cardiomyopathy produce similar clinical signs due to failing cardiac function and resultant pleural effusion and/or ascites. Lethargy, exercise intolerance, inappetence, weight loss, dyspnea, and respiratory distress are commonly seen. Coughing and abdominal enlargement (secondary to ascites) may also be present.

Diagnosis of cardiomyopathy can be made with an x-ray and ultrasound examination. While observation of cardiomegaly on x-ray is indicative of cardiomyopathy, cardiac ultrasound is required to determine the type of cardiomyopathy and the degree of damage present. Additional tests, such as an electrocardiogram, blood profiles, and thoracocentesis (using a thin needle to obtain fluid from the chest for microscopic examination) enable a more definitive diagnosis.

Treatment of cardiomyopathy involves medication to remove accumulated fluid, such as the diuretic furosemide. Vasodilators such as nitroglycerin or captopril to modulate blood pressure are also often used. Digitalis derivatives can be helpful to increase the strength and efficiency of the failing heart. The long-term prognosis for ferrets with cardiomyopathy is poor, but treatment can effectively reduce the symptoms and increase the quality of life for a period of many months. If diagnosed early and treated aggressively, ferrets can be stabilized for several months or years.

Dystocia

Dystocia is common in ferrets. Problems are typically caused by positional abnormalities or oversized feti. Congenitally malformed kits may also cause a delayed onset of labor. Kits remaining in utero beyond 43 days of gestation typically die. Medical intervention is indicated when a small litter size is the cause of delayed parturition. Parturition may be induced by injection of a prostaglandin (0.5–1.0 mg Lutalyse) followed by 0.3 mL of oxytocin (6 U) 3 hours later. If the jill does not deliver within 8 hours of this regimen, a cesarean section should be performed. Ideally, an inhaled anesthetic should be used.

Pregnancy Toxemia

Pregnancy toxemia is a life-threatening condition that may develop in late-term, pregnant females that undergo a negative energy balance, most frequently due to a large fetal load (>10 kits), feeding of an inadequate diet, or decreased food consumption as may occur following a change in diet. Primiparous or stressed jills are at highest risk. Hyperlipidemia, hypoglycemia, ketosis, and hepatic lipidosis are common sequelae. Clinical signs include lethargy, recumbency, altered mentation, dehydration, and melena. Fur may fall out in clumps when the animal is handled, and hypothermia is often evident. Toxemia should be suspected based on history and clinical signs. Additional diagnostics include CBC, chemistry, and urinalysis and may reveal a low blood glucose (<50 mg/dL), azotemia, and ketonuria. The only characteristic postmortem change is a fatty yellow liver. Treatment consists of IV fluids containing glucose, oral glucose, or high caloric supplement. Subcutaneous or intraosseous fluids may be given if an IV line cannot be placed. The ferret must be kept warm using a circulating water blanket, but caution must be taken not to cause heat prostration by overwarming the ferret. If diagnosed on day 40 of gestation or later, a cesarean section should be performed immediately under inhalant anesthesia. For early cases, nutritional support and supportive care must be provided until cesarean section becomes a viable option. Postoperatively, the jill should be provided supportive care including nutritional support, fluid therapy, and provision of an appropriate heat source. Prognosis is poor if liver damage is significant. The prognosis improves for animals that survive the first 24 hours after surgery. Supplemental feeding or cross-fostering of the kits may be required as agalactia of the jill is common.

Gastrointestinal Foreign Bodies

Because of their propensity to chew, ferrets frequently ingest inappropriate items that then obstruct the stomach or intestines. It has been reported that a gastrointestinal foreign body is the most common diagnosis in young, inappetent, or anorexic pet ferrets although foreign bodies may also occur in a research setting where animals are provided enrichment items or are allowed to exercise in inappropriate or unsupervised areas. Additionally, ferrets may develop trichobezoars that can obstruct the gastrointestinal tract. Clinical signs may include scant feces, a palpable mass in the stomach or intestines, depression, anorexia, dehydration, and sometimes vomiting. Diagnosis is made on history, clinical signs, physical examination with palpation, and abdominal radiographs. Contrast studies may help to pinpoint the location of the obstruction. Removal of items by use of an endoscope is possible in some cases. If not possible, surgical intervention should be taken.

Hair Loss

Alopecia in ferrets is common and can be associated with a number of conditions, including hyperadrenocorticism, biotin deficiency, ovarian tumor, persistent estrus, seasonal molting, flea bite hypersensitivity, and high environmental temperature and humidity. A bilaterally symmetrical pattern of hair loss is seen with endocrine-based alopecia. A random or patchy hair loss is seen with most other types of alopecia. Females usually molt following the first ovulation of the season, and males molt in October or November. At times, ferrets may lose their hair for undetermined reasons.

Infant Mortality

High infant mortality is a common problem for ferret breeders, with contributing causes including maternal lactation failure, maternal neglect, and inappropriate or unsanitary nesting boxes. Many of the deaths are attributable to failure of lactation. Spontaneous congenital malformations, including neuroschisis, gastroschisis, absence of limbs, and corneal dermoids, are also relatively common.

Lactation Failure

Postparturient females may not be able to produce enough milk to feed their kits. There are a number of reasons for this failure, including genetic predisposition, poor management, inadequate nutrition, systemic disease, or mastitis. Jills that are unable to nurse their kits frequently stop lactating quickly; thus for at least 5 days after parturition, jills and their kits should be left in a quiet environment. Food and water should be within reach of jill's nesting area so she can rest, nurse, and provide warmth to her kits. A diet with insufficient fat (25%–30%) or protein also leads to lactation failure as does metritis, cystitis, lymphosarcoma, or mastitis. If a nursing jill does become ill, providing food mixed with warm water or high-calorie supplements such as Nutrical can help support her nutritional requirements to maintain lactation.

Megaesophagus

A dilated esophagus is an uncommon but frequently fatal disorder of unknown etiology in ferrets. It is more commonly seen in middle-aged to older ferrets. Death is usually the result of aspiration pneumonia. Diagnosis is based on history, clinical signs, and radiographic evidence of an enlarged esophagus.

As a symptomatic treatment, ranitidine HCL (15 mg/mL) can be administered (0.1 mL twice daily, 30 minutes before feeding) to reduce gastric acid reflux into the esophagus. Cisapride may also help by enhancing gastrointestinal motility. When feeding the ferret with megaesophagus, it is important to elevate the head and maintain the neck in a straight alignment so that food can pass unobstructed into the stomach. This alternate positioning decreases the risk for aspiration pneumonia.

Renal Cysts

Renal cysts are relatively common in ferrets: one report gives an incidence of 10%–15%. The cysts may be single or multiple and may affect one or both kidneys. The identification of cysts is usually an incidental finding on physical examination or ultrasound with no induced clinical signs, but their presence may lead to renal failure if the cysts are large or numerous and impinge upon normal renal tissue. A CBC, serum chemistry, and urinalysis will help to assess renal function if polycystic kidneys are identified.

Splenomegaly

Splenomegaly is an extremely common physical exam finding in ferrets that is nonspecific and may be associated with several diseases, including neoplasia, adrenal disease, infection, and congestion secondary to cardiac disease (Box 12.4). The vast majority of enlarged spleens are benign conditions that do not threaten the ferret's health and are caused by the occurrence of extramedullary hematopoiesis (a massive proliferation of red and white blood cell precursors external to the bone marrow) in the spleen. About 5% of enlarged spleens are attributed to tumors, the most common being lymphosarcoma. Splenomegaly may also transiently develop in the anesthetized ferret due to splenic sequestration of red blood cells.

Box 12.4

Splenomegaly is an extremely common physical exam finding in ferrets that is nonspecific and may be associated with several diseases, including neoplasia, adrenal disease, infection, and congestion secondary to cardiac disease.

Diagnosis of splenomegaly includes abdominal palpation. On occasion, the splenomegaly is so pronounced that the outline of the spleen is visible when the ferret is dorsally recumbent. Additionally, blood work and fine needle splenic aspirates can help to differentiate hematopoiesis from lymphosarcoma. Hematology parameters are within normal limits in ferrets with benign splenomegaly. A splenectomy is recommended only if the ferret has become lethargic due to the presence of the enlarged spleen, and an infection is not identified.

Urolithiasis

Urolithiasis is not uncommon in ferrets, with neutered males most frequently affected. Magnesium ammonium phosphate (struvite) uroliths are most common and diet plays a large role in the production of stones. Animal protein diets result in acidic urine in which struvite is soluble. Ferrets fed a diet with plant protein have alkaline urine, and struvite tends to precipitate at this higher pH. The normal urine pH of ferrets should be around 6.0 when maintained on a high-quality, meat-based diet.

Clinical signs include frequent urination, licking of the perineum, urinary incontinence, hematuria, and dysuria. If obstructed, a ferret may show signs of straining to urinate and may vocalize in pain. If not promptly corrected, obstruction leads to life-threatening metabolic disturbances that result in coma and death. Treatment is similar to that for other mammals with this disease and includes reestablishment of urinary excretion, fluid therapy, and dietary management. Surgery is usually the treatment of choice for obstruction or if the uroliths in the bladder are of significant size. Long-term dietary management is based on a gradual switch to a meat-based diet to prevent stone formation. Diets used to decrease stone formation in dogs and cats generally have lower protein levels than is recommended for ferrets; therefore, their use is not advised.

BIBLIOGRAPHY

American Veterinary Medical Association (AVMA). 2013. *AVMA Guidelines for the Euthanasia of Animals*. Available at http://www.avma.org/KB/Policies/Documents/euthanasia.pdf [accessed June 18, 2018].

Autieri, C. R., C. L. Miller, K. E. Scott, et al. 2015. Systemic coronaviral disease in 5 ferrets. *Comp Med* 65(6): 508–516.

Batchelder, M. A., S. E. Erdman, X. Li, and J. G. Fox. 1996. A cluster of cases of juvenile mediastinal lymphoma in a ferret colony. *Lab Anim Sci* 46(3): 271–274.

Bell, J. A. 1997. *Helicobacter mustelae* gastritis, proliferative bowel disease, and eosinophilic gastroenteritis. In *Ferrets, Rabbits and Rodents: Clinical Medicine and Surgery*, E. V. Hillyer and K. E. Quesenberry (eds.), pp. 37–43. Philadelphia, PA: Saunders.

Besch-Williford, C. L. 1987. Biology and medicine of the ferret. *Vet Clin North Am Small Anim Pract* 17(5): 1155–1183.

Brown, S. A. 1993. Ferrets. In *A Practitoner's Guide to Rabbits and Ferrets*, J. R. Jenkins and S. A. Brown (eds.), pp. 43–111. Lakewood, CO: American Animal Hospital Association.

Brown, S. A. 1995. Ferret drug dosages. In *Exotic Animal Formulary*, L. Bauck, T. H. Boyer, and S. A. Brown, et al. (eds.), pp. 5–11. Lakewood, CO: American Animal Hospital Association.

Brown, S. A. 1999. Ferret drug dosages. In *Exotic Formulary*, pp. 43–61. Lakewood, CO: AAHA Press.

Buchanan, K. C. and D. A. Belote. 2003. Pancreatic islet cell tumor in a domestic ferret. *Contemp Top Lab Anim Sci* 42(6): 46–48.

Burgess, M. and M. M. Garner. 2002. Clinical aspects of inflammatory bowel disease in ferrets. *Exotic DVM* 4(2): 29–34.

Burke, T.J. 1988. Common diseases and medical management of ferrets. In: *Exotic Animals*, E.R. Jacobson and G.V. Kollias, Jr. (eds), pp. 247–260. New York, NY: Churchill Livingstone.

Cantwell, S. L. 2001. Ferret, rabbit, and rodent anesthesia. *Vet Clin North Am: Exotic Anim Pract* 4: 169–191.

Caplan, E. R., M. E. Peterson, H. S. Mullen, et al. 1996. Diagnosis and treatment of insulin-secreting pancreatic islet cell tumors in ferrets: 57 cases (1986–1994). *J Am Vet Med Assoc* 209 (10): 1741–1745.

Collins, B. R. 1995. Antimicrobial drug use in rabbits, rodents, and other small mammals. In *Antimicrobial Therapy in Caged Birds and Exotic Pets*, pp. 3–10. Trenton, NJ: Veterinary Learning Systems.

Dobromylskyj, P., P. A. Flecknell, B. D. Lascelles, et al. 2000. Management of postoperative and other acute pain. In *Pain Management in Animals*, P. Flecknell and A. Waterman-Pearson (eds.), pp. 81–145. London: WB Saunders.

Erdman, S. E., S. A. Brown, T. A. Kawasaki, et al. 1996. Clinical and pathologic findings in ferrets with lymphoma: 60 cases (1982–1994). *J Am Vet Med Assoc* 208(8): 1285–1289.

Evans, A. T. and K. Springsteen. 1998. Anesthesia in ferrets. *Sem Avian Exotic Pet Med* 7(1): 48–52.

Fazakas, S. 2000. Eosinophilic gastroenteritis in a domestic ferret. *Can Vet J* 41(9): 707–709.

Flecknell, P. A. 1987. *Laboratory Animal Anesthesia*. San Diego, CA: Academic Press.

Flecknell, P. A. 1997. Medetomidine and atipamezole: Potential uses in laboratory animals. *Lab Anim (NY)* 26(2): 21–25.

Flecknell, P. A. 2009. *Laboratory Animal Anaesthesia*, 3rd ed. London: Academic Press.

Fox, J. G. 1998. Neoplasia. In *Biology and Diseases of the Ferret*, pp. 275–277. Baltimore, MD: Williams and Wilkins.

Fox, J. G., P. Correa, N. S. Taylor, et al. 1990. *Helicobacter mustelae*–associated gastritis in ferrets: An animal model of *Helicobacter pylori* gastritis in humans. *Gastroenterology* 99: 352–361.

Goett, S. C. and D. A. Degner. 2003. Suspected adrenocortical insufficiency subsequent to bilateral adrenalectomy in a ferret. *Exotic DVM* 5(1): 6–9.

Graham, E., C. Lamm, D. Denk, et al. 2012. Systemic coronavirus-associated disease resembling feline infectious peritonitis in ferrets in the UK. *Vet Rec* 171(8): 200–201.

Harkness, J. E. and J. E. Wagner. 1995. *Biology and Medicine of Rabbits and Rodents*, 4th ed. Philadelphia, PA: Williams & Wilkins.

Heard, D. J. 1993. Principles and techniques of anesthesia and analgesia for exotic practice. *Vet Clin North Am Small Anim Pract* 23(6): 1301–1327.

Hillyer, E. V. and S. A. Brown. 1994. Ferrets. In *Saunders Manual of Small Animal Practice*, S. J. Birchard and R. G. Sherding (eds.), pp. 1317–1344. Philadelphia, PA: WB Saunders.

Hoefer, H. L., J. G. Fox, and J. A. Bell. 2012. Gastrointestinal diseases. In *Ferrets, Rabbits, and Rodents: Clinical Medicine and Surgery*, 3rd ed. K. E. Quesenberry and J. W. Carpenter (eds.), pp. 27–45. Philadelphia, PA: WB Saunders.

Hull, R. M. 1995. Guideline limit volumes for dosing animals in the preclinical stage of safety evaluation. *Hum Exp Toxicol* 14: 305–307.

Hutchinson, M. J., D. E. Jacobs, and N. Mencke. 2001. Establishment of the cat flea (*Ctenocephalides felis felis*) on the ferret (*Mustela putorius furo*) and its control with imidacloprid. *Med Vet Entomol* 15(2): 212–214.

Institute of Laboratory Animal Resources (ILAR). 2011. *Guide for the Care and Use of Laboratory Animals*, 8th ed. ILAR, National Research Council. Washington, DC: National Academies Press.

Johnson-Delaney, C. A. 1996. *Exotic Companion Medicine Handbook for Veterinarians*. Lake Worth, FL: Wingers.

Ko, J. C. H. and T. G. Heaton-Jones. 1997. Anesthetic effects of medetomidine, medetomidine–butorphanol, medetomidine–ketamine, and medetomidine–butorphanol–ketamine in the ferret. Abstracts from the 1996 Meeting of the American Association of Veterinary Anesthesiologists. Available at http://www.acva.org/professional/abstracts/abstract97a.html [accessed August 1, 2006].

Ko, J. C. H., L. S. Pablo, J. E. Bailey, and T. G. Heaton-Jones. 1996. Anesthetic effects of Telazol® and combinations of ketamine–xylazine and Telazol®–ketamine–xylazine in ferrets. *Contemp Topics* 35(2): 47–52.

Ko, J. C. H., T. A. Smith, W. C. Kuo, and C. F. Nicklin. 1998. Comparison of anesthetic and cardiorespiratory effects of diazepam–butorphanol–ketamine, acepromazine–butorphanol–ketamine, and xylazine–butorphanol–ketamine in ferrets. *J Am Anim Hosp Assoc* 34(5): 407–416.

Lewington, J. H. 2000. *Ferret Husbandry, Medicine & Surgery*. Edinburgh: Elsevier.

Lukas, V. 1999. Volume guidelines for compound administration. In *The Care and Feeding of an IACUC*, M. L. Podolsky and V. S. Lukas (eds.), p. 187. Boca Raton, FL: CRC Press.

Marini, R. P., L. R. Jackson, M. I. Esteves, et al. 1994. Effect of isoflurane on hematologic variables in ferrets. *Am J Vet Res* 55: 1479–1483.

Marini, R. P., J. G. Fox, N. S. Taylor, et al. 1999. Ranitidine bismuth citrate and clarithromycin, alone or in combination, for eradication of *Helicobacter mustelae*. *Am J Vet Res* 60(10): 1280–1286.

Martina, B. E., B. L. Haagmans, T. Kuiken, et al. 2003. Virology: SARS virus infection of cats and ferrets. *Nature* 425: 915.

Mayer, J., R. P. Marini, and J. G. Fox. 2015. Biology and diseases of ferrets. In *Laboratory Animal Medicine*, 3rd ed., J. G. Fox, L. C. Anderson, G. Otto, K. R. Pritchett-Corning, M. T. Whary (eds.), pp. 577–616 San Diego, CA: Elsevier.

Morrisey, J. K. and J. W. Carpenter. 2012. Formulary. In *Ferrets, Rabbits, and Rodents: Clinical Medicine and Surgery*, 3rd ed., K. E. Quesenberry and J. W. Carpenter (eds.), pp. 566–575. Philadelphia, PA: WB Saunders.

Murray, J., M. Kiupel, and R. K Maes. 2010. Ferret coronavirus-associated diseases. *Vet Clin North Am: Exotic Anim Pract* 13(3): 543–560.

Nwaokorie, E. E., C. A. Osborne, J. P. Lulich, et al. 2011. Epidemiology of struvite uroliths in ferrets: 272 cases (1981–2007). *J Am Vet Med Assoc* 239(10): 1319–1324.

Orcutt, C. 2001. Update on "Oxyglobin use in ferrets". *Exotic Veterinary Magazine* 3(3): 29–30.

Paul-Murphy, J. 2001. Melatonin use in ferret adrenal gland disease. *Proc North Am Vet Conf* 15: 897.

Payton, A. J. and J. R. Pick. 1989. Evaluation of a combination of tiletamine and zolazepam as an anesthetic for ferrets. *Lab Anim Sci* 39(3): 243–246.

Pollock, C. G. 2012. Disorders of the urinary and reproductive systems. In *Ferrets, Rabbits, and Rodents: Clinical Medicine and Surgery*, 3rd ed., K. E. Quesenberry and J. W. Carpenter (eds.), pp. 46–61. Philadelphia, PA: WB Saunders.

Richardson, J. A. and R. A. Balabuszko. 2001. Ibuprofen ingestion in ferrets: 43 cases (January 1996–March 2000). *J Vet Emerg Crit Care* 11(1): 53–59.

Rosenthal, K. L. and N. R. Wyre. 2012. Endocrine diseases. In *Ferrets, Rabbits, and Rodents: Clinical Medicine and Surgery*, 3rd ed., K. E. Quesenberry and J. W. Carpenter (eds.), pp. 86–102. St. Louis, MO: Elsevier Saunders.

Tanner, P. A., T. Tseggai, et al. 2000. Minimum protective dose and efficacy of a recombinant canine distemper virus vaccine for ferrets. In Proceedings of the 81st Annual Meeting of the Conference of Research Workers in Animal Diseases. Abstract 156.

Wade, L. L. 2018. Vaccination of ferrets for rabies and distemper. *Vet Clin North Am Exot Anim Pract* 21(1): 105–114

Weiss, C. A. and M. V. Scott. 1997. Clinical aspects and surgical treatment of hyperadrenocorticism in the domestic ferret: 94 cases (1994–1996). *J Am Anim Hosp Assoc* 33(6): 487–493.

Weiss, C. A., B. H. Williams, J. B. Scott, and M. V. Scott. 1999. Surgical treatment and long-term outcome of ferrets with bilateral adrenal tumors or adrenal hyperplasia: 56 cases (1994–1997). *J Am Vet Med Assoc* 215(6): 820.

Williams, B. H. 2000. Therapeutics in ferrets. In *Vet Clin North Am: Exotic Anim Pract* 3(1): 131–151.

Williams, B. H., M. Kiupel, K. H. West, et al. 2000. Coronavirus-associated epizootic catarrhal enteritis in ferrets. *J Am Vet Med Assoc* 217(4): 526–530.

Wills, S. E., H. H. Beaufrère, B. A. Brisson, et al. 2018. Pancreatitis and systemic coronavirus infection in a ferret (*Mustela putorius furo*). *Comp Med* 68(3): 208–211.

Zitzow, L. A., T. Rowe, T. Morken, et al. 2002. Pathogenesis of avian influenza A (H5N1) viruses in ferrets. *J Virol* 76: 4420–4429.

FURTHER READING

Hillyer, E. V. 1992. Ferret endocrinology. In *Current Therapy XI—Small Animal Practice*, R. W. Kirk and J. D. Bonagura (eds.), pp. 1185–1188. Philadelphia: WB Saunders.

Lavin, L. M. 2007. Avian and exotic radiography. In *Radiography in Veterinary Technology*, 4th ed., pp. 294–301. St. Louis, MO: WB Saunders.

Mitchell, M. and T. Tully. 2009. *Manual of Exotic Pet Practice*. St. Louis, MO: Saunders.

Quesenberry, K. E. and J. W. Carpenter. 2011. *Ferrets, Rabbits, and Rodents: Clinical Medicine and Surgery*, 3rd ed. St. Louis, MO: Elsevier Saunders.

CHAPTER 12 REVIEW

Matching

1. _____group of ferrets
2. _____male ferret
3. _____neutered male
4. _____young ferret
5. _____female ferret
6. _____spayed female
   A. hob
   B. kit
   C. clowder
   D. jill
   E. business
   F. gib
   G. pack
   H. sprite
7. Name two unique characteristics of ferrets and the two research uses that make them good models for this research.
8. How old are ferrets when they reach sexual maturity?
9. The ferret is a(an)
   A. carnivore
   B. strict herbivore
   C. omnivore
   D. vegetarian
10. Ferrets are seasonal breeders. How can you adjust the light cycle to take advantage of this to induce an earlier onset of estrus?

(Continued)

11. Which genus of bacteria associated with gastritis and ulcers is common in ferrets?
12. Which two viruses should ferrets be routinely vaccinated against?
13. Female ferret that is not bred and has a protracted estrus cycle can develop
    A. splenomegaly
    B. aplastic anemia
    C. eosinophilic gastroenteritis
    D. lymphoma
14. What is the causal organism of pedal mange?
    A. Demodex
    B. Ctenocephalides
    C. Sarcoptes
    D. Otodectes
15. Ferrets have a rapid GI transit time and do not have which section of the GI tract?
16. The wild-type coat color for ferrets is called
    A. agouti
    B. buff
    C. albino
    D. fitch
17. What is the most commonly reported neoplasm in ferrets?
18. What is an extremely common nonspecific physical exam finding in ferrets, necessitating caution when palpating the abdomen?

Critical Thinking

19. Ferrets are frequently utilized in toxicology testing. Why?

13 Primates

Nomenclature and classification of nonhuman primates are subject to periodic changes. Nevertheless, individuals concerned with the medical care or research use of these animals should be able to recognize the more frequently seen species and categorize them correctly. Nonhuman primates can be characterized by their unique biologic characteristics, regions of origin, environmental and nutritional requirements, and disease susceptibility. There is a vast range in size among different species of nonhuman primates from the smallest, the pygmy mouse lemur (*Microcebus myoxinus*) at 30–109 g, to the largest ape, the gorilla, weighing more than 200 kg.

TAXONOMY

Taxonomic classification of nonhuman primates is an ever-changing field. There is a long-standing debate regarding classification of certain nonhuman primates (NHPs), such as tarsiers, and both current and obsolete references are found in the literature. For the purposes of this book, we adopt the approach of classifying NHPs into two suborders: Strepsirrhini ("wet-nosed") and Haplorrhini ("dry-nosed"). Strepsirrhini translates from Greek into "having a curved nose" and includes lemurs, lorises, and galagos. Haplorrhini translates from Greek into "simple-nosed" and includes tarsiers, monkeys, and apes (Figure 13.1). This chapter focuses on the more prominently used research species within the Haplorrhini suborder.

Clinical Laboratory Animal Medicine: An Introduction, Fifth Edition.
Lesley A. Colby, Megan H. Nowland, and Lucy H. Kennedy.

Companion website: www.wiley.com/go/colby/clinical

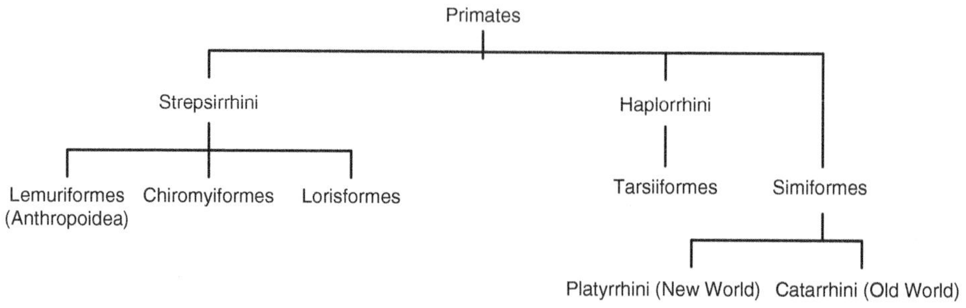

Fig 13.1. Phylogenetic tree of the order Primates. (*Source:* Adapted from Groves (2004).)

Strepsirrhini (Lemurs, Lorises, and Galagos)

Many strepsirrhine species superficially resemble dogs or rodents more than what we think of as primates. Their snouts are generally elongated and the moist nose (rhinarium) joins with the upper lip, which attaches to the gum, limiting their ability to make facial expressions. The brain-to-body ratio is smaller than that of haplorrhines. The olfactory lobes are large, indicating a greater reliance on smell. All lemuriformes (lemurs), with the exception of the aye-aye, have a dental comb made up of grouped incisors and canines as well as a specialized claw on the second toe, both adaptations for grooming purposes. The most medial digit of the foot is widely separated from the others, allowing a tight grip for locomotion. Most species are nocturnal and have sensitive hearing for night hunting. Their natural diet consists primarily of insects, but some species prefer a fruit diet and some are carnivorous. Strepsirrhines have a breeding season rather than a cycle, as is typical of haplorrhines. All species in this suborder possess a bicornate uterus, have one or two pairs of mammary glands in varying locations, and produce 1–3 offspring per pregnancy. Strepsirrhine species include lemurs, lorises, and galagos. All species of lemurs are classified as endangered; very few are used in biomedical research.

Haplorrhini (Tarsiers, Monkeys, and Apes)

No single anatomic feature distinguishes haplorrhines from other animals. Because the upper lip is not directly connected to the nose or gum, these primates can make a wide range of facial expressions. The brain-to-body ratio is significantly greater than that of the strepsirrhines. Vision is the dominant sense, and most species have some degree of dichromatic or trichromatic vision. A majority of the species are diurnal, or active in the daytime, with the exception of tarsiers and owl monkeys. The hands and feet are adapted more generally for locomotion. Some additional important characteristics are the presence of a simplex uterus (aside from tarsiers that have a bicornate uterus), paired pectoral mammae, a pendulous penis, scrotal testes, a clavicle, and a hallux (most medial toe of the foot). The suborder Haplorrhini is divided into nine families: Tarsiidae, Callitrichidae, Cebidae, Aotidae, Pitheciidae, Atelidae, Cercopithecidae (Old World monkeys), Hylobatidae (lesser apes), and Hominidae (great apes).

New World Primates (Family—Callitrichidae)

Marmosets and tamarins are among the smallest of the New World (Central and South American) primates. They have soft, silky hair and long tails that are not prehensile. Callitrichids have several unique characteristics: possessing claws rather than nails; having axillary rather than anterior mammary glands; and being biovulatory—thus twinning is normal. Representative species are common marmosets, pygmy marmosets, golden lion tamarins, and cotton-top tamarins. The cotton-top tamarin, *Sanguinus oedipus*, is endangered and thus can be used only in research that benefits the species. The average weight is 450–550 g. The common marmoset, *Callithrix jacchus*, is the callitrichid species that is most frequently used in research and has an average body weight of 300–350 g. Marmosets have a specialized set of glands in the anogenital region used for scent marking, an important method of communication within marmoset colonies. Marmosets are used in a variety of research applications, including infectious disease, viral oncology, pharmacokinetics, and behavioral and reproductive studies.

New World Primates (Family—Cebidae)

Squirrel monkeys, *Saimiri sciureus*, have short, dense hair coats varying in color from orange to gray; a dark, round muzzle; and white hairless patches around their eyes. They have long tails that are partially prehensile, meaning the tail can aid in locomotion and balance but cannot manipulate objects. Squirrel monkeys typically weigh 500–1500 g and are one of the most common neotropical primates used for research due to their small size, tractable nature, and tendency to breed well in captivity. Sexual dimorphism is marked primarily by body weight, with males weighing 25%–30% more than females. Both males and females undergo seasonal reproductive changes. They have been used in a variety of research applications and are particularly important in the study of atherosclerosis. Squirrel monkeys are widely distributed throughout the rain forests of South and Central America. Animals from different geographic areas are generally distinguished by having a "gothic arch" (*S. sciureus* group comprising three subspecies) or "Roman arch" (*Saimiri boliviensis* group comprising two subspecies) in reference to the slightly differing color and shape characteristics of the hair around the eyes.

Sapajus, formerly known as cebus monkeys, have also been referred to as capuchins because their coloration likens them to the Capuchin order of monks. The six species of *Sapajus* have medium-length, dense hair coats ranging from dark brownish-black to white with long and partially prehensile tails. Adults weigh on average 1–3 kg. *Sapajus apella*, the black-capped capuchin, has a unique appearance, with long, dark sideburns and tufts of dark hair arising from its brow and is occasionally used in research.

New World Primates (Family—Atelidae)

Spider monkeys, *Ateles* spp., are aptly named because of their long, gangly arms and legs and thick, rounded abdomens. These monkeys are anatomically unique, possessing four fingers but no thumb, and long, prehensile tails. In the wild, they are strictly arboreal. Adults weigh 5–7 kg. Females have an unusually long clitoris that can be mistaken for a penis. Spider monkeys are native to the rain forests of South and Central America. They are not commonly used in research.

New World Primates (Family—Aotidae)

Owl monkeys, *Aotus* spp., are one of only two nocturnal haplorrhine primates (the second are the tarsiers). They have short, dense hair coats varying in color from gray to red; a small, dark muzzle; large, owl-like eyes; and white crescents of hair around each eye. They have long, nonprehensile tails, weigh 900–1200 g, and are arboreal and monogamous. These primates are not as hardy as squirrel monkeys and do not adapt as well to the laboratory. Owl monkeys are one of the most important models for studies of human malaria (*Plasmodium* spp.) and viral oncology and are of special importance in vision research due to a unique eye structure. There are eight different species of owl monkeys with diploid chromosome numbers ranging from 46 to 56.

Old World Monkeys (Family—Cercopithecidae)

Rhesus monkeys, *Macaca mulatta*, are medium-sized, Old World, Asian monkeys that have short, reddish-brown hair coats and medium-length tails. The close-cropped head hair accentuates an expressive face. There is moderate sexual dimorphism; males are larger and weigh 6–11 kg, females weigh 4–9 kg. Similarly, males develop large canine teeth, whereas females do not. Rhesus monkeys tend to be one of the more aggressive macaque species. They are frequently used for vaccine testing, pharmacology and toxicology studies, and infectious disease research. *M. mulatta* are found across a wide range of Central Asia from Afghanistan to China. Due to destruction of their natural habitat as well as religious and political factors, the supply of rhesus monkeys from the wild is restricted.

Cynomolgus monkeys, *Macaca fascicularis*, also called crab-eating and long-tailed macaques, are slightly smaller than rhesus and have long, nonprehensile tails and medium-length, olive hair coats on the dorsum, with white to gray hairs on the ventrum and around the face. The hair around the face is longer and tends to form a small mane. Males have long, sharp, canine teeth and are slightly larger than females. They tend to be less aggressive than rhesus monkeys. Cynomolgus are frequently used in evaluation of new therapeutic compounds and in infectious disease research. They are found primarily in Southeast Asia; however, a population of *M. fascicularis* was introduced onto the island of Mauritius located in the Indian Ocean, just east of Madagascar.

Papio anubis, the olive baboon, and *Papio cynocephalus*, the yellow baboon, are the baboon species most commonly used in biomedical research. They are large, weighing 15–30 kg as adults. They have long hair coats, nonprehensile tails, and an elongate, prominent muzzle that gives them a dog-faced appearance. There is marked sexual dimorphism, with males exhibiting a shoulder mane; having large, sharp canine teeth; and weighing 50% more than females. They are found over a wide range of Africa and they tend to be agricultural pests. The baboon is occasionally used for surgery, for reproductive physiology research, and as an alternative model for acquired immunodeficiency syndrome (AIDS).

African green monkeys, *Chlorocebus aethiops*, formerly *Cercopithecus aethiops*, are small monkeys, with brownish-green hair coats and long nonprehensile tails. African greens are a species of guenon and are also commonly known as vervet or grivet monkeys. They weigh 2–6 kg. Male vervets have a distinct “red, white and blue display” made up of their bright blue scrotal areas, red penises and the white fur of their ventrum. They are occasionally used in biomedical research.

Mangabeys, *Cercocebus* spp. and *Lophocebus* spp., are slender primates with long legs and tails. *Cercocebus atys atys*, or sooty mangabeys, are susceptible to the organism that causes leprosy, *Mycobacterium leprae*, and act as asymptomatic carriers of the simian immunodeficiency virus (SIV). They have been used in leprosy and AIDS research, but their status as an endangered species now limits their use.

Lesser Apes (Family—Hylobatidae)

Lesser apes comprise several genera of gibbons, including *Hylobates* spp., *Hoolock* spp., *Nomascus* spp., and the largest gibbon or siamang, *Symphalangus* spp. These animals have exceptionally long arms and no tail; locomotion involves brachiating from branch to branch. They are monogamous and mate for life. They are arboreal, sleeping in a fork between branches, and principally eat fruits and vegetables. Gibbons are notorious for loud vocalizations, which are used in the wild to warn off other members of this species from their territory. They are listed as endangered.

Great Apes (Family—Hominidae)

The chimpanzee, genus *Pan*, is the highest form of nonhuman primate once used in significant numbers in biomedical research. Adults grow quite large, with average weights of 40 kg for females and 50 kg for males. They have historically been used for testing hepatitis B and C virus and AIDS vaccines, and for psychobiology research. In 2000, the Chimpanzee Health, Improvement, Maintenance, and Protection (CHIMP) Act (PL 106-551) was signed into law to provide support for the construction of chimpanzee sanctuaries and for the lifetime care of the animals used in government research through funding from the National Institutes of Health (NIH). In 2013, the NIH announced that chimpanzee research would no longer be supported. Soon thereafter, in 2015, the US Fish and Wildlife Service classified captive chimps as endangered, matching the designation of wild chimps. Since then, chimpanzee research has effectively ceased and animals are being moved into sanctuaries to provide for their well-being for the rest of their lives.

Orangutans, genus *Pongo*, are found in Borneo and Sumatra and appear to be approaching extinction. These animals are not used in biomedical research. Gorillas, genus *Gorilla*, are native to equatorial Africa. These primates are endangered and used only rarely in studies that are not detrimental to their health, such as for learning and behavioral research.

USES

Nonhuman primates share an unparalleled anatomic and physiologic proximity to humans, consequently serving a critical role in biomedical research. Historically, nonhuman primates have been primary models in the study of viral diseases, including smallpox and poliovirus. Today, they continue to be important models for the study

Box 13.1

The greatest numbers of nonhuman primates used in biomedical research are the macaques, primarily the cynomolgus and rhesus species.

of viral diseases such as AIDS, toxicological investigations, behavior, learning, neurological diseases such as Parkinson's and Alzheimer's, dentistry, reproduction, and infectious diseases.

The greatest numbers of nonhuman primates used in biomedical research are the macaques, primarily the cynomolgus and rhesus species (Box 13.1). These two species of macaques constitute more than 50% of the total number of nonhuman primates used in research. Squirrel monkeys, marmosets, baboons, African green monkeys, mangabeys, owl monkeys, and cebus monkeys are used in moderate to small numbers. Overall, nonhuman primates constitute less than 2% of the total number of animals used in biomedical research each year. Conservation of species has been a major concern; threatened and endangered species are not removed from wild populations. Research investigations using captive animals have led to a greater knowledge base of their biological requirements and methods to enhance conservation.

National Primate Research Centers

Seven National Primate Research Centers (NPRCs) are located throughout the country and provide animals, facilities, and expertise in all aspects of nonhuman primate biology and husbandry. These facilities and resources enable collaborative research among NPRC staff scientists, NPRC host institutions, and other NIH-funded researchers. Major areas of research include AIDS, avian flu, Alzheimer's disease, Parkinson's disease, diabetes, asthma, and endometriosis. The centers' specialized resources are also used by investigators funded by other federal, state, and local agencies, as well as by research foundations and the private sector. The primate centers house a dozen different primate species; the majority are macaques. More information about these resources, including access criteria, is available through the National Primate Research Centers (https://nprcresearch.org/primate).

BEHAVIOR

Due to complexity and species diversity, it is beyond the scope of this chapter to provide a detailed description of the behavior of nonhuman primates. Rather, this section provides an overview to familiarize the reader.

A majority of nonhuman primate species are extremely social animals. The most common social organization is that of a troop containing from 20 to 100 animals; however, some are primarily solitary or live in small family groups. Baboons and macaques aggregate in sizeable troops. Within these groups exists a definite hierarchical arrangement: one male is the dominant or alpha male and one female is the dominant or alpha female. Next in the hierarchy are a small number of males, followed by a group of high-ranking females, and finally a group of low-ranking males, females, and younger animals. An animal's rank has a high correlation to the rank of its mother. The hierarchical position of a female in a troop normally remains quite stable, whereas the position of a male seems to be more transitory, with changes in leadership every 4–5 years. Depending on the stability of the hierarchy and the species, fighting frequently occurs in social groupings. Subordinate members lipsmack and present their hindquarters to more dominant animals as a sign of submission. Direct eye contact is perceived as a threat and will often elicit aggressive behavior, including yawns, which reveal their large canines, as well as threatening facial expressions and postures. Nonhuman primates learn reproductive and social behaviors from adults; thus, they must be reared in a reasonably representative social situation to develop normal behavioral patterns. Hand-reared and isolated animals frequently develop behavioral abnormalities and rarely mate.

As highly social animals, grooming is a critical component of social bond formation. Primates usually exhibit fewer incidences of stereotypical behavior when housed in social groups and provided with environmental enrichment; this fosters the development of normal reproductive and social behaviors. Primary disadvantages to group housing include increased trauma from fighting, the inability to determine adequate food and fluid intake of individuals, and the inability to easily isolate individuals for treatment. Despite potential drawbacks, social housing is preferred for the psychological well-being of these animals; single housing must be scientifically justified by the principal investigator and approved by the IACUC.

ANATOMIC AND PHYSIOLOGIC FEATURES

Physical characteristics that distinguish Old World (OW) from New World (NW) primates are outlined in Table 13.1. OW primates are also classified as catarrhines, a Latin derivative for "narrow-nosed"; NW monkeys are also classified as platyrrhines, or Latin for "flat-nosed." Most nonhuman primates used in research are so similar to humans morphologically that human anatomy and surgery references can serve as excellent guides.

Rhesus and some other OW species have cheek pouches in which food is collected to be chewed and swallowed later. In a number of species, including macaques and

Table 13.1. Monkey physical characteristics: New World vs. Old World

New World Monkeys (Platyrrhines)	Old World Monkeys (Catarrhines)
Prehensile tails in some species	No prehensile tails
No ischial callosities	Ischial callosities in some species
Broad-nosed	Narrow-nosed
Require dietary vitamin D_3	Do not require dietary vitamin D_3
No cheek pouches	Cheek pouches in some species
No opposable thumbs	Opposable thumbs in all species
Three premolar teeth per quadrant	Two premolar teeth per quadrant

Box 13.2

Most mammals can synthesize vitamin C, but primates require a dietary source.

baboons, males have formidable canine teeth that may serve as vicious weapons. Some OW species possess ischial callosities on their buttocks; these hard, keratinized pads serve as protection for the bony prominence of the ischium.

There is marked sexual dimorphism of body structure, weight, hair coat, and size of the teeth in some species. Females have a simplex-type uterus, similar to the type found in humans. Most have placentas that are monodiscoid (one lobe) or bidiscoid (two lobes). Sexing is usually simple except in a few species such as spider monkeys; the females have a long clitoris that resembles a penis but may be differentiated by the absence of a urethral opening. All female OW primates have menstrual bleeding as a feature of their sexual cycle. This is absent in NW species. Twinning is extremely rare in OW monkeys, but it is the norm in some species of NW monkeys.

Most mammals can synthesize vitamin C, but primates require a dietary source (Box 13.2). NW primates cannot utilize vitamin D_2 and must be provided with a dietary source of vitamin D_3. NW species also require a higher percentage of protein in their diets than do OW species.

Blood parameters vary to some extent among species and may also vary depending on the methods used for sampling and on the housing conditions. It has been reported that baboon and chimpanzee hematologic and clinical chemistry values compare favorably with normal clinical values established for humans. Selected hematologic and biochemical values for several species of nonhuman primates are listed in Appendix 1, "Normal Values."

BREEDING AND REPRODUCTION

General biologic and reproductive data are listed in Table 13.2. The breeding and the reproductive biology of nonhuman primates varies across species. General breeding and reproductive indices, as well as some peculiarities for some of the more common nonhuman primates, are presented.

Puberty is marked in OW monkeys by the onset of menstrual cycling, or menarche, in the female and increased testicular size and spermatogenesis in the male. The average age of initiation of menarche in cynomolgus and rhesus macaques is between 2 and 3 years. The average age of sexual maturity of the female is between 2.5 and 3.5 years in these species, with the first birth usually occurring between 3 and 5 years. Males generally mature 1–2 years later than females.

Although most OW species are nonseasonally polyestrous (spontaneous ovulators), the rhesus macaque is a seasonal breeder, with most fertile cycles occurring in the winter months. The menstrual cycle lasts an average of 28–30 days in most OW species. Baboons, rhesus, and chimpanzees present with edema and color changes of the perineal or sex skin that cycles with the hormonal changes. In the rhesus, the sex skin has a corrugated appearance, whereas the sex skin of the baboon is smoother. Maximum turgescence and pinkish-red color intensity are associated with the follicular phase of the menstrual cycle, estrus, and ovulation. Deturgescence and decreased color intensity occur rapidly after ovulation and are associated with the luteal phase of the menstrual cycle. Optimal mating time can be determined for individuals who have regular cycle patterns by averaging three to four of their menstrual cycle lengths and mating them 3–4 days prior to deturgescence.

Many OW species, including the cynomolgus and rhesus macaques as well as chimpanzees, have a "placental sign" or vaginal bleeding indicating pregnancy. This occurs approximately the same time as menstruation would appear, but it is actually hemorrhage associated with implantation of the blastocyst. Gestation lengths for some of the more common species are listed in Table 13.2. Parturition in macaques frequently occurs in the late evening or early morning hours, with labor lasting 2–3 hours. Head-first presentation of the fetus is normal. Infants begin nursing immediately after birth and nurse frequently throughout the day. Infant macaques and baboons may begin ingesting solid food around 2–3 months of age. Weaning is variable by species and occurs at approximately 1 year of age.

Table 13.2. Biologic and reproductive data for select nonhuman primate species

	Rhesus	Cynomolgus	Baboon	Squirrel
Adult body weight: Male	6–11 kg	6 kg	22–30 kg	700–1100 g
Adult body weight: Female	4–9 kg	4 kg	11–15 kg	500–1000 g
Life span	30+ y	37 y	40–45 y	20 y
Body temperature	36°–40°C (96.8°–104°F)	36°–38°C (96.8°–100.4°F)	36°–39°C (96.8°–102.2°F)	33.5°–38.8°C (92.3°–101.8°F)
Heart rate	150–333 beats per minute	107–215 beats per minute	80–200 beats per minute	225–350 beats per minute
Respiratory rate	10–25 breaths per minute	32–44 breaths per minute	29 breaths per minute	20–50 breaths per minute
Breeding onset: Male	38 mo	42–60 mo	73 mo	60 mo
Breeding onset: Female	34–43 mo	46 mo	51–73 mo	36–46 mo
Estrous cycle length	28 d	28 d	31–36 d	18 d
Gestation period	167 d	162 d	175–180 d	170 d
Weaning age	210–425 d	365–547 d	180–456 d	182 d
Chromosome number (diploid)	42	42	42	44

Source: Adapted from Johnson-Delaney (1994) and Turnquist and Minugh-Purvis (1995).

HUSBANDRY

Housing and Environment

The most suitable housing system for nonhuman primates depends on species, use, climatic conditions, and a number of other factors. In research laboratories, animals are often housed in stainless steel cages with slotted or grid floors. The Animal Welfare Act (AWA) regulations and the *Guide for the Care and Use of Laboratory Animals* (the *Guide*; ILAR, 2011) give cage size specifications for nonhuman primates. Most macaque monkeys are less than 15 kg and can be housed in 0.56 m^2 (6.0 ft^2) cages with a height of at least 81.28 cm (32 in.). A cage with a built-in squeeze design is desirable when animals are to receive frequent injections or blood collections. Cage pans are frequently used beneath individual cages to collect feces and urine. Wood-chip bedding may be placed in the pans to help absorb moisture; alternatively, there may be a sloped floor beneath a row of cages that diverts the urine and feces into a sewage drain. Nonhuman primates are highly intelligent and frequently learn how to open cage doors; thus, a sufficiently secure lock, such as a padlock, should be used.

In housing nonhuman primates for research purposes, rigid control of room temperature, relative humidity, ventilation, and lighting are essential. A temperature range of 18°–29°C (64°–84°F), relative humidity range of 30%–70%, and 10–15 air changes per hour are recommended. Ventilation from nonhuman primate housing should be filtered and fully exhausted to prevent contamination of personnel areas. Typically, 12–14 hours of light per day should be provided, controlled by automatic timers.

Breeding colonies can be housed in a variety of ways, including indoor pens connected to outdoor runs, covered cylindrical enclosures called corn cribs, outdoor corrals with some form of protection from extreme weather conditions, and free range on islands.

Environmental Enrichment and Social Housing

The AWA regulations mandate that primates used in research must be provided with environmental enrichment to promote psychological well-being. An excellent reference on this topic, *The Psychological Well-Being of Nonhuman Primates*, is published by the Institute for Laboratory Animal Research (ILAR, 1998; see www.nap.edu). A detailed, written plan for environmental enhancement must be developed, documented, and implemented (Box 13.3); these should be reviewed and reapproved by the IACUC periodically. It is well documented that social interaction is the best form of enrichment, although if animals are incompatible, fighting and trauma may occur. Thus, compatibility must be determined by trial and observation. The *Guide* states, "Group housing is critical and numerous species specific factors such as age, behavioral repertoire, sex, natural social organization, breeding requirements, and health status

Box 13.3

A detailed, written plan for environmental enhancement must be developed, documented, and implemented.

should be taken into consideration when forming a group. In addition, due to conformational differences of animals within groups, more space or height may be required to meet the animals' physical and behavioral needs." Newly grouped animals should never be left unattended for long periods. Pair or group housing is most successful when animals are placed together at a young age, and this promotes normal behavior such as allogrooming. Numerous cage designs allow side-by-side or top and bottom cages to become one large social cage by simply removing the dividing panels. If individual primates are strongly socialized toward humans, positive human interaction can also be considered an additional form of enrichment. Personnel safety is important in these interactions and should be prioritized.

In addition to social housing, other forms of environmental enrichment should be provided to promote species-typical activities. Newer caging designs are available that allow occupants to select audio and video recordings and to alter lighting and temperature, and that provide a "social wheel" to permit or exclude visualization or contact with other animals (Figure 13.2). Portable exercise rooms are also available that allow for periods of more aerobic activity (Figure 13.3). Grooming and foraging boards and more complex problem-solving devices such as puzzle feeders or video games can be used to encourage species-typical behavior. A simple piece of wood with bark or coconut shells enables important foraging and grooming behavior. For arboreal species, a swing or perch is important to allow the animals to engage in climbing activities. Food treats such as fruit, peanuts, granola, flavored ice cubes, vegetables, popcorn, and seeds may also be used. Finally, manipulanda such as mirrors, balls, and chains can be offered as toys, but they must be nontoxic, safe, durable, easily cleaned, and designed for laboratory primate use. It is best to offer a varied schedule of

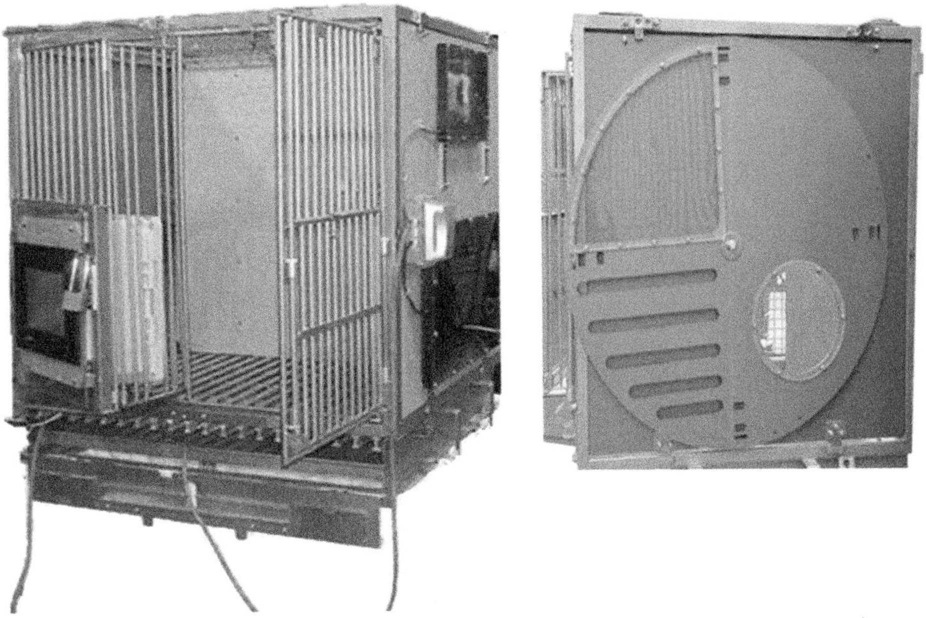

Fig 13.2. C.H.O.I.C.E Smart Cage and social wheel viewing access. (*Source:* Images courtesy of Britz and Company.)

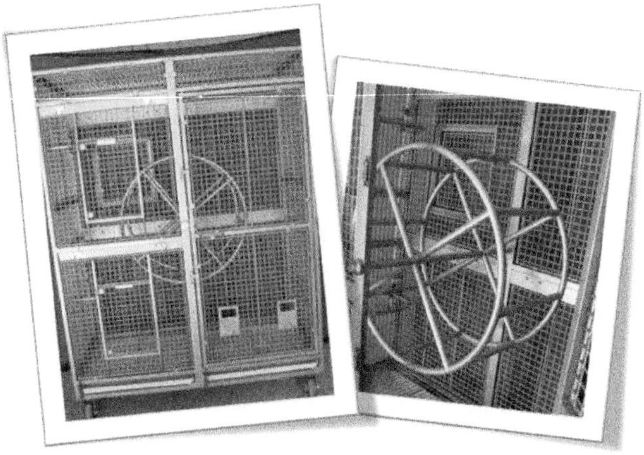

Fig 13.3. Play cage with wheel in the middle. (*Source:* Image courtesy of Britz and Company.)

enrichments so that the objects remain novel. Clear communication among veterinarians, principal investigators, and the IACUC regarding the introduction or standard use of enrichment items is necessary.

Feeding and Watering

Commercially milled, pelleted diets produced for specific types of laboratory primates adequately meet the nutritional needs if properly stored and if fed within 180 days of milling. Primates will consume an average of 3%–5% of their body weight in dry feed per day, but there is considerable waste; splitting portions into 2 or 3 daily feedings may reduce waste and more closely approximates natural behavior. Commercial diets prepared for NW primates usually contain 25% protein and 9% fat, supplemented with vitamin D_3; OW diets typically contain 15% protein and 5% fat. Some nutritionists recommend a 25% protein diet for pregnant, lactating, or juvenile OW monkeys. Protein-deficient animals are more susceptible to pneumonia, bacterial enteritis, and other illnesses. Diets may be supplemented with fresh fruits and vegetables, primarily as a form of environmental enrichment. Feeders or feeding stations should be physically distanced to prevent dominant animals from monopolizing the food supply.

Fresh, potable water should be provided *ad libitum* either through an automated watering system or in water bottles attached to the cage. Water bottles are more labor intensive but provide a route for the administration of medications or dietary supplements. Automated watering systems should be manually checked by the animal care staff daily to ensure the availability of water to each cage. Watering system malfunction should be suspected and investigated if otherwise healthy animals become suddenly anorexic.

Sanitation

Due to concerns regarding the potential transmission of zoonotic disease discussed later in this chapter, it is important to note that all work involving nonhuman primates must employ universal precautions, including a gown or other protective outer layer, splash-proof eye protection (or full face shield), cap, mask, shoe covers, and exam gloves. This protection is particularly important when working with soiled caging and other implements used with NHPs, particularly when spray may aerosolize biological material.

Housing requires a minimum of once-daily cleaning. In certain situations, such as group housing in a gang cage, a sufficient amount of urine and feces is produced to justify twice-daily cleaning. Generally, cage pans are removed, and the urine and feces are disposed of through a drain system or collected as contaminated waste. If suspended pans are not used, then the feces and urine must be rinsed from beneath the cages and to the drain. Care must be taken to avoid wetting the occupants when any spray-down method is used. Floors should be thoroughly rinsed or mopped to remove any adherent debris. Pans can be either replaced with clean pans or washed thoroughly and replaced. Racks, cages, pans, water bottles, and feed hoppers should be sanitized at least once every 2 weeks with chemicals, hot water 61.6°–82.2°C (143°–180°F), or a combination of both. Refer to Chapter 4 for more specific information on sanitization of caging.

TECHNIQUES

Handling and Restraint

One of the most striking features of primates is their great strength and agility. Chemical restraint is recommended for safe handling of all larger nonhuman primates. Individuals who handle NHPs must be adequately trained in order to minimize stress to the animal and to maximize safety for the handler. Personnel handling primates must wear protective clothing including a gown or other protective outer layer, splash-proof eye protection, cap, mask, shoe covers, and exam gloves (Figure 13.4). Great care must be taken with macaques as scratches from the animals or their caging, aerosolized biological material, mucous membrane splashes or bites have the potential to transmit *Macacine herpesvirus 1* (B virus), which induces a fatal encephalomyelitis in humans. The video "Working Safely with Nonhuman Primates," produced by the NIH Office of Animal Care and Use and available through the Office of Laboratory Animal Welfare, provides instruction and training in personal protection and primate behavior.

For primates weighing more than 2 kg, chemical restraint is strongly recommended. Administration of injections is greatly facilitated by restraint in a squeeze-back cage by staff who are trained to use this equipment. With patience and the use of positive reinforcement, animals can be trained to present themselves for an injection and greatly reduce the stress on both personnel and animals. Ketamine hydrochloride is the drug most frequently used for chemical restraint. Individual animals may have different responses to ketamine and may regain purposeful movement sooner than expected; a second dose should be available for quick response to these situations.

Manual restraint can be used for animals weighing less than 10 kg, but it should ideally be performed with at least two handlers. The risk for personal injury increases with manual restraint; in addition to protective clothing, elbow-length leather gloves

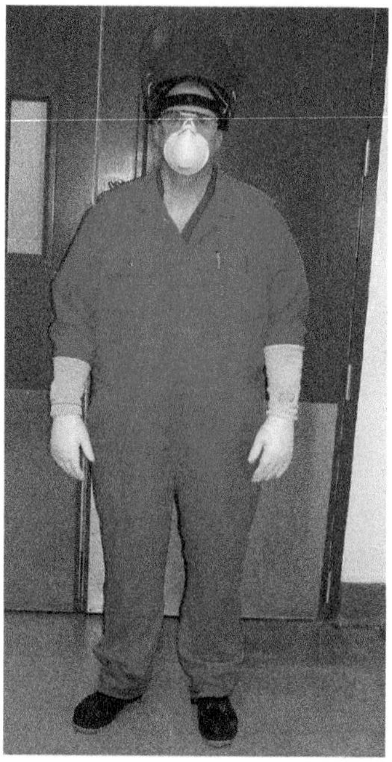

Fig 13.4. Protective clothing for working with macaque monkeys. (*Source:* Photo courtesy of *C. Medina.*)

should be worn but may not be impervious to sharp canine teeth. Manual restraint can be accomplished by squeezing the primate to the front of the cage to immobilize it; the cage may be opened and the upper arms just above the elbows can be grasped. The animal can then be removed by holding the arms behind the back so that the elbows nearly touch. The second handler is needed to release the squeeze mechanism, to operate the cage door, and for safety reasons. Primates restrained in this manner should be held away from the handler's body to avoid being grabbed or scratched by the animal's feet. The manual restraint of a small primate is depicted in Figure 13.5.

Another option for restraint is the pole-and-collar method. A small, lightweight plastic or aluminum collar with two small handles is secured around the neck of the anesthetized animal several days to weeks before restraint is actually necessary to permit acclimation. Depending on the primate's size and temperament, pole-and-collar restraint can be accomplished with one or two handlers. Once the animal is squeeze-restrained in the cage, the collar handles are grasped with poles and the primate is assisted from its cage and placed in a restraint chair or on a restraint table, where the neck collar is secured. Primates should be trained to this type of restraint with positive reinforcement and repetition. They can adapt well to this routine and will often walk to the restraint device.

Smaller primates can be restrained in specially made devices for some procedures, such as this marmoset undergoing an ultrasound (Figure 13.6). Animals placed in a restraint device should never be left unattended.

Restraint devices are specifically mentioned in the AWA regulations with the following specifications: (1) restraint devices are not to be considered a normal method

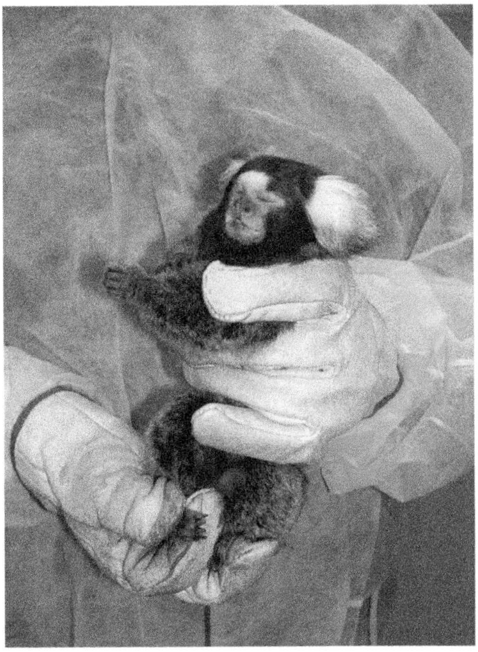

Fig 13.5. Manual restraint of a marmoset (*Callithrix jacchus*). (*Source:* Photo courtesy of *C. Medina.*)

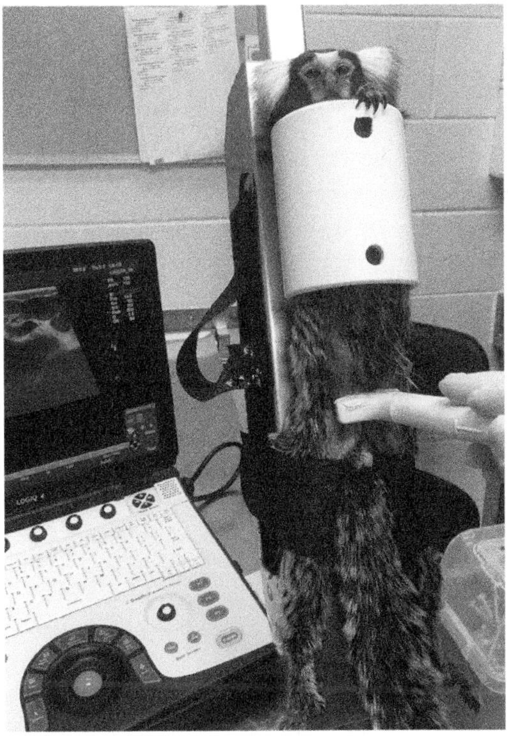

Fig 13.6. Specially designed restraint device for brief procedures such as an ultrasound. (*Source:* Photo courtesy of Wisconsin National Primate Resource Center.)

of housing; (2) restraint must be approved by the institutional animal care and use committee (IACUC); (3) restraint of animals should be kept to an absolute minimum amount of time; (4) restraint should not be used merely as a convenience but must be necessary to achieve research goals; and (5) restraint devices may require animals to be temporarily or permanently removed if they become ill, injured, or behaviorally altered from restraint. In instances where restraint over 12 hours is required, the animal must be provided the opportunity for daily unrestricted activity for at least one continuous hour during the period of restraint, unless continuous restraint is justified in the research proposal and approved by the IACUC.

Identification

Cage cards are used as a means of identifying individually caged animals but are never used as the sole means. Additional methods include chest or thigh tattoos, neck tags, ear tags, or electronic microchips. For group-housed animals, it is best to be able to identify individuals from a distance by means of a large identification tag placed around the neck. A unique pattern of clipped hair or marker or dye on the coat or skin can be used as methods for temporary identification.

Blood Collection

Approximate blood volumes for adults of several nonhuman primate species are listed in Table 13.3. Assuming the animal is mature, healthy, and on an adequate plane of nutrition, the blood volume of most species averages 7% of the body weight in grams. A typical rule of thumb for blood withdrawal suggests that up to 10% of the circulating blood volume can be withdrawn from normal, healthy animals every 2–3 weeks with minimal adverse effect. If larger volumes are required, collection intervals should be increased, hematocrits should be monitored, and fluid replacement therapy should be instituted to offset the volume depletion.

Blood samples can easily be obtained from percutaneous venipuncture of the femoral vein or artery. Sedation is required for larger animals, and the femoral triangle must be cleaned with alcohol or disinfectant. The needle should be introduced just medial to the femoral pulse to obtain a venous sample. Individuals performing this technique must be familiar with the typical anatomy of the femoral triangle. If an arterial sample is taken, apply direct pressure for a minimum of 3–5 minutes to prevent hematoma formation.

Other collection sites include the cephalic and saphenous veins. With a dedicated staff who can provide consistent training, primates can be trained using positive rein-

Table 13.3. Adult nonhuman primate blood volumes (mL)

	Rhesus	Cynomolgus	Baboon	Squirrel
Total blood	320–880	320–480	880–2400	40–120
Single sample	40–110	40–60	110–300	5–15
Exsanguination	120–330	120–180	190–330	15–45

Source: Adapted from Dysko and Hoskins (1995) and Johnson-Delaney (1994).
Notes: Values are approximate.

forcement (operant conditioning) to offer their arms or legs for blood collection. The use of training is encouraged in the 2011 edition of the *Guide*, which states, "Habituatring animals to routine husbandry or experimental procedures should be encouraged whenever possible as it may assist the animal to better cope with a captive environment by reducing stress associated with novel procedures or people. The type and duration of habituation needed will be determined by the complexity of the procedure. In most cases, principles of operant conditioning may be employed during training sessions, using progressive behavioral shaping to induce voluntary cooperation with procedures."

Surgically placed vascular access ports (VAPs) and tether systems allow for long-term blood collection and chronic dosing. The VAP can be maintained for many months with proper use of anticoagulants and sterile technique.

Urine Collection

Urine can be collected by cystocentesis, placement of a urinary catheter, or free-catch. When performing cystocentesis, the bladder should first be palpated to ensure urine is present and the abdomen cleaned with alcohol or disinfectant. Utilizing ultrasound guidance, the needle should enter perpendicular to the abdomen just cranial to the pubic bone. To use the free-catch method, a metabolism cage or a collection pan with a wire grid to separate the urine and the feces can be used.

Drug Administration

Maximum dosing volumes for various routes are listed in Table 13.4. Drug administration routes for NHPs are similar to those of most other large mammals. Oral dosing can be accomplished by placing the drug in a piece of fruit or on a piece of bread covered with peanut butter and jelly. Tablets can also be crushed or capsules opened to mix the drug in a favorite food. Primates, however, are adept at picking out the drug or eating around it. Many will accept drugs when mixed into a flavored yogurt or flavored syrup or juice; alternatively, animals can be trained to take juice from a syringe. Commercial vendors incorporate drugs into fruit-flavored tablets upon receipt of a prescription from a veterinarian. These tablets are well received and ensure accurate enteral dosing. Unpalatable drugs can be given to a lightly sedated animal through a nasogastric tube or orogastric tube using a bite block. Ensure proper placement of the stomach tube prior to administration.

Table 13.4. Maximum dosing volumes (mL/kg) in select species of nonhuman primates

Route	Macaque	Marmoset	Baboon
IP	10.0	20.0	5.0
SC	5.0	5.0	3.0
IM	0.5 (3.0 mL max)	0.5 (1.0 mL max)	0.5 (3.0 mL max)
IV	2.0 (bolus)/10.0 (infusion)	2.5 (bolus)/10.0 (infusion)	2.0 (bolus)/5.0 (infusion)
PO	15.0	15.0	15.0

Source: Adapted from Lukas (1999).

Subcutaneous (SC) injections can be administered under the loose skin over the dorsal cervical area. Intramuscular (IM) injections are usually given in the thigh muscles, using care to avoid the sciatic nerve. The triceps and gluteal muscles can also be used for IM injections of larger monkeys.

The cephalic, jugular, or saphenous veins can be used to deliver drugs intravenously. Larger volumes should be administered through an indwelling catheter. Surgical implantation of a vascular access port (VAP) is another alternative for long-term dosing. The VAP is implanted subcutaneously, usually on the back between the shoulder blades. Primates can be trained to present their VAP for injections into the port, or they can be restrained via a pole-and-collar system. Alternatively, the vascular system can be accessed through a tether system, which consists of a jacketed backpack pump or cage-top pump that allows for continuous infusion of drugs or saline. The vascular catheter exits through the skin on the back of the animal and enters the backpack pump or through a swivel that protects the catheter as it courses up to the cage-top pump. Osmotic minipumps may also be implanted for extended drug delivery.

Anesthesia, Surgery, and Postoperative Care

Due to a higher basal metabolic rate, NW primates often require higher dosages of anesthetics per kilogram of body weight compared with OW species. Due to the great diversity in nonhuman primate species, a discussion of anesthesia for the many different species is beyond the scope of this book. Presented here is a general overview of anesthesia, surgery, and postoperative care for the most common species used in biomedical research, the macaque (specifically *M. fascicularis*, *M. mulatta*). Agents commonly used for anesthesia and tranquilization are listed in Table 13.5. Macaques

Table 13.5. Anesthetic agents and tranquilizers used in macaques

Drug	Dose	Route	Reference
Inhalants			
Isoflurane	3%–4% induction, 1.5%–2.0% maintenance	Inhalation	Feeser and White (1992)
Sevoflurane	4%–8% induction, 1.25%–4% maintenance	Inhalation	Murphy et al. (2012)
Injectables			
Acepromazine	0.5–1 mg/kg	IM, SC, PO	Johnson et al. (1981)
Fentanyl	5–10 μg/kg IV bolus with 10–25 μg/kg/h continuous infusion	IV	Murphy et al. (2012)
Ketamine	10–15 mg/kg	IM	Carpenter (2017)
Ketamine	10 mg/kg	IM	Flecknell (2015)
+ xylazine	0.5 mg/kg	IM	
Propofol	5–10 mg/kg	IV	Sainsbury (1991)
	2.5–5.0 mg/kg followed by 0.3–0.4 mg/kg/min	IV	Sainsbury (1991)
Tiletamine–zolazepam	2–6 mg/kg; marked hypothermia	IM	Ialeggio (1989)

IM = intramuscular; IV = intravenous; PO = per os; and SC = subcutaneous.

are usually anesthetized with an injection of ketamine hydrochloride at 10 mg/kg IM to remove them from the cage safely. This dose may be adequate for endotracheal intubation; the animal can then be maintained by inhalation anesthesia. If the initial dose is inadequate, a small intravenous bolus of ketamine or propofol can be given to achieve intubation. Inhalants, including isoflurane and sevoflurane, are safe and commonly used in nonhuman primates. Animals should be premedicated with atropine or glycopyrrolate to minimize salivation and bradycardia.

Ketamine alone is not satisfactory for major surgery, since it does not provide adequate analgesia. The ketamine/xylazine combination, however, can be used for minor, short-term procedures. This injectable regimen usually provides about 30–45 minutes of anesthesia. Propofol at 5–10 mg/kg when given intravenously through an indwelling catheter provides a smooth induction and can be used to maintain anesthesia by constant-rate infusion, but it will induce a brief period of apnea and will not provide adequate analgesia for very invasive procedures. The depth of anesthesia is best gauged by the rate and depth of respiration, heart rate, and degree of jaw tension. The palpebral and pedal reflexes may also be used. Intraoperatively, body temperature should be maintained by use of a circulating water heating blanket. Warmed intravenous fluids are also helpful in preventing hypothermia. Placement of an intravenous catheter is important for longer duration anesthesia, allowing for administration of fluids and emergency drugs. Sterile technique is imperative.

Some of the most frequent surgeries performed on nonhuman primates include finger and tail amputations and laceration repair due to fight injuries. The use of a subcuticular suture pattern is recommended as it usually prevents the animal from removing the sutures and eliminates the need for suture removal.

Postoperatively, the animal should be placed in a recovery cage (or in the home cage if housed singly); supplemental heat such as a heat lamp should be provided to help prevent hypothermia. Frequent observation is required until the primate is able to maintain an upright position.

It is absolutely essential that pain be minimized through the use of analgesics in nonhuman primates that undergo painful procedures. Provision of analgesics prior to the painful stimulus, or preemptive analgesia, is the most effective method of pain management. The dosage and frequency of administration of all analgesic agents must be tailored to the animal, procedure, and anticipated level of pain. Table 13.6 lists analgesics for use in macaques. Buprenorphine is recommended for control of acute or

Table 13.6. Analgesic agents used in macaques

Drug	Dosage	Route	Reference
Bupivicaine	1–2 mg/kg locally	Infiltration	Murphy et al. (2012)
Buprenorphine	0.005–0.03 mg/kg q12h	IV, IM, SC	Murphy et al. (2012)
Butorphanol	0.5 mg/kg q8h	IM	APV (2018)
Carprofen	3–4 mg/kg q24h	SC	Flecknell (2015)
Ketoprofen	2 mg/kg q24h	IV, IM	APV (2018)
Meloxicam	0.1–0.2 mg/kg q24h	SC, PO	Flecknell (2015)

IM = intramuscular; IV = intravenous; PO = per os; and SC = subcutaneous.

chronic visceral pain but can cause sedation. Butorphanol can be used for mild postoperative discomfort. Nonsteroidal anti-inflammatory drugs (NSAIDs) such as carprofen and ketoprofen provide up to 24 hours of analgesia for mild-to-moderate pain. Local analgesics such as bupivicaine should also be considered to provide enhanced pain control with a nerve block for highly invasive procedures, such as thoracotomies. Combinations of opioids and NSAIDs are commonly used.

Euthanasia

All methods of euthanasia must conform to the most current *AVMA Guidelines on Euthanasia* (AVMA, 2013). After sedation with an IM injection of ketamine, primates can be euthanized by an intravenous overdose of a barbiturate or commercial euthanasia solution. Other methods of euthanasia are permissible if the animal is fully anesthetized, such as a bolus of potassium chloride or exsanguination and perfusion with a tissue fixative. Refer to Chapter 4 for more details regarding euthanasia guidelines.

THERAPEUTIC AGENTS

When considering therapeutics for nonhuman primates, it is important to carefully consider the diversity of species. The wide range of body size and types of primates makes extrapolation from one animal to another undependable, and it should be avoided. Whenever possible, the scientific literature or species experts should be consulted to determine the safest drugs and dosages. Antimicrobial and antifungal drug dosages for use with macaques are listed in Table 13.7; antiparasitic agents are listed in Table 13.8 and miscellaneous drugs are listed in Table 13.9.

INTRODUCTION TO DISEASES OF NONHUMAN PRIMATES

Improvements in husbandry, diagnostics, and therapeutics have led to the identification and control of a wide range of pathogenic organisms in closed colonies of nonhuman primates today. When housed in large colonies in outdoor corrals, the incidence of disease tends to increase, as there is a greater likelihood of pathogen exposure and often less environmental control. Basic knowledge of the agents that may infect a population is required to quickly and appropriately respond to a disease outbreak. The most common health problems of nonhuman primates are bacterial enteritis and bacterial pneumonia. These diseases may be latent in animals living in an unstressed state; however, active disease may be precipitated by the stress of transportation, a change in diet, or a new environment. Select vaccinations may be considered for all nonhuman primates, especially those housed in large colonies or outdoors. Vaccination against measles, rabies, and tetanus should be strongly considered for macaques housed under these conditions.

Nonhuman primates should be placed in quarantine and receive a thorough physical examination soon after their arrival at a new facility. Subsequent physical examinations should be conducted at least annually although more frequent

Table 13.7. Antimicrobial and antifungal agents used in macaques

Drug	Dosage	Route	Reference
Amoxicillin + clavulanic acid	6.5–13.5 mg/kg q8h	PO	Carpenter (2017)
Ampicillin	20 mg/kg q8h	PO, IM, IV	Johnson et al. (1981)
Cefazolin	20 mg/kg q8h	IM, IV	APV (2018)
Cephalexin	30 mg/kg q12h	PO	APV (2018)
Doxycycline	2.5 mg/kg q12h	PO	Johnson-Delaney (1994)
Enrofloxacin	5 mg/kg q24h for 10 d (to treat shigellosis)	PO, IM	Banish et al. (1993)
Erythromycin	75 mg/kg q12h for 10 d	PO	RPRC-WA (1987)
	15–20 mg/kg q12h	IM	APV (2018)
Fluconazole	2–3 mg/kg q24h for 30 d	PO	Carpenter (2017)
Metronidazole	12.5–15 mg/kg q12h	PO	Carpenter (2017)
	50 mg/kg q24h	PO	APV (2018)
Oxytetracycline	10 mg/kg q24h	SC, IM	Carpenter (2017)
Penicillin G, benzathine	20,000–60,000 IU/kg q24h	IM	APV (2018)
Penicillin G, procaine	20,000–40,000 IU/kg q12h	IM, SC	APV (2018)
Sulfamethazine	66 mg/kg q12h	PO	Carpenter (2017)
Tetracycline	20 mg/kg q8h	PO	APV (2018)
Trimethoprim	4 mg/kg q8h	SC, PO	APV (2018)

IM = intramuscular; IV = intravenous; PO = per os; and SC = subcutaneous.

Table 13.8. Antiparasitic agents used in macaques

Drug	Dosage	Route	Reference
Albendazole	25 mg/kg q12h for 3–5 d	PO	Murphy et al. (2012)
Fenbendazole	50 mg/kg q24h for 3 d, repeat in 3 wk., repeat in 3 mo	PO	APV (2018)
Ivermectin	0.2 mg/kg	PO, SC	APV (2018)
Piperazine	65 mg/kg q24h for 10 d	PO	Russell et al. (1981)
Praziquantel	5 mg/kg for one dose	PO, IM, SC	APV (2018)
Pyrantel	11 mg/kg for one dose	PO	Wolff (1990)
Sulfadimethoxine	50 mg/kg/d for the 1st day, then 25 mg/kg/d	PO	Wolff (1990)

IM = intramuscular; PO = per os; and SC = subcutaneous.

examinations may be warranted depending on health status, stage of life, and type of use. These animals tend to be quite stoic, making the accurate detection of clinical signs of illness or distress challenging.

A physical examination is performed in a manner similar to that for other species, with attention given to evidence of diarrhea, nasal or ocular discharge, dyspnea, conditions of the skin and hair coat, alertness, and nutritional state. Areas that should

Table 13.9. Miscellaneous agents used in macaques

Drug	Dosage	Route	Reference
Atropine	0.02–0.04 mg/kg	IM, IV, SC	APV (2018)
Bismuth subsalicylate	40 mg/kg q8–12h	PO	APV (2018)
Cimetadine	10 mg/kg q8h	IM, PO	APV (2018)
Cisapride	0.2 mg/kg q12h with meals	PO	Hotchkiss (1995)
Dexamethasone	≤2 mg/kg	IV, IM, PO	Johnson et al. (1981)
Diphenhydramine	5 mg/kg q6–8h	IV, IM, PO	APV (2018)
Dobutamine	2–10 μg/kg/min	IV	Popilskis and Kohn (1997)
Dopamine	2–5 μg/kg/min	IV	Popilskis and Kohn (1997)
Doxapram	2 mg/kg	IV	Flecknell (1987)
Epinephrine	0.2–0.4 mg/kg diluted in 5 mL sterile water	IT	Fortman et al. (2017)
	0.1–0.5 mg	SC, IM, IV	APV (2018)
Etomidate	1 mg/kg	IV	Carpenter (2017)
Flumazenil	0.02 mg/kg	IV	Murphy et al. (2012)
Furosemide	2 mg/kg	PO	Johnson et al. (1981)
Glycopyrrolate	0.005–0.01 mg/kg	IM	Carpenter (2017)
Lidocaine	0.7–1.4 mg/kg prn	IV	APV (2018)
Mannitol (25%)	0.25–1.0 g/kg bolus over 20 min	IV	Murphy et al. (2012)
Metoclopramide	0.2–0.5 mg/kg q8–24h	IM	APV (2018)
Naloxone	0.1 mg/kg as needed to reverse opioids	IV, IM, SC	APV (2018)
Omeprazole	0.4 mg/kg q12h	PO	Dubois et al. (1998)
Phenylephrine	One spray in each nostril q6h	Intranasal	Johnson et al. (1981)
Prednisolone sodium succinate	10 mg/kg	IM, IV	APV (2018)
Prednisone	0.5–1 mg/kg q12h for 3–5 d, then q24h for 3–5 d, then q48h for 10 d, then half the dose q48h	PO	Isaza et al. (1992)
Ranitidine	0.5 mg/kg q12h	PO	Carpenter (2017)
Vitamin C	25 mg/kg q12h for 5 d	PO	Ratterree et al. (1990)
Vitamin E + selenium	3.75 IU/kg + 1.15 mg/kg q 3d for 30 d	IM	Sainsbury (1991)
Yohimbine	0.1 mg/kg	IM, IV	APV (2018)

IM = intramuscular; IV = intravenous; PO = per os; SC = subcutaneous; and IT = intratracheal.

receive particular attention are body weight and body condition, the lymph nodes, the mouth, the palpable reproductive organs, and the digits. Body weights should be frequently monitored and considered in concert with a critical, hands-on examination of body condition so that unexpected changes can be quickly identified and investigated. Superficial lymph node enlargement or drainage can be suggestive of tuberculosis infection. Oral examination should include a thorough dental examination for detection of dental caries and broken teeth. Ulcers in a macaque are suggestive of the fatal zoonotic herpes B virus. Hemorrhage of the gums and gingivitis is characteristic of vitamin C deficiencies and gingivitis is associated with shigellosis in some species. The palpable reproductive organs (e.g., external genitalia, testicles, uterus, and ovaries) should be evaluated for evidence of trauma, neoplasia, and expected hormonal variations; digits should be evaluated for evidence of trauma such as may be incurred through fighting or entrapment in caging.

It is equally important that an animal is observed, ideally without the animal's awareness of the observer's presence, prior to disturbing the animal in any way. This provides the observer the opportunity to appreciate changes in an animal's activity, locomotion, and interaction with other nearby animals that may be affected by the observer's presence.

Zoonotic Diseases

One of the primary concerns in managing nonhuman primates is the protection of personnel from zoonotic, potentially fatal, diseases. All nonhuman primates must be regarded as potential sources of zoonotic disease (Box 13.4). Generally, the more closely related a species is to humans, the greater the danger for zoonotic disease transmission.

Some of the significant bacterial diseases transmissible to humans are tuberculosis, shigellosis, salmonellosis, melioidosis, and staphylococcal and streptococcal infections. Among the most significant viral diseases transmissible to humans from nonhuman primates are *Macacine herpesvirus 1* (herpes B), viral hepatitis, poxviruses, yellow fever, SV-40, poliomyelitis, rabies, and measles.

The most significant zoonotic parasites include protozoan and helminth parasites such as *Entamoeba histolytica* and *Enterobius vermicularis*. Malaria can also be transmitted if a vector is available. Many parasites of OW monkeys are transmissible to humans, while parasites of NW monkeys are more closely related to those of dogs and rodents and are generally not a zoonotic concern.

The following sections describe diseases that may likely be encountered in modern research colonies in the United States. They include infectious diseases that may spread quickly through a colony, often with fatal results, or that are caused by a zoonotic or anthropozoonotic (transmissible from humans to animal) organism. In addition, select, common, noninfectious disease conditions are described.

Box 13.4

All nonhuman primates must be regarded as potential sources of zoonotic disease.

Bacterial Diseases

Pneumonia and Respiratory Diseases

Nonhuman primates are susceptible to the human, bovine, and avian strains of *Mycobacterium* spp. The human strain, *Mycobacterium tuberculosis*, is by far the most frequent cause of simian tuberculosis. Although not the most common disease of nonhuman primates, it is one of the most devastating diseases likely to be encountered.

Tuberculosis is usually transmitted from humans to nonhuman primates in captivity, which underlies the importance of screening employees for subclinical tuberculosis infection. All nonhuman primate species are capable of contracting tuberculosis, but the disease is more prevalent in OW monkeys than in NW monkeys. Young macaques are the most susceptible group; rapid disease dissemination prior to the development of clinical signs is often seen. Disease development in older macaques, baboons, and apes is more similar to that in humans, with a slower progression. Experimentally induced tuberculosis has been observed to progress from initial infection to death within 6 weeks to 12 months. The primary route of transmission is through aerosols via the respiratory tract. Other routes include intestinal tract invasion; cutaneous infection such as by bites or tattoo needles; and exposure to the blood, sputum, excreta, cerebrospinal fluid, and exudates from lesions or tissues of infected animals.

The clinical signs of tuberculosis are usually not striking until the disease is in an advanced stage. The most commonly recognized signs are lethargy and weight loss. Other clinical signs are pneumonia, diarrhea, skin ulceration, and suppuration of lymph nodes. In some cases, no signs of illness are observed prior to sudden death of the animal.

Yellowish caseous nodules in the lungs and hilar lymph nodes are characteristic gross findings at necropsy. The liver, spleen, and lymph nodes of the abdominal, inguinal, and axillary areas are also frequently involved. Histologically, a classic presentation consists of tubercles with a central zone of caseous necrosis infiltrated with neutrophils and lymphocytes surrounded by a zone of epithelioid cells. Multinucleated giant cells of Langhans type may be seen. Mineralization and fibrosis of the tubercles are rare in nonhuman primates.

Diseases from which tuberculosis must be distinguished include lung mites, pulmonary nocardiosis, pseudotuberculosis, systemic mycoses, and neoplasms. No single premortem test is both sufficiently sensitive and specific to definitively diagnose tuberculosis infection (or lack of infection). As a result, although one test may be used in periodic colony screening, a combination of tests is recommended for more intensive screening or in the face of a potential disease outbreak. The intradermal tuberculin skin test (TST) remains one of the most commonly used screening tools. With this test, a known quantity of tuberculin is injected intradermally, usually in the upper palpebrae. The surrounding area is observed at 24, 48, and 72 hours postinjection for a delayed-type hypersensitivity response characterized by tissue edema, discoloration, ulceration, and necrosis. The eyelid is the preferred site as it facilitates reading of the test without recapturing the animal. Unfortunately, infected animals may not appropriately respond to this test (i.e., produce a false negative) due to anergy from repeated testing, recent measles vaccination, and immunosuppression such as may occur secondary to overwhelming tuberculosis infection or other concurrent disease. Alternatively, false-positive TST results may occur due to an animal's previous exposure to an organism antigenically similar to *Mycobacterium* spp., recent exposure to Freund's complete adjuvant, or traumatic injection technique. Other diagnostic methods developed for colony screening include *in vitro* assays to detect gamma interferon response or humoral immune response to tuberculin antigens.

Additional premortem and postmortem diagnostics are employed to confirm suspected *Mycobacterium* infections, including tissue, sputum, bronchoalveolar lavage, and gastric aspiration for acid-fast staining and cultures as well as polymerase chain reaction (PCR). Thoracic x-rays are occasionally employed to detect lung lesions in suspect animals. The lesions of nonhuman primate tuberculosis are often difficult to detect because calcium deposits within lymph nodes are rare and the heart blocks visualization of lesions around the hilar lymph nodes. Other factors that limit the value of thoracic radiographs are the small size of early lesions, lack of encapsulation, and the incidence of granulomas in many organs other than the lungs. Although treatment, such as long-term (approximately one year), systemic administration of isoniazid (alone or in combination with other drugs such as streptomycin) is possible for extremely valuable animals (e.g., great apes or select experimental animals), infected animals are most frequently euthanized due to the risk they present to humans and other animals within the colony. Disadvantages of using isoniazid include that it may (1) induce resistant strains, (2) mask the disease, (3) cause pyridoxine deficiency, and (4) alter experimental results. The most effective means of control is quarantine, testing, and elimination of reactors. Animals with a known or expected exposure to a tuberculosis-infected animal should be isolated and repeatedly tested for the disease or culled from the colony.

Another devastating pathogen of nonhuman primates is *Streptococcus pneumoniae*. *S. pneumoniae* is a common cause of fibrinopurulent pneumonia in OW primates that occasionally progresses to fibrinopurulent meningitis and arthritis with quick death. Transmission is by aerosol. Stress and waning passive immunity in neonates play a role in predisposing animals to infection and disease. *Bordetella bronchiseptica* has been reported to cause a high incidence of fibrinopurulent hemorrhagic bronchopneumonia in NW monkeys while it is less of a problem in OW primates. Other organisms often associated with pneumonia in primates include *Klebsiella pneumoniae*, *Pasteurella multocida*, *Haemophilus influenzae*, *Staphylococcus aureus*, and other *Streptococcus* spp.

Clinical signs of pneumonia are generally nonspecific and include fever, tachycardia, sneezing, coughing, mucopurulent nasal discharge, lethargy, anorexia, and dyspnea. In severe cases, cyanosis and prostration may be evident. With *S. pneumoniae*, meningitis with accompanying central nervous system signs is a frequent complication. The disease course may be several days to weeks.

Necropsy findings in cases of pneumonia typically include consolidated, red-to-gray lungs. A fibrinous pleuritis, pericarditis, and occasionally empyema are characteristic of infections with *S. pneumoniae*. Meningitis appears grossly as a diffuse gray opacity of the meninges with an accumulation of yellow–white viscous material in the sulci.

Culture and determination of antibiotic sensitivities are important in selection of the most effective antibiotic. Penicillins, cephalosporins, enrofloxacin, tetracycline, and chloramphenicol are some antibiotics commonly used to treat bacterial pneumonia. Supportive treatment includes maintaining the ambient temperature at a comfortable level and providing nutritional supplements and fluids if animals refuse food and water. Bronchial dilators and decongestants are often useful.

Moraxella catarrhalis is the causative agent for "bloody nose syndrome" in macaques. *M. catarrhalis* is a common cause of sinusitis in people although it is debated if an identical bacterial strain infects both nonhuman primates and humans. The organism can be isolated from the nasopharynx of clinically normal macaques and thus does not always induce disease. Clinical signs include epistaxis and occasionally periorbital edema. Diagnosis is by isolation of the diplococcal organism and response to select antibiotics (e.g., amoxicillin–clavulanic acid, extended spectrum cephalosporins, trimethoprim–sulfa, tetracyclines, and fluoroquinolones).

Bacterial Gastroenteritis

Three of the most common types of bacterial gastroenteritis in primates are campylobacteriosis, shigellosis, and salmonellosis.

Campylobacter jejuni is the organism most frequently isolated from active cases of campylobacteriosis diarrheal disease and is primarily found in OW primates. Asymptomatic carriers are common, and transmission is fecal–oral. Clinical signs include watery diarrhea, most frequently without blood or mucous, and severe dehydration. Diagnosis requires fecal culture on special media incubated in a 5%–10% CO_2 environment, although serologic tests have been developed. Treatment includes supportive care including rehydration and correction of electrolyte abnormalities. The use of antibiotics has been debated.

Clinically apparent shigellosis is most frequently due to *Shigella flexneri* although other *Shigella* species may also induce disease. The organism is zoonotic with transmission via the fecal–oral route. Stress may precipitate clinical disease from a silent infection. Though adult humans seldom become clinically ill, the disease can be severe or even fatal in children. Infections in nonhuman primates and humans range from asymptomatic carriers to acute fulminant dysentery. Clinical signs in nonhuman primates include depression; blood-tinged, mucoid diarrhea; weakness; emaciation; and dehydration. Abdominal pain is often evident, and the affected primate may bend forward in a sitting position with its hands folded across its abdomen. Typically, as the disease progresses, the animal becomes semicomatose; death may occur from 24 hours to 2 weeks after onset of illness. Alternatively, nonenteric *Shigella* infections may occur and clinical signs include gingivitis, abortion, and air sac infection. Culture is required for diagnosis although *Shigella* spp. can frequently be isolated from asymptomatic individuals. Strict environmental decontamination should be instituted.

Although less common than *Shigella* spp. and *Campylobacter* spp. infections, gastroenteritis from *Salmonella* spp. infections also occurs in nonhuman primates. Contaminated feed and contact with infected animals are the principal sources of infection with *Salmonella* spp. The clinical features of *Salmonella* spp. infection are similar to those of *Shigella* spp. infection except that vomiting is more common and the course of the disease is often less acute.

The gross lesions of shigellosis and salmonellosis are not readily distinguishable, and the two may exist as a mixed infection. In fatal cases of shigellosis, the colon is usually distended and contains mucus and occasionally blood. The mucosa is thickened, reddened, and may be ulcerated, and the surface covered by an exudate composed of fibrin and necrotic cells. Typical gross findings with salmonellosis are pasty-to-liquid intestinal contents, a swollen and reddened intestinal mucosa, and splenic congestion. *Salmonella* spp. infections frequently involve the ileum, whereas ileal involvement is infrequent with shigellosis.

It is often difficult to recover *Shigella* spp. organisms from rectal swabs; thus a negative culture is not conclusive. In culturing for intestinal pathogens, the swab should be inserted into the rectum and the surface of the mucosa scraped. The bacteria are very sensitive to drying, so swabs must be protected before presentation to the laboratory. Ideally, plates are streaked directly from rectal swabs immediately following specimen collection.

In general, treatment of bacterial gastroenteritis includes provision of supportive care and antibiotic administration based on culture and sensitivity testing. Antisecretory drugs such as diphenoxylate hydrochloride, kaolin, and pectin, or other intestinal absorbents may be indicated. Fluid and electrolyte replacement is essential in cases of severe diarrhea and are ideally administered intravenously although intraosseous or subcutaneous administration can be used if necessary. NW monkeys often require higher relative volumes of fluids compared with OW monkeys. Animals exposed to known infected animals should be evaluated for infection and considered for treatment.

Tetanus

Tetanus is caused by two neurotoxins produced by *Clostridium tetani*: tetanospasmin and tetanolysin. Old world and new world monkeys, as well as apes, are susceptible. Clinical signs include tonic muscle spasms, trismus (lockjaw), dysphagia, opisthotonos, seizures, respiratory paralysis, and death. Vaccines (e.g., tetanus toxoid) are recommended for primates housed outdoors with soil contact. Tetanus antitoxin can be effective in treating cases of tetanus.

Other Zoonotic Bacterial Organisms

Other bacterial organisms, including *Helicobacter pylori*, *Lawsonia intracellularis*, *Yersinia pseudotuberculosis*, *Yersinia enterocolitica*, and *Burkholderia pseudomallei*, known to infect humans have been shown to cause disease in nonhuman primates. To date, the natural transmission of these organisms from nonhuman primates to humans has not been documented. However, their zoonotic potential should be understood and appropriate precautions instituted to guard against their transmission between species.

Several species of OW monkeys, especially rhesus, harbor *H. pylori* in their stomachs. *Helicobacter* spp. have been identified as causative agents for gastritis and gastric ulcers in humans and many other species. There are usually no clinical signs in nonhuman primates aside from inappetence and occasional vomiting. Diagnosis is based on gastric biopsy and culture results. Histologically, a lymphocytic plasmacytic gastritis may be present. Treatment is similar to that of humans, including a multiday, multidrug regimen; however, eradication of the organism may not be successful.

L. intracellularis, the cause of proliferative enteritis in several species, has been isolated from young rhesus, 6–16 months of age, with fatal proliferative enteritis. Epizootics of the disease are usually confined to younger animals. Infection occurs primarily in weanlings, when passive maternal immunity declines. Transmission is fecal–oral. Organisms localize to and multiply in intestinal proliferating crypt epithelial cells. Clinical signs included depression, mild diarrhea, and abdominal distension. Anemia and hypothermia are reported in severely affected individuals.

Pseudotuberculosis is caused by *Y. pseudotuberculosis* or *Y. enterocolitica* and has been reported in both OW and NW monkeys. Wild rodents and birds are reservoir hosts, and transmission is by ingestion of contaminated feed. Acute yersiniosis typically occurs as enteritis primarily affecting the jejunum and ileum. Clinical signs may include diarrhea, depression, and dehydration, or simply acute death. In its chronic form, septicemia results in necropurulent lesions in the liver, spleen, and other organs and may be confused grossly with tuberculosis. Microscopic liver or lung lesions consist of a central area of necrosis with neutrophils and clumps of bacteria surrounded by a zone of macrophages.

Melioidosis is caused by *B. pseudomallei*, which is a soil and water saprophyte typically found in tropical areas, including Southeast Asia and select regions of Australia, Central and South America, Africa, and the Middle East. It is currently designated as a Tier 1 select agent (www.selectagents.gov) by the Centers for Disease Control and Prevention (CDC) and the US Department of Agriculture (USDA). The disease has been reported in OW monkeys and apes. The organism can remain clinically latent for years. Disease transmission typically results from contact with a contaminated environment via the integumentary, respiratory, or gastrointestinal system. The disease is not readily transmitted among individuals. The clinical course of melioidosis may be acute and fulminant or chronic. Clinical signs can be nonspecific or dependent on the affected organ system but may include bronchopneumonia, multiple subcutaneous abscesses, lymphadenitis, and swollen joints. Gross findings include suppurative or caseous nodules in tissues or organs—including the lungs, spleen, liver, and lymph nodes—and/or pneumonia. Infections are most frequently resistant to treatment.

Mycotic Diseases

Dermatophytosis

Ringworm in nonhuman primates can be caused by several *Microsporum* spp. and *Trichophyton* spp. Long-term, systemic antifungal treatment is recommended.

Systemic Mycoses

Candidiasis occurs in animals that are immunosuppressed, debilitated, or on long-term antibiotic therapy. Thrush is the most common presentation of *Candida albicans* infection and is seen as a white, velvety overlay in the mouth and throat.

Pneumocystis carinii is another fungal organism primarily seen as an opportunistic infection in immunosuppressed primates. Clinical signs include fever, dyspnea, and coughing. Fungal cysts can be identified with special stains such as Gomori's methenamine silver.

Histoplasma capsulatum var. *duboisii* is the etiologic agent of African histoplasmosis. Histoplasmosis has been reported in baboons maintained in outdoor colonies within the United States. Transmission is from dermal contact, inhalation, or ingestion of spores from contaminated soil as well as direct contact with infected primates. Organs affected include the skin, lymph nodes, and bones. Treatment includes appropriate antibiotic administration with or without surgical excision of affected areas.

Nocardiosis in nonhuman primates is most commonly seen as a granulomatous disease of the lungs resembling tuberculosis. Nocardiosis can be differentiated from tuberculosis by the absence of involvement of hilar lymph nodes.

Viral Diseases

Herpesviruses

Although a large number of herpesviruses have been isolated from different species of nonhuman primates, the pathogenic effects of many of these isolates have not been established. A number of specific alphaherpesviruses do produce highly fatal systemic diseases. In most alphaherpesvirus infections, there are two types of host: a reservoir or natural host, in which the virus exists as a subclinical or latent infection; and an aberrant or accidental host of a different species, in which the infection is usually fatal. These viruses and their natural and aberrant hosts are important to consider when selecting the physical placement and path of personnel and the movement of equipment between colonies of different primate species.

Herpes simplex virus (*Human herpesvirus 1*) is the cause of fever blisters or cold sores in humans. Humans are the reservoir hosts. Certain species of nonhuman primates (primarily marmosets, tamarins, and owl monkeys) are aberrant hosts that suffer fatal infections. Lesions in affected nonhuman primates include ulceration of the lips, tongue, and gastrointestinal tract, and hepatic necrosis.

The natural host of *Saimiriine herpesvirus 1* (SaHV1), previously known as Herpesvirus tamarinus, is the squirrel monkey, and infection in this species is asymptomatic. It can exist as a latent infection in squirrel, cebus, and spider monkeys. Host species may show oral vesicles or ulcers, similar to those of herpes simplex virus in humans and herpes B virus in macaques. Fatal infections most commonly occur in owl monkeys, tamarins, and marmosets. Lesions in fatally infected monkeys include facial swelling with self-trauma; ulceration of the lips, tongue, and gastrointestinal tract; and hepatic necrosis. The virus is not zoonotic.

Other select herpesviruses of note include *Cercopithecine herpesvirus 2* (formerly known as Simian agent 8), *Cercopithecine herpesvirus 9* (formerly Simian varicella virus), *Saimiriine herpesvirus 2* (formerly Herpesvirus saimiri), and *Ateline herpesvirus* (formerly Herpesvirus ateles). While these viruses are not recognized zoonotic agents, they do induce serious, often fatal, disease in their aberrant nonhuman primate host species.

Macacine herpesvirus 1, previously known as *Cercopithecine herpesvirus 1* and commonly referred to as herpes B virus, is an alphaherpesvirus that is an important zoonotic disease of macaques. Macaques are the natural hosts for herpes B in which infection is lifelong with intermittent reactivation and shedding of the virus in saliva or genital secretions, particularly during periods of stress or immunosuppression. Humans are one of the aberrant hosts of this virus. Transmission to humans is usually through bites and scratches from infected macaques although transmission may also occur through scratches or punctures from contaminated medical equipment, fomites,

Box 13.5

Because B virus is intermittently shed, persons in close contact with macaques must treat all macaques as potentially infectious carriers and wear appropriate protective clothing to prevent exposure.

or caging or through contact of an animal's infectious secretions with a person's mucous membranes. Infected macaques may develop conjunctivitis, vesicles or ulcers on the oral or genital mucosa, or may be asymptomatic. Obtaining macaques from herpes B–negative colonies is recommended but does not eliminate the possibility of disease. Because B virus is intermittently shed, persons in close contact with macaques must treat all macaques as potentially infectious carriers and wear appropriate protective clothing (e.g., gown, gloves, mask, full eye protection or face shield) to prevent exposure (Box 13.5). Universal precautions should be followed in handling all equipment and specimens that may be contaminated with macaque blood, urine, saliva, or tissues.

Personnel working with or around macaques must be educated about the clinical manifestations of herpes B infection. In humans, infection with the virus can frequently result in severe encephalomyelitis. Although the incidence of human disease is very low, the case fatality rate is approximately 80% with death occurring within 10–14 days. An expert panel of virologists and physicians have developed and published "Recommendations for prevention of and therapy for exposure to B virus" (Cohen et al., 2002). These recommendations state, "Materials including supplies used for first aid and specimen collection, copies of written instructional materials, and treatment protocols for exposures should be available in areas where exposure can occur. Signs that indicate the proper actions to take in the event of exposure should be posted in areas in which exposures to macaques may occur." Following an exposure to the herpes B virus, potentially exposed skin should be washed with a solution containing detergent soap for at least 15 minutes in an attempt to reduce or eliminate the number of viable viral organisms. Eyes or mucous membranes potentially exposed to B virus should be irrigated immediately with sterile saline solution or water for 15 minutes. Following the immediate washing, the exposed individuals must be evaluated by the designated occupation health physician knowledgeable about herpes B virus. The physician will then determine the need for additional wound cleaning and/or the initiation of antiviral treatment.

Paired sera should be obtained from the human and macaque on the day of exposure as well as approximately 3 weeks later. Viral cultures of the buccal mucosa, genital mucosa, and conjunctiva of each eye of the macaque and of the human exposure site should be collected to determine if virus is present. False negatives can occur. Viral cultures should be submitted to the B Virus Research and Reference Laboratory at Georgia State University. Clinical signs in humans may include vesicles, pain and itching at the exposure site, lymphadenopathy, fever, numbness, muscle weakness or paralysis in the exposed extremity, conjunctivitis, neck stiffness, sinusitis, headache, nausea, vomiting, altered mental state, and other central nervous system signs before death. Early treatment of humans with an antiviral agent, before they show central nervous system signs, has resulted in halting the disease progression but does not appear to eliminate the virus. Exposed individuals should be closely monitored by a physician until it can be safely assumed that the individual is free of infection. During the intervening time, the individual should be counseled to avoid activities that could result in disease dissemination to other humans.

Measles

Measles (rubeola), a human paramyxovirus, can infect both OW and NW monkeys and apes although it is not naturally found in wild populations removed from human contact. Humans serve as the disease reservoir for nonhuman primates. Measles is highly contagious with transmission by aerosol or direct contact with secretions. Measles commonly produces a mild upper respiratory infection in most species of OW primates. Macaques may exhibit a more severe respiratory illness, including pneumonia. Clinical signs most frequently seen in OW monkeys include nasal and ocular discharge, conjunctivitis, facial edema, blepharitis, and a papular skin rash. Occasionally, the infection will progress to depression, anorexia, coughing, and dyspnea in conjunction with giant cell pneumonia. Abortions and neurologic signs have also been reported. Morbidity is high and mortality, caused by secondary bacterial infections, is low in OW monkeys. The disease is much more severe in marmosets, owl monkeys, and colobines, in which hemorrhagic gastroenteritis predominates and respiratory tract lesions and the skin rash are absent or less significant. Active infection with measles produces a general immunosuppression that mutes the antigenic response to the tuberculin skin test, possibly resulting in a false-negative reading.

The most important preventive measure is avoiding exposure to infected humans, the primary source of nonhuman primate infections although the virus can be transmitted between nonhuman primates. Some facilities require measles vaccination or proof of serologic immunity of all humans who enter nonhuman primate facilities (e.g., animal caretakers, visitors, building support personnel). A monovalent human measles vaccine (Attenuvax) has been shown to be effective in protecting both OW and NW monkeys from the disease. It should be noted that this vaccination can cause immunosuppression that interferes with the intradermal tuberculin test, and animals may require up to 4 weeks to return to normal immunocompetency. Due to this complication as well as the high cost of the human vaccine, an alternative, less expensive but equally effective vaccine (e.g., canine distemper vaccine, Vanguard-2) had been used. Unfortunately, production of Attenuvax has been suspended, and the formulation of Vanguard-2 has been altered to eliminate the measles component. Though some trials have recently been performed to assess efficacy, an alternative measles vaccine has not yet been validated for use in nonhuman primates.

Poxviruses

Five different poxviruses are known to naturally infect nonhuman primates: monkeypox, Yaba-like disease virus (YLDV), Yaba monkey tumor virus (YMTV), cowpox, and *Molluscum contagiosum*. All five viruses can infect humans. In most cases, only epidermal changes are seen in NHPs and humans, and infections are self-limiting. The incidence of each virus should be extremely low in a modern nonhuman primate research facility.

Monkeypox is closely related to smallpox (variola) and vaccinia viruses and affects NW and OW monkeys and apes (including humans). Characteristic lesions associated with the disease in nonhuman primates are 1- to 4-mm circular papules that develop predominantly on the skin of the hands, feet, and face and that progress in approximately 10 days to vesicles, pustules, and scabs. The respiratory system may also be affected. No specific treatment exists. Human disease is seen mainly in Africa with clinical signs similar to early smallpox disease, including fatigue, fever, muscular and back pain, and disseminated pox skin lesions. A small percentage of fatalities have occurred in infected children. In 2003, in the United States there was an outbreak of monkeypox in people associated with pet prairie dogs. Immunization with vaccinia protects both human and nonhuman primates against the disease.

Yaba-like disease virus, once believed to be identical to the closely related *Tanapox virus*, is a benign cutaneous infection of humans. While NW primates are resistant, OW primates are susceptible to the disease and develop skin lesions that are circular, with umbilication and an adherent scab in the center. Papules initially appear similar to monkeypox lesions but do not progress to pustules. Histologically, there is hyperplasia of the epithelium of the skin and epidermal necrosis with little damage to the underlying dermis. A notable characteristic of this disease is that there are usually only a few epidermal lesions seen on each infected animal. The lesions usually regress spontaneously in 3–4 weeks. Human infections can occur and are characterized by pyrexia and skin papules and nodules that progress to pock lesions.

Yaba monkey tumor virus is an oncogenic virus originally isolated from rhesus monkeys at Yaba, Nigeria. Few natural outbreaks of disease have been reported in rhesus and baboons; NW primates are resistant to the disease. Transmission is unknown but is suspected to be through arthropod vectors, trauma, or nosocomial from the use of contaminated needles between animals. The virus can infect both NHPs and humans and is characterized by the presence of nodular lesions, primarily on the extremities, that progress up to multiple centimeters in diameter, may ulcerate, and then completely regress within approximately 6 weeks. Histologically, the tumors consist of proliferations of histiocytes, frequently with eosinophilic intracytoplasmic inclusions.

Cowpox virus has been identified in OW primates as well as in NW primates, in which the disease may be fatal. Transmission is through rodent vectors not present in the United States; therefore, while it is a zoonotic agent, the risk to personnel in US facilities is exceedingly low.

M. contagiosum is a poxvirus disease primarily of humans. Transmission is usually by direct contact. A similar, if not identical, viral infection has been reported in chimpanzees with skin lesions that appear as waxy papular cutaneous elevations, especially on the eyelid and groin. Histologically, there are large, basophilic intracytoplasmic inclusion bodies called molluscum bodies. It is unknown if the viral agent of nonhuman primates can directly infect humans.

Treatment of poxvirus lesions, if indicated, should be directed at prevention of self-trauma and secondary infection through the use of sedatives, antipruritic drugs, and antibiotics.

Hepatitis Viruses

Hepatitis A virus (HAV), a hepatovirus, causes a disease that was formerly known as infectious hepatitis. Naturally occurring infections have been reported in several nonhuman primate species, including rhesus, cynomolgus, African green monkeys, owl monkeys, chimpanzees, and marmosets. Transmission is fecal–oral. Humans and nonhuman primates are usually asymptomatic. Prevention involves attention to handwashing and personal hygiene as numerous cases of nonhuman primate-to-human transmission have been documented. Personnel working with experimentally infected HAV monkeys should be vaccinated with a commercially available HAV vaccine.

Hepatitis B virus (HBV), known as *Hepadnavirus B*, induces a significant viral hepatitis in humans in which approximately 8% of infected people become chronic carriers and may eventually develop hepatocellular carcinoma. Naturally occurring infections have been reported primarily in wild chimpanzees and gorillas, which remain asymptomatic. Transmission within these species is by parenteral inoculation; droplet exposure of mucous membranes; or contact exposure of broken skin with contaminated blood, saliva, semen, cerebrospinal fluid, or urine. Although disease transmission has not been documented between nonhuman primates and humans, the possibility remains. As such, personnel working with chimpanzees and gorillas should be vaccinated with a commercially available HBV vaccine.

Hepatitis C virus (HCV), a *Hepacivirus*, causes a hepatic disease that was previously called non-A, non-B hepatitis (NANBH). Transmission is parenteral and is similar to that for HBV. It appears that there are no naturally occurring cases of this viral disease in nonhuman primates, and only experimentally infected chimpanzees pose a zoonotic hazard to personnel. There is no vaccine available to prevent this disease.

Viruses Causing Hemorrhagic Fevers

Multiple hemorrhagic fever viruses (e.g., Ebola virus, Marburg virus, and simian hemorrhagic fever virus) can infect nonhuman primates and may induce seroconversion or often-fatal disease in humans. While these viruses are of specific concern when working with nonhuman primates (or their cells or tissues) imported from select foreign locations or with purposefully infected animals, the viruses are not expected in US facilities as they are heavily screened for in all nonhuman primates imported into the country.

Encephalomyocarditis Viruses

Encephalomyocarditis viruses (EMCV) are a collection of cardioviruses that have been shown to cause myocarditis in nonhuman primates, elephants, pigs, and other species. Various nonhuman primate species, including orangutans, chimpanzees, baboons, squirrel monkeys, rhesus macaques, tamarins, and lemurs have been affected, most commonly in zoo populations. Rodents, especially rats and mice, are believed to be the reservoir host. Sudden death and frothy exudate from the nose and mouth are the primary clinical signs seen in nonhuman primates. Gross findings include pericardial effusion and pale streaks in the myocardium. Histologically, there is necrosis of the myofibers with inflammation and edema. Controlling rodent populations around outdoor housing as well as protecting food and water sources from rodent contamination is important in preventing infections. EMCV detection by PCR is the most rapid, sensitive, and specific method for the diagnosis of this infection. PCR methodology can reduce the frequency of false-negative diagnoses of this virus. Although this virus can infect humans, human infections are exceedingly rare and the means of disease transmission are not understood.

Retroviruses

The *Retroviridae* family consists of two subfamilies: *Orthoretrovirinae* and *Spumaretrovirinae*. To date, only viruses within *Orthoretrovirinae* have been shown to cause clinical disease in nonhuman primates. There are endogenous and exogenous viruses within the *Retroviridae* family. *Endogenous viruses* have become incorporated into the host's genomic material and are transmitted vertically. *Exogenous viruses* exist outside of the host and are transmitted horizontally.

Simian T-cell leukemia virus (STLV) belongs to the genus *Deltaretrovirus* and is an exogenous type C oncovirus. It is 90%–95% homologous to the human T-cell leukemia virus (HTLV) that induces adult T-cell leukemia/lymphoma and other disorders. There are numerous strains of STLV, just as there are numerous strains of HTLV. Naturally occurring infections have been reported in baboons, patas monkeys, African green monkeys, macaques, and chimpanzees. Transmission is by sexual contact or parenteral inoculation. Most animals remain asymptomatic; however, a leukemia/lymphoma syndrome has been reported in baboons, African green monkeys, and macaques. Diagnosis is by serology and identification of the virus in tumor cells by molecular biologic techniques. The STLV infection is an important model for studying HTLV infections in humans. PCR can be used to identify monkeys that are positive for STLV viruses.

Two groups of simian retroviruses are of particular importance to nonhuman primates: simian retrovirus (SRV; formerly known as simian retrovirus type D) and simian immunodeficiency virus (SIV), which is closely related to the etiologic agent of human AIDS. SRV and SIV differ in the species of nonhuman primates they infect, their prevalence in captive populations, their clinical course in symptomatic individuals (often variants of immunodeficiencies), and their associated diseases. However, susceptible animal populations should be screened for these viruses as they may be significant confounders of study results. The zoonotic potential of the simian retroviruses is not fully understood but is suspected to be low, except possibly in severely immunocompromised humans.

Rabies

Rabies occurs occasionally in nonhuman primates. Animals housed outdoors are particularly at risk for contracting the disease due to their possible interaction with rabid wildlife. Clinical signs include irritability, aggression, hypersalivation, self-trauma, paralysis, and sudden death. Only killed vaccines should be administered to nonhuman primates as vaccination with a modified-live rabies vaccine has been suspected to induce the disease.

Miscellaneous Viral Infections

Other viral infections that have been reported less frequently in nonhuman primates include yellow fever, chicken pox, Epstein–Barr virus, adenovirus, papillomavirus, papovavirus, lymphocytic choriomeningitis, and cytomegalovirus.

Parasitic Diseases

Protozoa

Entamoeba histolytica is pathogenic for OW and NW monkeys and apes, including humans, in whom amebic dysentery is induced. *E. histolytica* must be differentiated from the nonpathogenic protozoan *E. dispar*, which is morphologically identical. Asymptomatic carriers are common although clinical diarrhea is occasionally seen. The most common lesions are gut ulceration and hepatic abscesses. Ulcers in the gut typically have a flask shape. Special techniques are needed to recover and identify the organism because it is not ordinarily detected by routine fecal flotation. Detection of specific *E. histolytica* antigens in stools is a fast, sensitive technique that should be considered the method of choice. Stool PCR is a highly sensitive and specific technique, but it is more costly. The utility of serologic tests in distinguishing *E. dispar* from *E. histolytica* is controversial. However, serology is still considered the method of choice for diagnosis of extraintestinal amebiasis. Recommended treatments include metronidazole, tetracycline, chloramphenicol, paramomycin, and diiodohydroxyquin.

Balantidium coli is frequently found in fecal specimens of various nonhuman primate species, especially the anthropoid apes. Asymptomatic infections are common. Transmission is fecal–oral through ingestion of contaminated food or water. The pathogenicity of the organism for nonhuman primates has not been clearly established, but ulcerative lesions in the large intestine have been reported and set the stage for systemic spread. Infections in humans may result in severe diarrhea and dysentery. Recommended treatments for elimination of *B. coli* include metronidazole, tetracycline, and diiodohydroxyquin.

Both OW and NW monkeys as well as apes can contract malaria through infection with various *Plasmodium* spp. Females of various species of anopheline mosquitoes transmit malaria. The life cycle in nonhuman primates occurs in the hepatocytes and red blood cells. Some *Plasmodium* spp. cause cyclic bouts of fever and anemia due to lysis of red blood cells caused by multiplication of the protozoan organisms. Infected animals may be a source of infection for humans if the required species of mosquito vectors are present or via parenteral inoculation. Gross findings include gray lungs, liver, and spleen due to malarial pigment in the macrophages as well as hepatosplenomegaly. Common treatment regimens include use of chloroquine and primaquine; however, chloroquine-resistant strains of malarial organisms are increasingly common.

Hepatocystis spp. are protozoans related to *Plasmodium* spp. These organisms infect African and Asian OW monkeys, primarily baboons, African green monkeys, and macaques. Transmission is through the bite of a midge, the intermediate host. Infected monkeys remain asymptomatic because replication of the organism occurs only in the hepatocytes. Gross findings include 2- to 4-mm opaque cysts or scars in the liver, and adhesions to the liver may be present. Neither treatment nor prophylaxis is commonly necessary as the intermediate host is not present in the United States. However, infections of imported nonhuman primates are common.

Nematodes

Oesophagostomum spp., or nodular nematodes, are the most common helminth parasites affecting OW monkeys and apes; they also infect multiple other species of primates, but rarely NW monkeys. The infection is usually asymptomatic, but heavy burdens can cause diarrhea, unthriftiness, weight loss, and intra-abdominal adhesions with parasite death or migration. The parasite produces firm, smooth, black or white nodules in the wall of the large intestine and cecum and mesentery that initially contained the viable adults. Premortem diagnosis is by observation of the eggs or adults in the feces, although this can be difficult as the eggs are indistinguishable from hookworm eggs. Postmortem diagnosis is by histologic observation of the characteristic nodules. Thiabendazole, levamisole phosphate, and mebendazole can be effective treatments. The parasite may infect humans, thus appropriate sanitation and animal handling procedures should be followed.

Strongyloides fulleborni and *Strongyloides cebus* are very common zoonotic parasites of nonhuman primates. Infections are frequently asymptomatic, but heavy infections can cause severe diarrhea and coughing from migration of the larvae through the lungs. Apes are more prone to develop severe clinical disease. Thiabendazole and ivermectin are effective in treating strongyloidiasis. Organisms are capable of penetrating human skin if appropriate personal protective equipment is not used when contacting infected animals and their feces.

Adult *Dipetalonema* spp. are commonly seen in the peritoneal cavity of NW monkeys and occasionally are found in OW monkeys. Midges serve as parasite vectors. Microfilariae appear in the blood of infected animals. Although often found in large numbers, the parasite appears to cause only mild proliferative lesions in the peritoneal cavity. Treatment is not indicated. Zoonotic transmission is possible.

Tapeworms

Larval cestodes, including cysticercus larvae (*Taenia* spp.), coenurus larvae (*Multiceps* spp.), hydatid larvae (*Echinococcus* spp.), and *Hymenolepis nana* larvae, are seen with some frequency. Transmission is by ingestion of infective eggs or intermediate hosts, such as arthropods. These are usually incidental findings at necropsy or surgery, as there are rarely clinical signs of infection. Larvae may be found in subcutaneous tissues, muscles, and in the abdominal, peritoneal, or cranial cavities. Select cestodes of nonhuman primates (e.g., *Hymenolepis nana* and *Echinococcus granulosus*) are infectious to humans.

Acanthocephalans

Prosthenorchis elegans and *P. spirula* are the thorny-headed helminths of NW primates. The cockroach and beetle serve as intermediate hosts. The adults burrow deeply into the mucosa of the terminal ileum, cecum, or colon, causing abscesses, granulomas, and occasionally peritonitis. A large population of adults can cause intestinal blockage. The use of praziquantel reduces the population of adults but will not eliminate all the parasites. Zoonotic infections have not been reported and are unlikely.

Arthropods

Ectoparasites of nonhuman primates include lice and mites. Several of the more common external parasites reported are *Sarcoptes scabiei*, *Demodex* spp., *Pedicinus* spp., and *Psorergates simplex*. Topical organophosphate insecticides and pyrethrins, as well as parenteral ivermectin, are effective in treating external parasites.

The lung mite, *Pneumonyssus simicola*, is an arthropod capable of infecting OW primates. Although previously a common finding in wild macaques, the use of anthelmintics in captive breeding programs has almost eliminated this mite. Affected animals are usually asymptomatic. At necropsy, pale yellow foci containing the mites are found throughout the lungs, and in some cases, cavitation of the lungs is seen. The lesions of lung mites may grossly resemble those of tuberculosis. Histologically, the presence of brown to black pigment and a focal bronchiolitis are characteristic of lung mite infestation. Radiographically, diffuse interstitial densities or discrete opaque densities may be seen throughout the lung lobes. Secondary bacterial bronchopneumonia may develop. Ivermectin appears to be an effective treatment. The parasite is not zoonotic.

Miscellaneous Conditions

Acute Gastric Dilation

Acute gastric dilation, with or without torsion, occurs with some frequency in macaques and baboons. The exact etiology is unknown. Chronic broad-spectrum antibiotic administration, anesthesia, excessive food intake, and excessive water intake are considered predisposing causes. Large amounts of raw vegetables or fruits may be particularly problematic. The condition is most often seen in animals that hoard food from cagemates or animals in which full feeding was resumed after a period of restricted feeding. Most deaths occur at night following the evening feeding. Gaseous distention of the stomach develops rapidly. The abdominal distention is extreme and may be accompanied by an accumulation of subcutaneous gas. Ingesta may be seen in the oral cavity, but neither frank vomiting nor bloody diarrhea is a feature of acute gastric dilation.

Mortality is high even when the condition is detected early and vigorous treatment is instituted. Recommended treatment consists of passing a gastric tube to relieve the gas and excess fluid contents until peristalsis is resumed. Supportive therapy in the form of intravenous fluids and analgesics should be administered. The use of antibiotics and steroids is also thought to increase the chances of survival. Bloat in primates is prevented by multiple feedings of small quantities of food plus full access to water.

Trauma

Bite wounds are the most frequent problem seen in group-housed primates. Wounds may be very extensive and often involve the extremities and face. Fresh lacerations should be thoroughly cleaned and, depending on the degree of tissue trauma, gross contamination, and time until treatment, sutured using a subcuticular pattern to decrease the chance of the animal disturbing the sutures. Thorough examination of traumatic wounds is necessary as the subcutaneous damage may be more severe than the wounds of the skin would indicate. Broad-spectrum antibiotics, such as enrofloxacin, are indicated, since the oral cavity carries a heavy microbial burden. Bandages are difficult, if not impossible, to keep in place, and self-trauma following injury often poses a problem. Crushing injuries of the muscles may release large amounts of methemoglobin, which can lead to acute renal failure if left untreated. Intravenous fluid therapy must be aggressive to help diurese the kidneys; otherwise, treatment is essentially the same as for other species. Primates should receive tetanus antitoxin after penetrating injuries if they have not been previously immunized.

Metabolic Bone Disease and Vitamin D Deficiency

Metabolic bone disease, referred to as simian bone disease, cage paralysis, or osteodystrophia fibrosa (secondary hyperparathyroidism), results from a deficiency of vitamin D and an imbalance in the calcium-to-phosphorus ratio (a much higher content of phosphorus than calcium), combined with inadequate exposure to direct sunlight. This disease syndrome is due to a nutritional secondary hyperparathyroidism, which results in bone resorption and fibrous replacement.

Vitamin D deficiencies, most frequently seen in NW primates, cause rickets in young animals and osteomalacia in adult animals. In rickets, calcification of the cartilage never occurs. In osteomalacia, calcium resorption causes decalcified bones. NW primates cannot utilize vitamin D_2 and thus require a diet containing vitamin D_3. Clinical signs include decreased activity, pain, paresis, osteomalacia, kyphosis, deformities of long bones, multiple fractures, and high levels of serum alkaline phosphatase. Radiographs show thinning of cortical bone. Treatment should be aimed at correcting the diet by providing vitamin D_3, calcium, and a proper calcium-to-phosphorus ratio. A full-spectrum light source will also aid in the production of adequate vitamin D_3 levels. Appropriate treatment with 5000 IU of vitamin D_3 per kilogram per week plus a diet high in calcium and protein will prevent further progression of metabolic bone disease. This disease should not occur in modern nonhuman primate research facilities as commercial, nutritionally complete diets are readily available for all primate species.

Scurvy

Without an adequate dietary supply of vitamin C, scurvy develops in nonhuman primates. The usual clinical signs are swelling of the epiphyses of long bones and hemorrhage of the gums, eyes, and periosteum. Cephalohematoma is a unique clinical manifestation seen in squirrel monkeys. Treatment of hypovitaminosis C consists of administration of 25 mg/kg per day of vitamin C until clinical signs disappear. Response to therapy is usually rapid, with clinical signs resolving in several weeks. Prevention of scurvy is dependent upon feeding diets formulated with appropriate vitamin C levels that have been stored at an appropriate temperature and for no longer than recommended by the feed manufacturer. As with metabolic bone disease, scurvy is largely a historical disease as nutritionally complete diets are readily available for all nonhuman primate species. There have been, however, recalls of primate diets by manufacturers due to errors in vitamin C. If suspicious clinical signs are present, diet recall information should be checked and the animal treated.

Endometriosis

Endometriosis is a condition in which endometrial glands and stroma are found in abnormal locations, most commonly on the serosal surface of pelvic organs. Endometriosis can be seen in middle-aged to older rhesus monkeys. Clinical signs may be absent or may consist of irregular menstrual cycles, infertility, periodic inactivity, or decreased food consumption. Abdominal masses may occasionally be palpable, especially when adhesions have developed. The pathogenesis of this disease in humans and nonhuman primates is unresolved. Treatment usually consists of surgical removal of the abnormally placed endometrial tissue, ovariectomy, hysterectomy, and possibly hormonal therapies such as medroxyprogesterone and leuprolide. Analgesic use should be strongly considered. Extremely advanced cases may warrant euthanasia.

Fatal Fasting Syndrome of Obese Macaques (Fatal Fatty Liver Syndrome)

Seen predominantly in obese female macaques, older animals, and in periods of anorexia, fatal fasting syndrome of obese macaques may be mechanistically similar to hepatic lipidosis of cats. Clinical signs include anorexia, lethargy, weight loss, and high mortality. Histologically, there is fatty change in both the liver and the kidney. Treatment using a percutaneous endoscopic gastrotomy (PEG) tube and enteral feeding has been described as an effective method to provide nutritional support until normal eating behaviors resume.

Amyloidosis

Amyloidosis, a condition in which extracellular accumulations of amyloid protein fibrils are deposited in various organs or tissues, is common. While amyloidosis can develop as a result of multiple underlying causes, the most frequently associated inciting cause is a chronic infectious or inflammatory process resulting in amyloid disposition primarily in the liver and intestines with subsequent weight loss with or without diarrhea. Clinical signs are dictated by the organ(s) or tissue(s) affected. Affected organs may be notably large on palpation. The condition is diagnosed through observation of the birefringent amyloid deposits seen with Congo Red stain of affected tissues collected through biopsy or at necropsy. For premortem diagnosis, assessment of Serum Amyloid A can be used as a screening test, with confirmation via biopsy. Most severely affected animals are euthanized without treatment.

Arthritis

Arthritis is a common disease of many species of older nonhuman primates and is commonly seen in macaques. Clinical signs include enlarged joints, limited joint mobility, muscle contracture, and wasting. Interphalangeal and knee joints are most commonly affected. Treatment with polysulfated glycosaminoglycans has been proposed by some to be beneficial in alleviating clinical signs. Analgesics and an increased opportunity for regular movement and exercise are recommended; human arthritis medications may be indicated for severe cases.

Marmoset Wasting Syndrome

Marmoset wasting syndrome is poorly understood but is characterized by marked and progressive weight loss, muscle atrophy, and hair loss concurrent with chronic diarrhea, colitis, and hemolytic anemia in both captive marmosets and tamarins. The syndrome's etiology is unknown but has been postulated to involve nutritional vitamin E deficiency and possibly protein deficiency as a sequela to chronic diarrhea. Treatment of affected animals has not been successful, but nutritional supplementation of vitamin E, selenium, zinc, and copper has been successful for disease prevention.

Dental Disease

Dental disease is a common condition of captive nonhuman primates, frequently involving excess tartar accumulation, gingivitis, tooth abscesses, dental caries, and dental trauma. Primary dental disease can progress to severe systemic disease (e.g., tooth root abscess progressing to cardiac valve disease). As such, the oral cavity and associated structures should be assessed at the time of each physical exam and routine dental cleaning. Abscesses of the upper canine teeth are common in squirrel monkeys. Diagnosis and treatment of severe dental disease in all species should be performed in collaboration with dental professionals.

Although once common, the routine extraction or blunting of canine teeth ("disarming") is no longer acceptable due to animal welfare concerns and the high incidence of severe, long-term complications (e.g., tooth root abscesses, unintended tooth migration resulting in malocclusion) induced by the procedure.

Extreme caution should be taken when performing dental work on nonhuman primates, especially macaques, because the possibility of aerosols, splatter of blood, and accidental self-injury (such as during tooth extraction) is significant. Personnel involved in the dental work must wear personal protective equipment (PPE) appropriate for all work with macaques. Additional PPE may be indicated based on the procedures to be performed (e.g., respirator use during ultrasonic dental scaling).

BIBLIOGRAPHY

Abee, C. R., K. Mansfield, S. Tardiff, and T. Morris (eds.). 2012. *Nonhuman Primates in Biomedical Research*. 2nd ed. San Diego, CA: Academic Press.

American Veterinary Medical Association (AVMA). 2013. *AVMA Guidelines for the Euthanasia of Animals*. Available at http://www.avma.org/KB/Policies/Documents/euthanasia.pdf [accessed May 29, 2018].

Association of Primate Veterinarians (APV). Nonhuman primate formulary. Available at https://www.primatevets.org/education--resources [accessed May 29, 2018].

Banish, L. D., R. Sims, M. Bush, et al. 1993. Clearance of *Shigella flexneri* carriers in a zoologic collection of primates. *J Am Vet Med Assoc* 203(1): 133–136.

Carpenter, J. W. 2017. *Exotic Animal Formulary*, 5th ed. St. Louis, MO: Elsevier Saunders.

Christe, K. L., and C. R. Valverde. 1999. The use of a percutaneous endoscopic gastrotomy (PEG) tube to reverse fatal fasting syndrome in a cynomolgus macaque (*Macaca fascicularis*). *Contemp Top Lab Anim Sci* 38(4): 12–15.

Christe, K. L., M. B. McChesney, A. Spinner, et al. 2002. Comparative efficacy of a canine distemper–measles and a standard measles vaccine for immunization of rhesus macaques (*Macaca mulatta*). *Comp Med* 52(5): 467–472.

Cohen, J. I., D. S. Davenport, J. A. Stewart, et al. 2002. Recommendations for prevention of and therapy for exposure to B virus. *Clin Infect Dis* 35: 1191–1203.

Dubois, A., D. E. Ber, N. Fiala, et al. 1998. Cure of *Helicobacter pylori* infection by omeprazole-clarithromycin–based therapy in nonhuman primates. *J Gastroenterol* 33: 18–22.

Dysko, R. C. and D. E. Hoskins. 1995. Collection of biological samples and therapy administration. In *Nonhuman Primates in Biomedical Research*, B. T. Bennett, C. R. Abee, and R. Henrickson (eds.), pp.270–271. Sandiego, CA: Academic Press.
Feeser, P., and F. White. 1992. Medical management of *Lemur catta*, *Varecia varegata*, and *Propithecus verreauxi* in natural habitat enclosures. In *Proceedings of the Annual Meeting of the American Association of Zoo Veterinarians*, pp. 320–323.
Flecknell, P. A. 1987. *Laboratory Animal Anesthesia*. London: Academic Press.
Flecknell, P. 2015. *Laboratory Animal Anaesthesia*, 4th ed. London: Academic Press.
Fortman, J. D., T. A. Hewett, and B. T. Bennett. 2017. *The Laboratory Nonhuman Primate*, 2nd ed. Boca Raton, FL: CRC Press.
Garcia, M. A., D. M. Bouley, M. J. Larson, et al. 2004. Outbreak of *Mycobacterium bovis* in a conditioned colony of rhesus (*Macaca mulatta*) and cynomolgus (*Macaca fascicularis*) macaques. *Comp Med* 54(5): 578–584.
Godeny, E. K. 2002. Enzyme-linked immunosorbent assay for detection of antibodies against simian hemorrhagic fever virus. *Comp Med* 52(3): 229–232.
Hainsey, B. M., G. B. Hubbard, M. M. Leland, and K. M. Brasky. 1993. Clinical parameters of the normal baboons (*Papio* species) and chimpanzees (*Pan troglodytes*). *Lab Anim Sci* 43(3): 236–243.
Hotchkiss, E. C. 1995. Use of cisapride for the treatment of intestinal pseudoobstruction in a stumptail macaque (*Macaca arctoides*). *J Zoo Wild Med* 26(1): 98–101.
Ialeggio, D. M. 1989. Practical medicine of primate pets. *Compend Contin Educ Pract Vet* 11: 1252–1259.
Institute for Laboratory Animal Research (ILAR). 1998. *The Psychological Well-Being of Nonhuman Primates*. Committee on Well-Being of Nonhuman Primates, ILAR, National Research Council. Washington, DC: National Academies Press. Available at www.nap.edu [accessed May 29, 2018].
Institute of Laboratory Animal Resources (ILAR). 2011. *Guide for the Care and Use of Laboratory Animals*, 8th ed. ILAR, National Research Council. Washington, DC: National Academies Press.
Isaza, R., B. Baker, and F. Dunker. 1992. Medical management of inflammatory bowel disease in a spider monkey. *J Am Vet Med Assoc* 200(10): 1543–1545.
Johnson, D. K., R. J. Russell, and J. A. Stunkard. 1981. *A Guide to the Diagnosis, Treatment, and Husbandry of Nonhuman Primates*. Edwardsville, KS: Veterinary Medicine.
Johnson-Delaney, C. A. 1994. Primates. *Vet Clin North Am Small Anim Pract* 24(1): 121–156.
Junge, R. E., K. G. Mehren, T. P. Meehan, et al. 1992. Hypertrophic osteoarthropathy and renal disease in three black lemurs (*Lemur macaco*). In *Proceedings of the Annual Meeting of the American Association of Zoo Veterinarians*, pp. 324–330.
Krasnow, S. W. 1987. Primate nutrition [ACLAM notes]. Privately published, January 12, 1987.
Krugner-Higby, L. A., A. Gendron, N. K. Laughlin, et al. 2001. Chronic myelocytic leukemia in a juvenile rhesus macaque (*Macaca mulatta*). *Contemp Top Lab Anim Sci* 40(4): 44–48.
Lukas, V. 1999. Volume guidelines for compound administration. In *The Care and Feeding of an IACUC*, M. L. Podolsky and V. S. Lukas (eds.), p. 187. Boca Raton, FL: CRC Press.

Marks, S. K. 1994. *Disease Review: Balantidiasis. A Report of the American Association of Zoo Veterinarians Infectious Disease Committee*. Philadelphia: American Association of Zoo Veterinarians.

Murphy, K. L., M. G. Baxter, and P. A. Flecknell. 2012. Anesthesia and analgesia in nonhuman primates. In *Nonhuman Primates in Biomedical Research, Volume I*, 2nd ed., C. R. Abee, K. Mansfield, S. D. Tardif, and T. Morris (eds.), pp. 403–436. San Diego, CA: Academic Press.

Parrot, T. 2016. Primates. In: *The Merck Veterinary Manual*, 11th ed., D.G. Allen, K.K. Carter, P.D. Constable, et al. (eds.). Available at https://www.merckvetmanual.com/exotic-and-laboratory-animals/nonhuman-primates [accessed May 29, 2018].

Payton, M. E., J. M. d'Offay, M. E. Prado, et al. 2004. Comparative transmission of multiple herpesviruses and simian virus 40 in a baboon breeding colony. *Comp Med* 54(6): 695–704.

Popiliskis, S. J. and D. F. Kohn. 1997. Anesthesia and analgesia in nonhuman primates. In *Anesthesia and Analgesia in Laboratory Animals*, D. F. Kohn, S. K. Wixson, W. J. White, and G. J. Benson (eds.), pp. 233–255. New York: Academic Press.

Popilskis, S. J., D. R. Lee, and D. B. Elmore. 2008. Anesthesia and analgesia in nonhuman primates. In *Anesthesia and Analgesia in Laboratory Animals*, 2nd ed. R. E Fish, M. J. Brown, P. J. Danneman, and A. Z. Karas (eds.), pp. 335–364. New York: Academic Press.

Ratterree, M. S., P. J. Didier, J. L. Blanchard, et al. 1990. Vitamin C deficiency in captive nonhuman primates fed commercial primate diet. *Lab Anim Sci* 40: 165–168.

Regional Primate Research Center, Univ. Washington (RPRC-WA). 1987. Antibiotics routinely used for treatment. [Privately published.] Regional Primate Research Center at the University of Washington, Colony Division, Seattle, WA.

Rice, K. A., E. S. Chen, K. A. M. Pate, E. K. Hutchinson, and R. J. Adams. (2013). Diagnosis of amyloidosis and differentiation from chronic, idiopathic enterocolitis in rhesus (*Macaca mulatta)* and pig-tailed (*M. nemestrina*) macaques. *Comp Med* 63(3), 262–271.

Rosenberg, D. P. 1991. Nonhuman primate analgesia. *Lab Anim (NY)* 20(9): 22–33.

Russell, R. J., D. K. Johnson, and J. A. Stunkard. 1981. *A Guide to Diagnosis, Treatment, and Husbandry of Pet Rabbits and Rodents*. Edwardsville, KS: Veterinary Medicine Publishing.

Smith, T. 2006. Individual olfactory signatures in common marmosets (*Callithrix jacchus*). *Am J Primatol* 68(6): 585–604.

Swenson, R. B. 1993. Protozoal parasites of great apes. In *Zoo and Wildlife Animal Medicine—Current Therapy*, Volume 3, M.E. Fowler (ed.), pp. 352–355. Philadelphia: WB Saunders.

Thorton, S. M. 2002. Primates. In *BSAVA Manual of Exotic Pets*, A. Meredith and S. Redrobe (eds.), pp. 127–137. Quedgeley, Gloucester, UK: British Small Animal Veterinary Association.

Turnquist, J. E. and N. Minugh-Purvis. 1995. Functional morphology. In *Nonhuman Primates in Biomedical Research*, B. T. Bennett, C. R. Abee, and R. Henrickson (eds.), pp.270–271. Sandiego, CA: Academic Press

Vervenne, R. A., S. L. Jones, D. van Soolingen, et al. 2004. TB diagnosis in non-human primates: Comparison of two interferon-gamma assays and the skin test for identification of *Mycobacterium tuberculosis* infection. *Vet Immunol Immunopathol* 100(1–2): 61–71.
Weld, K. P., J. A. Mench, R. A. Woodward, et al. 1998. Effect of tryptophan treatment on self-biting and central nervous system serotonin metabolism in rhesus monkeys (*Macaca mulatta*). *Neuropsychopharmacology* 19: 314–321.
Weller, R. E., J. F. Baer, C.A. Málaga, et al. 1992. Renal clearance and excretion of endogenous substances in the owl monkey. *Am J Primatol* 28(2): 115–123.
Wolf R. F., and G. L. White. 2012. Clinical techniques used for nonhuman primates. In *Nonhuman Primates in Biomedical Research*, C. R. Abee, K. Mansfield, S. Tardiff, and T. Morris (eds.), pp. 323–337. San Diego, CA: Academic Press.
Wolf, R. H., S. V. Gibson, E. A. Watson, and G. B. Baskin. 1988. Multidrug chemotherapy of tuberculosis in rhesus monkeys. *Lab Anim Sci* 38(1): 25–33.
Wolfensohn, S. 1998. *Shigella* infection in macaque colonies: Case report of an eradication and control program. *Lab Anim Sci* 48(4): 330–333.
Wolff, P. L. 1990. The parasites of New World primates: A review. In *Proceedings of the American Association of Zoo Veterinarians*, pp. 87–94.
Yee, J. L., NPRC Breeding Colony Management Consortium, M. B. McChesney, and K. L. Christe. (2015). Multicenter safety and immunogenicity trial of an attenuated measles vaccine for NHP. *Comp Med*, 65(5), 448–454.
Zeiss, C. J., and N. Shomer. 2001. Hepatocystosis in a baboon (*Papio anubis*). *Contemp Top Lab Anim Sci* 40(1): 41–42.

FURTHER READING

Archer, D. F. 2004. Role of the nonhuman primate for research related to women's health. *ILAR J* 45(2): 212–219.
Cawthon, K. A. 2005. Primate factsheets: Vervet *(Chlorocebus)* taxonomy, morphology, and ecology. October 28, 2005. Available at http://pin.primate.wisc.edu/factsheets/entry/vervet [accessed May 29, 2018].
Coleman, C., M. Bloomsmith, C. Crocket, and J. Weed. 2012. Behavior, management, enrichment, and psychological well-being in laboratory nonhuman primates. In *Nonhuman Primates in Biomedical Research: Biology and Management*, 2nd ed., C. Abee, K. Mansfield, S. Tardif, and T. Morris (eds.), pp. 149–176. San Diego, CA: Academic Press.
Crouthamel, B., and G. Sackett. 2004. Oral medication administration: Training monkeys to take juice from a syringe. *Lab Prim News* 43(1): 14.
DeMarcus, T. A., M. A. Tipple, and S. R. Ostrowski. 1999. US policy for disease control among imported nonhuman primates. *J Infect Dis* 179(Suppl 1): S281–S282.
Groves, C. 2001. *Primate Taxonomy*. Washington, DC: Smithsonian Institution Press.
Groves, C. 2004. The what, why, and how of primate taxonomy. *Int J Primatol* 25(5): 1105–1126.

Hara, M., T. Kikuchi, F. Ono, et al. 2005. Survey of captive cynomolgus macaque colonies for SRV/D infection using polymerase chain reaction assays. *Comp Med* 55(2): 145–149.

Hawk, C. T., S. L. Leary, and T. H. Morris. 2005. *Formulary for Laboratory Animals*. 3rd ed. Ames, IA: Iowa State University Press.

Hawkins, J. V., C. E. Jaquish, R. L. Carlson, et al. 1992. *Trichospirura leptostoma* infection in *Callithrix jacchus* (common marmoset): Disease and treatment [abstract]. *Contemp Topics* 31(4): 26.

Heard, D. J. 1993. Principles and techniques of anesthesia and analgesia for exotic practice. *Vet Clin North Am Small Anim Pract* 23(6): 1301–1327.

Jenkins, W. L. 1987. Pharmacologic aspects of analgesic drugs in animals: An overview. *J Am Vet Med Assoc* 191(10): 1231–1240.

Kramer, J. A., E. W. Ford, and S. Capuano. 2012. Preventative medicine in nonhuman primates. In *Nonhuman Primates in Biomedical Research, Volume I*, 2nd ed., C. R. Abee, K. Mansfield, S. D. Tardif, and T. Morris (eds.), pp. 293–322. San Diego, CA: Academic Press.

Lerch, N. W., J. L. Yee, S. V. Capuano, and J. L. Flynn. 2008. New approaches to tuberculosis surveillance in nonhuman primates. *ILAR* 49(2): 170–178.

Line, A. S. 1993. Comments on Baytril antimicrobial therapy and considerations for intramuscular antibiotic therapy in captive primates. *Lab Primate News* 32: 3.

Liu, S. K. 2002. Metabolic disease in animals. *Semin Musculoskelet Radiol* 6(4): 341–346.

Lowenstine, L. J., and K. G. Osborn. 2012. Respiratory system diseases of nonhuman primates. In *Nonhuman Primates in Biomedical Research, Volume II*, 2nd ed., C. R. Abee, K. Mansfield, S. D. Tardif, and T. Morris (eds.), pp. 413–482. San Diego, CA: Academic Press.

Martin, D. P. 1986. Primates: Feeding and nutrition. In *Zoo and Wild Animal Medicine*, M. E. Fowler (ed.), pp. 661–663. Philadelphia: WB Saunders.

Miller, A. D. 2012. Neoplasia and proliferative disorders of nonhuman primates. In *Nonhuman Primates in Biomedical Research, Volume II*, 2nd ed., C. R. Abee, K. Mansfield, S. D. Tardif, and T. Morris (eds.), pp. 325–356. San Diego, CA: Academic Press.

National Institutes of Health (NIH). Primate resources for researchers. National Primate Research Centers, Office of Research Infrastructure Programs, NIH, U.S. Department of Health and Human Services. Available at https://orip.nih.gov/comparative-medicine/programs/vertebrate-models#primates-nprc [accessed May 29, 2018].

Ostrowski, S. R., M. J. Leslie, T. Parrott, et al. 1998. B-virus from pet macaque monkeys: An emerging threat in the United States? *Emerg Infect Dis* 4(1): 117–121.

Paul-Murphy, J. 1992. Preventative medicine program for nonhuman primates. In *Proceedings of the North American Veterinary Conference*, pp. 736–738.

Pernikoff, D. S., and J. Orkin. 1991. Bacterial meningitis syndrome: An overall review of the disease complex and considerations of cross infectivity between great apes and man. In *Proceedings of the American Association of Zoo Veterinarians*, pp. 235–241.

Pritzker, K. P. H., and M. J. Kessler. 2012. Arthritis, muscle, adipose tissue, and bone diseases of nonhuman primates. In *Nonhuman Primates in Biomedical Research, Volume II*, 2nd ed., C. R. Abee, K. Mansfield, S. D. Tardif, and T. Morris (eds.), pp. 629–698. San Diego, CA: Academic Press.

Sanders, E. A., R. D. Gleed, and P. W. Nathanielsz. 1991. Anesthetic management for instrumentation of the pregnant rhesus monkey. *J Med Primatol* 20(5): 223–228.

Schou, S., and A. K. Hansen. 2000. Marburg and Ebola virus infections in laboratory non-human primates: A literature review. *Comp Med* 50(2): 108–123.

Shumaker, R. W., and B. B. Beck. 2003. *Primates in Question*. Washington, DC: Smithsonian Institute Press.

Simmons, J., and S. Gibson. 2012. Bacterial and mycotic diseases of nonhuman primates. In *Nonhuman Primates in Biomedical Research, Volume II*, 2nd ed., C. R. Abee, K. Mansfield, S. D. Tardif, and T. Morris (eds.), pp. 105–172. San Diego, CA: Academic Press.

Smith, D. G. 2012. Taxonomy. In *Nonhuman Primates in Biomedical Research: Biology and Management*, 2nd ed., C. R. Abee, K. Mansfield, S. D. Tardif, and T. Morris (eds.), pp. 57–86. San Diego, CA: Academic Press.

Soma, L. R., W. J. Tierney, and N. Satoh. 1988. Sevoflurane anesthesia in the monkey: The effects of multiples of MAC. *Hiroshima J Anesth* 24: 3–14.

Strait, K., J. G. Else, and M. L. Eberhard. 2012. Parasitic diseases of nonhuman primates. In *Nonhuman Primates in Biomedical Research, Volume II*, 2nd ed., C. R. Abee, K. Mansfield, S. D. Tardif, and T. Morris (eds.), pp. 197–298. San Diego, CA: Academic Press.

Thorton, S. M. 2002. Primates. In *BSAVA Manual of Exotic Pets*, A. Meredith and S. Redrobe (eds.), pp. 127–137. Quedgeley, Gloucester, UK: British Small Animal Veterinary Association.

Undar, A., H. C. Eichstaedt, F. J. Clubb Jr., et al. 2004. Anesthetic induction with ketamine inhibits platelet activation before, during, and after cardiopulmonary bypass in baboons. *Artif Organs* 28(10): 959–962.

Wachtman, L., and K. Mansfield. 2012. Viral diseases of nonhuman primates. In *Nonhuman Primates in Biomedical Research, Volume II*, 2nd ed., C. R. Abee, K. Mansfield, S. D. Tardif, and T. Morris (eds.), pp. 1–104. San Diego, CA: Academic Press.

White, G. L., and J. F. Cummings. 1979. A comparison of ketamine and ketamine–xylazine in the baboon. *Vet Med Small Anim Clin* 74(3): 392–394, 396.

Willy, M. E., R. A. Woodward, V. B. Thornton, et al. 1999. Management of a measles outbreak among Old World nonhuman primates. *Lab Anim Sci* 49(1): 42–48.

Wolf-Coote, S. 2005. *The Laboratory Primate: The Handbook of Experimental Animals*, pp. 3–15. San Diego, CA: Academic Press.

Yeager, J. J., P. Facemire, P. A. Dabisch, et al. 2012. Natural history of inhalation melioidosis in rhesus macaques (*Macaca mulatta*) and African green monkeys (*Chlorocebus aethiops*). *Infect Immun* 80(9): 3332–3340.

CHAPTER 13 REVIEW

Short Answer

1. What are the three characteristics that define New World vs. Old World primates?
2. Primates require a dietary source of vitamin C. What disease does this prevent and what are the clinical signs of that disease?
3. Give one other name for Herpes B virus. What clinical signs might it cause in animals? What signs might it cause in humans?
4. What PPE should be worn when working with primates?
5. What organism is the causative agent of tuberculosis in non-human primates?
6. This small New World Primate has a high incidence of twinning. What are its common and scientific names?
7. What group of primates is most commonly used in biomedical research?
8. Why do hand-reared monkeys frequently develop behavioral abnormalities?
9. What vaccinations should be considered when housing primates in large outdoor colonies?
10. True/False: Many parasites of Old World monkeys are more closely related to dog or rodent parasites and are not transmissible to humans.
11. What kind of caging facilitates examination and immobilization of nonhuman primates?
    A. Metabolic
    B. Gang
    C. Exercise
    D. Squeeze
12. Metabolic bone disease is caused by a deficiency of vitamin D and an imbalance of which two minerals?
13. What is the causative agent for "bloody nose syndrome" in macaques?
14. What are the signs of measles in nonhuman primates?

Critical Thinking

15. Your facility is housing primates for the first time, beginning next month. What are the two important safety topics that you want to ensure are covered in training staff to work with primates?

14

Cattle, Sheep, Goats, and Pigs

Cattle, sheep and goats are ruminants in the family Bovidae. Pigs share an order (Artiodactyla) with the ruminants but are classified within the family Suidae. Breeds of cattle are often specifically raised for meat or milk. Sheep and goat breeds may have good meat quality, highly desirable wool, or increased milk production. Pigs have been bred over time to be extraordinarily efficient at feed conversion, with remarkable growth rates. This chapter addresses specific considerations regarding these animals' use in biomedical research. Basic anatomy, biology, and diseases are well-covered in other texts so an in-depth exploration of these topics will not be included here.

USES

In addition to their use in animal production research (such as increased feed conversion or improvements in fiber production) agricultural animals are often used in biomedical research for various areas of study including cardiovascular modeling, joint replacement, organ transplant, and prosthesis development as well as other implantable medical devices (Box 14.1). These species lend themselves well to these areas of study due to their increased size over the more "traditional" laboratory species as well as some anatomical or physiological similarities between them and the human conditions they are modeling. Additionally, genetically modified livestock have been produced to express recombinant proteins in their milk, with the potential to serve as a source for therapeutic agents (such as antithrombin produced in goat's milk or recombinant albumin from cow's milk).

Clinical Laboratory Animal Medicine: An Introduction, Fifth Edition.
Lesley A. Colby, Megan H. Nowland, and Lucy H. Kennedy.

Companion website: www.wiley.com/go/colby/clinical

Box 14.1

Agricultural animals are often used in biomedical research for various areas of study including cardiovascular modeling, joint replacement, organ transplant, and prosthesis development as well as other implantable medical devices.

While this chapter provides a broad overview of the use of, and care for, these species in a biomedical research setting, the reader is referred to the "Further Reading" section at the end of this chapter for additional, in-depth coverage of species-specific biology, care, and clinical conditions.

BEHAVIOR

For all species, maintaining the psychological health of the animals is very important. Social housing whenever possible and breed-appropriate enrichment devices as well as positive human interaction can all be employed to reach this goal. Additionally, personnel safety and minimization of risk should be addressed when handling these animals. Intelligent facility design and appropriate equipment can facilitate this goal. Positive human interaction and acclimation to handling can assist in making research and routine husbandry and veterinary manipulations go smoothly. As a natural consequence of this, handlers will become extremely familiar with the animals under their charge, allowing subtle changes in attitude, appetite, or behavior to be detected early.

While dairy breeds tend to be more complacent and easier to handle, beef cattle may be more aggressive and difficult to control. When working with any breed of cattle, prioritize personnel safety. Specialized facilities or equipment, including appropriately sized pens and solid-walled chutes can provide safe and low-stress handling for cattle.

Sheep are generally docile. If threatened, they are likely to attempt escape rather than fight. They are prey animals and have strong flocking behavior. As such, they will attempt to maintain contact with their group as much as possible. A lone sheep separated from the flock (in a farm setting) can be a strong indicator of illness or injury. Handling sheep as a group (when possible) can be more successful than manipulating animals one at a time.

Highly social and intelligent, swine should be housed with conspecifics whenever possible. Their natural rooting behavior can be destructive if not given an appropriate outlet (toys, bedding, etc.). Pigs rely heavily on auditory, tactile, and olfactory cues; their eyesight is poor so additions of mirrors or murals for enrichment purposes may not be efficacious.

For further reading on the behavior of livestock species, Dr. Temple Grandin is an advocate of humane treatment of animals raised for human consumption and many of her precepts can be adapted to minimize stress in handling of these species in any setting, whether research or farm.

ANATOMIC AND PHYSIOLOGIC FEATURES

Ruminants have a four-compartment stomach. The rumen, reticulum, and omasum make up the forestomach while the abomasum is considered the true stomach. This large, fluid-filled organ can impact research due to changes in food metabolism, oral absorption of therapeutic or experimental compounds, and additional complications during anesthesia such as bloat or compromised venous return due to improper positioning.

Due to their rapid growth, size/weight of swine and cattle should be a consideration when planning research studies (Box 14.2). For long-term projects, a typical farm pig could become large enough to be difficult to house or to transport around the facility. To address this eventuality, careful timing of projects to minimize the time in-house should be considered. If research needs require extended housing of animals, one of the miniature swine breeds can provide a more manageable size over longer periods of time. Fixed meal feeding, rather than *ad libitum* feeding should be employed to manage obesity in these animals.

One anatomical characteristic of swine makes it an appealing model of human coronary artery disease. Swine have a left coronary artery that is larger and longer than the right, as well as minimal collateral circulation among the coronary arteries as a whole. This is similar to humans, and the reverse of other species such as dogs, which makes swine a good species for research involving surgical models of heart disease.

Unlike some other species, ruminants have a lymphocyte predominance on hematology assessment. Neutrophils are present, but in much lower relative quantities than other species. General physiological parameters for these species can be found in Table 14.1.

BREEDING AND REPRODUCTION

Ewes typically reach sexual maturity between 6 and 12 months of age, while rams reach sexual maturity at 5 to 7 months. Goats reach puberty between 4 and 12 months depending on breed, season, and overall animal health. Cattle can be bred between 9 and 12 months of age. Cattle and swine are polyestrous and will cycle year round. However, most breeds of sheep and goats are seasonally polyestrous (short-day breeders). If wanting to naturally breed flocks of sheep or goats, the light cycle should be manipulated appropriately to mimic the fall if animals are kept indoors.

With their high incidence of multiple births, sheep can be a useful model for reproductive studies, particularly those involving fetal surgery, as the unoperated fetus can

Box 14.2

Due to their rapid growth, size/weight of swine and cattle should be a consideration when planning research studies.

Table 14.1. Temperature, pulse, and respiratory rates in adult sheep and goats

Parameter	Sheep	Goats
Rectal temperature (°F)	102–103.5	100.5–103.5
Rectal temperature (°C)	39–40	38–40
Pulse (beats/minute)	70–80	70–90
Respiration (breaths/minute)	12–20	15–30

Source: Adapted from Pugh and Baird (2012).

serve as its sibling's control, and the fetus is large enough for in utero surgical manipulation.

Sheep, goats, and cattle have a bicornuate uterus as well as an epitheliochorial and cotyledonary placentation. The latter means that colostrum to newly born young is important for establishing passive immunity, as there is minimal passage across the placenta prior to parturition. Goats may exhibit pseudopregnancy, lasting just as long as their normal gestation (144–155 days) and resulting in the "delivery" of a large amount of fluid. Normal gestation for sheep is similar to goats at about 150 days, and for cattle ranges from 279 to 287 days.

Swine, which also have a bicornuate uterus but a diffuse, epitheliochorial placenta, reach sexual maturity around 5–6 months of age and are polyestrous with a 21-day cycle. Estrus lasts for approximately 48 hours. Gestation is "three months, three weeks, and three days" or 114 days. As a sign that farrowing is imminent, milk will flow from the sow 6–12 hours prior to the initiation of parturition. Sows can deliver large litters. On average, a piglet will be born every 15 minutes. If the inter-piglet interval becomes longer than 30–60 minutes, veterinary intervention is required. Piglets are born iron-deficient, thus should be administered 100–200 mg of iron dextran via intramuscular (IM) or subcutaneous (SC) injections within the first week of life.

A summary of reproductive information can be found in Table 14.2.

HUSBANDRY

Housing and Environment

Housing for agricultural species can vary from typical farmlike settings to highly controlled indoor facilities. Regardless of the setting, adequate space should be provided for each animal to perform normal species-specific behaviors without overcrowding.

Depending on how and where animals will be housed (indoors vs. outdoors, vivarium vs. barn vs. pasture vs. paddock) as well as duration of the housing of the colony, a routine preventive health routine should be developed. In consultation with the attending veterinarian, this program may include vaccination, deworming, pasture rotation, quarantine options, etc. Individual programmatic needs will drive much of this planning with long-term animals housed in a more natural setting likely needing more herd-based management similar to that of a typical farm, compared to animals

Table 14.2. Reproductive parameters for large animals

Species	Age at puberty (months)	Cycle type	Duration of cycle (days)	Length of estrus (hours)	Gestation (days)
Cattle	4–18	Polyestrus	18–24	10–24	270–292
Sheep	7–8	Seasonally polyestrus	14–19	24–30	147–150
Goat	4–8	Seasonally polyestrus	18–24	24–96	144–155
Swine	3–7 (4–6 for miniature swine)	Polyestrous	17–25	24–72	114–115

Source: Adapted from Helke et al. (2015) and Underwood et al. (2015).

Box 14.3

Sources of agricultural animals should be thoroughly vetted to gain a full appreciation for the health status and possible endemic issues that may be encountered.

housed in an indoor vivarium that may need to be managed on a more individual, case-by-case basis.

Sources of agricultural animals should be thoroughly vetted to gain a full appreciation for the health status and possible endemic issues that may be encountered (Box 14.3). Upon arrival, animals should be given a brief physical examination in order to ensure they are in good health prior to being admitted to the facility. A more thorough exam to assess any latent or stress-induced diseases should be performed within a few days to validate the animals as good research subjects. Purpose-bred vs. farm-raised animals may have very different health statuses. If more than one supplier is used per species, housing should be separated by vendor.

Transportation of agricultural animals is often associated with other regulatory and logistical requirements. Being familiar with any permits required for transportation as well as coming to an understanding with the vendor and transporter is important. Delineating temperature extremes (whether too hot or too cold) for animal transport and coming to agreement regarding refusal of unsuitable animals "at the dock" are all questions to be answered in advance of the truck arriving at the facility.

After arrival, animals should be provided with an acclimation period prior to enrollment in a research study. This period allows for adaptation of physiological and behavioral parameters that have been disrupted by shipping. Depending on the age, health status, or individual condition of the animals or source herd, acclimation periods may be extended.

All agricultural animals housed in an indoor vivarium should be provided with secure footing to prevent slipping and injury. A roughened surface will provide a surface for appropriate hoof wear, though if flooring is too rough, it can lead to foot trauma and skin lesions, particularly over bony prominences. If animals are housed on raised, slatted floors, ensure the design of the floor is such that hooves and claws are protected from slipping in between slats or from excessive stress upon the interdigital spaces. Housing on the floor of the room with appropriate bedding has its own set of pros and cons, including removal of bedding and manure (many plumbing systems are not designed for disposal of this type of waste). When designing the animal facility, these considerations should be taken into account if agricultural animals are to be housed.

When housed in a farm setting, parasite management is important for grazing animals. Various strategies for deworming have been used in order to control intestinal parasites. Intelligent use of anthelminthics will prevent development of resistance while maintaining a low level of worm burden and ensuring animal welfare. Strategic planning and use of the FAMACHA scoring system can help target animals in need of additional parasite treatment. For animals housed in more tightly controlled animal housing facilities, regular sanitation should minimize many parasite issues.

The type of housing can dictate what kind of ancillary equipment is necessary within the vivarium. For example, animals housed in pens with bedding and animals housed on raised slatted floors require different animal transport cages. Having transports that allow the animal to directly exit at floor level for pens, or at the height of the raised flooring for cages minimizes the need for animals to step up or down, thus reducing stress and trauma for all involved.

Vivarium layout, heating, ventilation, and air conditioning (HVAC) handling, and traffic flow need to be considered in all vivarium spaces, but agricultural animals have some unique concerns. Noise, smells, and disease transmission can all present challenges when housing these species. For example, if the vivarium houses dogs (which can be quite loud), sheep can become distressed if they can hear them barking. Air handling should be closely examined to ensure that odors and particulates are appropriately managed, both from an animal pheromone aspect and for comfort of the humans that interact with or may occupy spaces near the animal facility. If any animals carry zoonotic pathogens, appropriate personal protective equipment (PPE) practices and traffic flow patterns (such as handling/entering last) should be adopted.

As mentioned above, the process of digestion in ruminants can produce large amounts of gas. Thus, ventilation in vivaria housing these species is of particular importance both for the comfort of the human caretakers and to prevent the buildup of gases such as ammonia which can contribute to respiratory disease in these animals.

Sanitation

Maintaining a clean environment for large animals is just as important as for any other species. Providing a sanitary housing area ensures the minimization of opportunistic infections that can arise in dirty environments. Spraying down pens daily (taking care not to wet the animals) is an effective means of cleaning. This can generate a large amount of humidity within the room, necessitating the need for a robust HVAC system in order to manage the moisture and heat load appropriately.

For sheep or goats housed in a pasture setting, control of intestinal parasites is of importance. This includes monitoring flock parasite levels with fecal egg counts and subsequently addressing the most prevalent parasites with targeted selected treatment.

Use of the FAMACHA scoring system to identify anemic animals is an effective way to determine which animals will be best served by targeted deworming and which animals can be left untreated.

Environmental Enrichment and Social Housing

The social and environmental enrichment of farm animals is important to address. They are social animals and often have strong herding or flocking behaviors that should be satisfied when possible. Specific animals that need to be housed singly (rams, or to satisfy a research need) should be brought to the attention of the IACUC for approval. Visual or auditory contact should be maintained wherever possible and enrichment items should be increased and varied with single-housed animals, particularly when those animals are young.

Rooting is a strong behavioral urge in pigs. As such, they will often up-end food or water bowls that are not secured. This behavior can be safely expressed by providing the swine with large, durable balls or other rootable objects. Additionally, swine will often explore their environments with their mouths. Again, durability is key—ensuring that the animals will not destroy the objects provided (and thus possibly injure themselves) is important. Alternatively, purposefully destructible, edible objects can be used for enrichment purposes (Figure 14.1).

Sheep have a well-developed ability for facial recognition. Housing them in pairs, groups, or flocks is ideal. In cases where scientific justification exists for single-housed animals, visual contact with other animals is of particular importance in this species. When such a thing is not possible, the strategic placement of mirrors or photographs can help alleviate some of the stress generated by housing animals alone.

Feeding and Watering

Appropriate nutrition should be maintained for all animals, as species requirements dictate. Diets formulated for each species and appropriate life stage should be used thoughtfully. For example, swine grow rapidly. Using a grower-finisher diet for a

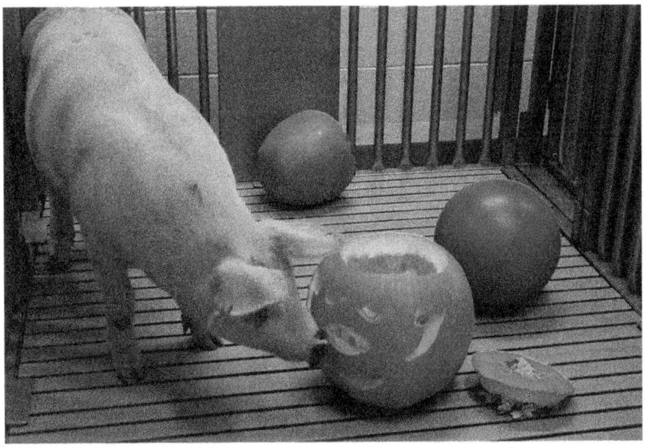

Fig 14.1. Purposefully destructible, edible objects can be used for swine enrichment. (*Source:* Photo courtesy of A. Puffenberger.)

long-term study may result in pigs that are too heavy or large for the facility caging, surgery tables, or other equipment.

Food can be provided to the animals in wall-mounted feeders or floor pans (for indoor vivaria) or troughs or bunks for more agricultural settings. For ruminants, hay can be supplemented for fiber and enrichment and may be provided via hanging nets. More detailed information regarding the specific nutritional requirements for each of these species can be found in the resources listed under "Further Reading" section.

Due to the tendency of pigs to root and explore their enclosures with their mouths, food bowls and water receptacles (if an automated watering system is not used) should be secured in order to prevent up-ending, which can result in inadequate food or water availability. Meal feeding of pigs is recommended in order to prevent over-conditioning during the experiment or study period.

Agricultural animals can be readily trained to use automated watering systems; during this training and transition time, a secondary water source (such as a bucket) is recommended to prevent dehydration. Knowledge of the watering system at the animal vendor/source is important so this transition can be managed appropriately. The source of water should also be known. For most vivaria, this will typically be treated city water. If housing on a farm, well water is more likely and should be regularly tested for contaminants. In rare cases, research buildings are entirely plumbed with highly conditioned water such as reverse osmosis. Feeding a well-formulated diet will replace any minerals that would ordinarily be supplied in the water.

TECHNIQUES

Handling and Restraint

Handling and restraint should be performed with a mind to minimize human and animal distress and risk of injury (Box 14.4). Two people are often needed in order to handle animals appropriately and minimize risk to both personnel and animals. Ensure all personnel are appropriately trained in all equipment (chutes, slings, etc.).

PPE will often differ in a research setting compared with an agricultural one. Research facilities are rarely able to be set up as an all-in-all-out facility and may house animals of various species, from various sources and of various health statuses in close proximity. As such, care should be taken to minimize the possibility of spreading pathogens from one group of animals to another. Gloves and protective disposable coats should be disposed of and boots should be sanitized between species and between groups of the same species with different sources or health statuses.

Practices that may be appropriate in an agricultural setting for pigs (such as snout tying, rear leg suspension of piglets) should not be used in a biomedical research setting,

Box 14.4

Handling and restraint should be performed with a mind to minimize human and animal distress and risk of injury.

since animals are often chronically housed and such techniques, when used over time, can result in stress, altering biomarkers and research parameters as well as breaking down the trust between the animals and their handlers. Pigs are intelligent and highly food-motivated so target training and other positive reinforcement techniques can be used to encourage animals to perform various tasks including holding for a blood draw, walking to a scale, or exiting a cage for routine cleaning. Pig boards can be used to great effect to safely redirect animals and they will readily acclimate to a sling for long-term restraint. This is exactly what it sounds like: a large piece of sturdy fabric, with holes to allow the animal's legs to pass through. The sling can then be raised to keep the animal's feet off the ground, providing gentle restraint and suspending the animal in the hammock of the sling. Monitor animals for any signs of distress while restrained, and never leave them unattended within the sling (Figure 14.2).

Handling agricultural animals should be done with an awareness of two concepts: flight zone and point of balance. An animal's flight zone determines how close a possible threat (read: human researcher) can come to the animal before it will be instigated to flee. This distance can be reduced with positive handling and acclimation to human presence. Point of balance is a point relative to the animal; if a possible threat (human) is in front of the point of balance, the animal will move backward. If the threat is behind the point of balance, the animal will move forward. These two concepts can be used in tandem to encourage a group of animals or a single animal to move away, forward, or backward. Use of these natural behaviors when possible can reduce stress on both the animals and their human handlers.

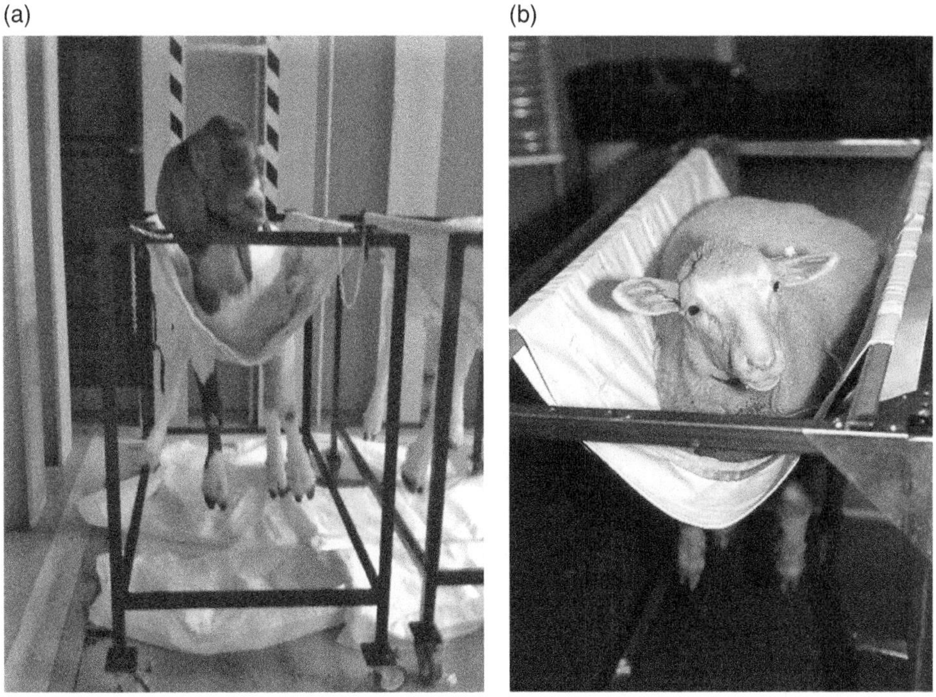

Fig 14.2. A goat (a) and a sheep (b) restrained in Panepinto Slings®. (*Source:* Photos courtesy of Panepinto and Associates, www.panepinto.com.)

Identification

Ear tags, ear tattoos, microchips or transponders, and ear notching (in swine) are common ways to identify agricultural animals. For single-housed animals, a cage card may be sufficient. Group-housed animals can also be distinguished by physical characteristics such as coat color or pattern. For some agricultural species, national eradication programs (such as scrapie for sheep and goats) may require that animals be permanently identified with their source flock and origin (Figure 14.3).

Blood Collection

With a large blood volume and large vessels, blood collection from swine, sheep, goats, and cattle is relatively straightforward. The jugular vein is a reliable source of blood though other locations may be used including the auricular, cephalic, and saphenous veins. Use of a butterfly catheter can assist with ease of blood collection, allowing for some movement if animals are not ideally restrained. For studies requiring large and repeated withdrawal of blood, consider implanting a vascular access port (VAP) to maintain ready access to the circulatory system.

Urine Collection

For unanesthetized animals, free-catch urine samples are the least complicated. A cup attached to a broom handle or dowel may facilitate catching of the sample midstream. If research needs dictate, indwelling urinary catheters or ultrasound-guided cystocentesis are used for sample collection.

Drug Administration

Pigs will readily eat many things. For oral administration of therapeutic or experimental compounds, often mixing with food or rolling into a treat will be sufficient for the animal to consume it voluntarily; if using this technique, verify that the drug has been consumed in its entirety. Due to the space between their incisors and molars (diastema), passage of a rumen tube in cattle, sheep, or goats is relatively simple and allows for administration of substances directly to the rumen.

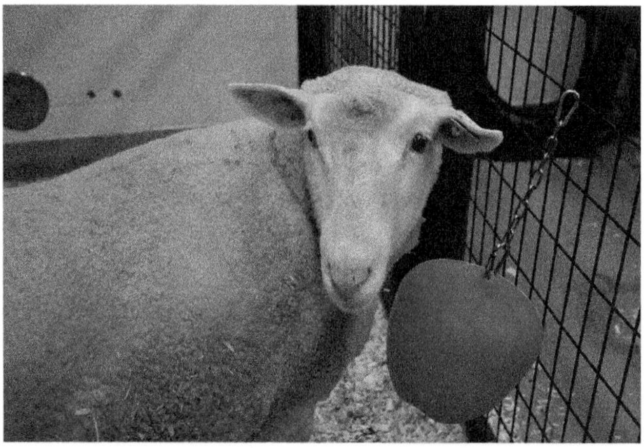

Fig 14.3. The tag in this sheep's left ear identifies it and its part in the scrapie eradication program. Information on the tag can be used to track the animal back to its farm of origin. (*Source:* Photo courtesy of A. Puffenberger.)

Intravenous drugs can be injected by any of the means listed for blood collection earlier. As with repeated blood collections, if multiple intravenous (IV) injections are planned over the course of the study, consider implantation of a VAP.

Intramuscular injections can be facilitated with a butterfly catheter in order to allow the animal some movement during the injection of the relatively large volumes that are required for animals of this size. Unlike in production medicine, research-related activities are less restrained in the possible locations for IM injection, since preservation of meat quality is not a consideration. Additionally, considerations such as withdrawal times are generally not of concern. As such, use of drugs off-label can be appropriate, with professional veterinary oversight.

Anesthesia, Surgery, and Postoperative Care

In a biomedical setting, standard surgery practices and aseptic techniques apply. For animals housed in an agricultural or farm setting, some procedures may be performed in the field, provided standard practices are observed as they relate to aseptic technique, surgeon preparation, and animal preparation.

Due to the large volume of the rumen, preanesthetic fasting times for sheep, goats, and cattle are often a prolonged 12–24 hours when compared with our typical monogastric species. This same anatomy can make surgical positioning difficult. In dorsal recumbency, the rumen may obstruct most or all of the organs of interest and the amount of material contained within can put pressure on the circulatory system, impeding venous return. Standing surgery, with appropriate restraint and a local anesthetic for pain management is not uncommon in a farm setting for rumenotomy or cesarean section.

Swine have a spiral colon that incorporates much of the cecum and colon itself, located in the upper left abdominal quadrant, but very similar digestion to humans. No extensive fasting is required for this species; 6–8 hours is sufficient.

Appropriate aseptic technique and postoperative monitoring and pain management should be provided for these species, just as any other research animal. As animals in a research setting are often managed on an individual basis, rather than as a herd, pain recognition and management is easier to accomplish and as such the expectations are more robust.

Euthanasia

All methods of euthanasia must conform to the most current American Veterinary Medical Association (AVMA) *Guidelines for the Euthanasia of Animals*. Injectable barbiturates are the acceptable methods for sheep, goats, cattle, and swine. Methods that may be acceptable with conditions can differ by species and can include gas or physical methods. Follow the *AVMA guidelines,* institutional policy, or an approved IACUC protocol when euthanizing animals and ensure all personnel are trained appropriately when using physical methods in order to ensure a rapid death for the animal and minimize the risk of human injury.

Euthanasia of large animals brings with it a set of logistical concerns. Given the size of the resultant carcasses, disposal can be difficult. There may be specific methods of packaging and shipping for disposal, or the facility may have on-site digesters for reduction of carcasses.

THERAPEUTIC AGENTS

Suggested anesthetic and analgesic agents are listed in Table 14.3.

INTRODUCTION TO DISEASES OF AGRICULTURAL ANIMALS OF PARTICULAR IMPORTANCE TO RESEARCH

As the primary goal in a research setting is to exclude common pathogens, the wide array of clinical conditions afflicting sheep, goats, cattle, and swine will not be addressed in detail here. Rather some general considerations and important causative agents by body system are listed next. Additionally, zoonotic diseases are often a particular concern in agricultural animals. A table of zoonoses and the associated species can be found in Table 14.4.

While exclusion of common pathogens is the goal, depending on the needs of the study, the source of the animals, and the availability of vendors, logistics may require the acceptance of some endemic disease within agricultural animals. Additionally, consideration of shipping stress is important as some agents which are asymptomatic or latent at the animal's home farm may cause the animal to present with disease upon arrival or shortly thereafter.

Neurological

In the United States, a comprehensive program to eradicate scrapie has been implemented. A transmissible spongiform encephalopathy (TSE), scrapie causes slowly progressing neurological signs, often beginning with subtle behavior changes and pruritus. This progresses to more severe locomotor issues and death. More common in Suffolk sheep, scrapie seems to have a genetic component to an animal's susceptibility. All sheep in the United States should have a scrapie identification tag. This information is used to trace back an animal's farm of origin; since scrapie is such a delayed-onset disease, this information may easily be lost otherwise. Other TSEs include bovine spongiform encephalopathy (mad cow disease) in cattle and variant Creutzfeldt-Jakob disease (vCJD) in humans. Ensure all sheep entering the facility are tagged appropriately in order to be in compliance with the eradication program requirements.

Cardiorespiratory

Transportation is an enormous stressor on animals. This stress can negatively impact the immune system, causing an increase in susceptibility to various viruses and bacteria. In agricultural animals, this often manifests as a respiratory disease colloquially known as "shipping fever." Shortly after arrival, animals may present with respiratory difficulty, coughing, lethargy, or nasal discharge. Appropriate antibiotic treatment is often effective.

The smallest free-living cells, *Mycoplasma* spp. can cause a variety of diseases including respiratory infections in agricultural animals. Though requiring special handling conditions due to its fastidious nature, culture is the best way to diagnose this bacterium. Affected animals may have coughing, nasal discharge, and reduced

Table 14.3. Anesthetics, tranquilizers, and analgesics used in sheep and goats

Drug	Sheep	Goats
Acepromazine maleate	0.05–0.10 mg/kg IM	0.05–0.10 mg/kg IM 0.2 mg/kg IM for tetany
Atipamezole	0.1–0.2 mg/kg IV slowly 0.005 μg/kg IV slowly after intrathecal or subarachnoid $alpha_2$-agonists	0.1–0.2 mg/kg IV slowly 0.005 μg/kg IV slowly after intrathecal or subarachnoid $alpha_2$-agonists
Buprenorphine	0.01 mg/kg IM every 6 hours 0.5 mg/kg SC 6 μg/kg IV	
Butorphanol	0.2–0.5 mg/kg IM or SC for sedation and analgesia	0.2–0.5 mg/kg IM for sedation and analgesia 0.1 mg/kg IV for reducing stress response
Detomidine	0.01 mg/kg intrathecally 0.01–0.02 mg/kg IM	0.01–0.04 mg/kg IM
Dexmedetomidine	0.005–0.020 mg/kg IV	0.005–0.020 mg/kg IV
Diazepam	0.3–0.4 mg/kg IV 1 mg/kg IV for tetany	0.3–0.4 mg/kg IV 1 mg/kg IV for tetany 0.06 mg/kg IV to stimulate appetite
Fentanyl transdermal patch on clean shaved skin	2 μg/kg/hour	
Flumazenil	20 μg/kg IV to reverse benzodiazepine effects	
Guaifenesin	50 mg/kg IV	
Guaifenesin–ketamine-xylazine	1.2 mL/kg/hour for induction, 2.6 mL/kg/hour for maintenance (guaifenesin, 50 mg/mL; ketamine, 1 mg/mL; xylazine, 0.1 mg/mL)	
Ketamine	1 mg/kg epidural for analgesia 4–7.5 mg/kg IV	4-5 mg/kg IV in combination with midazolam 10 mg/kg IV 0.03 mg/kg/minute constant-rate infusion for anesthesia
Midazolam	0.3–0.4 mg/kg IV for induction and analgesia	0.3–0.6 mg/kg IV for induction

(*Continued*)

Table 14.3. (*Continued*)

Drug	Sheep	Goats
Propofol	2.0–6.0 mg/kg IV for induction	2.0–6.0 mg/kg IV for induction
	0.3 mg/kg/minute IV for constant-rate infusion	0.3 mg/kg/minute IV for constant-rate infusion
Thiopental (thiopentone) sodium	13–20 mg/kg IV	6–8 mg/kg IV
Tiletamine–zolazepam (Telazol)	1.1–5.5 mg/kg IV	1.1–5.5 mg/kg IV
Xylazine	0.05–0.22 mg/kg IV or IM	0.05–0.22 mg/kg IV or IM
Yohimbine	0.2–0.25 mg/kg IV	0.2–0.25 mg/kg IV

Source: Adapted from Pugh and Baird (2012).
IM = intramuscular; IP = intraperitoneal; IV = intravenous; and SC = subcutaneous.

appetite or growth rates. *M. hyopneumoniae* is the organism found in swine while *M. ovipneumoniae* affects sheep. Arthritis, resulting in lameness, is another possible presentation of infection with mycoplasma.

Dermatological

Orf, known also as sore mouth or contagious ecthyma, is a viral disease that causes a pustular dermatitis in sheep, with lesions commonly arising around mucocutaneous junctions; pustules or vesicles are seen around the muzzle, genitals or coronary bands of the hooves. As it is a zoonotic disease, proper PPE should always be worn when working with sheep, especially those presenting with lesions consistent with orf. Treatment is based on supportive care—ensuring animals eat, maintain hydration, and aren't painful. Affected animals should be isolated from the rest of the flock, and handled last in order to prevent spread throughout the colony.

Gastrointestinal

A common problem among young piglets is diarrheal disease. Different organisms are more likely based on the age of the animal. A summary can be found in Table 14.5.

Proliferative enteritis in pigs is caused by *Lawsonia intracellularis*. This intracellular bacterium is associated with abundantly proliferative lesions in the ileum of post-weaning piglets. Animals with clinical infections may present with anorexia and/or diarrhea. Due to the proliferation of intestinal tissue, nutrient absorption is adversely affected and as such, animals grow at slower-than-expected rates. While animals may resolve spontaneously within several weeks, antibiotic treatment is often attempted in order to control clinical signs, but good culture and sensitivity data are difficult to attain, due to the microaerophilic nature of the organism.

Rectal prolapse is not uncommon in sheep, goats, and cattle, particularly in young animals that may have been straining due to high parasitic loads, diarrhea, or other inflammatory processes involving the large intestine. Additionally, urolithiasis causing urinary obstruction can also result in rectal prolapse due to straining. Treatment

Table 14.4. Zoonotic agents associated with cattle, sheep, and swine

	Cattle	Sheep	Swine
Actinobacillus lignieresii	X		
Arcanobacterium pyogenes	X		
Bacillus anthracis	X	X	
Borrelia burgdorferi	X		
Brucella spp.	X	X	X
Burkholderia pseudomallei	X		X
Campylobacter fetus	X	X	
Campylobacter jejuni	X	X	X
Chlamydophila abortus		X	
Clostridium difficile	X		X
Corynebacterium pseudotuberculosis		X	
Coxiella burnetii (Q fever)	X	X	
Cryptosporidium spp.	X		X
Dermatophilus congolensis	X		
Entamoeba hystolytica	X		
Erysipelothrix rhusiopathiae		X	X
Escherichia coli	X		X
Fasciola spp.	X		
Giardia intestinalis	X		X
Gongylonema pulchrum	X		
Leptosopira spp.	X	X	X
Listeria monocytogenes	X	X	X
Microsporum spp.	X	X	X
Mycobacterium spp.	X	X	X
Parapoxvirus (Orf)		X	
Rabies	X	X	X
Salmonella spp.	X	X	X
Sarcocystis spp.	X		X
Shigella spp.	X		
Staphylococcus aureus	X	X	X
Streptococcus spp.	X		X
Swine influenza			X
Taenia spp.	X		X
Toxoplasma gondii	X		X
Trichophyton spp.	X	X	X
Trichostrongylus spp.	X		
Yersinia pseudotuberculosis	X		X
Yersinia enterocolitica	X		X

Source: Adapted from Ganter (2015) and McDaniel et al. (2014).

Table 14.5. Diarrheal disease in piglets based on age and clinical signs

Disease	Clinical signs	Age	Etiology
Balantidiasis	Asymptomatic to severe ulcerative enterocolitis	Any age	*Balantidium coli*
Clostridial enteritis	Acute death, pink mucoid to severe hemorrhagic diarrhea	Newborn to postweaning	*Clostridium perfringens*
Coccidiosis	Asymptomatic to severe diarrhea	1–2 weeks of age	*Isospora suis*
Colibacillosis	Acute death, clear watery to white–yellow or hemorrhagic, diarrhea	Newborn to postweaning	*Escherichia coli* ETEC, EPEC (AEEC), EHEC
Giardiasis	Asymptomatic to anorexia with diarrhea	Any age	*Giardia intestinalis*
Proliferative enteropathy	Acute death, anorexia, loose watery to hemorrhagic diarrhea	Postweaning	*Lawsonia intracellularis*
Rotavirus	Profuse watery, white/yellow diarrhea, fever and vomiting	Most severe within days of birth	Porcine rotavirus
Salmonella enterocolitis	Watery, yellow diarrhea with fever, anorexia, depression	Postweaning	*Salmonella typhimurium, S. choleraesuis*
Small intestinal threadworms	Asymptomatic to severe diarrhea with mortality	Nursing pigs	*Strongyloides ransomi*
Swine dysentery	Watery, mucoid, and hemorrhagic diarrhea, rarely acute deaths	1 week and older	*Serpulina hyodysenteriae*
Transmissible gastroenteritis	Vomiting, severe diarrhea, high mortality	Any age	TGE virus
Whipworms	Asymptomatic to severe mucoid or hemorrhagic diarrhea with mortality	Postweaning	*Trichuris suis*

Source: Adapted from Helke et al. (2015).

involves cleaning and assessment of the prolapsed tissue. If the tissue looks healthy and intact, the prolapse should be replaced and held in using a purse-string suture around the anus. For more severe or chronic prolapses, the exposed tissue may require amputation. An investigation into the underlying cause for the prolapse should also be performed.

Bloat can be caused by excessive buildup of gas within the rumen, typically instigated by a sudden and abundant intake of grain or succulent plants. Whether the bloat is purely gas or what's known as "frothy" bloat can inform which course of treatment to take. Free-gas bloat can be released/decompressed via rumen tube, providing a ready exit for the gas to escape. Frothy bloat is more troublesome, requiring administration of a surfactant or other substance via rumen tube in order to break down the foam and allow the gas to escape. If decompression is not possible via rumen tube, a trochar in the paralumbar fossa directly into the rumen or a rumenotomy may be indicated. Once the immediate resolution of decompression is achieved, investigation into the root cause of the bloat should be undertaken. This may be of particular concern in research requiring prolonged anesthetic periods.

Musculoskeletal

White muscle disease, found in all large animals, is due to a nutritional deficiency in vitamin E and selenium. While exceptionally uncommon in animals on a commercially available feed, animals housed in a farm setting or on pasture may be susceptible.

Lameness can be caused by a variety of bacteria, should they invade the joint spaces, but the most common cause of lameness or limping in agricultural animals is trauma of some kind. Providing a sturdy floor surface to prevent slippage is a primary point of prevention. Routine hoof examination and trimming or other care as appropriate can help address issues before they become serious problems.

Reproductive and Genitourinary

Q fever, caused by *Coxiella burnetii*, is a bacterial disease associated with pregnant ewes, though it can also infect goats and cattle. While typically asymptomatic in sheep, it is zoonotic, so care should be taken and appropriate PPE worn when dealing with late-term ewes and in the immediately postparturient period. Birthing tissues or fluids as well as feces and milk of infected animals can carry the organism. Human infection is a result of inhalation, so an appropriate and well-fitting respirator and eye protection should be worn.

Resulting from a negative energy balance in late-stage pregnancy, pregnancy toxemia can affect ewes or does. This can occur in over-conditioned animals as well as in thin animals. Simply put, the pregnant animal cannot (whether due to decreased rumen capacity because of large fetal mass, lack of good-quality forage, or a concurrent issue such as malocclusion) take in enough nutrition to keep up with the metabolic demand required for proper development of the fetus (or fetuses). Diagnosed via increased ketones in the blood or urine, initial signs typically arise in the last 2–4 weeks of pregnancy and may include weakness, lethargy, or anorexia. This may progress to neurological signs including incoordination or star-gazing. The goal of treatment for affected animals should be to correct the nutritional and metabolic imbalances. Glucose should be given along with slow IV infusion of calcium borogluconate if hypocalcemic. Supportive care such as B vitamins and flunixin meglumine may encourage a return of the appetite and result in more favorable outcomes.

The anatomy of cattle as well as sheep and goats predisposes them to urinary blockage by uroliths. In male cattle, the urethra narrows significantly at the sigmoid flexure while rams and bucks have a urethral process, which is prone to catching stones. Clinical signs include expressions of pain (vocalization, kicking at the belly, etc.) as well as straining to urinate and reduced urine output. Surgical removal of the vermiform appendage can relieve the problem in sheep and goats. Surgical treatment for cattle is more involved and often the prognosis is poor.

Neoplasia

While several cases of various types of neoplasia have been reported in swine, most research projects are of a short enough time-course that animals do not develop this condition. Neoplasia has been reported in sheep and goats but is particularly rare.

Miscellaneous Conditions

Salt poisoning is of a concern with pigs. When deprived with water for a period of time (usually about 24 hours, though clinical signs can appear after deprivation for only a few hours), animals will drink profusely upon reintroduction of water. This rehydration process causes an osmolality imbalance in the neural tissues resulting in water diffusing into the CNS, which causes swelling and edema. This in turn causes neurological signs, typically leading to death. Ensuring swine have access to water (bucket, functioning lixit, or other source) is therefore of prime importance. Be particularly cognizant of this if research requires water restriction or manipulation.

Pigs possessing a mutation in their ryanodine receptor (RYR) are susceptible to porcine stress syndrome, also referred to as malignant hyperthermia. When exposed to stressful situations, or some anesthetics (such as halothane, isoflurane, and others), their skeletal muscles are unable to keep an appropriate calcium balance, resulting in a broad array of clinical signs. Muscle rigidity is one of these signs as well as tachypnea, tachycardia, and hyperthermia. If an animal displays these signs, anesthesia administration should be immediately ceased and 100% oxygen provided. Cooling the animal with IV fluids (including sodium bicarbonate to reverse the accompanying acidosis), air circulation, and ice packing can help bring the animal's body temperature under control. Dantrolene should also be administered as soon as signs are recognized.

BIBLIOGRAPHY

American Veterinary Medical Association (AVMA). 2013. *AVMA Guidelines for the Euthanasia of Animals*. Schaumburg, IL: AVMA. Available at: http://www.avma.org/KB/Policies/Documents/euthanasia.pdf.

Federation of Animal Science Societies (FASS). 2010. *Guide for the Care and Use of Agricultural Animals in Research in Teaching*, 3rd ed. Champaign, IL: FASS.

Ganter M. 2015. Zoonotic risks from small ruminants. Vet Microbiol 181(1–2):53–65.

Helke, K. L., P. C. Ezell, R. Duran-Struuck, and M. M. Swindle. 2015. Biology and diseases of swine. In *Laboratory Animal Medicine*, 3rd ed., J.G. Fox, L.C. Anderson, G. Otto, K.R. Pritchet-Corning, M.T. Whary (eds.), pp. 695–771. San Diego, CA: Elsevier.

McCrackin M. A. and M. M. Swindle. 2015. Biology, Handling, Husbandry and Anatomy. In *Swine in the Laboratory: Surgery, Anesthesia, Imaging, and Experimental Techniques*, 3rd ed., M.M. Swindle and A.C. Smith (eds.), pp. 1–39. Boca Raton, FL: CRC Press.

McDaniel, C. J., D. M. Cardwell, R. B. Moeller, and G. C. Gray. 2014. Humans and cattle: A review of bovine zoonoses. Vector Borne Zoonotic Dis 14(1): 1–19.

Pugh, D. G. and A. N. Baird. 2012. *Sheep and Goat Medicine*, 2nd ed. Maryland Heights, MS: Elsevier.

Uddin Khan S., K. R. Atanasova, W. S. Krueger, et al. 2013. Epidemiology, geographical distribution, and economic consequences of swine zoonoses: A narrative review. Emerg Microbes Infect 2(12): e92.

Underwood, W. J., R. Blauwiekel, M. L. Delano, et al. 2015. Biology and diseases of ruminants (sheep, goats, and cattle). In *Laboratory Animal Medicine*, 3rd ed., J.G. Fox, L.C. Anderson, G. Otto, K.R. Pritchet-Corning, and M.T. Whary (eds.), pp. 623–694. San Diego, CA: Elsevier.

FURTHER READING

Grandin, T. 2017. *Temple Grandin's Guide to Working with Farm Animals: Safe, Humane Livestock Handling Practices for the Small Farm.* North Adams, MA: Storey.

National Academies of Sciences, Engineering & Medicine. 2016. *Nutrient Requirements of Beef Cattle: Eighth Revised Edition.* Washington, DC: National Academies Press.

National Research Council. 2012. *Nutrient Requirements of Swine: Eleventh Revised Edition.* Washington, DC: National Academies Press.

National Research Council. 2007. *Nutrient Requirements of Small Ruminants: Sheep, Goats, Cervids, and New World Camelids.* Washington, DC: National Academies Press.

National Research Council. 2001. *Nutrient Requirements of Dairy Cattle: Seventh Revised Edition.* Washington, DC: National Academies Press.

Pugh, D. G. and A. N. Baird. 2012. *Sheep and Goat Medicine*, 2nd ed. Maryland Heights, MS: Elsevier.

Swindle, M. M and A. C. Smith, (eds.) 2015. *Swine in the Laboratory: Surgery, Anesthesia, Imaging, and Experimental Techniques*, 3rd ed. Boca Raton, FL: CRC Press.

CHAPTER 14 REVIEW

Short Answer

1. Agricultural animals are often used for research projects involving prosthesis development, joint replacement, and other implantable medical devices. Why is this?
2. What should be the priority when handling large animals in any setting?
3. Sheep and goats are typically seasonally polyestrous. What strategy can be employed if year-round breeding is desired?
4. What factors may influence the preventive medicine program for agricultural animals developed at an institution? (describe two)
5. What is the purpose of an acclimation period?

(Continued)

6. If animals need to be housed singly for research purposes, what group should be consulted for approval?
7. Why should meal feeding of pigs be considered for long-term studies?
8. Define flight zone.
9. Define point of balance.
10. Describe how you could use flight zone and point of balance in order to encourage an animal to move willingly out of one pen and into another.
11. Why are preanesthetic fasting periods often extended in ruminants?
12. What is "shipping fever"?
13. How can you prevent salt poisoning in swine?

Critical Thinking

14. A researcher in your institution needs weekly weights on the swine involved in her project. The pig room is down the hall from the scale. What are some strategies to minimize stress and maximize safety for both humans and animals when moving the pigs down the hallway?

15

Research Variables, Biosecurity, and Colony Health Surveillance

RESEARCH VARIABLES

In a research setting, it is important to keep nonexperimental variables to a minimum. Otherwise, a variety of factors can confound experimental results and lead to erroneous conclusions from the data collected. These factors can be grouped into two general classifications: *intrinsic factors* inherent to the animal, such as genotype, age, and sex; and *extrinsic factors* that are external to the animal, such as environment, diet, and infectious agents. Both intrinsic and extrinsic factors can influence an animal's physiology and behavior. Figure 15.1 depicts intrinsic and extrinsic factors that can act as unintended experimental variables and affect the biologic responses of laboratory animals.

Intrinsic Factors

Genotype and Genetic Integrity: When designing a research project, the genotype of the animal used is an important intrinsic consideration, as genetic composition often determines the biologic responses of individual animals within a species. Animal strains or stocks may respond differently to pharmaceutical drugs or generate dissimilar immune responses to pathogenic organisms. For example, administration of chloramphenicol succinate induces leukopenia in the BALB/c inbred strain of mice,

Clinical Laboratory Animal Medicine: An Introduction, Fifth Edition.
Lesley A. Colby, Megan H. Nowland, and Lucy H. Kennedy.

Companion website: www.wiley.com/go/colby/clinical

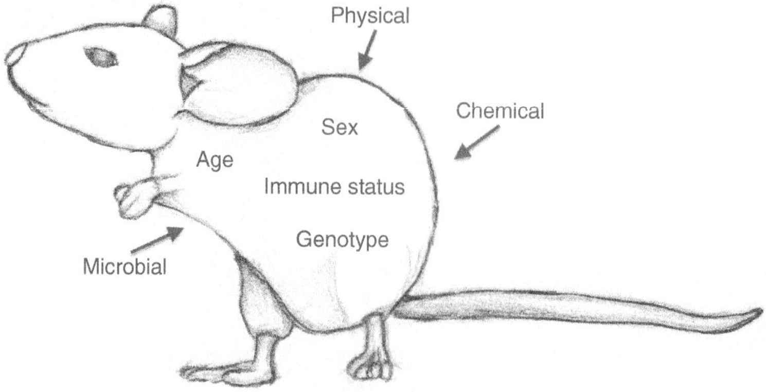

Fig 15.1. Intrinsic (e.g., genotype, age, sex, and immune status) and extrinsic factors (e.g., physical, chemical, and microbial) that can act as nonexperimental variables. (*Source:* Illustration by Tess Keller.)

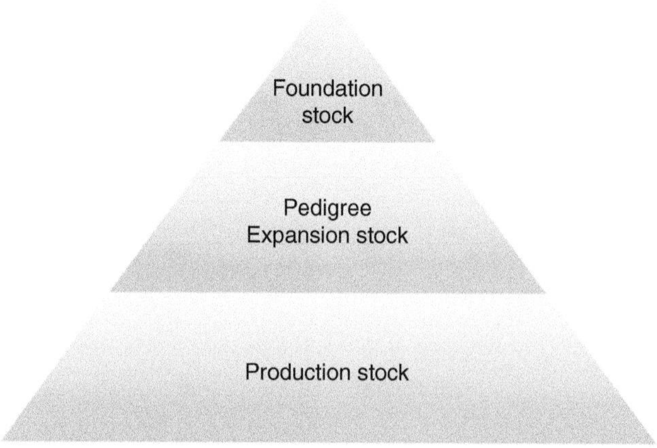

Fig 15.2. Hierarchical breeding scheme used in the production of inbred animals.

but not in the CD-1 outbred stock of mice. The DBA/1J mouse strain is highly susceptible to Sendai virus, whereas the SJL mouse strain is highly resistant to developing clinical disease. Likewise, LEW rats are more susceptible to infection with sialodacryoadenitis virus than are F344 rats.

In addition to selecting the most appropriate species, strain, or stock for use in a research study, it is critical that the genetic integrity of the animals be maintained to the greatest extent possible to minimize unintended experimental variability. Inbred animals are frequently selected for use as their nearly identical genetic composition reduces experimental variability both within and across experiments. Inbred animals are produced through a hierarchical breeding scheme involving foundation stock, pedigree expansion stock, and production stock to maintain animal homogeneity (Figure 15.2). Despite this, genetic differences will always exist between animals of the same inbred strain due to the occurrence of spontaneous genetic mutations and chromosomal aberrations (Box 15.1). Unfortunately, human error resulting in

Box 15.1

Genetic differences will always exist between animals of the same inbred strain due to the occurrence of spontaneous genetic mutations and chromosomal aberrations.

Box 15.2

Genetic drift cannot be entirely prevented, but should be minimized.

mismatings and inadvertent outcrossings with other strains is often a significant and unrecognized cause of genetic variability within an animal colony. For this reason, it is advisable to institute multiple methods to help avoid errors, such as housing different strains of breeding mice with the same coat color in separate rooms and ensuring all cages are clearly labeled with complete animal identification information. In contrast to inbred animals, outbred animals are produced from large breeding colonies strategically bred to maintain heterogeneity. In order to ensure this variability, outbred stocks must be managed just as carefully as inbred strains to reduce genetic drift.

Genetically modified animals present additional concerns for unintended experimental variability. For instance, the background strain of these animals may influence their phenotypic expression of genetic modifications, thereby affecting animal physiology and behavior. Depending on the method used to induce the modification, changes in the genetic code may increase or disrupt other anatomic or physiologic functions that are difficult or impossible to detect.

Genetic drift, the change in frequency of genes in a population over time, is a natural occurrence and cannot be entirely prevented. However, when managing a colony of inbred, outbred, or genetically modified animals, the goal is to minimize the effect of genetic drift, therefore maintaining consistency of the same stock or strain of animals in different colonies despite the fact that one may be housed at an institution in Seattle and another may be housed in London (Box 15.2). Methods to monitor genetic drift are centered predominantly on the use of molecular-based testing. Nevertheless, careful observation of the physical characteristics and behavior of colony animals is also paramount and requires knowledge of the normal characteristics of a strain or stock. Expected coat color, frequency of inherited medical conditions such as microphthalmia or hydrocephalus, and behavior patterns such as aggression can all be used in colony monitoring.

DNA-based assays that can distinguish extremely subtle genetic alterations, such as polymerase chain reaction (PCR), single nucleotide polymorphism (SNP), and microsatellite panels, form the cornerstone of genetic monitoring programs. Typically, PCR is used to determine the presence or absence of a gene of interest in a genetically modified animal. Quantitative PCR, also called real-time PCR, enables both detection and quantification of a targeted DNA molecule including determination of homozygosity or heterozygosity and gene copy number. Microsatellites are short segments of DNA that have repeat sequences. SNP and microsatellite marker panels are available to validate the genetic status of an animal and identify specific genes.

Samples for genetic testing can be taken from a variety of sources, including oral mucosa (obtained by buccal swabs), tail or ear tissue, saliva, fecal pellets, and hair follicles. Significant differences can exist in the quality of genetic samples obtained from separate anatomic locations. Similarly, locations may differ in the amount of extraneous genetic material (e.g., fecal bacteria) that may be inadvertently collected and complicate testing results. Due to welfare considerations, the use of least invasive and stressful methods for reliable sample collection is advocated.

Age, sex, and immune status: In addition to animal genotype, other equally important intrinsic factors that should be considered include animal age, sex, and immune status. Age can influence such things as animal respiratory rate, blood pressure, demand for oxygen, drug metabolism capacity, renal concentration and dilution ability, and the ability to thermoregulate. Compared with adults, neonates are more sensitive to various carcinogenic compounds. Older animals frequently have decreased cardiovascular, hepatic, and kidney functions that can confound experimental results. Marked differences may be seen in differing sexes of the same population due to sex-linked hormonal variations. As an example, male rats are significantly more sensitive to the analgesic properties of morphine than are females. Immune function is another important intrinsic factor that plays a role in response to experimental manipulations. Nude, severe combined immunodeficient (SCID), and many transgenic strains of animals lack specific components of a complete immune system, thereby eliciting a different response to antigens than immunocompetent animals.

Extrinsic Factors

Extrinsic factors can be generally divided into three categories: physical, chemical, and microbial.

Physical: Physical factors include the *microenvironment* (an animal's immediate surroundings, such as the cage), *macroenvironment* (the area surrounding the microenvironment, such as the housing room), and physiologic and behavioral stressors. The microenvironment can be directly influenced by the cage or housing system, the macroenvironment, and the animals themselves. For instance, a high animal cage density and the presence of polyuric animals (e.g., diabetic mice) can each induce high ammonia levels within a cage. Alternatively, the macro- and microenvironment may differ substantially, largely as a result of the caging system used. For example, humidity and ammonia levels may significantly differ in housing rooms (the macroenvironment) containing mice in open-top caging, static microisolation caging, or individually ventilated microisolation cages (IVC).

Multiple environmental variables can affect both the micro- and macroenvironment including temperature, relative humidity, lighting, ventilation, noise, and vibration (Box 15.3). The *Guide for the Care and Use of Laboratory Animals* (the *Guide*; ILAR, 2011) has established guidelines for the macroenvironment to help assure the well-being of animals. According to the *Guide*, regulation of body temperature within normal variation is necessary for the well-being of homeotherms. Exposure of unadapted animals to temperature extremes above 29.4°C (85°F) or below 7.2°C (45°F)

Box 15.3

Multiple environmental variables can affect both the micro- and macroenvironment including temperature, relative humidity, lighting, ventilation, noise, and vibration.

may produce life-threatening physiologic effects. Furthermore, elevation of the macroenvironmental temperature of breeding rodents can cause sterility or reduced milk production.

Relative humidity can significantly influence animal well-being and affect experimental outcomes. Humidity levels affect thermoregulation, food consumption, transmission of infectious agents, and skin absorption studies. Low environmental humidity has been associated with the development of ringtail in rat pups and epistaxis in some species of nonhuman primates. High environmental humidity contributes to gerbils developing greasy and unkempt haircoats. High relative humidity can promote the growth of ammonia-producing fecal bacteria resulting in elevated ammonia levels within an animal's environment, especially in static microisolation cages or other enclosed areas.

Light intensity and duration can impact animal behavior and physiology. Excessive light intensity for a prolonged period can cause retinal degeneration in albino rodents. Animals exposed to varying light levels within a room have been shown to confound long-term carcinogenicity studies. Thus light intensity and cage position are important variables for consideration. Light cycles are also extremely important in most species for maintenance of circadian rhythms and breeding production.

The *Guide* recommends a room ventilation rate of 10–15 air changes per hour. However, as the *Guide* promotes use of performance standards in place of stringent engineering standards, this rate is not strictly required. Rather, the determination of room ventilation rates should take into account the many variables that can affect air quality, such as the density of animals within a room, caging type, and the amount of heat generated by animals and equipment. Mechanical engineers can assist in determining room ventilation requirements necessary to accommodate animal needs.

Noise generation is inherent in an animal facility, and can have differing effects across animal species. For example, intraspecies communication at the ultrasonic level is of particular importance to rodents and can easily be affected by environmental noise. Cage-changing activities, cleaning and movement of equipment, fire alarm activation, and construction noise are of particular concern. Use of ventilated racks, laminar flow hoods, and biological safety cabinets can generate noise perceptible by animals. Noise produced in animal facilities is often outside the range audible to humans, but may be clearly perceived by some animal species. Low-frequency sounds can alter blood pressure and excess noise levels can cause audiogenic seizures in a number of mouse strains, such as the DBA strain. Noise can even induce effects post-exposure, as demonstrated by the reduced learning ability of mouse pups exposed to noise during pregnancy. Noise generated by the animals themselves should also be considered. This is particularly important in facilities housing different species of animals, especially when one species is a recognized predator of another species. In these situations, measures should be taken to prevent noise transmission between animal-occupied areas.

Multiple sources of vibration exist within a facility including housing room equipment (e.g., IVC rack blowers and laminar flow hoods) and movement of wheeled equipment, personnel, and animal cages. Vibrations may also originate external to a facility but transfer into an animal-occupied area. Common sources include nearby construction activities and transportation corridors such as roads, tracks, and tunnels. Exposure to intermittent or continuous vibrations can influence animal behavior, breeding, physiological responses, and stress. Facilities should be located and designed to minimize the creation and transmission of vibrations. Vibration suppression systems should be used to isolate or dampen vibrations that cannot be eliminated.

Physiologic and behavioral stressors influenced by housing methods, cage population, and transportation can directly affect animals and must not be overlooked. Cage designs should take into account an animal's space, health, and social needs in order to create a minimally stressful environment. Specific factors have been studied extensively to gain an understanding of the needs of a particular species, or a specific strain. Different species will require different cage parameters, based on normal anatomic and physiologic factors. For example, gerbils frequently adopt a semi-erect posture, so cage height needs to be sufficient to allow this movement. Similar species differences exist when considering flooring type, bedding type and depth, food delivery systems, air exchange rates, and cage density. Understanding the social needs of a species is particularly important for reducing stressors; social species should be housed in groups whenever research and animal health and behavior allow, while species that prefer single housing can experience significant stress or impacts to animal health when housed socially. Transportation of animals also contributes to physiologic stress in almost all species. All animals should be provided a minimum period of acclimation prior to starting an experiment to allow animal stress levels and physiologic values to stabilize and adapt to the new environment. The length of acclimation period is partially dependent on the animal species, the duration and complexity of transportation, and needs of the anticipated research project. Minimizing these physiologic and behavioral stressors is important to both animal welfare and experiment validity and integrity.

Chemical: Xenobiotics, chemicals that are foreign to a biological system, can impact animals through their macro- and/or microenvironment. Air, diet, bedding material, caging materials, and cleaning agents are potential sources of chemical exposure. Their effect or toxicity is partially based on the dose and disposition of the chemical. Chemicals may cause direct damage to animal tissues and organs or may have indirect effects through biotransformation and the production of metabolites. Chemicals or their metabolites may cause physiologic alterations in animals, affecting the immune response or acting as a mutagen and/or as a teratogen.

Animal food, drinking water, and bedding materials are important potential sources of chemicals or compound exposure. Each is discussed in detail in the **Biosecurity and Exclusion of Contaminants** section.

Another area of chemical exposure that is often overlooked is exposure to pharmaceutical agents. Drugs are administered to anesthetize animals, relieve pain, prevent or treat disease, or as part of a protocol to activate promoters that turn on or off specific genes. Administration of these pharmaceutical agents is usually a necessary step in the scientific process; however, these agents may produce different or confounding physiologic effects that alter the experiment. Cardiovascular depression and respiratory depression are two common side effects of anesthetic agents; these biologic effects could clearly impact an animal's response to an experimental manipulation. Chemical variables must be monitored and eliminated when possible.

Microbial: Microbes are one of the most obvious factors that can affect research integrity. Pathogenic organisms frequently cause disease that directly impacts the biologic responses of affected animals. Many organisms cause latent or subclinical infections in animals. Although there are no overt clinical signs of illness, latent microbial infections often cause subtle changes in the physiologic responses of infected animals.

An infection can be transmitted to a susceptible host directly through vertical or horizontal transmission or indirectly through fomites or vectors. Vertical transmission is the transfer of a pathogen from a parent, usually the dam, to the offspring and occurs in utero—or at birth (Figure 15.3). Horizontal transmission is the transfer of a pathogen from an infected animal to a susceptible animal (Figure 15.4) and occurs through multiple routes, including respiratory aerosols and by direct contact. Fomites (inanimate objects that may transmit infectious organisms) transfer contaminated material via food, water, bedding, and equipment that then contacts the animal. Vectors such as mites, lice, and flies may be a part of the life cycle of the organism, or

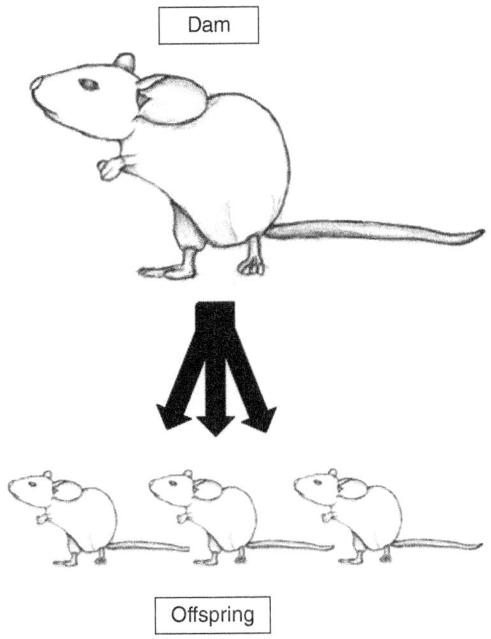

Fig 15.3. Vertical transmission of infection. (*Source:* Illustration by Tess Keller.)

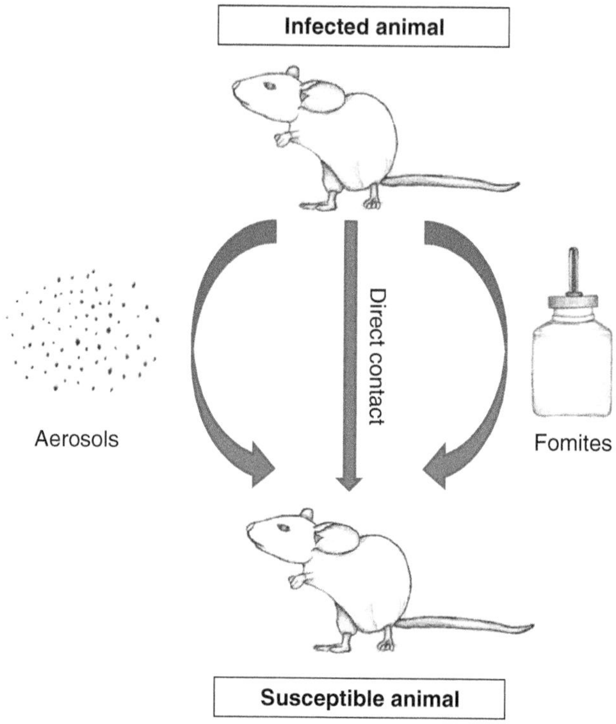

Fig 15.4. Horizontal transmission of infection. (*Source:* Illustrations by Tess Keller.)

they can mechanically transmit the organism from one animal to another. The mode of transmission varies with the infectious agent; for example, mouse hepatitis virus is transmitted primarily via feces, whereas lymphocytic choriomeningitis virus is transmitted via urine, saliva, and milk.

In addition to potentially pathogenic organisms, the microbiome of animals must also be considered. The microbiome is the aggregate of microorganisms that live on or within an animal. The influence of the microbiome on animal health and experimental outcomes is only now being recognized. Disruption of an animal's native microbiome can not only influence its susceptibility to disease, but also result in changes to its physiologic and behavioral functions. In fact, current research suggests that an animal's microbiome may play a key role in multiple diseases including inflammatory bowel disease, cancer, autoimmune disease, and hypertension.

Animals with dissimilar microbiomes can be an important source of experimental variability within a study. Differences can be induced by animals' exposure to unique food or water sources, environments, medications, and numerous other factors. As a result, the microbiome of animals housed at or obtained from separate institutions may be distinct. In fact, the microbiome of both inbred strains and outbred stocks of rodents may be of markedly different composition in animals obtained from independent commercial vendors. Therefore, the potential influence of the microbiome on experimental results must be considered and addressed, when necessary.

BIOSECURITY AND EXCLUSION OF CONTAMINANTS

Animal health and the integrity of research results require that *adventitious agents*, organisms that are unintentionally introduced into animals or their environment, and other contaminants be excluded from animal research colonies and their environment. When exclusion practices fail, it is equally important that contaminants and affected animals be reliably identified. To achieve these objectives, institutions should establish formal biosecurity programs composed of procedures or processes used to prevent the introduction or spread of harmful biological organisms within an area, as well as colony-level animal health monitoring programs. Adventitious agents and other contaminants may originate from multiple sources including animals introduced to a facility; food, bedding, and water; fomites; biological materials; vermin; and personnel.

Animals intended for transfer into a facility should be assessed for both symptomatic and asymptomatic infection with agents purposefully excluded from the facility. The list of excluded agents will vary among research facilities and should be consistent with research needs and facility design and operation. The health and microbial status of animals designated for receipt may be assessed by multiple means. While direct testing of each individual animal may be possible, alternate methods are more frequently employed due to convenience, financial and time constraints, and testing limitations such as a lack of reliable premortem testing methods. Receiving institutions routinely review the institutional health monitoring program of animal source facilities as well as months or years of health surveillance testing results to evaluate the overall health of the source facility's animal populations. Receiving institutions may also require the testing of all or a subset of animals for specific organisms within a defined time period prior to transfer.

Institutions may elect to place animals that meet their exclusion criteria in areas of the facility occupied by established colony animals. Institutions receiving animals from commercial rodent vendors commonly do this. Alternatively, institutions may initially house all new animals in quarantine areas for additional testing and observations. Facilities with strict biosecurity programs may require that animals be introduced into the facility only through embryo or cesarean rederivation. When animals are shown or suspected to be infected with an excluded organism, receiving facilities may deny transfer of the animals and require animal rederivation. Alternatively, institutions may accept the animals into specially designated isolation areas in which they will either remain throughout their life or be treated to eliminate the organism. Use of microisolation housing and segregation of animal shipments between housing areas are recommended to help prevent the potential spread of infectious organisms between groups of quarantined animals. Likewise, strict operational procedures should be followed to preclude transfer of infectious agents to established colonies.

Animal food, bedding, and drinking water are potential sources of adventitious agents or contaminants. According to the *Guide*, laboratory animals should be fed palatable, uncontaminated, and nutritionally adequate food unless the protocol in which they are being used requires otherwise. Diets may contain either natural or synthetic compounds that can affect experimental outcomes by altering animal physiologic processes. Heavy metals, nitrosamines, aflatoxins, estrogenic compounds, organophosphates, and polychlorinated biphenyls are examples of dietary contaminants. Exposure to heavy metals such as lead and cadmium lowers disease resistance in rodents. Nitrosamine contamination can have a carcinogenic effect. Diets can also be contaminated with estrogenic compounds during formulation of the product or by aflatoxin during storage of various cereal grains. Organophosphate and polychlorinated biphenyls are dietary contaminants from agricultural residues.

Bedding materials can directly cause biologic changes or can become contaminated with chemicals and indirectly affect studies. Softwood bedding materials such as cedar are not recommended because they emit aromatic hydrocarbons that induce hepatic microsomal enzymes and cytotoxicity. Mice housed on cotton bedding have been shown to have lower intestinal humoral immune responses than those housed on hardwood bedding.

Food and bedding should be purchased from reputable vendors whose production, storage, and transportation processes are consistent with the strict quality levels required for research. The conduct of independent quality assurance assessments may be advisable for food and bedding products produced by noncommercial entities or entities that do not routinely supply the research industry. Assessments should consider microbial and amicrobial (e.g., chemicals, metals) contaminants, as well as the nutritional formulation of food. When microbial levels must be controlled, as is commonly desired in rodent colonies, food and bedding can be autoclaved to render a sterile product. A special formulation of the food may be required if the autoclaving process would inactivate or degrade nutritional elements below their minimally required levels. Alternatively, rodent chow pretreated with gamma irradiation is widely available; however it should be noted that unless irradiation levels used are higher than those employed by most rodent food vendors, irradiated diets are not sterile, although their microbial levels are markedly reduced. This is an important distinction for food provided to germ-free or gnotobiotic animals. Within a facility, food and bedding should be stored in a manner to prevent their contamination with chemicals (e.g., cleaning solutions) or by vermin.

According to the *Guide*, animals should have access to potable, uncontaminated drinking water. There is substantial variation in water quality depending upon locality, source, and treatment prior to consumption. Drinking water can be contaminated by a variety of agents that can alter experimental outcomes, including pesticides, heavy metals, volatile organics, asbestos fibers, polychlorinated biphenyls, and radionuclides. The level of microbial control and purity required will vary by animal species, animal immune status, and research needs. Water may be filtered to remove particulate including larger microbial organisms (e.g., bacteria). Water may be further treated with ultraviolet radiation, reverse osmosis membrane filtration, chlorination, acidification, or autoclaving to remove potential contaminants and/or to inhibit microbial growth during storage or when accessible by animals (e.g., in rodent water bottles). Treatments, however, can also produce physiologic changes in animals and indirectly alter experimental outcomes. For example, chlorine may cause changes in the immune response, and acidification can cause decreased water intake and weight gain. The delivery system used can also impact studies. Autoclaving glass bottles can cause formation of silicon crystals, and rubber stoppers used to cap the bottles can leach minerals into the water.

Sanitation and effective control of movements within a facility are key to preventing the introduction of adventitious organisms or contaminants into a facility by fomites. Here, fomites are defined as inanimate objects or substances that can carry an infectious organism or contaminant. Items brought into a facility as well as items moved within a facility can serve as fomites and present a health risk to animal colonies. For instance, laboratory equipment (e.g., scales) previously used with research animals unknowingly infected with a pathogen or parasite may be contaminated with that same organism. The external surface of animal shipping containers or food bags may be contaminated by wild rodents with access to shipping vehicles or loading docks. All items brought into a facility should be sanitized prior to their entry into the facility. When effective sanitation methods are not possible, then operational procedures should be enacted to prevent the transfer of an organism or contaminant into a facility. For instance, with plastic-lined food bags with a paper exterior, the paper can be removed and the plastic bag chemically disinfected. Objects within a facility may also serve as fomites. Examples include animal restrainers, carts, and soiled caging. Material movement within an animal facility should always flow from the cleanest to the dirtiest areas of the facility. Items moved between areas should either be sanitized or be protected from potential contamination (e.g., enclosed in plastic with replacement of the plastic between uses). Clean and soiled items should be isolated from each other and, ideally, both should be covered when not in use to prevent inadvertent transfer of contaminants. Sterilization of clean caging, caging materials (food, bedding, and water), and other items to which animals may have direct contact (e.g., enrichment items) may be warranted for some animal colonies, such as with rodents and immunocompromised animals. Procedures should be in place to ensure that the sanitation and sterilization processes are effective. Adenosine triphosphate (ATP) bioluminescent technology and replicate organism detection and counting (RODAC) plates can be used when assessing the efficacy of sanitation of inanimate objects or surfaces.

Biological materials such as cells, cell cultures, tissues, and blood and blood products administered to animals have been a source of infectious agent transmission to animal colonies on multiple occasions (Box 15.4). Biological materials freshly derived from animals or humans, including those repeatedly passaged in animals, as well as those from cold storage or obtained from active cell cultures may be unknowingly contaminated. Groups involved in animal research should screen all biological materials for contamination, such as through PCR testing, prior to administration to animals or use in any way.

Intrusion of wild animals and insects into all animal-use areas should be prevented as both can be sources of disease transmission to research colonies. Wild animals may transmit disease through direct contact with research animals as well as through contamination of the environment, such as through urine and fecal deposits. Insects

Box 15.4

Biological materials have been a source of infectious agent transmission to animal colonies on multiple occasions.

may serve as mechanical vectors, simply transporting an infectious organism to a susceptible host, or as an intermediate host, in which an organism develops from a noninfectious to an infectious form. Institutions should implement an integrated pest management program (IPM) designed to prevent intrusion of vermin into animal facilities, to monitor for and identify signs of intrusions or attempted intrusions, and to control and eradicate intrusions, if they occur. Although not part of an IPM, methods should also be in place to identify, quickly capture, and then handle any research animals that may escape from their enclosures. This is especially pertinent to rodent colonies where escaped animals can be a source of genetic contamination (e.g., if an animal moves to a different cage to breed) or can become contaminated with organisms present in the animal room that may negatively affect research findings.

Lastly, personnel must be considered as a potential source of animal contamination. This may occur if personnel do not follow facility operational procedures for the flow of movements within the facility (e.g., working in soiled cage wash immediately before handling immunocompromised animals), for equipment sanitation, or for proper use of equipment including personal protective equipment. The latter may result in transfer of organisms between animal colonies, such as if personnel do not change gloves between handling animals from both colonies. Alternatively, personnel may directly transmit organisms to animals, such as transfer of the normal bacterial flora of human skin (e.g., *Staphylococcus aureus*) to severely immunocompromised animals. In addition, personnel have the potential of inadvertently transmitting infectious agents acquired through contact with animal populations maintained outside of the research environment. As a result, some institutions prohibit their personnel from interacting with select groups of animals outside of work. For instance, commercial rodent vendors may prohibit personnel from interacting with pet rodents; personnel who work with dog colonies may be prohibited from interaction with any unvaccinated dogs or young puppies. Personnel must recognize the importance of preventing the movement and transmission of potential contaminants within a facility and understand the processes they must follow to achieve it.

Prevention is the key! Research animals should be of the healthiest status possible and come from vendors that monitor and ensure their microbial and genetic status. Attention should be given to potential sources and means of transmission of adventitious infectious agents. Minimizing risk factors will protect animal health and safeguard experimental outcomes.

ANIMAL COLONY HEALTH SURVEILLANCE

Every effort should be made to exclude adventitious agents from research animal colonies as their presence can negatively affect animal (and possibly human) health and introduce unwanted experimental variables in biomedical research. Each institution must determine the list of agents (e.g., bacteria, viruses, fungi, and parasites) to be excluded from their facility. Factors to consider when determining this list include animal species and populations, research requirements (e.g., need for adenovirus-naïve animals for study involving adenoviral vector administration), and the potential for an agent to affect research results.

Agent exclusion requires that animals transferred into an existing colony be free of infection with excluded agents. In addition, colony animals should be periodically assessed for evidence of infection with excluded agents so that affected animals are identified and the agent contained or eradicated from the colony.

A well-trained staff, capable of recognizing signs of illness, is an important component of these efforts. Unfortunately, many excluded agents induce no or only nonspecific clinical signs. Animals exhibiting signs of illness as well as observed changes in animal production (e.g., percentage of successful matings, litter size, and body weight) or behavior should be evaluated for possible infectious causes. When animals exhibiting clinical signs are observed, it is often prudent to examine both clinically affected animals and asymptomatic animals of differing ages as disease may manifest differently in these animals.

Without prompt detection, some agents may quickly spread within and between animal colonies and/or introduce uncontrolled experimental variability, thereby invalidating research results. Therefore, a formal animal health surveillance program should be instituted to periodically assess the health of colony animals. An example list of excluded agents and testing frequencies for an academic rodent colony maintained in IVC housing is provided in Table 15.1.

In general, two methods are most frequently used for colony health monitoring: testing of animal-derived samples (e.g., blood, feces, or fur) and testing of animal environments.

Testing of Animal-Derived Samples

The selection of animals whose health accurately reflects the colony's health is key to the success of this surveillance method. This is especially noteworthy as most modern

Table 15.1. Example of colony health testing frequencies for agents excluded from an academic institution's barrier rodent colony housed in individually ventilated caging

Pathogen	Testing Frequency
Minute Virus of Mice (MVM)	Every 4 mo
Mouse Hepatitis Virus (MHV)	
Mouse Parvo Virus (MPV)	
Murine Rotavirus (MRV/EDIM)	
Pinworms (*Syphacia obvelata*, *Aspiculuris tetraptera*)	
Fur mites (*Myobia musculi*, *Radfordia affinis*, and *Myocoptes musculinus*)	
Mycoplasma pulmonis	Annually
Ectromelia Virus	
Lymphocytic choriomeningitis virus (LCMV)	
Mouse Adenovirus-1, Mouse Adenovirus-2 (MAV 1 & 2)	
Murine Cytomegalovirus (MCMV)	
Pneumonia Virus of Mice (PVM)	
Reovirus (Reo3)	
Sendai virus	
Theiler's Murine Encephalomyelitis Virus (TMEV)	

husbandry practices and housing systems are designed to segregate cages or subsets of animals from the larger colony both to prevent transmission of adventitious agents and to isolate experimental groups. The number of animals to be tested should be based on the estimated prevalence of an agent within a colony, the sensitivity of the diagnostic method, and the level of certainty desired of the testing results.

Animals selected for testing must be compatible with the diagnostic testing systems employed. For example, the use of diagnostic tests that detect an immunologic response to infection requires that the animals tested be capable of mounting a detectable immune response. Animals with spontaneous or purposeful genetic mutations may not be suitable as they may be fully or partially immunodeficient. Young and aged animals may produce only muted immune responses. In addition, diagnostic samples must be collected within the period of time an animal would mount an immune response to infection, not before a significant response could develop or after a response has subsided. Testing methods that specifically detect an infectious organism and do not require the presence of an immune response may also be employed, and can be especially useful with immunodeficient animals.

In some situations, selection of existing colony animals (e.g., breeders, offspring, or experimental animals) for testing may be appropriate. However, this is rarely possible in large rodent colonies as sufficient quantities or ages of animals may not be available and their use may negatively impact research goals. Furthermore, they may have minimal-to-no exposure to animals outside of their own cage/housing enclosure or isolated experimental group and therefore not be representative of the whole colony.

Specially purposed animal sentinels are most commonly used to monitor the health status of rodent colonies. Sentinel animals should be free of all excluded agents for the area they are used to monitor. They are most commonly obtained from an external source, such as a commercial vendor, immediately prior to use. Use of colony-derived animals as sentinels can be acceptable, but is infrequently done due to the severe consequences that would occur if they were unknowingly infected with an agent prior to their distribution throughout a facility. Most institutions purchase young (approximately 3–5 weeks of age), outbred, female sentinel animals as young outbred animals may have the most pronounced immunologic response and are less expensive than inbred strains. However, different aged animals may be necessary for transmission and detection of some agents. Females are less prone to fighting and can be easily identified if unintended breeding occurred with colony animals. After being distributed within the facility, sentinels are exposed to colony animals in some way and then sampled. Multiple methods of colony exposure can be employed. Methods infrequently used include cohousing or housing animals in open-topped cages (i.e., static cages without microisolation filter tops) positioned in close proximity to similarly housed colony animals. More commonly, sentinel animals are exposed to the colony through systematic transfer of soiled bedding material (5–15 mL) from colony animal cages to the sentinel's cage at the time of each cage change. Although many infections are transmitted most efficiently through animal-to-animal contact, the transfer of soiled bedding material to sentinel cages can be effective with agents normally transmitted by the fecal–oral route. Organisms predominantly transmitted by aerosols and some ectoparasites are rarely transmitted to sentinels through soiled bedding transfer.

In an attempt to improve agent detection (especially agents transmitted by aerosol) and to decrease the labor required for soiled bedding transfers, methods have been developed to expose sentinels to the air exhausted from colony animal cages on individually ventilated rodent racks. This method has not been widely adopted, largely due to the questionable efficiency of agent transmission to the sentinel animals, the need for costly modification of ventilated caging racks to divert air to the sentinel cage(s), and the continued requirement of live animal sentinels.

Rodent sentinels require approximately 7–14 days to develop an antibody response following exposure to an infectious agent. Therefore, when sentinels are assessed through serologic testing for antibodies, sampling should occur 2–3 weeks after the last exposure to soiled bedding, although seroconversion to some agents, such as mouse norovirus, can take 8 weeks or longer. Sentinels should not be kept longer than 3–6 months as the sensitivity to agents such as mouse parvovirus decreases with age.

Following exposure to colony animals, premortem and/or postmortem samples are taken from sentinel animals and tested. Numerous diagnostic methods may be used including serology; molecular-based testing (e.g., PCR); gross and histopathological examination; parasitological exams including pelage and skin exams, direct examination of the gastrointestinal tract, fecal floatation, and perianal adhesive tape tests; and microbiological culture and identification.

Serologic testing using either serum or plasma is a common means of assessing rodent colony sentinels. It provides an indirect measure of past exposure to an infectious agent and is most useful for viral and mycoplasmal infections. Serologic tests are generally sensitive and specific, and allow for screening of multiple infectious agents with one sample. Both antibody and antigen assays are available for serologic testing. As antibody assays determine whether the serum sample contains antibodies to a particular infectious agent, they are considered an indirect test. Animals used for indirect serologic monitoring must be immunocompetent, allowed adequate time to seroconvert, and of an appropriate age to be capable of an acceptable immune response. Antibody assay methods include the microbead-based assay, enzyme-linked immunosorbent assay (ELISA), and indirect immunofluoresence assay (IFA). Microbead assays are most commonly used because they are extremely sensitive, require a minute sample size, and allow for high throughput volume. Beads are coated with a purified antigen, such as from a virus or a bacterium that will react with its specific antibody, if present in the sample. This testing involves a multiplex format, where beads are used to detect multiple agents and/or strains of a single agent, and use of multiple controls for accuracy. ELISAs are used if no microbead assay is available for the agent or as a confirmatory test, while IFAs are employed for parasitology, some bacteria, and also as confirmation of other test results. Serologic antibody testing, however, can fail to identify an animal with an acute illness and does not provide information about the current infection status of an animal.

Polymerase chain reaction assays directly test for the presence of nucleic acids from an infectious agent. PCR detects DNA, and reverse transcriptase PCR (PCR-RT) detects RNA. Fecal pellets, tissue, skin, fur and lung swabs, saliva, buccal swabs, and serum can be used as the test sample. PCR assays are extremely sensitive and are available for most prevalent rodent viruses. These assays are excellent tests to detect current infection in immunodeficient animals that are incapable of mounting an immune response and recently received animals (e.g., in quarantine) without sufficient time to mount an immune response to an agent exposure during the shipping process. PCR can be used to identify a particular serotype of virus, such as parvovirus, and is also useful for agents that persist in tissues such as lymph nodes and biological materials. Samples can be pooled from across multiple animals and assays can be performed quickly in automated systems with low frequencies of error.

Microbiologic monitoring involves inoculating agar and/or broth with animal or environmental samples. The nasopharynx and cecum are routinely used in monitoring rodents for bacterial pathogens.

Testing of Animal Environments

Over the past decade, significant advances have been made in detecting the presence of adventitious agents within the animal's environment. Most methods utilize PCR technology to identify the distinctive genetic composition of agents. Early testing methods involved personnel manually sampling individual items, such as rodent cage interiors, and has since evolved to more refined systems such as specially designed filters mounted within exhaust air ducts of rodent individually ventilated cage (IVC) racks. Such systems allow simultaneous sampling of all animals housed on the rack without effort by animal care personnel aside from the placement and removal of the filters. Once removed, filter material is tested by PCR for excluded agents. Detection of genetic material suggests that one or more animals housed on the rack since the rack was last sanitized had been exposed to, and likely infected with, that agent. It should be recalled that genetic material can be recovered and identified from nonviable (and therefore noninfectious) organisms. False-positive results can result if genetic material persists within rack air ducts and racks are not sufficiently cleaned between successive filter placements. Confirmatory testing, such as direct testing of animal-derived samples or PCR evaluation of individual cages, is required when an excluded agent is detected on IVC air exhaust filters.

One of the greatest advantages of environmental testing is elimination or at least significant reduction in the number of sentinel animals required (Box 15.5). This is a significant advance in one of the 3R's of animal experimentation: reduction of animal use.

There are advantages and disadvantages both of testing animal-derived samples and testing animal environments. Often, facilities employ each to some extent. Regardless of the method(s) used, the frequency of testing must be determined and will be influenced by the source and frequency of animals transferred into the colony, housing methods within the facility, and the level of personnel compliance with facility biosecurity practices. As testing can be costly, it is best to prioritize a list of agents for monitoring based on the prevalence and potential animal or human health impact.

Box 15.5

The number of sentinel animals used for animal colony health surveillance can be significantly reduced through strategic use of environmental testing.

The impact of specific pathogens to ongoing research must also be considered. In conventional rodent facilities, monitoring is usually done on a quarterly or semiannual basis. Established protocols should be followed when collecting and processing samples for testing to minimize errors and sample contamination.

No diagnostic test is completely accurate and precise. Unexpected or unusual test results should always be confirmed by an alternative test; test results should be interpreted using scientific and professional judgment. Most diagnostic laboratories provide their customers access to experts who can provide guidance on the interpretation of and response to test results. Table 15.2 provides a partial listing of commercial comprehensive animal diagnostic laboratories. Table 15.3 presents a partial listing of laboratories that perform nonhuman primate diagnostic testing, while Table 15.4 presents the same for zebrafish. The information provided is strictly a point of reference and in no way indicates author preferences. Other diagnostic laboratories may be available in your area.

Table 15.2. Rodent comprehensive diagnostic testing laboratories

Company Contact Information	Comments
Charles River Laboratories 251 Ballardvale St. Wilmington, MA 01887 Phone: 781-222-6000 http://www.criver.com	Comprehensive health monitoring, serology, genetic testing, pathology services, environmental testing, and serology reagents and test kits
Envigo 8520 Allison Pointe Blvd., Suite 400 Indianapolis, IN 46250 Phone: 800-793-7287 https://insights.envigo.com	Comprehensive health monitoring, serology, genetic testing, and pathology services
Taconic Biosciences 1 Discovery Drive, Suite 304 Rensselaer, NY 12144 Phone: (518) 697-3900 http://www.taconic.com	Comprehensive health monitoring, serology, genetic testing, and pathology services
IDEXX BioAnalytics Research Animal Diagnostic Laboratory 4011 Discovery Drive Columbia, MO 65201 Phone: 800-554-5205, option 1 http://www.idexxbioanalytics.com	Comprehensive health monitoring, serology, genetic testing, and pathology services
VRL Laboratories P.O. Box 40100 7540 Louis Pasteur, Suite 200 San Antonio, TX 78229 Phone: 877-615-7275 http://www.vrlsat.com	Comprehensive health monitoring, serology, clinical pathology, environmental testing, microbiology, molecular biology assays, and pathology services

Table 15.3. Nonhuman primate diagnostic testing laboratories

Company	Comments
Charles River Laboratories 251 Ballardvale St. Wilmington, MA 01887 Phone: 781-222-6000 http://www.criver.com	Comprehensive health monitoring, serology, microbiology, and histopathology services
National B Virus Resource Center Viral Immunology Center Georgia State University 161 Jesse Hill Jr. Drive Atlanta, GA 30303 Phone: 404-413-6550 bvirus@gsu.edu	B-virus screens for nonhuman primates and humans
Primate Assay Laboratory Core California National Primate Research Center University of California, Davis One Shields Avenue Davis, CA 95616-8542 Phone: 530-752-0447 https://cnprc.ucdavis.edu/primate-assay-laboratory-core	Comprehensive diagnostic testing, serology, virus assays, hormone analysis, clinical pathology, and pathology services
VRL Laboratories P.O. Box 40100 7540 Louis Pasteur, Suite 200 San Antonio, TX 78229 Phone: 877-615-7275 http://www.vrlsat.com	Comprehensive health monitoring, clinical pathology, microbiology, and molecular biology assays

Table 15.4. Zebrafish diagnostic testing laboratories

Company	Comments
Charles River Laboratories 251 Ballardvale St. Wilmington, MA 01887 Phone: 781-222-6000 http://www.criver.com	Comprehensive health monitoring, bacteriology, histopathology, and molecular biology assays
IDEXX BioAnalytics Research Animal Diagnostic Laboratory 4011 Discovery Drive Columbia, MO 65201 Phone: 800-554-5205, option 1 http://www.idexxbioanalytics.com	Comprehensive health monitoring, bacteriology, histopathology, and molecular biology assays
Zebrafish International Resource Center Health Services 1307 Franklin Blvd. 5274 University of Oregon, Eugene, Oregon 97403-5274 (541) 346-6028, ext. 14 https://zebrafish.org/health/index.php	Histopathology, bacteriology, necropsy, and molecular biology assays

BIBLIOGRAPHY

Baker, D.G., and N. S. Lipman. 2015. Factors that can influence animal research. In *Laboratory Animal Medicine*, 3rd ed., J. G. Fox, L. C. Anderson, G. M. Otto, K. R. Pritchett-Corning, and M. T. Whary (eds.), pp. 1441–1495. San Diego, CA: Academic Press.

Bauer B. A., C. Besch-Williford, R. S. Livingston, et al. 2016. Influence of rack design and disease prevalence on detection of rodent pathogens in exhaust debris samples from individually ventilated caging systems. *JAALAS* 55(6):782–788.

de Bruin W. C., E. M. van de Ven, and C. R. Hooijmans. 2016. Efficacy of soiled bedding transfer for transmission of mouse and rat infections to sentinels: A systematic review. *PLoS One* 11(8):e0158410.

Cicero, T. J., B. Nock, and E. R. Meyer. 1996. Gender differences in the antinociceptive properties of morphine. *J Pharmacol Exp Ther* 279: 767–773.

Compton, S. R., F. R. Homberger, F. X. Paturzo, and J. MacArthur Clark. 2004. Efficacy of three microbiological monitoring methods in a ventilated cage rack. *Comp Med* 54(4): 382–392.

Crim M. J., C. Lawrence, R. S. Livingston, et al. 2017. Comparison of antemortem and environmental samples for zebrafish health monitoring and quarantine. *JAALAS* 56(4):412–424.

Institute of Laboratory Animal Resources (ILAR). 1991a. *Companion Guide to Infectious Diseases of Mice and Rats*. Committee on Infectious Diseases of Mice and Rats, ILAR, Commission on Life Sciences, National Research Council. Washington, DC: National Academies Press.

Institute of Laboratory Animal Resources (ILAR). 1991b. *Infectious Diseases of Mice and Rats*. Committee on Infectious Diseases of Mice and Rats, ILAR, Commission on Life Sciences, National Research Council. Washington, DC: National Academies Press.

Institute of Laboratory Animal Resources (ILAR). 2011. *Guide for the Care and Use of Laboratory Animals*, 8th ed. ILAR, National Research Council. Washington, DC: National Academies Press.

Pritchett-Corning, K. R., J. Cosentino, and C. B. Clifford. 2009. Contemporary prevalence of infectious agents in laboratory mice and rats. *Lab Anim* 43: 165–173.

FURTHER READING

Bailoo J.D., T. S. Reichlin, and H. Würbel. 2014. Refinement of experimental design and conduct in laboratory animal research. *ILAR J* 55(3):383–91.

Charles River. 2011. *Guidebook on Mouse and Rat Colony Management*. Wilmington, MA: Charles River Laboratories. Available at https://www.criver.com/resources/charles-river-guidebook-series [accessed December 30, 2018].

Charles River. 2011. *International genetic standardization (IGS) program technical sheet*. Available at www.crj.co.jp/cms/cmsrs/pdf/company/rm_rm_r_igs.pdf [accessed December 27, 2018].

Charles River. 2014. *A Guide to Modern Strategies for Infection Surveillance of Rodent Populations: Beyond Sentinels*. Wilmington, MA: Charles River Laboratories.

Available at https://www.criver.com/resources/charles-river-guidebook-series [accessed December 30, 2018].

Jackson S. J., N. Andrews, D. Ball, et al. 2017. Does age matter? The impact of rodent age on study outcomes. *Lab Anim* 51(2):160–169.

Marx, J. O., D. J. Gaertner, and A. L. Smith. 2017. Results of survey regarding prevalence of adventitial infections in mice and rats at biomedical research facilities. *JAALAS* 56(5):527–533.

Miller M., and M. Brielmeier. 2018. Environmental samples make soiled bedding sentinels dispensable for hygienic monitoring of IVC-reared mouse colonies. *Lab Anim* 52(3):233–239.

Pritchett-Corning K. R., J. B. Prins, R. Feinstein, et al. 2014. AALAS/FELASA working group on health monitoring of rodents for animal transfer. *JAALAS* 53(6):633–40.

Shek, W. R., A. L. Smith, and K. R. Pritchett-Corning. 2015. Microbiological quality control for laboratory rodents and lagomorphs. In *Laboratory Animal Medicine*, 3rd ed., J. G. Fox, L. C. Anderson, G. M. Otto, K. R. Pritchett-Corning, and M. T. Whary (eds.), pp. 463–510. San Diego, CA: Academic Press.

Strobel, M. C., L. G. Reinholdt, R. D. Malcolm, and K. Pritchett-Corning. 2015. Genetic monitoring of laboratory mice and rats. In *Laboratory Animal Medicine*, 3rd ed., J. G. Fox, L. C. Anderson, G. M. Otto, K. R. Pritchett-Corning, and M. T. Whary (eds.), pp. 1403–1416. San Diego, CA: Academic Press.

CHAPTER 15 REVIEW

Fill in the Blank

Each of the following is a factor that may induce research variables. Indicate if each is an example of an extrinsic factor (E) or an intrinsic factor (I).

1. ____ Immunodeficiency
2. ____ Age
3. ____ Diet
4. ____ Room temperature
5. ____ IVC housing system
6. ____ Female or male
7. ____ Inbred strain
8. ____ Cage density
9. ____ Mouse hepatitis virus
10. ____ Vibrations

Multiple Choice

11. Chemicals that are foreign to a biological system are
    A. probiotics.
    B. xenobiotics.
    C. antibiotics.
    D. radiobiotics.
12. Adventitious agents, by definition,
    A. are the aggregation of microorganisms that live on or within an animal.
    B. cause a latent or subclinical infection with no overt clinical signs of illness.
    C. are organisms that are unintentionally introduced into animals or their environment.
    D. are inanimate objects or substances that can carry an infectious organism or a contaminant.
13. One means of vertical transmission of a pathogen is
    A. by a fomite.
    B. through fecal–oral transmission.
    C. from mother to offspring in utero.
    D. by direct contact with another animal.
14. A RODAC plate is used to
    A. irradiate rodent chow.
    B. filter drinking water.
    C. assess the effectiveness of sanitation.
    D. count pinworm larvae.
15. Each of the following may serve as a fomite *except*
    A. personal protective equipment.
    B. caging.
    C. environmental enrichment.
    D. high-intensity lighting.
16. Which of the following is *not* a component of an integrated pest management program?
    A. methods to prevent intrusion of insects into animal facilities
    B. methods to detect wild rodents' attempts to enter a facility
    C. eradication of insects within a facility
    D. recapture of research mice that have escaped from their cages
17. Produced to maintain heterogeneity:
    A. transgenic
    B. outbred stocks
    C. nude
    D. inbred strains
18. After shipping, rodents should be allowed an acclimation period of what minimum duration prior to their use in a research protocol?
    A. 12 hours
    B. 24 hours
    C. 48 hours
    D. an amount that reflects the unique needs of both the animal subjects and the research project

(*Continued*)

19. Common water treatment methods include
    A. filtration.
    B. gamma irradiation.
    C. iodine supplementation.
    D. centrifugation.
20. When used for colony health monitoring, polymerase chain reaction (PCR) assays
    A. directly test for antibodies produced by infected animals.
    B. are useful in detecting current infections in immunodeficient animals.
    C. are not suitable in the evaluation of tissue samples.
    D. have low sensitivity.

Critical Thinking

21. A researcher has received a grant to study the microbiome of wild mice. She explains that, pending IACUC approval of her submitted animal use protocol, she wishes to capture wild mice from a nearby field and house them in your institution's rodent facility. What additional information do you want and how will you acquire it? What, if any, diagnostic testing would you want to perform on the captured animals? How and where would you house them? What other precautions or disease surveillance activities do you wish to pursue?

Appendix 1 Normal Values

Tables A.1–A.4 provide "normal" hematologic and biochemical data for each species covered in the text. The values should be used as guidelines, for there are many inherent variables in reporting such data. Sample collection method; the breed, strain, or stock; health status; age; sex; environment; and analytic techniques are but a few of the many variables that can affect specific clinical laboratory values.

Table A.1. Hematologic data: erythrocytes and platelets

Species	RBC ($10^6/\mu L$)	PCV (%)	Hb (g/dL)	Platelets ($10^3/mL$)
Mouse[a]	7.0–12.5	39–49	10.2–16.6	800–1100
Rat[a]	7–10	36–48	11–18	500–1300
Gerbil[a]	8–9	43–49	12.6–16.2	400–600
Hamster[a]	6–10	36–55	10–16	200–500
Guinea pig[a]	4.5–7	37–48	11–15	250–850
Chinchilla[b]	3.8	37	13.1	—
Rabbit[a]	4–7.2	36–48	10–15.5	200–1000
Ferret[c]	6.8–12.2	42–61	15–18	297–910
Rhesus macaque[d]	4.5–6	39–43	12.7	130–144
Squirrel monkey[d]	7.1–10.9	43–56	12.9–17.0	112

Hb = hemoglobin; PCV = packed cell volume; and RBC = red blood cells.

[a] From Harkness and Wagner (1995).

[b] Adapted from de Oliveira Silva et al. (2005).

[c] From Bernard et al. (1984).

[d] From Johnson-Delaney (1994).

Clinical Laboratory Animal Medicine: An Introduction, Fifth Edition.
Lesley A. Colby, Megan H. Nowland, and Lucy H. Kennedy.

Companion website: www.wiley.com/go/colby/clinical

Table A.2. Hematologic data: leukocytes

Species	WBC (10^3/L)	Neutrophils (%)	Lymphocytes (%)	Monocytes (%)	Eosinophils (%)	Basophils (%)
Mouse[a]	6–15	10–40	55–95	0.1–3.5	0–4	0–0.3
Rat[a]	6–17	9–34	65–85	0–5	0–6	0–1.5
Gerbil[a]	7–15	5–34	60–95	0–3	0–4	0–1
Hamster[a]	3–11	10–42	50–95	0–3	0–4.5	0–1
Guinea pig[a]	7–18	28–44	39–72	3–12	1–5	0–3
Chinchilla[b]	5.2	40	35	11.5	5.8	5.3
Rabbit[a]	7.5–13.5	20–35	55–80	1–4	0–4	2–10
Ferret[c]	4–19	11–84	12–54	0–9	0–7	0–2
Rhesus macaque[d]	11.5–12.4	20–56	40–76	0–2	1–3	0–1
Squirrel monkey[d]	5.1–10.9	36–66	27–55	0–6	0–11	<1

WBC = white blood cells.

[a] From Harkness and Wagner (1995).

[b] Adapted from de Oliveira Silva et al. (2005).

[c] From Bernard et al. (1984).

[d] From Johnson-Delaney (1994).

Table A.3. Serum biochemical data

Species	BUN (mg/dL)	Creatinine (mg/dL)	Glucose (mg/dL)	ALT (IU/L)	AST (IU/L)	AP (IU/L)	Total bilirubin (mg/dL)	Cholesterol (mg/dL)
Mouse[a, b]	12–28	0.3–1	62–175	26–77	54–269	45–222	0.1–0.9	26–82
Rat[a–c]	15–21	0.2–0.8	50–135	16–89	192–262	16–125	0.2–0.55	40–130
Gerbil[a, d]	17–27	0.6–1.4	50–135	—	—	12–37	0.2–0.6	90–150
Hamster[a, b]	12–25	0.91–0.99	60–150	22–128	28–122	45–187	0.25–0.6	25–135
Guinea pig[a–c]	9–31.5	0.6–2.2	60–125	10–25	45.5–48.2	18–28	0.3–0.9	20–43
Chinchilla[b, e]	10–25	0.4–1.3	60–120	10–35	96	3–47	0.6–1.28	40–100
Rabbit[a, e]	15–23.5	0.8–1.8	75–150	14–80	14–113	4–16	0.25–0.74	35–60
Ferret[f]	12–43	0.2–0.6	62.5–134	78–149	57–165	30–120	0–0.1	119–209
Rhesus macaque[e, g]	14.2–19.6	0.1–2.8	53–87	145–171	20–34	—	0.1–0.66	94–162
Squirrel monkey[e]	23–39	—	52–108	59–99	56–118	—	0.1–0.53	127–207

ALT = alanine transferase; AST = aspartate transferase; AP = alkaline phosphate; and BUN = blood urea nitrogen.

[a] From Harkness and Wagner (1995).

[b] From Anderson (1994).

[c] Adapted from Loeb and Quimby (1989).

[d] From Canadian Council on Animal Care (1980).

[e] From Carpenter et al. (1996).

[f] Adapted from Fox et al. (1986) and Lee et al. (1982).

[g] From McClure (1975).

Table A.4. Serum biochemical data

Species	Protein (g/dL)	Albumin (g/dL)	Globulin (g/dL)	Calcium (mg/dL)	Phosphorus (mg/dL)	Sodium (mEq/L)	Potassium (mEq/L)	Chloride (mEq/L)
Mouse[a, b]	3.5–7.2	2.5–4.8	0.6	3.2–8.5	2.3–9.2	112–193	5.1–10.4	82–114
Rat[a–c]	5.6–7.6	3.8–4.8	1.8–3	5.3–13	5.3–8.3	135–155	4–8	94–116.3
Gerbil[a, b, d]	4.3–12.5	1.8–5.5	1.2–6	3.7–6.2	3.7–7	144–158	3.8–5.2	93–118
Hamster[a, b, e]	4.5–7.5	2.6–4.1	2.7–4.2	5–12	3.4–8.2	128–144	3.9–5.5	93–98
Guinea pig[a, b]	4.6–6.2	2.1–3.9	1.7–2.6	5.3–12	3–12	132–156	4.5–8.9	98–115
Chinchilla[f, g]	3.8–5.6	2.3–4.1	0.9–2.2	5.6–12.1	4–8	130–155	5–6.5	105–115
Rabbit[a, h]	2.8–10	2.7–4.6	1.5–2.8	5.6–12.5	2.7–7.3	131–155	3.6–6.9	92–112
Ferret[i]	5.3–7.2	3.3–4.1	1.8–3.1	8.6–10.5	5.6–8.7	146–160	4.3–5.3	102–121
Rhesus monkey[j]	4.9–9.3	2.8–5.2	1.2–5.8	6.9–13	3.1–7.1	102–166	2.3–6.7	84–126
Squirrel monkey[k]	6.6–7.8	3.5–4.5	2.6–3.6	9.5–10.5	3.2–6.6	143.1–152.9	3.6–5.4	107.6–118.4

[a] From Harkness and Wagner (1995).

[b] From Anderson (1994).

[c] Ringler and Dabich (1979).

[d] From Canadian Council on Animal Care (1980).

[e] Mitruka and Rawnsley (1977).

[f] Adapted from Merry (1990).

[g] From Carpenter et al. (1996).

[h] From Quesenberry (1994).

[i] Adapted from Fox et al. (1986) and Lee et al. (1982).

[j] McClure (1975).

[k] Adapted from Manning et al. (1969).

BIBLIOGRAPHY

Anderson, N. J. 1994. Basic husbandry and medicine of pocket pets. In *Saunders Manual of Small Animal Practice*, S. J. Birchard and R. G. Sherding (eds.), pp. 1368–1369. Philadelphia: WB Saunders.

Bernard, S. L., J. R. Gorham, and L. M. Ryland. 1984. Biology and diseases of ferrets. In *Laboratory Animal Medicine*, J. G. Fox, B. J. Cohen, and F. M. Loew (Eds.), pp. 387. New York: Academic.

Canadian Council on Animal Care (CCAC). 1980. *Guide to the Care and Use of Experimental Animals*, Volume 1, p. 87. Ottawa, Ontario: Canadian Council on Animal Care.

Carpenter, J. W., T. Y. Mashima, and D. J. Rupiper. 1996. *Exotic Animal Formulary*, pp. 204, 225, 243, 278. Manhattan, KS: Greystone.

Fox, J. G., L. Hotaling, B. O. Ackerman, and K. Hewes. 1986. Serum chemistry and hematology reference values in the ferret (Mustela putorius furo). *Lab Anim Sci* 36: 583.

Harkness, J. E. and J. E. Wagner. 1995. *The Biology and Medicine of Rabbits and Rodents*, 4th ed. Philadelphia: Williams & Wilkins.

Johnson-Delaney, C. A. 1994. Primates. *Vet Clin North Am Small Anim Pract* 24: 121–156.

Lee, E. J., W. E. Moore, H. C. Fryer, et al. 1982. Haematological and serum chemistry profiles of ferrets (Mustela putorius furo). *Lab Anim* 16: 133.

Loeb, W., and F. Quimby. 1989. *The Clinical Chemistry of Laboratory Animals*, pp. 429–431. Elmsford, NY: Pergamon.

Manning, P. J., N. D. M. Lehner, M. A. Feldner, and B. C. Bullock. 1969. Selected hematologic, serum chemical, and arterial blood gas characteristics of squirrel monkeys (Saimiri sciureus). *Lab Anim Sci* 19: 831–837.

Mayer, J., R. P. Marini, and J. G. Fox. 2015. Biology and diseases of ferrets. In *Laboratory Animal Medicine*, 3rd ed., J. G. Fox, L. C. Anderson, G. Otto, K. R. Pritchett-Corning, M. T. Whary (eds.), pp. 577–616. San Diego, CA: Elsevier.

McClure, H. M. 1975. Hematologic, blood chemistry and cerebrospinal fluid data for the rhesus monkey. In *The Rhesus Monkey*, Volume 2, G. H. Bourne (ed.), pp. 409–429. New York: Academic.

Merry, C. J. 1990. An introduction to chinchillas. *Vet Tech* 11(5): 315–321.

Mitruka, B. M. and H. M. Rawnsley. 1977. *Clinical Biochemical and Hematological Reference Values in Normal Experimental Animals*. New York: Mason.

de Oliveira Silva, T., L. C. Kruetz, L. J. G. Barcellos, et al. 2005. Reference values for chinchilla (*Chinchilla laniger*) blood cells and serum biochemical parameters. *Ciencia Rural Santa Maria* 35(3): 602–606.

Quesenberry, K. E. 1994. Rabbits. In *Saunders Manual of Small Animal Practice*, S. J. Birchard and R. G. Sherding (eds.), p. 1346. Philadelphia: WB Saunders.

Ringler, D. H., and L. Dabich. 1979. Hematology and clinical biochemistry. In *The Laboratory Rat, Volume I, Biology and Diseases*, H. J. Baker, J. R. Lindsey, and S. H. Weisbroth (eds.), pp. 105–121. New York: Academic.

Appendix 2 Comparative Biologic and Reproductive Values by Species

BIBLIOGRAPHY

Bennett, B. T., C. R. Abee, and R. Henrickson (eds). 1995. *Nonhuman Primates in Biomedical Research*. San Diego, CA: Academic Press.

Fox, J. G. 1998. *Biology and Diseases of the Ferret*. Baltimore, MD: Williams and Wilkins.

Harkness, J. E. and J. E. Wagner. 1995. *Biology and Medicine of Rabbits and Rodents*, 4th ed. Media, PA: Williams and Wilkins.

Harkness, J. E., P. V. Turner, S. VandeWoude, and C. L. Wheler. 2010. *Harkness and Wagner's Biology and Medicine of Rabbits and Rodents*, 5th ed. Ames, IA: Wiley-Blackwell.

Johnson-Delaney, C. A. 1994. Primates. *Vet Clin North Am Small Anim Pract* 24(1): 121–156.

Mulder, G. B. 2012. Management, husbandry, and colony health. In *The Laboratory Rabbit, Guinea Pig, Hamster, and Other Rodents*, M. A. Suckow, K. A. Stevens, and R. P. Wilson (eds.), pp. 765–777. San Diego, CA: Academic Press.

Quesenberry, K. E. and J. W. Carpenter. 2004. *Ferrets, Rabbits, and Rodents: Clinical Medicine and Surgery*. St. Louis, MO: WB Saunders.

Clinical Laboratory Animal Medicine: An Introduction, Fifth Edition.
Lesley A. Colby, Megan H. Nowland, and Lucy H. Kennedy.

Companion website: www.wiley.com/go/colby/clinical

Table B.1. Comparative biologic and reproductive values by species

	Mouse	Rat	Gerbil	Syrian Hamster	Guinea Pig	Chinchilla	Rabbit	Ferret	Rhesus Macaque	Cynomolgus Macaque	Baboon	Squirrel Monkey
Adult body weight: Male	20–40 g	450–520 g	80–130 g	85–130 g	900–1200 g	400–500 g	2–5 kg	1–2 kg	6–11 kg	6 kg	22–30 kg	700–1100 g
Adult body weight: Female	25–40 g	250–300 g	55–85 g	95–150 g	700–900 g	400–600 g	2–6 kg	600–950 g	4–9 kg	4 kg	11–15 kg	500–1000 g
Life span	1.5–3 y	2.5–3.5 y	3–4 y	18–24 mo	5–7 y	9–18 y	5–6 y or more	5–11 y	30+ y	37 y	40–45 y	20 y
Body temperature	36.5°–38°C (97.7°–100.4°F)	35.9°–37.5°C (96.6°–99.5°F)	37°–38.5°C (98.6°–101.°F)	37°–38°C (98.6°–100.4°F)	37.2°–39.5°C (99°–103.1°F)	37°–38°C (98.6°–100.4°F)	38.5°–40°C (101.3°–104°F)	37.8°–40°C (100°–104°F)	36°–40°C (96.8°–104°F)	36°–38°C (96.8°–100.4°F)	36°–39°C (96.8°–102.2°F)	33.5°–38.8 °C (92.3°–101.8 °F)
Heart rate (beats per minute)	325–780	250–450	360	250–500	230–380	100–150	130–325	200–400	150–333	107–215	80–200	225–350
Respiratory rate (breaths per minute)	60–220	70–115	90	35–135	40–130	40–80	30–60	33–36	10–25	32–44	29	20–50
Tidal volume	0.09–0.23 mL	0.6–2 mL		0.6–1.4 mL	2.3–5.3 mL/kg		4-6 mL/kg					
Food consumption (per day)	12–18 g/100 g	5–6 g/100 g	5–8 g/100 g	8–12 g/100 g	6 g/100 g	30–40 g/d; 5.5 g/100 g	5 g/100 g	140–190 g/d (semimoist diet)				
Water consumption (per day)	1 mL/100 g	10–12 mL/100 g	4–7 mL/100 g	Male, 4.5–5 mL/100 g; female, 13.6–14 mL/100 g	10 mL/100 g	10–20 mL/d; 8–9 mL/100 g	5–12 mL/100 g	75–100 mL				

(Continued)

Table B.1 (Continued)

	Mouse	Rat	Gerbil	Syrian Hamster	Guinea Pig	Chinchilla	Rabbit	Ferret	Rhesus Macaque	Cynomolgus Macaque	Baboon	Squirrel Monkey
Breeding onset: Male	50 d	65–110 d	70–85 d	10–14 wk	3–4 mo (600–700 g)	7–9 mo	6–10 mo	8–12 mo	38 mo	42–60 mo	73 mo	60 mo
Breeding onset: Female	50–60 d	65–110 d	65–85 d	6–10 wk	2–3 mo (350–450 g)	4–5 mo	4–9 mo	7–10 mo	34–43 mo	46 mo	51–73 mo	36–46 mo
Estrous cycle length	4–5 d	4–5 d	4–6 d	4 d	15–17 d	30–50 d	Induced ovulator	Continuous until intromission	28 d	28 d	31–36 d	18 d
Gestation period	19–21 d	21–23 d	24–26 d	15–16 d	59–72 d	105–120 d	29–35 d	42 + 2 d	167 d	162 d	175–180 d	170 d
Postpartum estrus	Fertile	Fertile	Fertile	Infertile	Fertile	Fertile	48 h	Occasional				
Litter size	6–12	6–12	3–7	5–9	1–6	1–6	4–10	8, avg. (1–18 range)				
Weaning age	21–28 d	21 d	20–26 d	20–25 d	14–21 d	6–8 wk	4–6 wk	6–8 wk	210–425 d	365–547 d	180–456 d	182 d
Breeding duration	7–9 mo	350–440 d	12–17 mo	10–12 mo	18–48 mo	3 y	1–3 y	2–5 y				
Chromosome number (diploid)	40	42	44	44	64	64	44	40	42	42	42	44

Source: Adapted from Bennett et al. (1995), Fox (1998), Harkness et al. (2010), Harkness and Wagner (1995), Johnson-Delaney (1994), Mulder (2012), and Quesenberry and Carpenter (2004).

Answers to Review Questions

Chapter 1

1. J, 2. I, 3. H, 4. D, 5. K, 6. G, 7. A, 8. E, 9. F, 10. B, 11. C, 12. L, 13. M, 14. Refinement, 15. Replacement, 16. Replacement, 17. Replacement, 18. Replacement, 19. Replacement, 20. Reduction, 21. Replacement, 22. Refinement, 23. Replacement, 24. Refinement, 25. Reduction, 26. Refinement, 27. Reduction

Chapter 2

1. H, 2. Q, 3. R, 4. N, 5. S, 6. I, 7. G, 8. F, 9. C, 10. A, 11. J, 12. K, 13. M, 14. P, 15. O, 16. No, 17. Yes, 18. Yes, 19. Yes, 20. Yes, 21. Yes, 22. Yes, 23. Yes, 24. No, 25. No

Chapter 3

1. A, 2. D, 3. C, 4. C, 5. C, 6. B, 7. C, 8. D, 9. B, 10. C, 11. B, 12. D, 13. B, 14. B, 15. D, 16. False, 17. D, 18. B, 19. A, 20. C, 21. 6 rats [(8.5 × 17) = 144.5 in.^{2}; 144 ÷ 23 = 6.2]

Chapter 4

1. Outbred stocks are heterogeneous—every mouse is genetically different. Inbred strains are genetically identical and should have no genetic variation between mice.
2. Germ-free mice, specific pathogen-free mice
3. Food and Drug Administration (FDA)
4. False—mammary tissue can be found all around the mouse body, including the sides and back.

Clinical Laboratory Animal Medicine: An Introduction, Fifth Edition.
Lesley A. Colby, Megan H. Nowland, and Lucy H. Kennedy.

Companion website: www.wiley.com/go/colby/clinical

5. Whitten effect
6. Cotton nesting material, it can cause damage to their eyes (due to a lack of eyelashes) or can wrap around their toes.
7. True
8. In gene targeting, a chimera is a mouse that has tissues or cells derived from two different embryonic stem cell sources—the ES cells that are being modified and implanted and the ES cells from the pseudopregnant recipient mouse.
9. Clustered Regularly Interspaced Short Palindromic Repeats
10. Ear punching
11. N
12. K
13. M
14. E
15. A
16. C
17. B
18. G
19. I
20. F

Chapter 5

1. A, C, D, 2. C, 3. B, 4. A, 5. C, 6. B, 7. C, 8. D, 9. D, 10. A, 11. B, 12. F, 13. B, 14. A, 15. G, 16. N, 17. J, 18. L, 19. H, 20. M, 21. C, 22. E, 23. D, 24. I, 25. K

Chapter 6

1. They have an incomplete circle of Willis, which supplies blood to the base of the brain. Due to this, carotid ligation is very effective at producing a stroke.
2. The midventral, abdominal sebaceous gland—twice as large in the male as it is in the female.
3. Adrenal glands
4. 24-26 days
5. False, they are altricial, similar to mice and rats
6. Gerbils are desert animals and produce very little urine compared to other rodent species. Their fecal pellets are also small and dry.
7. Burrowing
8. Degloving of the tail
9. Lateral saphenous vein, lateral tail vein, or submandibular vein
10. They produce very little urine—recommendation is to use a metabolic cage!
11. True
12. False—they do not have the same antibiotic sensitivity
13. Tyzzer's disease—caused by Clostrium piliforme
14. *Dentostomella translucida*
15. Using sand as a bedding material or providing a sand bath
16. They can have epileptiform seizures in response to loud noises.

Chapter 7

1. The shortest of any common lab animal—16 days
2. The Syrian (golden) hamster
3. BIO 1.50 and BIO 14.6
4. False: hamsters are better housed singly due to aggression and territorial natures
5. Low light intensity, short day lengths, quietness, and cooler temperatures of approximately 8°C (46°F) induce hibernation
6. They are immunologically privileged—meaning no immune cells from the hamster will come and cause the foreign tissue to be rejected
7. Sebaceous glands—used for marking territory and mating behavior
8. The female can be successfully mated in the evening of the third day after the observance of the postovulatory discharge.
9. True
10. Deep bedding for burrowing, wheels for exercising, huts or tubes for decreasing aggression, and materials for building nests
11. Cannibalism
12. Enterocolitis
13. Wet tail
14. Amyloidosis
15. Fasting
16. Tyzzer's disease/Clostridium piliforme
17. Hamster polyomavirus; trichoepitheliomas; lymphoma
18. Demodex
19. Seeds
20. Atrial thrombosis
21. Several husbandry related changes would help: moving to opaque housing boxes, adding more bedding for burrowing, adding nesting material or huts to create better nests, make sure the cage is in a quiet area, and disturb the cage as little as possible once the pups are born. Additionally, the PI should consider setting up new breeding pairs, as efficient breeding drops around 14 months of age.

Chapter 8

1. Preferring to maintain contact with the cage periphery
2. False
3. Whistle—anticipation of feeding; purr—social interactions; squeal/scream—injury or fear
4. Sudden changes in food or drink can result in dehydration and decreased/absent food intake.
5. Large tympanic bullae
6. Long narrow pharynx, palatal ostium
7. Vitamin C, scurvy
8. Seminiferous vesicles
9. Heterophils instead of neutrophils, Foa Kurloff cells with large intracytoplasmic inclusions

10. Dystocia due to fusion of the pelvic symphysis
11. Unsuccessful straining for 20 minutes or intermittent straining over 2 hours. Give oxytocin. If no delivery within 10-15 minutes, cesarean section
12. Fully haired, eyes open, can begin eating solid food and drinking water within the first week of life
13. Lumbar musculature or quadriceps muscle
14. Guinea pigs retain a significant amount of food in their cheek pouches which can be aspirated while under anesthesia if not cleared out prior to induction.
15. Ill guinea pigs tend to progressively decline rather than recover and do not tolerate clinical procedures well
16. Danger of intra-and interspecies spread as well as zoonotic potential
17. Conjunctival scraping
18. Trixacarus caviae and Chirodiscoides caviae
19. Cheek teeth (molars and premolars)
20. Obesity
21. Neophobia! Introducing all the new conditions early in the life of the animals will be important so as to not stress the animals unduly or risk inappetance or dehydration with novel presentation of food and/or water.

Chapter 9

1. Large tympanic bullae, lack of naturally occurring middle ear infections, less presbycusis
2. Age-related hearing loss
3. External genitalia of males and females look very similar
4. Lymphocytes
5. 111 days on average
6. They can be easily heat-stressed
7. Several times weekly, to absorb skin oils
8. Streptococcus and Staphylococcus
9. Gram-positive spectrum antibiotics
10. Pseudomonas aeruginosa
11. Selective appetite progressing to anorexia, excessive drooling (wet chin, chest & forepaws)
12. Behavioral reasons (fighting); Research reasons: close monitoring of food or water input or fecal or urinary output, a multitude of answers could be appropriate here, provided the student has thought about them carefully.

Chapter 10

1. The large number of embryos a single female can produce in one spawning, the small size of the embryos, the rapid 3-4 day development from fertilized egg to larval stage, the transparent nature of the embryo during development, and the ease of both manipulating those embryos to create mutations and then observing the effects of those manipulations
2. At least 5 fish per tank
3. False: Zebrafish do not have a stomach.

4. The cranial portion of the kidney.
5. Shallow areas and a light cycle of 14 hrs light : 10 hrs dark
6. Recirculating system
7. Flow through system
8. They are part of the nitrogen cycle—processing ammonia to nitrite and then further to nitrate, which is much less toxic to fish and is removed from the water by water exchanges.
9. Hardness measures divalent ions, while conductivity measures all dissolved ions.
10. *Artermia nauplii, Paramecium*, and rotifers
11. Clips from a fin
12. Rapid chilling followed by immersion in dilute bleach
13. Keep new fish on a separate water system (quarantine), bleach any embryos prior to raising them in the facility, get complete information from the sending institution on their pathogen status
14. *Mycobacterium marinum*
15. *Edwardsiella ictaluri*
16. It can transfer horizontally and vertically, and can even pass through embryo bleaching
17. True

Chapter 11

1. New Zealand White rabbit (albino), Dutch belted (not albino), Flemish Giant (not albino)
2. The Watanabe heritable hyperlipidemic rabbit has a spontaneous mutation in the low-density lipoprotein receptor, making it an ideal model for hypercholesterolemia in humans.
3. Rabbits have an extra set of incisors, called the peg teeth, just behind the incisors on the maxilla only
4. B vitamins and electrolytes
5. They have intracytoplasmic eosinophilic granules, making them resemble eosinophils instead of other neutrophils.
6. Calcium carbonate and/or ammonium magnesium phosphate crystals
7. True
8. Fur plucking from their dewlaps and sides to build a nest
9. False: Rabbit kits only need to nurse one time a day
10. Rabbits are heat sensitive and need lower temperatures than rodents—rabbits should be kept at 61-72 Fahrenheit, as opposed to rodents at 68-79 Fahrenheit.
11. The hind limbs and back need to be supported when lifting, carrying, or handling in any way
12. The marginal ear vein
13. Skin lesions that may include small nodules, diffuse swelling, and open abscesses or scabbing.

14. They have a small oral cavity and the larynx is difficult to visualize.
15. C
16. D
17. A
18. B
19. B
20. D
21. No, neither the floor space nor height is acceptable. The rabbits need a minimum of 3 ft^2, these measurements equal 2.625 ft^2. The minimum height required is 16 in, as well, so these 14 in cages will not suffice.

Chapter 12

1. E
2. A
3. F
4. B
5. D
6. H
7. Strong emesis response, similar anatomy to allow for intubation access, sensitive to influenza
8. 9-12 months
9. A
10. Extend light, shorten dark (16h and 8h respectively)
11. Helicobacter
12. Rabies and distemper
13. B
14. C
15. Cecum
16. D
17. Pancreatic Beta Cell Tumors (Insulinomas)
18. Splenomegaly
19. Alternative carnivore (to dogs and cats)—smaller than either of those species

Chapter 13

1. See Table 13.1 for list
2. Prevents scurvy (hypovitaminosis C). Clinical signs include swelling of epiphyses of long bones, hemorrhage of the gums, eyes and periostium. Cephalohematoma in squirrel monkeys.
3. Macacine herpesvirus 1 or (old name) Cercopithecine herpesvirus 2 Typically asymptomatic in animals, but may show "cold sore" type lesions on mucocutaneous junctions. In people, can cause a fatal encephalitis.
4. Gown, two pairs of exam gloves, mask, full eye protection or face shield, some places also require a hair bonnet, depending on a risk assessment.
5. *Mycobacterium tuberculosis*
6. Common marmoset, *Callithrix jacchus*
7. Macaques

8. Primates learn reproductive and social behaviors from adult animals.
9. Measles, rabies and tetanus
10. False. This is true of New World primates, however.
11. d
12. Calcium and phosphorus
13. *Moraxella catarrhalis*
14. Mild upper respiratory infection in most Old World primates, more severe in macaques including pneumonia. May see nasal & ocular discharge, conjunctivitis, facial edema, blepharitis and popular skin rash.
15. Zoonotic disease, appropriate handling

Chapter 14

1. Their size and similar anatomical or physiological similarities
2. Minimizing human and animal distress and risk of injury
3. Manipulate the light cycle to mimic the fall (short day/longer night)
4. Duration of housing, location of housing (indoors/outdoors/vivarium/barn/pasture)
5. Adaptation of physiological and behavioral parameters that have been disrupted by shipping
6. IACUC
7. Manage/prevent obesity
8. How close a possible threat can come to the animal before they will be instigated to flee
9. A point relative to the animal at which a threat in front of that point, the animal will move backward; if the threat is behind the animal, it will move forward
10. From behind the animal's point of balance, enter the flight zone so that it moves forward into the new pen
11. Large rumen volume
12. Colloquial name for respiratory disease resulting from stress incurred by shipping.
13. Ensuring swine have access to water (providing a bucket if lixit use is in question)
14. Condition the swine to human contact, use of food treats to reward animals when they display the desired behavior, use of pig boards and other equipment in order to guide the animal while maintaining human safety.

Chapter 15

1. I, 2. I, 3. E, 4. E, 5. E, 6. I, 7. I, 8. E, 9. E, 10. E, 11. B, 12. C, 13. C, 14. C, 15. D, 16. D, 17. B, 18. D, 19. A, 20. B

Index

Page numbers in bold represents figures and page numbers in italics represents tables.

Clinical Laboratory Animal Medicine: An Introduction, Fifth Edition.
Lesley A. Colby, Megan H. Nowland, and Lucy H. Kennedy.

Companion website: www.wiley.com/go/colby/clinical